Professional Issues in Nursing: Challenges & Opportunities

Professional Issues in Nursing: Challenges & Opportunities

Carol J. Huston, RN, MSN, MPA, DPA
Professor, School of Nursing
California State University, Chico
Chico, California

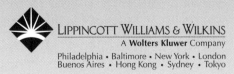

LIPPINCOTT WILLIAMS & WILKINS
A **Wolters Kluwer** Company
Philadelphia • Baltimore • New York • London
Buenos Aires • Hong Kong • Sydney • Tokyo

Acquisitions Editor: Quincy McDonald
Developmental Editor: Deedie McMahon
Editorial Assistant: Marivette Torres
Project Manager: Cynthia Rudy
Senior Production Manager: Helen Ewan
Senior Managing Editor / Production: Erika Kors
Art Director: Carolyn O'Brien
Senior Manufacturing Manager: William Alberti
Production Services / Compositor: Schawk, Inc.
Printer: Courier–Kendallville

9 8 7 6 5 4 3 2 1

Library of Congress Cataloging-in-Publication Data

Huston, Carol Jorgensen.
   Professional issues in nursing : challenges & opportunities / Carol J. Huston.
      p. ; cm.
   Includes bibliographical references and index.
   ISBN 0-7817-4875-5 (alk. paper)
    1. Nursing—United States. I. Title.
   [DNLM: 1. Nursing—trends. 2. Ethics, Nursing. 3. Nurse's Role. 4. Nursing—manpower.
    5. Professional Competence. WY 16 H972p 2006]

RT82.H87 2006
610.73—dc22   2005015351

LWW.com

I dedicate this book to our nursing leaders (past, present, and future) who have demonstrated the vision, courage, and tenacity to assure that nursing and quality health care are synonymous and that the conditions in which nurses work further that goal.

I also dedicate this book to the many mentors I have had in my nursing career: Bessie Marquis, Sherry Fox, Nancy-Dickenson Hazard, Clarann Weinert, Dan Pesut, and Carol Picard. Your influence, encouragement, and wisdom inspire me.

Contributors

Marjorie Beyers, RN, PhD, FAAN
Consultant, Bon Secours Health System, Inc.
Barrington, Illinois

(Chapter 23)

Catherine Dodd, RN, MS, FAAN
District Director
House Democratic Leader
Representative Nancy Pelosi
San Francisco, California

(Chapter 22)

Sherry D. Fox, PhD, RN
Director, School of Nursing
California State University
Chico, California

(Chapter 2)

Charmaine Hockley
Director
Charmaine Hockley & Associates
Strathalbyn, South Australia
Research Fellow
University of South Australia
Adelaide, Australia

(Chapter 12)

Jennifer Lillibridge, PhD, RN
Associate Professor
California State University, Chico
School of Nursing
Chico, California

(Chapter 16)

Jeanne Madison, PhD, RN
Head of School, School of Health
University of New England
Armidale, Australia

(Chapter 4)

**Catherine Wilde McPhee,
MSN, RN, FNP-C**
Director, RN to BSN Accelerated Degree Program
Azusa Pacific University
Azusa, California

(Chapter 7)

Suzanne S. Prevost, PhD, RN
Nursing Professor and
National HealthCare Chair of Excellence
Middle Tennessee State University
Murfreesboro, Tennessee

(Chapter 3)

Margaret J. Rowberg, DNP, APN
Certified Adult Nurse Practitioner
University of California, Irvine
Irvine, California

(Chapter 21)

Reviewers

Teresa Aprigliano, EdD, RN
Director, RN/Dual Degree/LPN–BS Program
Molloy College
Rockville Centre, New York

Margaret Blauvelt, MSN, MSE, RN
Associate Professor of Nursing
University of Saint Francis
Fort Wayne, Indiana

Harlene Caroline, RN, MS
Professor of Nursing
Curry College
Milton, Massachusetts

Janis C. Childs, RN, PhD
Associate Professor of Nursing and
Director of the Learning Resource Center
University of Southern Maine
Portland, Maine

Marlys Eggum, MSN, FNP-C, RN
Nursing Instructor
Miles Community College
Miles City, Montana

Connie S. Heflin, MSN, RN
Professor
West Kentucky Community and Technical College
Paducah, Kentucky

Nikole Anderson Hicks, MSN, RN,C
Assistant Professor
Kentucky Christian College
Grayson, Kentucky

Marilyn Jaffe-Ruiz, EdD, MA, RN
Professor of Nursing
Lienhard School of Nursing, Pace University
New York, New York

Nadine Mason, CEN, MSN, CRNP, RN
Assistant Professor
Cedar Crest College
Allentown, Pennsylvania

Carol Manning, MS, CCRN, ARNP, RN
Assistant Professor
Rivier College
Nashua, New Hampshire

Elinor M. Nugent, PhD, APRN-BC
Professor of Nursing
Curry College
Milton, Massachusetts

Jennifer D. Pearce, BSN, MSN, CNS, RN
Associate Professor
University of Cincinnati Raymond Walters College
Cincinnati, Ohio

Roy Ann Sherrod, BSN, MSN, DSN
Professor of Nursing
The University of Alabama
Capstone College of Nursing
Tuscaloosa, Alabama

Nancy E. Smith
Chair, Nursing Department
Southern Maine Community College
South Portland, Maine

Karen S. Ward, PhD, RN, COI
Professor and Associate Director
for Online Programs
Middle Tennessee State University
Murfreesboro, Tennessee

Patricia D. Wilcox, MSN, RN
Professor of Nursing
Owens State Community College
Toledo, Ohio

Linda Wilson, RN, PhD, CPAN, CAPA, BC
Drexel University College of Nursing
and Health Professions
Philadelphia, Pennsylvania

Preface

As a nursing educator for more than 25 years, I have taught many courses dealing with the significant issues impacting the nursing profession. I often felt frustrated that textbooks that were supposed to be devoted to professional issues in the field instead deviated into nursing research, theory, and leadership concepts. In addition, while many of the existing professional issues books dealt with the enduring issues of the profession, it was difficult to find a book for my students that incorporated those with the "hot topics" of the time.

Professional Issues in Nursing: Challenges & Opportunities is an effort to address both of these needs. It is first and foremost a professional issues book. While an effort has been made to integrate research, theory, and leadership into chapters where it seemed appropriate, these topics in and of themselves are too broad to be fully addressed in a professional issues book. This book also is directed at what I and my expert nursing colleagues have identified as both enduring professional issues as well as the most pressing contemporary issues facing the profession. It is my hope, then, that this book fills an unmet need in the current professional issues text market. It has an undiluted focus on professional issues in nursing and includes many timely issues not addressed in other professional issues texts.

The book has been designed primarily for the baccalaureate level, but is also appropriate for the graduate level. It is envisioned that this book will be used as a primary textbook or as a supplement for a typical two- to three-unit professional issues course. It would also be appropriate for most RN–BSN bridge courses and may be considered by some faculty as a supplemental reader to a Leadership/Management course that includes professional issues. The book can be used in both the traditional classroom and in online courses because the discussion question format works well for both small and large groups onsite as well as in bulletin board and chat room venues.

The book is edited with the primary author contributing 14 chapters and guest contributors with expertise in the specific subject material contributing the remaining nine chapters. The book is divided into five units, representing contemporary and enduring issues in professional nursing. The five sections include: *Furthering the Profession, Workforce Issues, Workplace Issues, Legal and Ethical Issues*, and *Professional Power*. Each unit has four to five chapters.

Each chapter begins with an overview of the professional issue being discussed. Multiple perspectives on each issue are then identified in an effort to reflect the diversity of thought found in the literature as well as espoused by experts in the field and varied professional nursing and health care organizations. "Discussion Points" encourage readers to pause and reflect on specific questions (individually or in groups), and "Consider" features encourage active learning, critical thinking, and values clarification by the users. In addition, at least one research study is profiled in every chapter in an effort to promote evidence-based analysis of the issue. Each chapter concludes with questions for additional discussion, a comprehensive and current reference list, and an expansive bibliography of resources for further exploration (electronic links, news media, and print resources). Each chapter also includes multiple displays, boxes, figures, and tables to help the user visualize important concepts.

Finally, support materials have been created for faculty using this book. A graphic-rich PowerPoint bank of more than 560 images has been included on a CD for faculty. In addition, the CD includes an instructor's manual outlining key terms and concepts, learning objectives, and teaching strategies for each chapter in the book, as well as a test bank of multiple choice questions.

Carol J. Huston, RN, MSN, MPA, DPA

Contents

Unit 3   **Workplace Issues   187**

Unit 4 Legal and Ethical Issues 293

Furthering the Profession

1

Entry Into Practice: An Elusive Dream or a Critical Professional Need?

1

Carol J. Huston

F
ew issues have been as long-standing or as contentious in nursing as the entry into practice debate. Although the debate dates back to the 1940s with the publication of Esther Lucille Brown's classic *Nursing for the Future*, the debate came to the forefront with a 1965 position paper by the American Nurses Association (ANA) (1965a; 1965b). This position paper suggested an orderly transition from hospital-based diploma nursing preparation to nursing education in colleges or universities based on the following premises:

- The education of all those who are licensed to practice nursing should take place in institutions of higher education.
- Minimum preparation for beginning professional nursing practice should be baccalaureate education in nursing.
- Minimum preparation for beginning technical practice should be associate education in nursing.
- Education for assistants in the health care occupations should be short, intensive, pre-service programs in vocational education institutions rather than on-the-job training programs.

In essence, two levels of preparation were suggested for registered nurses: *technical* and *professional*. Persons interested in technical practice would enroll in junior or community colleges and earn associate degrees in two-year programs. Those interested in professional nursing would enroll in four-year programs in colleges or universities (Donley & Flaherty, 2003). Hospital-based diploma programs were to be phased out.

The curriculums for the two programs were to be very different, as were each program's foci. The two-year technical degree was to result in an associate degree in nursing (ADN). This degree, as proposed by Mildred Montag (Figure 1.1) in her dissertation in 1952, with direction and support from R. Louise McManus, would prepare a "beginning, technical practitioner who would provide direct, safe nursing care under the supervision of the professional nurse in an acute-care setting" (Dillon, 1997, p. 21). In a typical program, approximately half of the credits needed for the associate degree are fulfilled by general education courses such as English, anatomy, physiology, speech, psychology, and sociology; the other half are fulfilled by nursing courses (Ellis & Hartley, 2004).

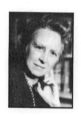

FIGURE 1.1
Mildred
Montag

The four-year degree would be a bachelor of science in nursing (BSN) and would encompass coursework taught in ADN programs as well as more in-depth treatment of the physical and social sciences, nursing research, public and community health, nursing management, and the humanities (AACN, 2003a). The additional course work was intended to enhance the students' professional development, prepare them for a broader scope of practice, and provide a better understanding of the cultural, political, economic, and social issues affecting patients and health care delivery (AACN, 2003a).

The ANA 1965 position statement was reaffirmed by a resolution at the ANA House of Delegates in 1978, which set forth the requirement that the baccalaureate degree would be the entry level into professional nursing practice by 1985. Associate degree and diploma programs responded strongly to what was viewed as inflammatory terminology and clearly stated that not being considered "professional" was unacceptable. The end result was that both programs refused to compromise title or licensure. Dissension ensued both within and among nursing groups and little movement occurred to make the position statement a reality.

Almost 40 years later, entry into practice at the baccalaureate level has not been accomplished. Even the strongest supporters of the BSN for entry into practice cannot deny that despite efforts spanning more than 50 years, registered nurse (RN) entry at the baccalaureate level continues to be an elusive goal.

▶ PROLIFERATION OF ADN EDUCATION

During the 1960s, ADN programs expanded so rapidly that at times, "a new ADN program was opening somewhere in the country every week" (Haase, 1990, p. 86). From 1974 to 1994, associate degree programs witnessed an increase of 103%; more than 56,000 individuals graduate from ADN programs each year (Tagliareni, Mengel, & Speakman, 1999). While 75% of nurses were educated in diploma schools of nursing in the early 1960s, only 16% were educated in baccalaureate programs, and associate degree programs were just beginning. By the year 2000, diploma education had decreased to just 6%, while BSN doubled to 30%, but ADN education now represented nearly 60% of all graduates (Gosnell, 2002).

ADN education has now become the primary model for nursing education in this country. Currently, more than 880 ADN programs operate in the United States (National Organization for Associate Degree Nursing, 2003a) and ADN graduates reflect 34% of the nursing workforce (Spratley, Johnson, Sochalski, et al. 2000). Associate degree nursing programs in many areas of the country are actively expanding enrollments and increasing the number of RNs with associate degrees (Auerbach, Buerhaus, & Staiger, 2000).

The American Association of Colleges of Nursing (AACN) states that as of 2003, 43% of the registered nursing workforce possessed a baccalaureate, master's, or doctoral degree; however, the number of nurses with just a baccalaureate degree drops that figure to 32.7% (U.S. Newswire, 2003; Spratley et al., 2000). Furthermore, according to the latest national sample survey of registered nurses conducted by the U.S. Department of Health and Human Services, only 16% of associate degree–prepared nurses obtain post-RN nursing or nursing-related degrees (U.S. Newswire, 2003).

*CONSIDER: Critics of BSN entry into practice argue that ADN, diploma and BSN educated nurses all take the same licensing examination and therefore have earned the title of registered nurse. In addition, nurses prepared at all three levels have successfully worked side by side, under the same scope of practice, for more than 50 years.

According to Tagliareni et al. (1999, p. 42), "graduates of ADN programs have a clear history of being safe and effective practitioners of nursing who serve the public trust" and these graduates have successfully worked for more than five decades in acute-care and long-term care settings. Tagliareni et al. suggest that the reality is that since ADN programs began to incorporate community-based care in their curricula, the differences between ADN and BSN nurses have become less clear and that community college–prepared nurses are actually ideally suited to care for the greater community because they are intrinsically community-based and are more diverse in age, gender, socioeconomic status, and race than their BSN counterparts. In addition, ADN graduates typically live, work, and complete their education within the local community, with 80% of graduates remaining in the local area after graduation.

◗ LICENSURE AND ENTRY INTO PRACTICE

Many employers state they are unable to differentiate roles for nurses based on education, because both ADN- and BSN-prepared nurses hold the same license. In addition, many employers provide no incentives for BSN education in terms of pay, recognition, or career mobility and are afraid to do so, fearing that this will impair their ability to fill nursing positions (Nelson, 2002). Also, state boards have asserted their inability to develop a different licensure system given the fact that employers have not developed different roles (Bednash, 2001a).

Critics of BSN as a requirement for entry into practice argue there is no need to raise entry levels because passing rates for the National Council Licensure Examination (NCLEX) show no significant differences between ADN, diploma, and BSN graduates (Table 1.1). While some might argue that this suggests similar competencies across the educational spectrum, the AACN (2003a) is quick to point out that the NCLEX is a test that measures minimum technical competencies for safe entry into basic nursing practice and, as such, does not measure performance over time or test for all of the knowledge and skills developed through a BSN program.

Cathcart (2003) agrees that the purpose of the regulatory examination is to keep unqualified practitioners from walking through the gate to begin practice rather than to distinguish different levels of education. Cathcart goes on to say that it is unlikely that the NCLEX accurately captures the skills, knowledge, and abilities of nurse candidates prepared in baccalaureate educational programs, but argues that the licensure examination is the wrong vehicle to argue for what should by now be a foregone conclusion: that the complex nature of professional nursing practice in today's health care environment necessitates preparation at the baccalaureate or higher degree level.

Long (2003) suggests, however, that one must ask why, in the case of RN licensure, there has been a failure to recognize educational preparation as a minimum qualification for different levels of practice. She notes that this already has been accomplished successfully in the case of practical nurses, registered nurses, and advanced practice nurses. She argues further that there seems no reason to contend that additional levels of nursing practice could not be identified with corresponding competencies, licenses, and legal scopes of practice. "Continuing to deploy a homogenized RN workforce, using a single scope of practice for those with substantively different entry-level preparation, is dangerous for patients and demoralizing for nurses" (Long, 2003, p. 124).

Complicating the picture is that both ADN and BSN schools preparing graduates for RN licensure meet similar criteria for state board approval and have roughly the same

TABLE 1.1	NCLEX-RN Passage Rate per Educational Program Type, January–December 2000		
	Program Type	**Number of Graduates**	**NCLEX-RN Passage Rate**
	Diploma	2,679	83.4%
	Associate degree	42,665	83.8%
	Baccalaureate degree	26,048	83.9%

Sources: National Council of State Boards of Nursing, 2000; National Organization for Associate Degree Nursing, 2003a.

Discussion Point

Should separate licensing examinations be developed for ADN-, diploma-, and BSN-prepared nurses?

number of nursing coursework units. All of these factors contributed to confusion about differentiations between ADN- and BSN-prepared nurses and resulted in an inability to move forward on implementing the BSN as the entry level for professional nursing.

Research also suggests that there are differences in the demographics of BSN and ADN graduates. Associate degree program graduates are approximately five years older than graduates of BSN programs, following the trend that older graduates are more likely to seek associate degrees than bachelor's degrees (Auerbach et al., 2000). Auerbach et al. report that older-aged RN graduates of ADN programs are a major cause of the rapidly aging RN workforce, a trend believed to have begun with the swift increase in the number of these programs over the past four decades.

It is also generally believed that ADN graduates represent greater diversity in race, gender, age, and educational experiences than BSN-prepared nurses. Critics of the BSN requirement for entry into professional nursing suggest that diversity is greatly needed in nursing, and it may be lost if entry levels are raised. However, Barter and Lenihan (2001) suggest that recent research shows minimal differences in terms of diversity and that associate degrees provide educational entry for more white women than for women of color (Almanac Issue, 1999).

▶ EDUCATIONAL LEVELS AND PATIENT OUTCOMES

Perhaps the most common argument against raising the entry level in nursing is an emotional one, with ADN-prepared nurses arguing that "caring does not require a baccalaureate degree." Many ADN-prepared nurses argue passionately that patients don't know or care what educational degree is held by their nurse as long as they receive high-quality care by the nurse at their bedside. ADN-prepared nurses also frequently claim that BSN-prepared nurses are too theoretically oriented, not in touch with real practice, and deficient in basic skills mastery and conclude that care provided by ADN-prepared nurses is at least as good as, if not better than, that provided by their BSN counterparts.

*CONSIDER: Most ADN-prepared nurses argue that significant differences exist between their practice and that of a licensed vocational/practical nurse, despite there often being only 12 months difference in educational preparation. Yet, many ADN educated nurses argue that the additional education that BSN educated nurses have makes little difference in their practice over that of their ADN counterparts.

An increasing number of studies, however, report differences between the performance levels of ADN- and BSN-prepared nurses. Research overwhelmingly supports better outcomes for patients cared for by BSN-prepared nurses than those with associate degrees. Fagin (2001) reviewed two separate studies, one in New York and another in Texas, that showed significantly higher levels of medication errors and procedural violations by nurses prepared at the associate-degree and diploma levels than those prepared at

BOX 1.1

Research Study Fuels the Controversy

Effect of Education on Patient Outcomes

A recent study of 232,342 surgical patients in 168 Pennsylvania hospitals over a 20-month period provided stinging evidence that educational entry level makes a difference in patient outcomes.

> Aiken, L., Clarke, S. P., Cheung, et al. (September, 2003). Educational levels of hospital nurses and surgical patient mortality. *Journal of the American Medical Association (JAMA)*, 290(12), 1617–1623.

Study Findings

This study found that patients experienced significantly lower mortality and failure to rescue rates in hospitals where more highly educated nurses were providing direct patient care. Indeed, the study indicated that a 10% increase in the proportion of nurses holding BSN degrees decreased the risk of patient death and failure to rescue by 5%. Furthermore, patient mortality and failure to rescue were predicted to be 19% lower in hospitals where 60% of nurses had BSNs or higher degrees than in hospitals where only 20% of nurses were educated at that level. Finally, the study demonstrated that if the proportion of BSN nurses in all hospitals was 60% rather than 20%, 17.8 fewer deaths per 1,000 surgical patients would be expected (AACN, 2003b; Aiken et al., 2003).

N-OADN Objects; Refutes Findings

The Aiken study resulted in an immediate rebuttal by the National Organization for Associate Degree Nursing (NO-ADN), (2003b), arguing that Aiken's research samples were far from pure with BSN research subjects also including those with earned master's and doctoral degrees. In addition, NO-ADN argued that several factors were unclear, including severity of the patient's condition and the surgeon's skill and education level. In addition, NO-ADN argued that data were based on hospital statistics and not on who actually cared for the patient and that hospitals deemed "BSN in nature" could in reality, have different care data internally.

the baccalaureate level. These findings echo those reported by Delgado (2002) that nurses prepared at the associate and diploma levels make the majority of practice-related violations. Phillips, Palmer, Zimmerman, and Mayfield (2002) added to the discussion with research showing that RN-to-BSN graduates demonstrated higher competency in nursing practice, communication, leadership, professional integration, and research/evaluation upon completion of their BSN program than upon entry (Box 1.1).

Discussion Point

If indeed employers prefer hiring BSN-prepared registered nurses, why don't more employers offer pay differentials for nurses with BSN degrees?

▶ EMPLOYERS' VIEWS AND PREFERENCES

Nursing employers are divided on the issue of entry into practice. The academic requirements of associate degree, diploma, and baccalaureate programs vary widely, yet health care settings that employ nursing graduates often make no distinction in the scope of practice among nurses who have different levels of preparation (Cathcart, 2003).

Employers, however, appear to be increasingly aware of purported differences between BSN and ADN graduates and this may be reflected in their hiring preferences. In a survey of chief nursing officers at university health systems, more than 70% of respondents noted better critical thinking skills and leadership abilities in BSN-prepared nurses (AACN, 2003a).

Similarly, a survey by the National Council of State Boards of Nursing (2001) revealed that employers have a clear preference for hiring experienced BSN graduates for nursing-management and RN-specialty positions. In addition, a study by Goode et al. (2001) showed that chief nursing officers in academic medical centers preferred employing BSN-prepared nurses. In a recent survey of deans of BSN programs, however, less than 10% of the deans believed that their BSN graduates enter work environments where roles are differentiated meaningfully on the basis of education (AACN, 2001).

A University Health Systems Consortium survey, however, found that chief nursing officers at university health systems prefer at least 70% of their staff nurses to be BSN prepared (Dorsman, 2002). The Veterans Administration (VA), with its 35,000 nurses on staff has gone a step further, requiring the BSN as the minimum education level for new hires and that all nonentry level nurses will have at least a BSN by 2005. The VA has committed $50 million over a five-year period to help VA nurses obtain baccalaureate or higher degrees.

▶ SHIFTING HEALTH CARE DELIVERY SITES AND REQUIRED COMPETENCIES

In the year 2000, approximately 59% of U.S. registered nurses worked in hospitals (Spratley et al., 2000). Although hospitals continue to be the main site of employment for nurses, there is an ongoing shift in health care from acute-care settings to the community and integrated health care settings. This shift will clearly require more highly educated nurses who can function autonomously.

> ***CONSIDER:** Baccalaureate and graduate level skills in research, leadership, management, and community health are increasingly needed in nursing as health care extends beyond the acute care hospital.

Joel (2002) argues that today's health care delivery systems challenge nurses with increased technology, the mandate for cost containment, a new consumerism and growing demand for self-care, diminished use of in patient facilities, and the continual call for counseling and health education. In addition, nurses need more skills in utilization review, case management, and quality assurance as well as in independent decision-making (Joel, 2002).

The National Advisory Council on Nurse Education and Practice (NACNEP) suggests that nursing's role for the future calls for RNs to manage care along a continuum, to work as peers in interdisciplinary teams, and to integrate clinical expertise with knowledge of community resources. This increased complexity of scope of practice will require the capacity to adapt to change; critical thinking and problem solving skills; a social foundation in a broad range of basic sciences; knowledge of behavioral, social, and management sciences; and the ability to analyze and communicate data (AACN, 2003a)—all are integral components of BSN education.

Some nurse leaders have even suggested that a BSN degree may not be adequate preparation for these expanded roles and that instead, master's or doctoral degrees should be required for entry into practice for registered nursing. "While raising the educational bar even higher can possibly be justified in terms of the knowledge base needed for advancing professional practice, we need to pay attention to past lessons and view with caution any proposed solution that would further split the profession and separate nurses with college degrees from the ranks of bedside caregivers" (Nelson, 2002, p. 9).

▶ ENTRY LEVEL AND PROFESSIONAL STATUS

"Nursing is currently involved in the same painful sequence of events experienced by other disciplines as they emerged to full professional status" (Joel, 2002, para. 11).

However, nurses have resisted the normal course of occupational development. As a result, nurses are the least educated of the health care professionals, with most health care professions now requiring graduate degrees for entry. Bednash (2001b, p. 18) goes so far as to say, "Although other health care disciplines are moving actively toward the clinical doctorate as entry level preparation, nursing is fixed in a 'moribund state of inaction' around requirements for entry into practice."

Anderson (2000b, p. 197), responding to advocates of certification as a replacement for BSN or higher academic preparation for entry, sounds a similar theme in the following question:

> ▶ *"Isn't it interesting that members of a profession who have refused to make a college degree prerequisite to practice are enamored with other letters that signify they have passed some kind of test that sets them apart from others?"*

*CONSIDER: Nursing is the only health care "profession" that does not require at least a bachelor's or higher degree for entry into practice.

Similarly, in a stirring editorial letter, Rabetoy (2003, para 1) argues:

> ▶ *The lack of a mandatory BSN entry level is the heart of the poor nursing image, nursing shortage, attrition for students entering nursing, and poor retention of seasoned nurses. It is also the reason why bright, career-oriented students and second career individuals should be directed away from entering nursing education in its present format. These individuals are being deceived and mistakenly led to believe that they are entering into a profession when, indeed, nursing is a vocational trade group.*

The primary identity of any group is based on the established education entry level. Attorneys, physicians, social workers, engineers, clergy, physical therapists, to list a few examples, have in common an essential education at the bachelor's level. Advanced degrees are required in many professions for entry positions at the professional level. Only nursing continues the hypocrisy of pretending that education is unimportant and does not make a difference. Only nursing allows individuals with no college course work, or with limited college study that lacks a well-rounded global college education, to lay claim to the same licensure and identity as that held by nurses having a baccalaureate education.

TABLE 1.2	Entry Level Degrees for the Health Professions	
	Health Profession	**Entry Level Degree**
	Medicine	Doctorate
	Pharmacy	Doctorate
	Social work	Master's
	Speech pathology	Master's
	Physical therapy	Master's
	Occupational therapy	Master's
	Nursing	Associate

Indeed, the educational gap between nursing and other health professions continues to grow (Table 1.2). Disciplines such as occupational therapy, physical therapy, speech therapy and social work now require master's degrees. Pharmacy has also raised its educational standards. Christman (1998) notes that at the point of care delivery, where most impressions of nurses are formed, most nurses encountered by patients and physicians and other health care providers do not have college degrees.

Discussion Point

Is nursing in danger of losing its designation as a "profession" if it fails to maintain educational entry levels comparable to those of the other health professions?

11

Some critics of the BSN requirement for entry to practice suggest that requiring a BSN for entry into practice is elitist. Bronson-Gray (1999) suggests the contrary, arguing that a bachelor's degree now does what a high school degree did early in the 20th century. "Teaching, accounting, medicine, pharmacy, occupational therapy, social work, physical therapy—all have the great benefit of having a shared and seamless educational foundation" (Bronson-Gray, 1999, p. 4), with at least a bachelor's degree for entry to practice. "Making sure nurses begin their career with a broad based and excellent education is not about putting people down, but rather about building them up, giving them the best chance to pursue new opportunities as time goes by" (Bronson-Gray, p. 4).

Anderson (2000a) concurs, arguing that the nursing profession is seriously under-educated and that a better-educated profession is necessary if nurses are to become full partners in health care and intellectual equals with other health care professionals. She concludes that "to remain less educated than our colleagues foretells a future of continued marginalization and absence from the decision table," and in a real sense, "not changing predicts a continuing oppression" (Anderson, 2000a, p. 54).

Joel (2002) agrees, arguing that while no one would debate nursing's service orientation, as we compete for full status in liberal arts institutions, the applied science nature of nursing has often become a liability. Traditional sciences accord the highest priority to the creation and expansion of knowledge, often with little regard to usefulness.

The opposite often occurs in nursing. As a result, "we resist many of the developmental patterns that have been common to all professional fields: recognition of the need for assisting categories of technical manpower, educational up-grading, and the application of the products of scientific investigation to practice" (Joel, 2002, p. 4). Consequently, any progress toward educational standardization or up-grading could jeopardize a substantial workforce for the health care industry and it is to no one's benefit to accomplish these things except nurses themselves (Joel, 2002).

▶ THE TWO-YEAR ADN PROGRAM?

Many ADN-prepared nurses argue that the "two-year" ADN program does not exist anyway. Many ADN students follow nontraditional education paths and almost all ADN programs currently require three or more years of education, not two, with a minimum of 12 to 24 months of prerequisites and a full two years of nursing education. Most associate's degrees require approximately 60 semester units or 90 quarter units of coursework. Despite the fact that the National League for Nursing Accreditation Commission (NLNAC) (1999) suggests that the maximum number of credits for an ADN program should be 108 quarter units or 72 semester units, many ADN schools struggle to meet these criteria.

[*CONSIDER: The two-year ADN program is a myth.]

Indeed, a report from the Center for the Health Professions at the University of California, San Francisco (Coffman, Spetz, Seago, et al. 2001), revealed that California ADN programs have widely divergent curriculums, with anywhere from 65 to 115 required units to graduate from what is supposed to be a two-year program. Bednash (2001a) concurs, reporting that it is virtually impossible to graduate from an ADN program in less than three years and often four or more years are required. Given that most BSN programs require approximately 120 semester units for graduation, the question must be asked whether requiring so many units at the associate degree level, without granting the upper division credit that could lead to a BSN degree, is an injustice to ADN graduates.

This extension of educational time in ADN programs has generally been attributed to the need to respond to a changing job market; that is, the need to prepare ADNs to work in more diverse environments (nonhospital) and to increasingly assume positions requiring management skills. While Montag clearly intended a differentiation between level of education and level of practice between ADN- and BSN-prepared nurses, many ADN programs have added leadership, management, research, and home health and community health courses to their curriculums in the past two decades. Bednash (2001a) refers to this as a "credit creep" and suggests that this is "clearly a dramatic shift from the original view of associate degree education as a two-year fast-track preparation for nurses who would be employed in acute-care settings, providing care for individuals with conditions that were both predictable and routine" (Bednash, 2001a, p. 193).

One must ask then what part of the curriculum should be cut to add these new experiences. What should the balance be between community and acute-care experiences in ADN programs? How much management content do ADN-prepared nurses need and what roles will they be expected to assume? If no content is deleted from the ADN programs to accommodate the new content, how can ADN education reasonably be completed within a two-year framework?

Montag expressed concern that when ADN programs add content inappropriate for technical practice, appropriate content may have to be deleted to maintain the estimated time for completion (National League for Nursing Council of Associate Degree Programs, 1985). The question that follows then is: if ADN education now incorporates much of what was meant to be BSN content, and if the time needed to complete this education is near that of a bachelor's degree, why are ADN graduates being given associate's degrees, which reflect expertise in technical practice, rather than BSN degrees, which reflect achievement of these higher-level competencies?

▶ SHORTAGES AND ENTRY-LEVEL REQUIREMENTS

"In times of shortage, there is always a call to reduce educational requirements and to change licensing and accreditation standards for professional nursing practice" (Donley & Flaherty, 2003, para 1). Indeed Montag's original project to create ADN education had two primary goals: (1) to alleviate a critical shortage of nurses by decreasing the length of the education process to two years, and (2) to provide a sound educational base for nursing instruction by placing the program in community and junior colleges (NO-ADN, 2003a).

Clearly, the immediate short-term threat of raising the entry level to the bachelor's degree may be to exacerbate the existing shortage. In the long run, however, raising the entry level may increase recruitment to and retention in the field. Bednash (2001a) argues that the failure to clarify role expectations and educational outcome differences for ADN and BSN education continues to hinder efforts to recruit the best and the brightest to nursing. In addition, research conducted by Rambur, Palumbo, McIntosh, and Mongeon (2003) suggests that increasing the proportion of BSN-prepared nurses in the registered nursing population may actually be essential to stabilizing the nursing workforce because nurses prepared at the BSN level were found to have higher levels of job satisfaction; a key to nurse retention.

> * **CONSIDER:** The impact of raising the entry level in nursing to the baccalaureate level on the current, profound nursing shortage is not known.

Barter and McFarland (2001) further argue that a chronic shortage of nursing personnel has persisted despite the proliferation of ADN programs and that the common wisdom that ADN programs are necessary to prevent or alleviate nursing shortages should be re-examined.

Nelson (2002) concurs, arguing that the current nursing shortage should not be used as an excuse for postponing action to raise educational standards. A nursing shortage existed at the time of the 1965 ANA proposal and has occurred intermittently since that time. Clearly, nursing has been swept along by a host of social, economic, and educational circumstances that have little to do with nursing or the clients we serve. Perhaps, then, the decision to raise the entry-to-practice level in nursing should be made because it is the right and necessary thing to do and not as a result of the influence of external communities of interest.

> * **CONSIDER:** Nurses, professional health care and nursing organizations, credentialing programs, and employers are divided on the entry into practice issue.

Debate over entry into practice is as varied among professional health care and nursing organizations, credentialing programs, and employers as it is among individual nurses. Getting support for the BSN as the entry-level requirement for nursing will be difficult because the overwhelming majority of nurses are currently ADN prepared and there are inadequate workplace incentives to increase entry requirements to the BSN degree.

▶ PROFESSIONAL ORGANIZATIONS AND ADVISORY BODIES SPEAK OUT

Some professional organizations have attempted to support both ADN and BSN education. The AACN, the American Organization of Nurse Executives (AONE), and the National Organization for Associate Degree Nursing (NO-ADN) formed a collaborative project in 1985 supporting both ADN and BSN education (Bednash, 2001a). These organizations suggested that the health care system required both types of nurses and that while the competencies of the ADN and BSN graduates were different, both were valued. This position, however, was never operationalized and each of these organizations has since refined its position.

Currently, a number of professional nursing organizations espouse support for the BSN requirement for entry into professional nursing. The ANA, however, is no longer the standard bearer in this effort. Instead, organizations such as AACN and the Association of California Nurse Leaders (ACNL) have published position statements supporting BSN entry. The mantra created by ACNL of "BSN by 2010" reflects ACNL's position that the baccalaureate degree be the credential for entry into practice as a registered nurse in the state of California by 2010 (Barter & McFarland, 2001).

The National Advisory Council on Nurse Education and Practice, which advises the Secretary of the U.S. Department of Health and Human Services and the U.S. Congress on policy issues related to nurse workforce supply, education and practice improvement, also urges that a minimum of two-thirds of working nurses hold baccalaureate or higher degrees in nursing by 2010 (Dorsman, 2002; AACN, 2003a; NACNEP, 2003).

Similarly, the Pew Health Professions Commission, in a 1998 report, called for a more concentrated production of BSN and higher degreed nurses. The Helene Fuld Health Trust, the nation's single largest private foundation devoted exclusively to nursing education and student nurses, announced in 2001 that it would give funding preference to programs that offer BSN and higher degrees in nursing (AACN, 2003a).

The National Black Nurses Association (NBNA) (2003) is particularly committed to increasing the number of Black nurses with baccalaureate-and-higher degrees. Toward that end, NBNA advocates for the support of baccalaureate and advanced education and practice as essential to the delivery of quality nursing.

Federal and state regulation of entry into practice has, for the most part, not occurred. Just one state became successful in changing the nurse practice act so that baccalaureate education was necessary for registered nurse licensure. That state, North Dakota, however, repealed this act in 2003, once again allowing nonbaccalaureate entry into practice. California does, however, require a BSN for certification as a public health nurse in that state. In addition, New York is currently considering a proposal to require registered nurses to earn a bachelor's degree to retain their certification (State Weighs Proposal..., 2004). Under the State Board of Nursing proposal, RNs with an associate's degree would have to earn a bachelor's degree within 10 years or their RN certification would be downgraded to a licensed practical nurse.

Certification programs are also divided on the entry into practice issue. The American Nurses Credentialing Center (ANCC) now confers the RN,C (certified) credential for diploma and associate degree nurses who demonstrate competency at that practice level, and the RN, BC (board certified) credential for nurses with a bachelor's or higher degree in nursing and who demonstrate competency at that particular level (Dorsman, 2002).

The American Legal Nurse Consultant Certification Board (ALNCC), on the other hand, announced the elimination of the baccalaureate in nursing requirement scheduled to take effect in 2004 for the Legal Nurse Consultant Certified (LNCC) certification examination (Auerbach et al., 2000). This change is a result of restructuring within the American Board of Nursing Specialties, which has revised its standards and will no longer require accredited certification programs to necessitate a BSN.

COLLABORATION AND CONSENSUS BUILDING: IS IT POSSIBLE?

Silva and Ludwick (2002) suggest that dissension among nurses, professional organizations, and employers poses several ethical issues. "Respect for persons is violated when nurses and student nurses denigrate each other over credentials and over who are the competent nurses. Nurse educators and administrators violate respect for persons when they bicker and dispute each other over educational preparation and hiring practices" (para 7). In both cases, the principle of respect for persons, as identified in the ANA *Code of Ethics for Nurses with Interpretive Statements* (ANA, 2001), is violated. Silva and Ludwick suggest that the ethical solution is not to participate in verbal sparring but to speak against it when it is heard and to engage in conversation about entry into practice with each other based on mutual respect and concern for what is best for the profession.

Bednash (2000a, p. 193) suggests that "discussions about entry into practice are most often received as a denigration of either option for education rather than a search for clarity." She goes on to say that the health care system in this nation cannot deliver high-quality care without a very large cadre of individuals prepared to deliver some form of nursing care and that providing this level of care is not facilitated by a system that fails to recognize that education makes a difference and the roles should be not only different, but also valued for those differences.

Similarly, Silva and Ludwick argue that collaboration, another goal identified in the ANA code, has failed regarding entry into practice. "Each entry level has its proponents, and each group of proponents has tended to put forth an agenda without consideration of other groups. Each entry-level group seems to lack the trust, recognition and respect that are vital to collaboration" (para 8). Silva and Ludwick suggest that ethical solutions at the individual level are to become involved and/or stay involved with professional associations and to push for collaboration on ending the stalemate on entry into practice.

GRANDFATHERING ENTRY LEVELS

Traditionally, when a state licensure law is enacted, or when a current law is repealed and a new law enacted, a process called "grandfathering" occurs. Grandfathering allows an individual to continue to practice his or her profession or occupation after new qualifications have been enacted into law (Ellis & Hartley, 2004). Should the entry level requirement for nursing be raised to a bachelor's or higher degree, debate will undoubtedly occur as to how and when grandfathering should be applied.

*CONSIDER: "Grandfathering" current ADN nurses as professional nurses smoothes political tensions between current educational entry levels but threatens the essence of the goal.

Several organizations have actively advocated that all RNs should be grandfathered if the entry level is raised. The American Nephrology Nurses Association (ANNA) is one such organization. ANNA (2003) supports the position that the minimum preparation for beginning professional practice is the bachelor's degree in nursing and that the minimum preparation for beginning technical nursing practice is the associate's degree in nursing, but only if a grandfather clause is incorporated in raising the educational level for entry into practice. Similarly, ACNL's position of "BSN by 2010" includes a transition plan that would grandfather all nurses who are licensed as RNs as of 2010 (Barter & McFarland, 2001).

Other professional organizations have argued that it should not occur at all. Still others believe that grandfathering should be conditional. For example, all RNs licensed at the time of the law would be allowed to retain their current title for a certain time, but would be required to return to school to increase their educational preparation if it did not meet the new entry level.

Joel (2002) suggests that determining how titling will be handled is a significant issue in the entry-to-practice debate. "Nurses have traditionally derived their identity from their statutory titles rather than their academic degrees. The result is possessiveness of the title *registered nurse* and reticence for any one group to relinquish continuing right to this title" (Joel, 2002, p. 7–8).

▶ LINKING ADN AND BSN PROGRAMS

Currently, 620 RN to BSN programs build on the education provided in diploma and ADN programs (AACN, 2003a). In addition, statewide articulation agreements exist in many states, including Florida, Connecticut, Texas, Iowa, Maryland, South Carolina, Idaho, Alabama, and Nevada, to facilitate advancement to the baccalaureate level.

*CONSIDER: A broad new system, composed of direct transfer, linkage, and partnership programs, is needed between community college and baccalaureate institutions to ensure a smooth transition from ADN to BSN as the entry-level requirement for professional nursing practice. This transition will be costly.

Coffman et al. (2001) suggest, however, that even in states such as California, where significant resources are dedicated to the education and training of new nurses, there is little integration, standardization, or cooperation between the three public systems of education (community colleges, California State University, and the University of California). Such integration, standardization, and cooperation will be essential for transition to BSN entry levels.

The NBNA (2003) suggests that transition programs or services for non–baccalaureate-prepared nurses must be designed to facilitate entry into baccalaureate and advanced education and practice programs. In addition, they advocate increasing funding for colleges and universities sponsoring baccalaureate and advanced practice nursing education programs.

Clearly, barriers for educational re-entry must be removed if the educational entry level in nursing is to be raised to a bachelor's or higher degree. Alternative pathways for RN education must be developed to create opportunities for learners who might not otherwise be able to pursue additional nursing education (Huston, 2003).

Finally, raising the entry level in professional nursing practice will be costly. University education simply costs more than education at community colleges and significant increases in federal and state funding for baccalaureate and graduate nursing education will need to occur. Given the significant budget deficit currently faced by almost all states, the likelihood of funding increases for nursing education is directly related to the public and legislative understanding of the complexity of roles nurses assume each and every day and the educational level they perceive is needed to accomplish these tasks.

▶ AN INTERNATIONAL ISSUE

The entry-into-practice debate in nursing is not limited to the United States. Canada, Australia, and England have already selected a date for implementing new entry requirements, grandfathering all those with a license before that date, and then creating new educational systems to make it easier to get the degree (Bronson-Gray, 1999). This does not mean the issue has been resolved for these countries. In 2003, the Royal College of Nursing's efforts to establish policy aiming for an all-graduate profession was defeated by members at its 2003 congress (RCN Delegates Against..., 2003).

▶ CONCLUSIONS

The entry-into-practice debate in the United States is one of the oldest and hottest professional issues nurses face as we enter the 21st century and experts are divided as to the progress that has actually been made on the issue. Donley and Flaherty (2003) suggest that if the 1965 ANA statement is viewed as a call to close hospitals' schools of nursing and move nursing education inside the walls of universities or colleges, then it was successful. If, however, the position is viewed as a mandate for a more educated nurse force to provide better patient care, the goal has not been achieved.

Achieving the BSN as the entry degree for professional nursing practice will take the best thinking of our nursing leaders. It will also require courage, as well as a respect for persons not seen in the entry debate, and collaboration of the highest order. It will also require nurses to depersonalize the issue and look at what is best for both the clients they serve and the profession, rather than for them individually.

Long (2003) argues that courage and leadership should not be squandered in tackling the old issue of entry level for professional practice. Rather, it is time to focus on meaningful differentiation that uses every nurse effectively to improve patient care. "This is not a time for the fainthearted. It requires the full and courageous involvement of nursing leaders in all spheres: education, practice, and regulation" (Long, 2003).

Margaret McClure (2003, p. 151), the 2003 President of the American Academy of Nursing (AAN), stated: "The time has come for the nursing profession to put its educational house in order. We have the ability and the commitment to confront this difficult problem and to solve it."

Even the most patient planned-change advocate would agree that 40 years is a long time for implementation of a position. Clearly, the driving forces for such a change have not yet overcome the restraining forces (Lewin, 1951), although movement is apparent. The question seems to come down to whether the nursing profession wants to spend another 40 years debating the issue or whether it wants to proactively take the steps necessary to make the goal a reality.

1. What are the greatest driving and restraining forces for increasing entry into practice to a bachelor's or higher level?
2. Are the terms "professional" and "technical" unnecessarily inflammatory in the entry-into-practice debate? Why do these terms elicit such a "personal" response?
3. Is calling the associate degree in nursing a two-year vocational degree an injustice to its graduates?
4. What is the legitimacy of requiring so many units at the community college level for an ADN degree? Why can't community colleges award bachelor's degrees?
5. How does the complexity of nursing roles and responsibilities compare to that of other health professions with higher entry levels?
6. What is the likelihood that nurses and the organizations that represent them will be able to achieve consensus on the entry-into-practice issue?
7. If the entry level is raised, should grandfathering be used? If so, should this grandfathering be conditional?
8. Is the goal of BSN entry by 2010 a realistic goal? If not, when?

REFERENCES

Aiken, L., Clarke, S. P., Cheung, R. B., et al. (September, 2003). Educational levels of hospital nurses and surgical patient mortality. *Journal of the American Medical Association*, *290*(12), 1617–1623.

Almanac Issue (1999). *The Chronicle of Higher Education*, *46*(1), 24–32.

American Association of Colleges of Nursing (AACN). (2001). *Task Force on Education and Regulation for Professional Nursing Practice Survey*. Unpublished.

American Association of Colleges of Nursing (AACN). (2003a). *Fact sheet: The impact of education on nursing practice*. Available at: http://www.aacn.nche.edu/edimpact/. Accessed February 15, 2005.

American Association of Colleges of Nursing (AACN). (2003b). *AACN applauds new study that confirms link between nursing education and patient mortality rates*. (Sept. 23, 2003). Available at http://www.aacn.nche.edu/Media/NewsReleases/2003AikenStudy.htm. Accessed October 28, 2003.

American Nephrology Nurses Association (ANNA). (March 2003). *Minimum preparation for entry into nursing practice: Position statement*. Available at: http://anna.inurse.com/. Accessed May 16, 2004.

American Nurses Association (ANA). (1965a). *A position paper*. New York: American Nurses Association.

American Nurses Association (ANA). (1965b). *Educational preparation for nurse practitioners and assistants to nurses: A position paper*. New York: American Nurses Association.

American Nurses Association (ANA). (2001). *Code of Ethics for Nurses with Interpretive Statements*. Washington, DC: American Nurses Publishing. Available at: www.nursingworld.org/ethics/ecode.htm. Accessed May 16, 2004.

Anderson, C. A. (2000a). Undereducated, aging, and... a cycle of decline? *Nursing Outlook*, *48*(2), 53–54.

Anderson, C. A. (2000b). Overstating the ordinary. *Nursing Outlook*, *48*(5), 197–198.

Auerbach, D., Buerhaus, P., & Staiger, D. (2000). Associate degree graduates and the rapidly aging RN workforce. *Nursing Economics*, *18*(4), 178–185.

Barter, M. & McFarland, P. L. (2001). BSN by 2010: A California initiative. *Journal of Nursing Administration*, *31*(3), 141–144.

Bednash, G. (2001a). A nursing leader speaks out on the nursing shortage: Creating a career destination of choice. *Policy, Politics, & Nursing Practice*, *2*(3), 191–195.

Bednash, G. (2001b). New directions. In: J. C. Clifford (Ed.), *Workforce challenges in the 21st century: Implications for health care and nursing*. Boston: The Institute for Nursing Healthcare Leadership.

Bronson-Gray, B. (1999). It's not elitist—The bachelor's degree is about opportunity. *Nurseweek*, *12*(24), 4.

Cathcart, E.B. (May/June 2003). Using the NCLEX-RN to argue for BSN preparation: Barking up the wrong tree. *Journal of Professional Nursing*, *19*(3), 121–122.

Christman, L. (1998). Who is a nurse? *Image: Journal of Nursing Scholarship*, *30*(3), 211–214.

Coffman, J., Spetz, J., Seago, J. A., et al. (January, 2001). *Nursing in California: A workforce crisis*. San Francisco, CA: University of California, San Francisco Center for the Health Professions California Workforce Initiative.

Delgado, C. (2002). Competent and safe practice: A profile of disciplined registered nurses. *Nurse Educator*, *27*(4), 159–161.

Dillon, P. (1997). The future of associate degree nursing. *N & HC: Perspectives in Community, 18*(1), 20–24.

Donley, S. R. & Flaherty, M. J. (2003). Entry into practice: Revisiting the American Nurses Association's first position on education for nurses. *Online Journal of Issues in Nursing.* Available at: http://nursingworld.org/mods/mod524/ceenabs.htm. Accessed April 6, 2005.

Dorsman, J. (2002). BSN: The new staffing standard? *Nursing Management, 33*(3), 50.

Ellis, J. R. & Hartley, C. L. (2004). *Nursing in today's world* (8th ed.). Philadelphia: Lippincott Williams & Wilkins.

Fagin, C. (2001). *When care becomes a burden: Diminishing access to adequate nursing.* New York: Milbank Memorial Fund.

Goode, C. J., Pinkerton, S. E., McCausland, M. P., et al. (February 2001). Documenting chief nursing officers' preferences for BSN-prepared nurses. *Journal of Nursing Administration, 31*(2), 55–59.

Gosnell, D. J. (May 31, 2002). Overview and summary: The 1965 entry into practice proposal—is it relevant today? Nursing World/ *Online Journal of Issues in Nursing, 7*(2). Available at: http://www.nursingworld.org/ojin/topic18/tpc18ntr.htm.

Haase, P. (1990). *The origins and rise of associate degree education.* Durham: Duke University Press.

Huston, C. (2003). Quality health care in an era of limited resources: Challenges and opportunities. *Journal of Nursing Care Quality, 18*(4), 295–301.

Joel, L.A. (May 31, 2002). Education for entry into nursing practice. *Online Journal of Issues in Nursing, 7*(2). Available at: http://www.nursingworld.org/ojin/topic18_4.htm.

Lewin, K. (1951). *Field theory in social sciences*; Selected theoretical papers. D. Cartwright (ed.). New York: Harper & Row.

Long, K. A. (May/June 2003). Licensure matters: Better patient care requires change in regulation as well as education. *Journal of Professional Nursing, 19*(3), 123–125.

McClure, M. L. (July/August 2003). Another look at entry into practice. *Nursing Outlook, 51*(4), 151.

National Advisory Council on Nurse Education and Practice (NACNEP) (2003). Available at: http://bhpr.hrsa.gov/nursing/nacnep/default.htm. Accessed October 26, 2003.

National Black Nurses Association (NBNA). (2003). NBNA *Position statement: Nursing education.* Available at: http://www.nbna.org/. Accessed October 28, 2003.

National Council of State Boards of Nursing (NCSBN). (2000). *Number of candidates taking NCLEX examination and percent passing, by type of candidate.* Retrieved April 11, 2005 from http://www.ncsbn.org/pdfs/Table_of_Pass_Rates_2000.pdf. Accessed October 26, 2003.

National League for Nursing Accreditation Commission (NLNAC). (1999). *Interpretive guidelines for standards and criteria 1999: Associate degree programs in nursing.* New York: NLN Press.

National League for Nursing Council of Associate Degree Programs (1985). *Associate degree education for nursing 1985–1986.* New York: NLN Press.

National Organization for Associate Degree Nursing (NO-ADN). (2003a). Associate degree nursing facts. Available at: http://www.noadn.org/adn_facts.htm. Accessed April 6, 2005.

National Organization for Associate Degree Nursing (NO-ADN). (2003b). *Talking points for JAMA article: Educational levels of hospital nurses and surgical patient mortality, September 23, 2003.* Available at: http://www.noadn.org/JAMA_talking_points.pdf. Accessed October 26, 2003.

Nelson, M.A. (2002). Education for professional nursing practice: Looking backward into the future. *Online Journal of Issues in Nursing, 7*(3). Available at: http://www.nursingworld.org/ojin/topic18tpc18_3.htm. Accessed April 6, 2005.

Phillips, C. Y., Palmer, C. V., Zimmerman, B. J. & Mayfield, M. (2002). Professional development: Assuring growth of RN-to-BSN students. *Journal of Nursing Education, 41*(6), 282–284.

Rabetoy, C. P. (January 21, 2003). Response to *The 1965 entry into practice proposal–is it relevant today?* by D. J. Gosnell, (May 31, 2002). *Online Journal of Issues in Nursing.* Available at: http://www.nursingworld.org/ojin/letters/t18e6.htm. Accessed October 30, 2003.

Rambur, B., Palumbo, M. V., McIntosh, B. & Mongeon, J. (2003). A statewide analysis of RNs' intention to leave their position. *Nursing Outlook, 51*(4), 182–188.

Scott, H. RCN votes that nursing should not become all-graduate. (May 8–21, 2003). *British Journal of Nursing, 12*(9), 524.

Silva, M. & Ludwick, R. (August 30, 2002). Ethics column: Ethical grounding for entry into practice: Respect, collaboration, and accountability. *Online Journal of Issues in Nursing.* Available at: http://www.nursingworld.org/ojin/ethicol/ethics_9.htm. Accessed May 16, 2004.

Spear, H. J. (May, 2003). The baccalaureate degree for entry into practice: It's time for nursing to take a stand. *Nurse Education Today, 23*(4), 243–245.

Spratley, E., Johnson, A., Sochalski, J., et al. (2000). *The registered nurse population*: *Findings from the national sample survey of registered nurses.* Washington, DC: U.S. Department of Health and Human Services. Available at: http://bhpr.hrsa.gov/healthworkforce/reports/rnsurvey/rnss1.htm#2. Accessed July 6, 2004.

State weighs proposal to require more RN schooling. (April 13, 2004). Boston.comNews. Available at: http://www.boston.com/news/education/continuing/articles/2004/04/13/state_weighs_proposal_to_require_more_rn_schooling?mode=PF. Accessed May 16, 2004.

Tagliareni, M. E., Mengel, A., & Speakman, E. (1999). Associate degree nursing education today: Myths and realities. *NSNA/Imprint, 46*(2), 42–45.

U.S. Newswire. (September 23, 2003). *AACN applauds study confirming link between nursing education, patient mortality rates; Education is key to patient safety, preventing deaths.* Available at: http://releases.usnewswire.com/GetRelease.asp?id=155-09232003. Accessed July 7, 2004.

American Association of Colleges of Nursing (AACN). (Sept. /Oct. 2001). The baccalaureate degree in nursing as minimal preparation for professional practice. *Journal of Professional Nursing*, *17*(5), 267–269.

American Association of Colleges of Nursing (AACN). (2002). *Fact sheet: Associate degree in nursing programs and AACN's support for articulation*. Available at: http://www.aacn.nche.edu. Accessed October 28, 2003.

American Association of Colleges of Nursing (AACN). (2002). White paper. *Hallmarks of the professional nursing practice environment*. Available at: http://www.aacn.nche.edu. Accessed April 6, 2005.

Blegen, M. A., Vaughn, T. E. & Goode, C. J. (January 2001). Nurse experience and education. Effect on quality of care. *Journal of Nursing Administration*, *31*(1), 33–39.

Boyce, C. A, Brow, M. B., Cote, K. C., et al. (April 31, 2001). End the debate. Entry level into practice should be the master's degree. *Journal of Nursing Administration*, *31*(4), 166–168.

Clark, J. D. & Booth, B. (March 23-30, 2000). Should nursing become a graduate-entry profession? *Nursing Times*, 96(12), 18.

Entry into practice. (March 2003). *American Journal of Nursing*, *103*(3), 69–70.

Fitzpatrick, J. J. (February 2003). Joint Commission on Accreditation of Health Care Organizations white paper: Health care at the crossroads: Strategies for addressing the evolving nursing crisis. *Policy, Politics & Nursing Review*, *4*(1), 71–74.

Garner, C., Brzytwa, E. C. & Gugerty, B. (Sept. /Oct. 2002). The future for nursing education: Three leaders respond. *Nursing Education Perspectives*, *23*(5), 214–215.

Gennaro, S. & Lewis, J. A. (March/April 2000). Is the goal of a BSN as the criteria for entry into professional nursing still worthwhile and realistic? *MCN American Journal of Maternal Child Nursing*, *25*(2), 62–63.

Goode, C. J., Pinkerton, S., McCausland, M. P. et al. (2001). Documenting chief nursing officers' preference for BSN-prepared nurses. *The Journal of Nursing Administration*, *31*, 55–59.

McClure, M. L. (2003). Another look at entry into practice. *Nursing Outlook*, *51*(4), 151.

Mehigan, S. (March 2000). Future practitioners.... advancing nursing practice in the perioperative setting. *British Journal Perioperative Nursing*, *10*(3), 153–156.

RN education: Readers respond. (May 2004). *Nursing*, *34*(5), 46–47.

Spear, H. J. (2003). The baccalaureate degree for entry into practice; It's time for nursing to take a stand. *Nurse Educator Today*, *23*(4), 243–245.

Williams, J. (2003). The 1965 entry into practice proposal—Is it relevant today? *Online Journal of Issues in Nursing*, *8*(2), 4p following 8.

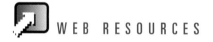 WEB RESOURCES

American Association of Colleges of Nursing	http://www.aacn.nche.edu/
American Association of Community Colleges	http://www.aacc.nche.edu/
American College of Nurse Practitioners	http://www.nurse.org/acnp/
American Nephrology Nurses Association	http://anna.inurse.com/
American Nurses Association	http://www.ana.org/
American Nurses Foundation	http://nursingworld.org/anf/
American Organization of Nurse Executives	http://www.aone.org/
Association of California Nurse Leaders	http://www.acnl.org/
Emergency Nurses Association	http://www.ena.org/
National Black Nurses Association	http://www.nbna.org/
National Council of State Boards of Nursing	http://www.ncsbn.org/
National League for Nursing	http://www.nln.org/
National Organization of Nurse Practitioner Faculties	http://www.nonpf.com/
National Organization for Associate Degree Nursing	http://www.noadn.org/

Differentiated Nursing Practice: Maximizing Resources or Dividing an Already Divided Profession?

2

Sherry D. Fox

D ifferentiated nursing practice, as explored in this chapter, refers to "structuring nursing roles on the basis of education, experience, and competence" (American Association of Colleges of Nursing [AACN], American Organization for Nurse Executives [AONE], & National Organization for Associate Degree Nursing [NO-ADN], (1995, p. 1). A major premise of differentiated nursing is that different levels of nursing education (diploma/associate, bachelor's, and master's) provide preparation for different competencies in practice. An additional premise is the recognition that nurses continue to develop competencies beyond the minimal level indicated by their licensure and educational levels. Differentiation of nursing roles based on education and competency is designed to allow registered nurses (RNs) to practice to the full extent of their capabilities and to structure work roles so that the most appropriate nurse is performing the most appropriate services, in a cost-effective manner.

Nursing has always had to deal with different levels of care providers, whether licensed or not, and has developed many ways to determine who should deliver what type of care. Brown (1948) and Montag (1951) described differentiation criteria in the mid-20th century primarily in terms of delineating licensed nurses from unlicensed assistive personnel. As the concept evolved in the 1980s, differentiation was used primarily to distinguish between the roles of the associate degree nurse and the baccalaureate degree nurse. Later evolutions of differentiated practice models added delineations of roles for vocational nurses and master's-prepared nurses.

The reality today is that four types of education (diploma, associate degree, bachelor's degree, and entry-level master's degree) prepare nurses for one license: registered nurse. State licensing requirements establish minimum initial competency levels for safe practice, but do not test for competencies beyond those required for entry-level positions in nursing. Beyond the minimum competence tested for licensure, working nurses have additional individual competencies that contribute to quality nursing care based on different educational and experiential backgrounds. However, such variability is not recognized in many settings.

Many nurses see differentiated practice as an efficient and cost-effective way to best utilize the abilities of nurses with varying levels of preparation and competence. The implementation of differentiated practice, in the form of clinical role definitions that acknowledge education, experience, and competence, provides a structured guidepost that RNs can use to map their professional careers, allowing them to purposefully develop the competencies required for a specified role. The National Commission on Nursing Implementation Project (NCNIP) (DeBack, 1987) suggested differentiated practice was a means to improve patient care, use resources effectively, and improve satisfaction in work environments.

For some, differentiated practice is seen as a way to heal the dissension in nursing over the issue of entry into practice, as well as other divisions based on variations in educational preparation, by explicitly valuing the contribution of multiple levels of nursing preparation and by designating how each level of preparation contributes to the whole of nursing care delivery. Others, however, see differentiation as a mechanism to devalue the contribution of the majority of nurses prepared at the associate degree level, causing even more division in the profession (Costello, 1998).

◗ ORIGINS OF DIFFERENTIATED NURSING PRACTICE

Current differentiated practice models derive from the formation of the associate degree nursing role, pioneered by Mildred Montag (Montag, 1951). In the mid-20th century, the majority of nurses were trained in diploma programs, with only 6% of nursing students in college degree programs (Brown, 1948). Associate degree programs did not yet exist. Although there was a sufficient supply of practical nurses and attendants, advances in public health and preventive medicine led to an extreme shortage of public health nurses, known then as professional nurses.

Major health care issues (similar concerns as those seen today, such as an aging populace requiring more care for the elderly, the growth in chronic diseases, and increased acuity of hospitalized patients) demanded more and higher levels of nursing care (Montag, 1951). Montag asserted that an intermediate level of nurse was needed to both relieve the professional nurses of the less demanding services in hospital settings and provide a higher level of care than practical (vocational) nurses.

Montag's doctoral dissertation outlined the concept of the associate degree nurse (which she labeled the "technical nurse") as a needed component of nursing practice to resolve a shortage of qualified nursing personnel. Montag proposed that the training for the technical nurse be provided at community colleges, which had long provided training for other technical fields. Montag outlined a compact and tidy curriculum, lasting exactly two years, composed of 65 units, and designed for associate degree completion. Her plan clearly elaborated concepts of differentiated practice:

> *The differentiation of nursing functions into assisting, technical, and professional functions, would make it possible to set up appropriate programs for the preparation of each group of workers. The preparation of workers for rather specific functions would make it possible to organize nursing care programs around these functions. Such an organization of nursing care should, then, insure better care for the patient and increase the job satisfaction of each worker. Each worker would be given the opportunity to perform those functions which require her most highly developed abilities. The nurse who works in the highest range of her abilities for the greatest part of the time is the happiest and most efficient worker.*
>
> *A differentiation in the programs of preparation for each group of workers would also be desirable from the standpoint of economy. There would be an economy in the time spent by the learner, in the amount of money spent by the school in the preparation of the worker, and in the money spent on salaries by the employing agency. The salaries would be adjusted according to the investment made by the learner in preparing to do the job (Montag, 1951, pp. 7–8).*

CONSIDER: The original precepts of the associate degree model provided clear-cut guidelines for the associate degree nursing role and for differentiation of two levels of nursing.

Differentiating Educational Levels

Nurse educators generally agree that associate degree programs prepare nurses for direct patient care in structured settings such as acute and long-term care. Baccalaureate programs add competencies in providing care across the continuum of health care, based on expanded content on health promotion and lifestyle management, epidemiology and public health, multiple cultures, quantitative reasoning (statistics), research, and foundations for collaborative communication and higher levels of leadership/management (AACN, 1998). Yet, despite these differences in basic preparation, many nursing positions have a "one-size-fits-all" quality.

> *CONSIDER: Typically, the differences in basic nursing education are not acknowledged or recognized in the practice arena.

Using basic licensure as the main common denominator for most nursing positions without regard to the educational pathway contributes to dissension and confusion among nurses and nursing educators. Expecting similar performance from nurses with varying educational preparation can lead to role confusion, stress, and burnout, as nurses struggle to develop role competencies for which they have not been prepared. Conversely, nurses who have been educated for role competencies they can't apply often feel underutilized, frustrated, and unfulfilled.

Yet, nurse educators are confronted by demands from the service arena for all graduates to function at higher and higher levels, as health care demands become more complex. More content is crammed into time-limited curricula, further blurring the distinctions between associate and baccalaureate levels of education. One result is the growth of content in associate degree programs, so that most are no longer 2-year programs, but in fact require 3 or more years to produce an RN who can meet the entry-level job demands.

Discussion Point

Are associate degree nurses being educated beyond the typical associate degree level? What are the benefits and disadvantages of prolonging the educational courses at community colleges versus advancing students to colleges/universities for baccalaureate level credit? (Consider the perspectives of community colleges, baccalaureate nursing programs, nursing faculty, and students.)

To bridge the gap between associate and baccalaureate degree programs, RN to bachelor degree in nursing (BSN) programs have proliferated. However, the confusion inherent in generic nursing roles does not provide adequate incentives and rewards for nurses to continue their education at a time when the growing complexity of health care demands more education for all nurses (Fox, Walker, Bream, & Education/Industry Interface Work Group of the California Strategic Planning Committee for Nursing/Colleagues in Caring, 1999). Enrollment in RN to BSN programs declined between 1999 and 2003, from 24,129 to 21,474, an average loss of 691 enrollees per year, although a slight rise was noted in 2003 (Berlin, Stennett, & Bednash, 2004 p. 2, 43).

Not the least of the difficulties inherent in so many types of education for one generic nursing role, is the human division—the rancor between nurses educated at different levels. Differentiated practice was conceived as a solution to these problems, and many nursing leaders contributed to the evolution of the concept. Institutions that have implemented it have reported many positive benefits. However, despite many projects in the latter half of the 20th century to implement differentiated practice models, the concept has not achieved widespread acceptance, and the future for differentiated practice is not clearly charted.

The Growth of Associate Degree Programs

Associate degree programs quickly became positioned for rapid growth, supported in part by foundations and federal funds, responding to the nursing shortage of that time (Haase, 1990). Within 20 years, associate degree programs constituted 42% of all basic nursing education programs (Haase). By the year 2000, there were over 800 programs, producing approximately 42,715 graduates, nearly 60% of total nursing graduates (U.S. Department of Health and Human Services [USDHHS], 2002).

Despite the rapid growth of programs, the service sector was slow to understand the differences among the new graduates of associate degree programs, the more traditional diploma programs, and the baccalaureate programs. Communication between educators and the service sector was inadequate to clarify the expectations for the new level of nurse.

At the same time, acuity levels in hospitals were rising and nursing shortages made it difficult to fill positions with qualified individuals. Hospitals took a uniform, "one-size-fits-all" approach to assigning nurses. Accustomed to the apprentice-type preparation common to diploma programs, orientation programs for new nurses were minimal, leading to general employer dissatisfaction with the new graduates' ability to move into clinical roles. Associate degree graduates were often thrown in over their heads, while baccalaureate graduates were assigned to positions that did not fully use their skills (Haase, 1990).

An Era of Projects

In the midst of confusion about how to use the new level of nurse, the Kellogg Foundation offered support by funding a national project (National Commission on Nursing Implementation Project—[NCNIP]) to develop consensus between service and education regarding the nursing workforce for the future (DeBack, 1987). The project identified characteristics of the professional and technical nurses of the future, as well as models of nursing management to deliver cost-effective quality care. It was envisioned that the vocational and diploma levels of nursing would be phased out (transitioning to collegiate programs where feasible), and the associate degree and baccalaureate levels of education would be refined to produce the technical degree nurse and the professional degree nurse of the future. The transition was to be complete by 2010 (Deback).

Demonstration projects subsequently defined the expected competency levels of graduates of the different programs, established common curricular content, and built job descriptions and clinical ladder programs to demonstrate differences in the work roles of the nurse. A major undertaking by the Midwest Alliance in Nursing (MAIN) was to outline differences in the service setting to make full use of the different competence levels (Primm, 1987).

The groundbreaking work of MAIN formed the foundation for today's differentiated practice models. Three basic overlapping components of the practice role of the nurse were designated: provision of direct care, communication with and on behalf of the client, and management of client care (Primm, 1987, p. 220).

Both associate degree and bachelor degree roles were derived from these common role components, sharing common functions. The ADN role was focused on common, well-defined nursing diagnoses for the individual client within a family in a structured health care setting with established policies, protocols, and procedures. The BSN role added a focus on clients with complex interactions of nursing diagnoses; clients might include individuals, families, groups, aggregates, and communities in structured and unstructured health care settings (see Table 2.1). The model was subsequently expanded to include master's level nursing. The model was successfully implemented in five states, through partnerships among hospitals and educational programs.

TABLE 2.1

Differentiated Nursing Roles from the MAIN Project

Role of the Associate Degree Nurse (ADN)	Role of the Baccalaureate Degree Nurse (BSN)
The ADN is a licensed nurse who provides direct care that is based on the nursing process and focused on individual clients who have common, well-defined nursing diagnoses. Consideration is given to the client's relationship within the family. The ADN functions in a structured health care setting that is a geographical or situational environment where the policies, procedures, and protocols for provision of health care are established. In the structured setting there is recourse to assistance and support from the full scope of nursing expertise.	The BSN is a licensed registered nurse who provides direct care that is based on the nursing process and focused on clients with complex interactions of nursing diagnoses. Clients include individuals, families, groups, aggregates, and communities in structured and unstructured health care settings. The unstructured setting is a geographical or situational environment that may not have established policies, procedures, and protocols and has the potential for variations requiring independent nursing decisions.
The ADN uses basic communication skills with focal clients and coordinates with other health team members to meet focal clients' needs. The ADN recognizes the individual's need for information and modifies a standard teaching plan. The ADN recognizes that nursing research influences nursing practice and assists in standardized data collection.	The BSN uses complex communication skills with focal clients. The BSN collaborates with other health team members and assumes an accountable role in change. The BSN assesses the need for information and designs comprehensive teaching plans individualized for the focal client. The BSN collaborates with nurse researchers and incorporates research findings into nursing practice.
The ADN organizes for focal clients those aspects of care for which she or he is responsible. The ADN maintains accountability for his or her practice and for aspects of nurse care she or he delegates to peers, licensed practical nurses, and ancillary nursing personnel. Within a specified work period, the ADN plans and implements nursing care that is consistent with the overall admission to postdischarge plan. The ADN practices within accepted ethical and legal parameters of nursing.	The BSN manages comprehensive nursing care for focal clients. The BSN maintains accountability for his or her practice and/or aspects of nursing care delegated to other nursing personnel consistent with their levels of education and expertise. The BSN plans for nursing care based on identified needs of the focal client from admission to postdischarge. The BSN practices within accepted ethical and legal parameters of nursing.

Adapted from Primm, 1987, p. 222.

Discussion Point

Consider the differentiation described in Table 2.1. What are the key differences in the associate and bachelor levels? Do these characteristics accurately describe the preparation received in your basic nursing education? Is there overlap in the characteristics? Is there enough clarity and distinction between the two levels?

Novice to Expert

Although Primm's model focused on educational levels as the differentiating factor, Benner's (1984) seminal work on the development of clinical competence appeared in the same decade and contributed critical new perspectives about the growth of competence, from novice to expert, within the actual practice of nursing. Benner's competence levels were subsequently incorporated into differentiated practice models and clinical ladder models (McClure, 1990).

Many differentiated practice models build on the convergence of competence attained through education and competence growth through practice. The acknowledgment of competence derived through experience defused some of the critics of differentiated practice who did not believe that competence was attained solely through formal educational pathways, and allowed for more flexibility in designing the differentiated role criteria.

This flexibility resulted in continued blurring of the distinction between the ADN and the BSN in the service setting, as nurses placed in positions were able to develop individual competence to fulfill their role demands, despite the fact that their education had not prepared them to do so. Because many RNs could meet job expectations without advancing their formal education, the value of advanced nursing education was questioned.

Discussion Point

What is the relative contribution of education and practice (experience) to your own nursing-skill mix? Which competencies can be more efficiently attained through education, rather than through practice? Which competencies can be more efficiently attained through practice, rather than through education?

Demonstration Projects

Sioux Valley Hospital in South Dakota was one of the early demonstration sites putting Primm's model into practice (Koerner, Bunkers, Nelson, & Santema, 1989). Building on the educational competencies previously defined by MAIN, job descriptions for two differentiated roles were developed. The associate role was comparable to generic staff nursing roles, with responsibility for the shift care of the client focused on short-term goals. A new role was designed to implement BSN level competencies by establishing responsibility for the client and family from preadmission to postdischarge, with home follow-up and appropriate referrals (Koepsell et al., 1994).

BOX 2.1   Outcomes of the Sioux Valley Project

Nursing Benefits

Increased satisfaction
Empowerment resulting from greater autonomy and control over nursing
    practice
Ability to choose a role that offered the most satisfaction
Greater autonomy in their roles as roles continued to grow
Increased autonomy under a shared governance system
Emotional compensation from patient and family satisfaction
Increased trust and respect from physicians as well as physician
    satisfaction
Monetary benefits on meeting identified goals

Patient and Family Benefits

Continuity of care
Participative care
Patient-centered care
Lower costs, primarily from decreased lengths of stay
High levels of patient satisfaction

Physician Benefits

Better continuity of care for patients
Organized discharge planning saves time and efforts
Increased patient satisfaction

Organizational Benefits

Enhanced recruitment and retention of nurses
Improved patient, family, and physician satisfaction
Cost containment resulting from continuity of care

Community Benefits

Recognition of need for outreach programs by RN case managers
Increased utilization of community services due to referrals
More collaborative care across the care continuum
High-quality, low-cost care

Source: Baker et al., 1994.

In describing criteria for distinct nursing roles, individual nurses' abilities and initiative were acknowledged to be as critical as educational background. The Sioux Valley model (Box 2.1) used all three components in its differentiated roles. The recognition that educational level alone does not necessarily determine competence was a distinction between the Sioux Valley Project and other models of differentiated practice (Koerner et al., 1989).

Critical understandings were added to the basic differentiated practice model that made the Sioux Valley project monumental in its impact—shifting the paradigm. Koerner explained the philosophy: "An evolutionary paradigm shift required of all nurses is the awareness that each nurse is not the whole of nursing, but rather each nurse contributes to the whole of nursing" (Koerner, 1992, p. 335). Differentiated roles required mutual valuing, and could be achieved only through a profound cultural shift of the service setting. The model was implemented through shared governance and consensus building.

These components were major contributions to the healing qualities that differentiated practice was envisioned to bring to a divided nursing profession. The Sioux Valley team believed this model provided the best opportunity to mend divisions in nursing

(Koerner et al., 1989). The Sioux Valley Hospital project provided some of the strongest documentation of the widespread benefits of their differentiated practice model, detailing the beneficiaries of the change, including patients and families, nurses, physicians, the organization, and the regional community (Baker, Aman, Dietz, & Miller, 1994).

The Healing Web

The work of the Sioux Valley project subsequently evolved into the Healing Web Partnership, involving several states, associate and baccalaureate degree educators, and nursing services (Fosbinder et al., n.d.). These partnerships promoted collaboration among educational levels and service in the design of work roles and educational experiences. As nursing roles in practice were differentiated, the clinical learning experiences for students were differentiated as well. ADN and BSN students shared clinical experiences with different roles in differentiated practice settings. BSN students were able to actually see role models and learn an expanded role, and at the same time work with and value the role of associate degree students. Fosbinder stated that the partnerships yielded the following benefits:

> ... ADN programs do not have to stretch their education time or curriculum beyond the intended scope to prepare their graduates for work demands that exceed that scope. Baccalaureate programs have the opportunity to provide students with experiences that incorporate the full scope of their curricular outcomes. Organizations that hire new graduates from these baccalaureate programs have a better grasp of the real range of abilities that each type of graduate has gained and, therefore, can expect that range in the graduates' performance. (Fosbinder et al., n.d., p. 6)

Fosbinder, Ashton, and Koerner (1997) proposed that differentiated nursing practice offered a superior paradigm for health care, and would contribute to effective responses to the dynamic health care needs of society.

By the latter half of the 20th century, a groundswell of interest in differentiated practice was evident, culminating in a national conference focused on many aspects of differentiated practice, including theoretical bases, the variety of nursing settings in which it had been implemented, cost analyses, frameworks for outcome evaluation, and challenges for the future (Goertzen, 1990). Despite the reported progress and interest in differentiated practice, McClure (1990) cautioned in her introduction to the conference that implementation of differentiated practice was slow in coming and long overdue, and would take high levels of commitment and perseverance.

"Valuing Differences, Creating Community"

Three major nursing organizations (AACN, NO-ADN, and AONE) worked together to develop a broad-based coalition of educational organizations and service leaders that would bring about change related to differentiated practice (AACN et al., 1995). This coalition built on the work of previous demonstration models. The task force report "A Model for Differentiated Nursing Practice" carried a logo composed of "ADN," "BSN," and "MSN," with the phrase "Valuing Differences, Creating Community," an apparent effort to focus on the model's potential to heal differences in nursing and create a unified approach (AACN et al., 1995) (Figure 2.1).

The task force determined that separate and distinct roles could be delineated for ADN, BSN, and MSN levels, with each role needed and valued for comprehensive health care delivery. The task force recognized that skills could be attained through experience

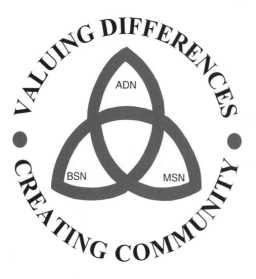

FIGURE 2.1 AACN/AONE/NOADN Differentiated Practice Logo

Source: American Association of Colleges of Nursing, American Organization for Nurse Executives, & National Organization for Associate Degree Nursing, 1995.

as well as education, but foresaw a future where the educational pathways would define the entry into the three differentiated practice roles (ADN, BSN, and MSN). The task force recommended that differentiated nursing practice be implemented in all health care practice settings and differentiated roles be taught in ADN and BSN education settings (AACN et al., 1995, p. 15). Many demonstration sites were developed over the next several years, implementing many of the recommendations of the AACN/AONE/NO-ADN task force (Barra & Johnsen, 1998; Nelson, Howell, Larson, & Karpiuk, 2001).

Statewide Models of Differentiated Practice

The scope and regulation of nursing practice and educational standards are controlled individually by each state, so true institutionalization of differentiated practice concepts must occur at the statewide level. Colorado developed the first voluntary statewide plan to improve articulation among educational levels in 1988, along with a model for differentiated nursing practice to facilitate appropriate utilization of nurses (AACN et al., 1995). Detailed competency statements and job descriptions for licensed practical nurses (LPN), ADN, and BSN levels were developed, to serve as guidelines for nurse educators, employers, and consumers (Table 2.2). The Colorado model set a standard and informed the work of many subsequent efforts.

In addition, many states participated in, and were partially funded by, the Robert Wood Johnson Foundation Colleagues in Caring Project, 1995–2003 (AACN, 2002a). Its purpose was to help develop nursing workforce coalitions that could analyze nursing workforce needs, address nursing shortages, enhance career mobility for nurses, and influence public policy and decisions (AACN, 2002a). More than 40 coalitions were formed nationwide, including major stakeholders in each region—all levels of nursing education, all categories of nursing employers, professional associations and state boards of nursing, policy bodies, consumers, payers, and businesses. Many of these coalitions concluded that the workforce projections documented the need for higher levels of education for nurses, and focused on differentiated practice models as one way to achieve better utilization of the existing workforce, as well as to provide incentives for ongoing education. Several of these collaboratives developed statewide models for differentiated practice (Eichelberger, 1997; Fox et al., 1999). A summary of presumed differentiated practice benefits derived from statewide discussions among educators and nursing service representatives is provided in Table 2.3.

TABLE 2.2

Sample Differentiated Competency Levels from the Colorado Alliance

LPN Provider Role	ADN Provider Role	BSN Provider Role
Assessment	Assessment	Assessment
Assists in the identification of a data base for the individual, family, or group, based on a holistic assessment of health needs.	Establishes a data base for the individual, family, or group based on a holistic assessment of needs.	Establishes and coordinates a comprehensive data base derived from a holistic assessment of the individual, family, group, or population, with complex and often unpredictable needs.
Evaluation	Evaluation	Evaluation
Participates in the evaluation of outcomes and in implementing the necessary changes.	Uses established indicators for evaluation of outcomes. Identifies alternate methods of meeting the individual, family, or group needs and modifies plan of care as necessary, documenting changes.	Develops indicators for evaluation of outcomes. Uses interdisciplinary resources for evaluation and revision of the plan of care for the individual, family, group, or population.

Source: Colorado Council on Nursing Education, 2000, pp. 10–12.

TABLE 2.3

Proposed Benefits of a Differentiated Practice Framework

Enables the Nurse to	Employers Will Have	Educators Will
• Work at an identified level of professional development • Evaluate own clinical performance and identify professional development needs • Direct professional growth • Pursue professional interests • Receive objective, competency-based performance evaluations • Decide whether to work toward advancing expertise or prepare for future roles • Decide whether higher education will enhance role performance • Have the opportunity for a defined framework for practice • Have the opportunity for recognition and potential for salary based on actual nursing performance and role	• A greater ability to target hiring practices to meet specific roles • More efficient use of the existing competencies of the nursing staff • The ability to recognize, reward, and promote the development of specific competencies needed in a specific work setting • The ability to work in partnership with nursing education to assure that a common understanding on practice and education competencies is maintained	• Be able to target educational resources to a core set of competencies that are desired, understood, and applied in nursing service • Decrease overlap among programs • Facilitate educational mobility of nurses • Work in partnership with nursing service to assure that a common understanding on practice and education competencies is maintained

Source: Adapted from Fox, Walker, & Bream, et al., 1999, pp. 23–24.

Differentiated Practice at the End of the Century

By the end of the 20th century, it appeared that great headway had been achieved in resolving the divisions in nursing education and allowing nurses to practice to their fullest capability. Baker et al. (1997) summarized the state of the science, noting the positive benefits demonstrated in 21 research studies (Box 2.2). Despite a good beginning, however, they cautioned that much more research was needed.

Accord (1999, p. 264) also applauded the achievements in differentiated practice. She described the movement as happening systematically and appropriately, respectful of the different levels of nursing because ". . . employers, administrators, educators, regulators, consumers, and nurses at all levels" worked to make it happen. It appeared the time for differentiated practice had come:

> *With the changing health care system and the need for a better-educated nursing work force, it has become imperative that nurses be employed according to their education and competency levels, not only for the sake of the public but for the sake of nurses who are being asked to function either above or below their areas of expertise. . . . In the long run, differentiating the work of registered nurses can only be viewed as positive. Nurses will be allowed to function at their level of competency and will have opportunities to increase their competency levels through further education and/or certification. Employers will benefit from knowing what competencies each nurse brings to the workplace (Accord, 1999, p. 264).*

BOX 2.2

Research Study Fuels the Controversy

The State of the Science
Baker et al. (1997) reviewed the research related to differentiated practice outcomes, critiquing 21 databased articles related to implementation of differentiated practice.

> Baker, C., Lamm, G., Winter, A., et al. (1997). Differentiated nursing practice: Assessing the state-of-the-science. *Nursing Economics, 15*(5), 253–261.

Study Findings
Many positive outcomes were reported, including increased nurse satisfaction, increased participatory management, improved documentation, and decreased RN overtime. Patient satisfaction improved, length of stay decreased, patient referrals increased, and modest improvements in patient falls and medication errors were reported. Although cost savings were reported, the costs of implementation in terms of organization investment were not fully addressed in the studies reviewed. Many of the outcomes reported were anecdotal, and methodological concerns were evident.

Baker et al. concluded that although there was evidence of positive outcomes, the state of the science was in its "infancy." Recommendations were made for refining future research approaches and reporting methods, including replication studies and cost-benefit analyses. However, the authors also acknowledged that the turbulent health care arena, demands on nurse administrators, and inadequate research funding would impact the likelihood of expanded research in this area. (*Note: These caveats proved to be prophetic, as following this extensive research review, few new studies on differentiated practice were published.*)

Accord did, however, acknowledge inherent difficulties; for example, nurses might experience identity threats and fear of change, despite the value-neutral language of the models; employers might resist if they believed the model would eliminate choice in their hiring practices; and the "nurse is a nurse is a nurse" mentality would be hard to change at all levels.

> ***CONSIDER:** Differentiation requires a high degree of integration or collaboration among the individuals and units, and requires extensive corporate support (Koerner, 1992).

> **Discussion Point**
>
> How might nursing shortages impact the implementation of differentiated practice? (Consider the impact if certain roles specified BSN preparation as a requirement, yet BSN shortages persisted.)

Opposing Views

Detractors of differentiated practice were evident in the late 20th century, though not widely prominent in the major nursing publications. A union representative categorically rejected differentiating practice, claiming, "There is a hidden agenda to differentiated practice. It is that of differentiated pay attached to the various envisioned levels. . . . It represents a hierarchical stratification model with no sound clinical basis and will be used to divide direct care registered nurses by pay and status . . ." (Costello, 1998, p. 25). This union ultimately rejected the use of educational preparation in clinical ladders, certification, and recognition of clinical expertise (California Nurses Association, 1999). McClure (1990) predicted that unionized settings would have the most difficulty implementing differentiated practice models, as unions traditionally have rejected programs in which anything other than seniority is rewarded with added compensation.

> **Discussion Point**
>
> In light of health care's needs for a better-educated workforce, does the union position that educational preparation should not be used as one of the elements of role descriptions seem defensible? What rationale might unions have for wishing to ignore educational achievement in clinical practice?

On the other side were those who believed higher educational levels were needed for all of nursing, and that differentiation did not resolve that issue. Bronson-Gray (1998), in a *Nurseweek* editorial, claimed:

> *The overall goal [of differentiated practice] is laudable: encourage nurses to seek higher education and put nurses in roles where they can best apply their education and experience. . . . but it doesn't go far enough. It doesn't say the bachelor's degree is so valuable that every nurse should get it. . . . All entry-level*

nurses should have equal status and standing in the eyes of the patient, the public, and the hospital. The only way to achieve that is to have one educational level for entry into the practice of nursing. No other profession has created a two-tiered system, and nursing's current model won't work for the future (Bronson-Gray, 1998).

Bronson-Gray advocated for the BSN as the basic minimum education requirement, echoing the entry-into-practice debate that was experiencing a resurgence at the time (see Chapter 1).

▶ DIFFERENTIATED PRACTICE IN THE 21ST CENTURY

Despite a promising entry into the 21st century, the prognosis for widespread implementation of differentiated practice remains guarded. As nursing shortages intensified, major nursing organizations applied their energies to workforce data collection, recruitment strategies, and efforts to enhance funding for basic nursing education at all levels, along with efforts to address emerging faculty shortages. Evidence of differentiated practice discussions in statewide collaboratives and in the literature diminished markedly. However, promising achievements were evident, including the positions of the Pew Commission designating 21st century competencies, accrediting bodies, use of differentiation in clinical ladders, and the growth of employers' recognition of the benefits of BSN preparation.

Competencies for the 21st Century

The Pew Commission, a leader in workforce policy development for health professions, challenged educational programs for all levels of health care providers to prepare providers for the expanding needs of health care, recommending that Pew's delineation of health care competencies for the 21st century be used as benchmarks for educators (Brady, Leuner, Bellack, et al., 2001).

A South Carolina Colleagues in Caring project developed a model to analyze the utility of the Pew competencies for nursing. The Pew competencies were differentiated across four levels of nursing education: LPN, ADN, BSN, and MSN—with recommended teaching–learning strategies for each level. The South Carolina model provides a guide for both educators and employers to transform the structure of nursing to attend to emerging nursing roles, managed care, quality and performance measures, new technologies, and complex patient problems (Brady et al., 2001).

Accrediting Agencies and Differentiation

Through the accreditation process, nursing education programs have been supported in clearly defining the competencies of their graduates in a manner consistent with defined standards (Felton, Abbe, Gilbert, & Ingle, 1999). To the extent that nursing programs adhere to national accreditation standards, adherence to principles of differentiation are supported. However, not all programs seek national accreditation, leading to continuing incongruence in educational approaches to differentiation among different program levels.

Use of Clinical Ladders

The clinical ladder concept for designating career progression within the work setting developed concurrently with many differentiated practice models as one way of expressing

UNIT 1   Furthering the Profession

competencies in terms relevant to service settings. Many clinical ladders clearly reflect differentiated practice competencies (Froman, 2001). An effective clinical ladder is currently seen as a means to enhance recruitment and retention of staff and to improve nurse satisfaction (Beyers, 1998; McClure, 1990). Many service organizations market their clinical ladders as part of their recruiting strategies, reflecting the presumed attractiveness of these systems for nurses. Implementation of clinical ladders may occur without a full-scale differentiated practice approach, but can achieve some of the same goals—encouraging continued formal education and purposeful development of competencies valued by the work setting. The value of clinical ladders that acknowledge education, level of training, and experience is reaffirmed by the Joint Commission on Accreditation of Healthcare Organizations (JCAHO) in its recommendations to bolster the nursing education infrastructure (JCAHO, 2002).

*CONSIDER: Strong support for hospitals to recognize education in their career ladders will help to further institutionalize differentiation in the service setting.

Discussion Point

Does your service setting acknowledge any difference between educational levels, such as educational requirements for specific positions or to advance to certain levels? If so, are financial rewards attached?

Employers' Preference for BSN

The actual determinant of how nurses are employed and the value placed on their educational background occurs at the point of service (Pesut, 2002). It appears that major inroads in differentiation have been made in this arena, based on surveys of chief nursing officers (Goode et al., 2001) and agencies employing RNs (Sechrist, Lewis, Rutledge, & Keating, 2002) (see Chapter 1). Employers who understand the differences in the competencies of the diverse levels of nursing preparation are more likely to design roles that will maximize the application of those competencies, and to hire those most likely to be able to assume those roles. To the extent that these practices occur, differentiation will become increasingly evident.

Fear and Fighting

Many nursing leaders, nursing administrators, educators, and nurses believe differentiated practice is a good idea. Its origins were logical and compelling. But, despite some inroads, many barriers to differentiated practice are evident at the beginning of the 21st century.

The nursing workforce culture is not highly supportive of RNs attaining higher degrees. The workforce is deeply divided on the issue of educational preparation, as seen by letters to the editor of major publications whenever the issue of educational levels is presented. A major division can be seen between those who proclaim the baccalaureate degree enhances practice and those who vehemently claim the BSN adds nothing. A major argument is that bedside nursing does not require a BSN, and that associate degree nurses are better prepared for bedside nursing. However, nurses who have not experienced baccalaureate or higher education are limited in their ability to determine what it

BOX 2.3

Research Study Fuels the Controversy

Impact of Education

Lillibridge and Fox (in press) conducted a qualitative descriptive study of RNs' perceptions on the impact of RN-BSN education. Six RNs were interviewed within two years of completion of the BSN. All respondents were women, aged 35 to 52 years, with 4 to 15 years of experience in nursing.

Lillibridge, J., & Fox, S. (2005). RN to BSN education: What do RNs think? *Nurse Educator, 30*(1), 12–16.

Study Findings

These RNs elected to advance their education because they wanted to have an edge on jobs and career mobility, and some saw the need for advancing their competencies. For example, one RN noted "While I had . . . good leadership skills, they weren't appropriate and they didn't work for what I was now being asked to do." Although the RNs were negative about their experiences at the beginning of the program, their attitudes became positive as they began to identify benefits in areas of learning they had been unaware of before entering the program. Benefits included "an expanded world view," "seeing the bigger picture," becoming knowledgeable about research findings, developing more confidence, and looking at things differently. Notably, they felt they could apply new thinking skills in the workplace; for example, implementing change in a specific nursing practice based on research and knowledge of the change process. One RN noted: ". . . while I think that I was a very, very clinically astute RN . . . you don't know what you don't know . . . I can remember feeling at first . . . how much different can it be?" RNs in this study overwhelmingly found benefits in attaining their BSNs, both personally and professionally. Most attained more than they expected, expressing amazement that they actually did change their perspectives, saw a bigger picture, or enhanced their critical thinking.

Although this was a small study focused on alumni of one program, findings indicate that RNs who experience both sides of the academic perspective—ADN preparation and practice and BSN preparation and practice do see a difference.

can offer for their practice. Recent research indicates that RNs who have completed an RN to BSN program do see added value from their education (Lillibridge & Fox, 2005) (Box 2.3).

> ***CONSIDER:** Nurses spend a lot of time trying to determine whether BSN or ADN programs produce the better nurse, rather than recognizing the differences in the competencies each program is geared to produce, and valuing the differences.

The predominance of associate degree and diploma nurses in the workforce poses a major barrier to changing the status quo. Associate degree and diploma nurses constitute 70% of the workforce (Spratley, Johnson, Sochalski, et al., 2002). In an undifferentiated model, RNs with diverse educational backgrounds hold many positions in nursing management, and are in the decision-making bodies that govern the structure of practice in their agencies. Lack of education may be a limitation in how these nurses envision the structure of nursing practice. Changes in nursing roles to incorporate competencies that associate degree and diploma nurses do not possess might pose overwhelming threats, as these nurses fear devaluing of their own education and status in the institution.

Proponents of differentiated practice propose that BSN graduates are socialized into a work setting dominated by associate degree nurses, and in settings that are not structured for the BSN to use all capabilities. Efforts to apply higher level skills in the practice of bedside nursing would likely lead to resistance to incorporating skills not held by the majority of nurses.

> *CONSIDER: Despite health care's increasing demands for a more educated workforce, only 16% of associate degree RNs and 24% of diploma RNs have gone on to attain a higher education (USDHHS, 2002).

Discussion Point

Would widespread implementation of differentiated practice provide greater incentives and rewards for nurses to continue their formal education?

The identity issue related to education in nursing is so dominant that nursing is one of the few professional fields that has not increased educational requirements corresponding to the growth in complexity of health care technology (see Chapter 1) (AACN, 2003). Many RNs feel the need to affirm that their basic education was adequate, and remains sufficient. Somehow, formal education has been separated from practice in the eyes of many nurses. They assert that more education does not make a "better" nurse.

Notably, recent debate over whether an RN's education affects the quality of patient care elicited an angry response from the president of the NO-ADN, affirming the organization's recent position that there is no value added when a graduate of an ADN program attains a BSN degree, finding the BSN "expensive and redundant" (Bernier, 2004). (This position is in marked contrast to the NO-ADN position less than a decade earlier, supporting differentiated practice models [AACN et al., 1995].)

Conversely, the president of AACN countered that education makes a difference in reducing medical errors and disciplinary actions. Lack of differentiation results in inadequate patient care and high nursing turnover (Long, 2003). Long further asserted that "continuing to deploy a homogenized RN workforce, using a single scope of practice for those with substantively different entry-level preparation, is dangerous for patients and demoralizing for nurses" (Long, 2003, p. 124).

Entry Into Practice: A Recurring Issue

The need for better-prepared nurses has led some, despite the nursing shortage, to firmly assert that the multiple entry points for one license are incompatible with today's health care needs. A major nursing organization in California, the Association of California Nurse Leaders (ACNL) proposed a "BSN by 2010" initiative for California (ACNL, 2002; Barter & McFarland, 2001). Along similar lines, the New York State Board for Nursing (Webber, 2004) proposed that nurses who graduate from diploma or associate degree programs be required to attain a baccalaureate degree in nursing within 10 years for license renewal in New York. RNs educated prior to an as yet unspecified date would be grandfathered and exempt from meeting this requirement. Both of these proposals have generated active discussion.

Organizational Resistance

Another major barrier to the implementation of differentiated practice is the implication that major structural changes in the organization of nursing care must occur. Many nursing administrators do not have advanced nursing education themselves, so envisioning a system-wide change to incorporate differentiated practice would be a daunting task. Additionally, organizations rely heavily on maintaining the status quo, unless outside forces such as accrediting agencies or third-party payers mandate change.

The type of structural changes demonstrated by the Sioux Valley project took seven years, requiring an extremely high level of institutional commitment and the cooperation of many outside of nursing (Koerner & Karpiuk, 1994). Not many institutions would be willing to make such a commitment, particularly in a time of nursing shortage when priority issues are recruitment and retention of nurses. However, institutions that have incorporated differentiated practice models would counter that the model effectively addresses recruitment and retention issues, by enhancing nurses' job satisfaction.

Discussion Point

Given that transformational leadership and extensive planning are critical to implementation of differentiated practice, how widespread is differentiated practice likely to become in the near future?

An Entirely New Nurse?

A large part of the discussions on differentiated practice focus on the escalating demands in health care for better-educated providers as one rationale for the model—to facilitate baccalaureate graduates to apply their complete spectrum of competencies. It is not surprising that, ultimately, nursing leaders would begin to question even the baccalaureate level as the minimal entry-level education. Yeaworth (1990) posed the question near the end of the 20th century:

> *We have had so much difficulty getting the baccalaureate-level nurse accepted as a professional that I wonder if we have been aiming too low? . . . Differences in practice are easy to distinguish between RNs with the various undergraduate levels of preparation and RNs with master's preparation in nursing. . . . Perhaps our goal should be the generic master's and the RN-to-master's, thus making a clear distinction between two levels of practice—associate degree and master's degree (Yeaworth, 1990, p. 20).*

Over a decade later, Joel (2002) echoed this sentiment, describing the complex challenges of today's health care and concluding:

> *The requirement for highly sophisticated providers and more independent decision-making is obvious. Given a supportive environment, the more educated practitioner will be the most cost-efficient. This means commitment to a longer and more demanding education than the baccalaureate degree.*

> *Moreover, the increased demand for nursing services, as evidenced by the growing presence of chronic illness and aging population, sustains the case for associate degree education. . . .. Contrasting the nurse prepared at the graduate level to the associate degree nurse demonstrates a significant difference in competency, one that is obvious to nurses, and additionally to the consumer, the industry and allied health care interests (Joel, 2002, p. 7).*

Along similar lines, in its Vision 2020 for Nursing, the Nursing Practice and Education Consortium (N-PEC) (a collaboration among 10 major national nursing organizations) proposed a marked revision in nursing roles and scopes of practice, suggesting four possible scopes of practice: an unlicensed provider; two intermediate licensed levels, with separate and distinct licensures; and one master's educated level. They charged the profession to continue work on delineating scopes of practice with corresponding competencies for each type of nursing care provider, developing appropriate licensure and certification mechanisms, and enacting new roles in practice settings (AONE, 2004, p. 3).

Concurrently, the AACN Task Force on Education and Regulation (TFER) revisited the progress on differentiated practice, concluding that the AACN/AONE/NO-ADN consensus statement of 1995 on differentiated practice resulted in very limited implementation of differentiated practice roles (AACN, 2002b). A major barrier was seen as the lack of separate licensure for different roles. The TFER concluded that a circle of inaction existed, in which "each side of the discussion—the practice community and the regulatory community is unwilling to change the status quo (AACN, 2002b, p. 5). In addition, the TFER stated that recurrent cycles of nursing shortages would never be broken unless profound changes occurred in nursing education, practice, and licensure.

Subsequently, the task force proposed a new nursing role—the clinical nurse leader (CNL), to meet health care delivery needs (AACN, 2003). The description of this nurse is:

> *. . . a leader in the health care delivery system across all settings in which health care is delivered, not just the acute care setting. The implementation of the CNL role, however, will vary across settings. The CNL role is not one of administration or management. The CNL assumes accountability for client care outcomes through the assimilation and application of research-based information to design, implement, and evaluate client plans of care. The CNL is a provider and a manager of care at the point of care to individuals and cohorts or populations. The CNL designs, implements, and evaluates client care by coordinating, delegating and supervising the care provided by the health care team, including licensed nurses, technicians, and other health professionals (AACN, 2003, p. 5).*

Preliminary discussions indicated the CNL would be educated beyond the baccalaureate level, with a new license and legal scope of practice (AACN, 2003). A new round of discussions on differentiation will result from this initiative. As the discussion evolves, differentiated practice concepts will continue to be a foundational part of the debate. However, discussions will expand beyond the efforts to differentiate the four educational pathways sharing one licensure.

Efforts to achieve a separate licensure for advanced positions requiring master's preparation will be a necessary part of the discussion. Thus, we begin the 21st century revisiting some of the arguments that led to the initial discussions on differentiated practice, but proposing to expand the number of roles and the education required, along with changes in licensure. Many of the same dilemmas found in the 20th century will be reencountered. Certainly foundation funding and demonstration projects will be needed, as will visionary leadership. Nursing unity will also be needed for widespread implementation. It is uncertain how that unity will materialize, as it has not been evident in the preceding decades.

Discussion Point

As attempts are made to categorize specific advanced functions in care coordinator or case manager roles as master's level functions, will BSN-prepared nurses begin to feel invalidated and threatened? Or, will more BSNs pursue graduate education to attain the advanced competencies needed? Will baccalaureate educators in colleges without master's degree programs likewise feel threatened? Will opponents of such changes declare that there are too few master's prepared nurses, too few graduate programs, and too few doctorally prepared faculty to be able to meet the demands for a new level of advanced practitioner? Will corporate executives declare that a master's level nurse will be too costly to employ in positions that might formerly have been filled by RNs without graduate education?

Reframing the Issue of Differentiation

Many professions recognize the value of education in providing the most expeditious path to advancing competencies. Experience also contributes to competence development, enhancing skills through practice, repetition, and the like. The general body of nurses appears to value the knowledge acquired through experience over the knowledge attained through formal education, the difference between knowing "how" versus knowing "why." Knowing how limits the nurse to functioning in the status quo, whereas knowing why allows for adaptation and innovation as circumstances change. The value of formal education must be paramount for nursing to grow to meet health care challenges. The ongoing debate in nursing over the value of education echoes Brown's epochal observation that the sights of nursing have not been lifted because education almost always is put in second place (Brown, 1948, p. 129).

Some lessons are clear from nursing's experiments with differentiated practice. Nursing roles and the competencies needed for those roles must be clearly defined; the appropriate education for those roles must be clearly linked to attaining the competencies; education pathways must be clearly outlined, with facilitation of nurses to enter those pathways; and legal scope of practice must agree with the education requisites. For differentiation to truly work, nurses with widely different education paths will need access to roles that match their preparation, and mechanisms to expand their preparation. Regardless of the role definitions that will ultimately result, all nurses will need to be prepared to expand their competencies through lifelong learning, as health care issues continue to escalate in complexity.

Whatever the initial educational level of the nurse, ongoing education can enhance practice. Perhaps the schism over educational levels can be reconceptualized so that all nurses embrace the value of all levels of education, without devaluing the foundational entry-level nursing education. Rather (1993, p. 114) speaks eloquently to the issue of how much education is needed, asserting:

> ◆ *"every nurse should obtain as much formal education as he or she possibly can"*. . . . *In the language of possibilities, more education is a positive thing in and of itself . . . more education is "better" for all of us, and it is better for the whole nursing community when one RN returns to school.*

---
*⁕**CONSIDER:** Most nurses, educators, and accrediting bodies support the notion of lifelong learning for nurses.

D i s c u s s i o n   P o i n t

How should lifelong learning occur? What are the pros and cons of such learning occurring through formal education versus individual initiative? How should the nurse provide evidence of such learning? Should ongoing learning be rewarded with advanced education credit?

◆ CONCLUSIONS

The evidence is overwhelming that health care delivery demands a high level of nursing competency. The logic of acknowledging, using, and rewarding advanced competency through differentiated practice is compelling; the logistics of widespread implementation and acceptance are daunting. Over three decades of discussion, projects, statewide collaboratives, and supportive research, differentiated practice has not attained widespread implementation. Extensive efforts have achieved better understanding of the differences among educational levels and the need for competency-based roles in service.

State and regional collaboratives have achieved broad-based dialogue and unified action, which have been particularly effective in bringing nurses and nursing organizations together to work on the most serious threat to health care delivery—critical nursing shortages. These accomplishments have served to unite the profession. However, to the extent that many nurses feel invalidated and disenfranchised by the concept of differentiated practice, the issue continues to be divisive. It appears that a well-planned, massive change in hospital culture can occur with enlightened leadership, overcoming individual resistance. However, such change requires great resolve, and is greatly enhanced by funding to support the change.

Many of the caveats of nurse leaders who promoted differentiated practice high-light many of the difficulties inherent in achieving widespread implementation, and help to explain the recent lack of noticeable progress. The need for a profound cultural shift (Koerner, 1992) has not materialized; the need for high levels of commitment and perseverance (McClure, 1990) have not been widespread; and identity threats and fear of change (Accord, 1999), which are widespread have prevented the full implementation of differentiated practice. Critical nursing shortages and a turbulent health care arena have also diverted the attention of nurses.

Currently, critical dialogue on nursing shortages overwhelms the issue of differentiation. When nursing resources are scarce, maximizing their use becomes more an issue of doing the best we can with what we have, even though this is a shortsighted approach. The nursing profession is united behind resolving nursing shortages, but will continue to disagree on how. Differentiated practice will continue to offer one possible solution, uniting in some ways, dividing in others. As more nurses advance their education, will the nature of this debate change?

Regardless of how differentiation occurs, it will always be needed, unless it becomes feasible for every patient to have access to one practitioner educated to the maximal level and able to provide comprehensive care. Given the resource constraints in the real world, the most efficient organization of health care delivery requires that those practitioners with the highest level of specialized competencies be used to their fullest capabilities. These specialists can serve the greatest number of clients if the functions that can be carried out by lower levels of workers are differentiated. For nursing to maintain control over care of the whole patient, the patient's family, groups, and the health care environment, it will have to be positioned to embrace and manage the necessary changes.

Effective differentiation in nursing will always require three things:

▶ Nurses who value lifelong education, and continue to advance their knowledge and competence, no matter what their initial nursing education is.
▶ Practice roles designed to use a nurse's full spectrum of competencies, based on full understanding of the educational preparation for each level of education.
▶ Educational systems that are in touch with rapid changes in practice.

The first requires the open, questing attitude of each individual nurse—one who does not resist change but embraces his or her continued growth and development. The service and educational components require continual communication, understanding, and responsiveness to health care demands on the part of service leaders and educational leaders.

FOR ADDITIONAL DISCUSSION

1. In a differentiated practice work environment, does increasing education require the nurse to move away from the patient?
2. In what ways are health care demands becoming more complex? What educational content will be needed to prepare nurses for these demands?
3. Who or what should determine the appropriate competence and required preparation for nursing roles? (state licensing boards? nursing employers? nurse educators? hospital accrediting bodies? educational accrediting bodies? nursing unions?)
4. Does an agency's support for differentiated practice depend on the educational level of the chief nursing officer and other administrators? Why or why not?
5. Differentiated practice models have outlined competencies for the clinical nurse. Are there competencies for nurse administrators? Should these be linked to education?
6. If the majority of nurses currently held a bachelor's degree, would differentiated practice achieve more widespread acceptance?
7. Would working RNs be more likely to pursue advanced formal education if they perceive that it is valued in the workplace, and an important aspect of progress in clinical ladders?
8. Do you have career ladders in your work setting? Is education considered a part of clinical career ladders? Should it be?
9. Do RNs in your work setting plan to continue their formal education, with either a BSN or an MSN?

REFERENCES

Accord, L. (1999). The case for differentiated practice. *Journal of Professional Nursing, 15*(5), 264.

American Association of Colleges of Nursing. (1998). *The essentials of baccalaureate education for professional nursing practice*. Washington, DC: Author.

American Association of Colleges of Nursing. (2002a). *Colleagues in caring project: General information*. Washington, DC: Author.

American Association of Colleges of Nursing. (2002b, April). *Report of the task force on education and regulation for professional nursing practice I*. Washington, DC: Author. Available at: http://www.aacn.nche.edu/Education/edandreg02.htm. Accessed January 14, 2004.

American Association of Colleges of Nursing. (May 2003). *Working paper on the role of the clinical nurse leader*. Available at: http://www.aacn.nche.edu/NewNurse/. Accessed November 7, 2004.

American Association of Colleges of Nursing, American Organization for Nurse Executives, & National Organization for Associate Degree Nursing. (1995). A model for differentiated nursing practice. Washington, DC: American Association of Colleges of Nursing.

American Organization of Nurse Executives. (2004). Vision 2020 for nursing. Retrieved March 31, 2004, from http://www.hospitalconnect.com/aone/advocacy/npec.html.

Association of California Nurse Leaders. (2002). A better educated nursing workforce. Retrieved March 29, 2004, from www.acnl.org.

Baker, C., Lamm, G., Winter, A., et al. (1997). Differentiated nursing practice: Assessing the state-of-the-science. *Nursing Economics, 15*(5), 253–261.

Baker, E., Aman, S., Dietz, R., & Miller, D. (1994). Compensation. In J. Koerner & K. Karpiuk (Eds.), *Implementing differentiated practice: Transformation by design* (pp. 290–305). Gaithersburg, MD: Aspen.

Barra, J. & Johnsen, V. (1998). The Healing Web: Implementation for education. *Journal of Nursing Education, 37*(7), 329–331.

Barter, M. & McFarland, P. (2001). BSN by 2010: A California initiative. *Journal of Nursing Administration, 31*(3), 141–144.

Benner, P. (1984). *From novice to expert: Excellence and power in clinical nursing practice*. Menlo Park, CA: Addison-Wesley.

Berlin, L., Stennett, J., & Bednash, G. (2004). 2003–2004 enrollment and graduations in baccalaureate and graduate programs in nursing. Washington, DC: American Association of Colleges of Nursing.

Bernier, S. (2004). RN education: A matter of degrees. *Nursing 2004, 34*(3), 48–51.

Beyers, M. (1998). About improving clinical ladders. *Nursing Management, 29*(10), 96.

Brady, M., Leuner, J., Bellack, J., et al. (2001). A proposed framework for differentiating the 21 Pew competencies by level of nursing education. *Nursing and Health Care Perspectives, 22*(1), 30–35.

Bronson-Gray, B. (June 7, 1998). What's different about differentiated practice? Available at: http://www.nurseweek.com/ednote/98/980607.html. Accessed March 2, 2004.

Brown, E. (1948). Nursing for the future: A report prepared for the National Nursing Council. New York: Russell Sage Foundation.

California Nurses Association. (1999). CNA's position on differentiated practice/competency based role differentation in nursing. Available at: http://www.calnurse.org/cna/np/np6101599.html. Accessed March 2, 2004.

Colorado Council on Nursing Education. (2000). The Colorado nursing articulation model. The Colorado Trust. Available at: www.uchsc.edu/ahec/cando/nursing/. Accessed March 31, 2004.

Costello, K. (1998). Differentiated practice—the recycled professional vs. technical debate. *Revolution: The Journal of Nurse Empowerment, 8*(3–4), 24–25.

DeBack, V. (1987). The National Commission on Nursing Implementation Project: Report to the participants of Nurses in Agreement conference. *Journal of Professional Nursing, 3*(4), 226–229.

Eichelberger, L. W. E. (1997). *The Mississippi competency model*. Jackson, MS: Office of Nursing Workforce Redevelopment.

Felton, G., Abbe, S., Gilbert, C., & Ingle, J. (1999). How does NLNAC support the concept of differentiated practice? *Nursing and Healthcare Perspectives, 20*(5), 275.

Fosbinder, D., Ashton, C., Karpiuk, K., et al. (n.d.). History of the Healing Web partnership: A national network. Pamphlet from the National Healing Web Conference.

Fosbinder, D., Ashton, C., & Koerner, J. (1997). The National Healing Web partnership. *Journal of Nursing Administration, 27*(4), 37–41.

Fox, S., Walker, P., Bream, T., & Education/Industry Interface Work Group of the California Strategic Planning Committee for Nursing/Colleagues in Caring. (1999a). *California's framework for competency-based role differentiation in nursing*. Sacramento, CA: Association of California Nurse Leaders.

Froman, R. (2001). Assessing the credibility of a clinical ladder review process: An interrater reliability study. *Nursing Outlook, 49*(1), 27–29.

Goertzen, I. (Ed.). (1990). *Differentiating nursing practice: Into the twenty-first century*. Kansas, MO: American Academy of Nursing.

Goode, C., Pinkerton, S., McCausland, M., et al. (2001). Documenting chief nursing officers' preference for BSN-prepared nurses. *Journal of Nursing Administration, 31*(2), 55–59.

Haase, P. T. (1990). *The origins and rise of associate degree nursing education.* Durham, NC: Duke University Press.

Joel, L. (2002, May 31). Education for entry into nursing practice: Revisited for the 21st century. *Online Journal of Issues in Nursing, 7*(2), Retrieved February 26, 2004, from http://www.nursingworld.org/ojin/topic18/tpc18_4.htm

Joint Commission on Accreditation of Healthcare Organizations. (2002). Health care at the crossroads: Strategies for addressing the evolving nursing crisis. Available at: http://www.jcaho.org/news+room/press+kits/executive+summary.htm. Accessed September 16, 2004.

Koepsell, P., Jensen, R., Reisdorfer, J., et al. (1994). Continuity. In J. Koerner & K. Karpiuk (Eds.), *Implementing differentiated nursing practice: Transformation by design* (pp. 129–187). Gaithersburg, MD: Aspen.

Koerner, J. (1992). Differentiated practice: The evolution of professional nursing. *Journal of Professional Nursing, 8*(6), 335–341.

Koerner, J., Bunkers, L., Nelson, B., & Santema, K. (1989). Implementing differentiated practice: The Sioux Valley Hospital experience. *Journal of Nursing Administration, 19*(2), 13–20.

Koerner, J. G., & Karpiuk, K. L. (1994). *Implementing differentiated nursing practice: Transformation by design.* Gaithersburg, MD: Aspen.

Lillibridge, J. & Fox, S. (2005). RN to BSN education: What do RNs think? *Nurse Educator, 30*(1), 12–16.

Long, K. (2003). Licensure matters: Better patient care requires change in regulation as well as education. *Journal of Professional Nursing, 19*(3), 123–125.

McClure, M. (1990). Introduction. In I. Goertzen (Ed.), *Differentiating nursing practice: Into the twenty-first century* (pp. 1–11). Kansas City, MO: American Academy of Nursing.

Montag, M. L. (1951). *The education of nursing technicians.* New York: G.P. Putnam's Sons.

Nelson, M., Howell, J., Larson, J., & Karpiuk, K. (2001). Student outcomes of the Healing Web: Evaluation of a transformative model for nursing education. *Journal of Nursing Education, 40*(9), 404–412.

Pesut, D. (2002). Differentiation: Practice versus services. *Journal of Professional Nursing, 18*(3), 118–119.

Primm, P. (1987). Differentiated practice for ADN- and BSN-prepared nurses. *Journal of Professional Nursing, 3*(4), 218–224.

Rather, M. (1993). "Harbingers of entry into practice": The lived experience of returning RN students. In N. L. Diekelmann & M. L. Rather (Eds.), *Transforming RN Education: Dialogue and Debate*, pp. 97–120. New York: National League for Nursing.

Sechrist, K., Lewis, E., Rutledge, D., & Keating, S. (2002). *Planning for California's Nursing Work Force: Phase III Final Report.* Sacramento, CA: Association of California Nurse Leaders.

Spratley, R., Johnson, A., Sochalski, J., et al. (2002). The registered nurse population: Findings from the national sample survey of registered nurses. Available at: http://bhpr.hrsa.gov/healthworkforce/reports/rnsurvey/rnss1.htm. Accessed March 31, 2004.

United States Department of Health and Human Services. (2002). Projected supply, demand, and shortages of registered nurses: 2000–2020. Available at: ftp://ftp.hrsa.gov/bhpr/nationalcenter/rnproject.pdf. Accessed March 31, 2004.

Webber, N. (2004). State nursing board proposes 'advancement of the profession' initiative. Available at: http://www.nysna.org/departments/communications/publications/report/2004/may/initiative.htm. Accessed May 31, 2004.

Yeaworth, R. (1990). An educator's response to models of differentiated practice. In I. Goertzen (Ed.), *Differentiating nursing practice: Into the twenty-first century* (pp. 415–421). Kansas City, MO: American Academy of Nursing.

BIBLIOGRAPHY

American Association of Colleges of Nursing. (1996). *The Essentials of Master's Education for Advanced Practice Nursing.* Washington, DC: Author.

American Association of Colleges of Nursing. (1999). Position statement. A vision of baccalaureate and graduate nursing education: The next decade. *Journal of Professional Nursing, 15*(1), 59–65.

American Nurses Association. (2002). *Nursing's Agenda for the Future.* New York: Author.

Board of Nurse Examiners for the State of Texas & Texas Board of Vocational Nurse Examiners. (2002). *Differentiated Entry Level Competencies of Graduates of Texas Nursing Programs.* Austin, Texas: Author.

Bunkers, S. (1992). The healing web: A transformative model for nursing. *Nursing and Health Care, 12*(2), 68–73.

Cleland, V., Forsey, L., & DeGroot, H. (1993). Computer simulations of the differentiated pay structure model. *Journal of Nursing Administration, 23*(3), 53–59.

Coffman, J., Spetz, J., Seago, J., et al. (2001). *Nursing in California: A workforce crisis.* San Francisco, CA: UCSF Center for the Health Professions California Workforce Initiative.

DeGroot, H., Forsey, L., & Cleland, V. (1992). The nursing practice personnel data set: Implications for professional practice systems. *Journal of Nursing Administration, 22*(3), 23–28.

Devaney, S. Kuehn, A., Jones, R., & Ott, L. (2003). Tackling the nursing shortage in rural America: Linking of education and service in a differentiated practice environment. *Nursing Leadership Forum, 8*(1), 13–17.

Forsey, L., Cleland, V., & Miller, B. (1993). Job descriptions for differentiated nursing practice and differentiated pay. *Journal of Nursing Administration, 23*(5), 33–40.

Keating, S., Rutledge, D., Sargent, A., & Walker, P. (2003). A test of the California competency-based differentiated role model. *Managed Care Quarterly, 11*(1), 40–46.

Keating, S. & Sargent, A. (2001). Testing California's differentiated practice model through industry and education partnerships. *Nursing Administration Quarterly, 26*(1), 24–28.

National Advisory Council on Nurse Education and Practice. (2002). Second report to the Secretary of Health and Human Services and the Congress. Rockville, MD: U.S. Department of Health and Human Services.

National League for Nursing Accrediting Commission. (2003). *Interpretive Guidelines by Program Type*. New York: Author.

Nelson, M. (2002, May 31). Education for professional nursing practice: Looking backward into the future. *Online Journal of Issues in Nursing, 7*(3). Available at: http://www.nursingworld.org/ojin/topic18/tpc18_3.htm.

New Mexico Consortium for Nursing Workforce Development. (1998). *Standards For Differentiated Competencies of the Nursing Workforce at Time of Entry/Advanced Beginner*. Albuquerque, NM: Author.

O'Neil, E. & Pew Health Professions Commission. (1998). *Recreating Health Professional Practice for a New Century*. San Francisco: Pew Health Professions Commission.

O'Rourke, M. (2002). A better educated nursing workforce: BSN 2010 initiative. Available at: www.acnl.org.

Pew Health Professions Commission. (1995). *Critical Challenges: Revitalizing the Health Professions for the Twenty-First Century*. San Francisco: UCSF Center for the Health Professions.

Poster, E. (2004). Nursing education and nursing practice: Collaboration essential to current differentiated entry level competencies of Texas nursing programs. *Nursing Outlook, 52*(1), 67–68.

Rick, C. (2003). Differentiated practice: Get beyond the fear factor. *Nursing Management, 34*(1), 11.

WEB RESOURCES

American Association of Colleges of Nursing	www.aacn.nche.edu
American Organization of Nurse Executives	http://www.aone.org/aone/index.jsp
Board of Nurse Examiners for the State of Texas	www.bne.state.tx.us
California Strategic Planning Committee for Nursing (archive)	www.ucihs.uci.edu/cspcn/
Colorado Alliance for Nursing Workforce Development Opportunities	www.uchsc.edu/ahec/cando/
National Advisory Council on Nurse Education and Practice	http://bhpr.hrsa.gov/nursing/nacnep/default.htm
National League for Nursing	www.nln.org
National Organization of Associate Degree Nursing	www.noadn.org
United States Department of Health and Human Services (nursing statistics)	http://bhpr.hrsa.gov/healthworkforce/reports/default.htm
University of California San Francisco Center for Health Professions (Pew competencies for nursing)	http://www.futurehealth.ucsf.edu

Defining Evidence-Based Best Practices

Suzanne S. Prevost

3

Nurses and other health care providers constantly strive to provide the best care for their patients. As new medications and health care innovations emerge, determining the best options can be challenging. This process has become more difficult in recent years, as health care administrators, insurance companies and other payers, accrediting agencies, and consumers demand the latest and greatest health care interventions. Nurses and physicians are expected to evaluate the care they provide and show evidence that care is not only clinically effective, but also cost-effective, and satisfying, to patients. In light of these challenges, the term *best practice* has emerged as a descriptor of the clinical practices that result in the best outcomes as well as the processes used to select those clinical practices.

This chapter begins with various definitions of best practices. The concept of best practice is compared to a similar concept, *evidence-based practice*. Examples of when and where nurses are using best practices are provided as are strategies for determining and applying best practices. In addition, the *who* of best practice is addressed regarding how nurses in various roles can support the use of best practices. Finally, future implications are discussed.

▶ WHAT IS BEST PRACTICE?

The term *best practice* is defined and used in various ways; and nurses should consider both the ends and the means behind the term. The concept of best practice arose from quality improvement initiatives in industries beyond health care (Hamill, 2000). Various other industries have used the concept to describe the strategies or methods that work most efficiently or achieve the best results. The term is often associated with *benchmarking*, which involves identifying the most successful companies or institutions in a particular sector of an industry, examining their methods of doing business, using their approach as the goal or gold standard, then replicating and refining their methods.

Green (2001) describes the origin of best practice in health care as a component of the process of translating the medical research findings into usable clinical interventions that are practical in an array of settings and populations. He suggests that best practice is that *process* of translating the research findings into useful interventions, rather than the actual intervention that is ultimately selected.

Perleth, Jakubowski, and Busse (2001) describe best practice as an approach to organizational process improvement that involves using research findings to change organizational policies to improve the delivery of health care. They also emphasize the importance of monitoring the effects of those policy changes over time to promote continuous improvements.

While best practice is often used to describe processes, best practice and evidence-based practice can also be used to describe actual clinical practices, interventions, or treatments. Smith and Labriola (2001) describe both an implementation process and a procedure for best practice in arterial sheath removal after interventional cardiac procedures. Best practices have also been defined as services or functions that are best from a contextual perspective; that is, best for a specific patient, group, community, or system, in that a given practice will help individuals or groups to achieve their benchmark goals (Driever, 2002).

Cherry and Jacob (2002) depict best practices as an approach to standardized care procedures that is based on research. Ignatavicius (2003) suggests that in addition to research, consensus statements, case reports, guidelines, standards, protocols, procedures, and federal mandates can help to define guidelines for best practices. Devlin, Czaus, and Santos (2002) describe best practice guidelines as evidence-based statements that assist practitioners and patients in making decisions in specific health care situations.

> ***CONSIDER:** Best practices can be processes of organizational change and also of specific clinical procedures.

The concept of best practices has also been used to describe optimal approaches to nursing administration and education, as well as nursing practice. For example, Ponte et al. (2003) describe cross-institutional collaboration as a method of achieving administrative best practice. Finally, according to Ling (2004, p. 1), "best practices are simply ideas that work."

▶ WHAT IS EVIDENCE-BASED PRACTICE?

The term *evidence-based practice* is being used with increasing frequency among health care providers—and often interchangeably with best practice. While these concepts are similar, there are some subtle differences.

Like best practice, evidence-based practice has a variety of definitions and interpretations. The term evidence-based practice evolved when discussions of evidence-based medicine were expanded to apply to an interdisciplinary audience, which included nurses. Sackett, Strauss, Richardson, Rosenberg, and Haynes defined evidence-based medicine as "the integration of best research evidence with clinical expertise and patient values in making decisions about the healthcare of patients" (Sackett et al., 2000, p. 1). Sigma Theta Tau International, the honor society for nurses (DiCenso et al., 2004, p. 69), expanded upon Sackett's definition to address a broad nursing context with the following definition of evidence-based nursing practice:

> ▶ *...integration of the best evidence available, nursing expertise, and the values and preferences of the individuals, families and communities who are served. This assumes that optimal nursing care is provided when nurses and healthcare decision-makers have access to a synthesis of the latest research, a consensus of expert opinion, and are thus able to exercise their judgment as they plan and provide care that takes into account cultural and personal values and preferences.*

> ***CONSIDER:** Most nurse experts agree that the best practices are also evidence-based practices.

Driever (2002) describes some similarities, differences, and relationships between best practice and evidence-based practice. She suggests that best practice more accurately describes an organizational concept or framework that promotes the incorporation of evidence into clinical practice. She also describes best practice as an organizational level of agreement about how research will be accessed, evaluated, and used to improve practice. She mentions that benchmarking, continuous monitoring, and process improvement are typical components of a best practice approach.

Although there are slight nuances in the comparison of best practice and evidence-based practice, the ultimate goal of both concepts is similar: to provide optimal patient care that is based on reliable evidence, with the goal of enhancing practice, and in turn, improving patient or system outcomes.

Discussion Point

Are there situations in which an evidence-based practice might not be considered a best practice? If yes, give an example and explain why.

WHY, WHEN, AND WHERE BEST PRACTICES ARE USED

Each week, new developments and innovations occur in health care—not only in research findings, but also in the public media. Contemporary health care consumers are knowledgeable and demanding. They expect the most current, effective, and efficient interventions.

Why Are Best Practices Important?

In their quest to provide the highest quality care for their patients, nurses are challenged to stay abreast of new developments in health care, even within the limits of their own areas of specialization. Simultaneously, with the growth of health care knowledge, health care costs increase and patient satisfaction takes on greater importance. Administrators expect health care providers to satisfy their customers, and do it in the most clinically effective and cost-effective manner. Control of health care costs was one of the initial drivers of the best practice movement (Larrabee, 2004). As the prospective reimbursement system decreased revenue to hospitals and providers, it became increasingly apparent that some providers were capable of providing high-quality care in a more efficient and cost-effective manner than their peers provided. These industry leaders were quickly identified and emulated for their best practices. Within the current litigious and cost-conscious health care environment, there remains a sense of urgency to select and implement the best interventions, as quickly and efficiently as possible. Nancy Brent (2001), a nurse attorney, advises that ignoring best practice changes can put health care agencies at legal and financial risk.

In today's health care environment, nurses are increasingly accepted as essential members, and often as leaders, of the interdisciplinary health care team. To effectively participate and lead a health care team, nurses must have knowledge of the most effective and reliable, evidence-based approaches to care. And as nurses increase their expertise in critiquing research, they are expected to apply the evidence of their findings to selecting optimal interventions for their patients.

The processes and tools of evidence-based best practice can help nurses respond to these challenges. This approach to care is based on the latest research, and other forms of evidence, as well as clinical expertise, and patient preferences. All of these factors contribute to providing quality care that is clinically effective, cost-effective, and satisfying to health care consumers.

Discussion Point

What type of knowledge and education do nurses need to prepare them for leading best-practice initiatives as described?

When and Where Are Evidence-Based, Best Practices Used?

In recent years, the implementation of evidence-based, best practices has been identified as a priority across nearly every nursing specialty. During the late 1990s, Sigma Theta Tau International conducted a strategic planning process to establish future directions for the organization. In a poll of membership, Sigma Theta Tau International learned that the most frequently cited request and recommendation from practicing nurses was a desire for support systems and resources to help them implement evidence-based practices. This feedback was consistent across nursing specialties and across nursing roles and positions. Initiatives to help nurses understand and implement evidence-based best practices have become a priority for the society since that time. A review of recent literature yields case studies and recommendations for best practice implementation across nursing specialties. These are shown in Table 3.1.

In addition to the universal application across nursing specialties, the concept of evidence-based best practice is also valued across nursing roles and responsibilities. Klardie et al. (2004) describes evidence-based approaches in the nurse practitioner role. Ponte et al. (2003) discuss collaboration across facilities as a mechanism for fostering administrative best practice among nurse executives. Krugman (2003) and Pape (2003) advocate for the realization of evidence-based practice by nurse educators; and Maramba, Richards, Myers, and Larrabee (2004) describe evidence-based practice as a model for discharge planning.

A commitment to evidence-based best practice is not limited to the United States. A few countries, in particular, Canada and the United Kingdom, adopted this approach to care several years before it became a preferred approach to care in the United States. Buchan (2002) described the application of evidence-based interventions to address the nursing shortage in Scotland. Devlin et al. (2002) used best practice guidelines to address pressure ulcers in Ontario. Zietz and McCutcheon (2003) describe the application of evidence-based practice for the care of postoperative patients in Australia. Gerrish and Clayton (2004) conducted research to assess the use of evidence-based practice as an organizational approach among nurses in the United Kingdom.

*CONSIDER: Within one decade, the concept of evidence-based practice has evolved and been embraced by nurses in nearly every clinical specialty, across a variety of roles and positions, and in locations around the globe.

How Do Nurses Determine Best Practices?

Craig and Smyth (2002) assert that best practice begins by asking good questions. Nurses must be empowered to ask critical questions in the spirit of looking for opportunities to improve nursing practice and patient outcomes. In any specialty or role, nurses can regard their work as a continuous series of questions and decisions.

In a given day, a staff nurse may be called to ask and answer questions, such as "Should I give the analgesic only when the patient requests it? Or, should I encourage

TABLE 3.1

Evidence-Based, Best Practices Across Nursing Specialties

Area of Specialization	Author and Year	Title or Theme	Type of Report
Critical care	Fulbrook (2003)	Care bundles in critical care: a practical approach to evidence-based practice	Recommendation for combining multiple best practices in a bundle or protocol
Gerontology	Hinrichs, Huseboe, J. Tang, & Titler (2001)	Management of constipation	Research-based protocol
Home care	Benefield (2003)	Implementing evidence-based practice in home care	Reviews a model of quality improvement to guide system changes
Informatics	Bakken, Cimino, & Hripcsak (2004)	Promoting patient safety and enabling evidence-based practice	Describes the infrastructure and application of informatics to support best practices
Long-term care	Brazil, Royle, Montemuro, et al. (2004)	Moving to evidence-based practice in long-term care	Report of a feasibility study and demonstration project
Medical-Surgical	Ardery, Herr, Titler, et al. (2003)	Assessing and managing acute pain in older adults: A research base to guide practice	Review of related research
Mental health	Geanellos (2004)	Nursing-based evidence: Moving beyond evidence-based practice	Overview and future projections
Obstetrics and neonatology	Maloni, Albrecht, Thomas, et al. (2003)	Implementing evidence-based practice: Reducing risk for low birth weight through pregnancy smoking cessation	Describes implementation process for an evidence-based protocol
Occupational health	Rogers (2004)	Putting research evidence into practice	Overview article
Pediatrics	Melnyk (2000)	Evidence-based practice: Past, present, and future	Strategies for implementation
Perianesthesia	Windle (2003)	Understanding evidence-based practice	Overview article
Primary care	Mosca, Appel, Benjamin, et al. (2004)	Evidence-based guidelines for cardiovascular disease prevention in women	Report of research review process and detailed clinical practice guidelines
Trauma	Bond, Draeger, Mandleco, & Donnelly (2003)	Needs of patients with severe traumatic brain injury: Implications for evidence-based practice	Report of descriptive research project

TABLE 3.1

Evidence-Based, Best Practices Across Nursing Specialties (continued)

Area of Specialization	Author and Year	Title or Theme	Type of Report
Women's health	Mason (2002)	Who says it's best practice?	Discussion of changes in prescribing of hormone replacement therapy
Applicable across specialties	Metheny & Titler (2001)	Assessing placement of feeding tubes	Review of research, practice guidelines, and algorithms

him to take it every four hours? Will aggressive ambulation expedite this patient's recovery, or will it consume too much energy? Will open family visitation help the patient feel supported; or will it interrupt her rest?"

A nurse manager or administrator might ask, "Who is the most qualified care provider for our sickest patient today? What is the optimal nurse-to-patient ratio for a specific unit? Do complication rates and sentinel events increase with less-educated staff? Do longer shifts result in greater staff fatigue and medication errors? Will higher quality and more expensive mattresses decrease the incidence of pressure ulcers? What benefits promote nurse retention? How does the use of supplemental (or agency) staffing affect the morale of existing staff? Can this population be treated on an outpatient, rather than inpatient, basis? What is the optimal length of time for a comprehensive home care assessment? Or, how many patients can a nurse practitioner see in 8 hours?"

Likewise, a nurse educator may ask, "Is it more effective to teach a procedure in the laboratory or on an actual patient? What are the most efficient methods of documenting continued competency? Do web-based students perform as well on standardized tests as students in traditional classrooms?"

Each type of question can lead to important decisions that affect outcomes, such as patient recovery, organizational effectiveness, and nursing competency. The best answers and consequently, the best decisions come from informed, evidence-based analysis of each situation. See Box 3.1 for a list of questions to assist the nurse in the process of evidence-based decision-making for various nursing scenarios.

BOX 3.1

Key Questions to Ask When Considering Best Practices

- Why have we always done "it" this way?
- Do we have evidence-based rationale? Or, is this practice merely based on tradition?
- Is there a better (more effective, faster, safer, less expensive, more comfortable) method?
- What approach does the patient (or the target group) prefer?
- What do experts in this specialty recommend?
- What methods are used by leading, or benchmark, organizations?
- Do the findings of recent research suggest an alternative method?
- Is there a review of the research on this topic?
- Are there nationally recognized standards of care, practice guidelines, or protocols that apply?
- Are organizational barriers inhibiting the application of best practices in this situation?

▶ FINDING EVIDENCE TO ANSWER NURSING QUESTIONS

Nurses rely on various sources to answer clinical questions such as those cited previously. A practicing staff nurse might consult a nurse with more experience, more education, or a higher level of authority to get help answering such questions. Institutional standards or policy and procedure manuals are also a common reference source for nurses in practice. Nursing coworkers or other health care providers, such as physicians, pharmacists, or therapists, might also be consulted. While all of these approaches are extremely common, they are more likely to yield clinical answers that are *tradition-based*, rather than *evidence-based*.

If evidence-based best practices are truly based on "...the integration of the best evidence available, nursing expertise, and the values and preferences of the individuals, families and communities ..." (DiCenso et al., 2004, p. 69), then local expertise and tradition is not sufficient. However, the optimal source of best evidence is a matter of controversy.

Research is generally considered a more reliable source of evidence than traditions or the clinical expertise of individuals. However, many experts argue that some types of research are better, or stronger, forms of evidence than others. In medicine and pharmacology, the *randomized controlled trial* (RCT) has been considered the gold standard of clinical evidence. RCTs yield the strongest statistical evidence regarding the effectiveness of an intervention in comparison to another intervention or placebo. For many clinical questions in medicine and pharmacy, there may be multiple RCTs in the literature addressing a single question, such as the effectiveness of a particular drug. In such situations, an even stronger form of evidence is an *integrative review or meta-analysis* wherein the results of several similar research studies are combined or synthesized to provide the most comprehensive answer to the question.

In nursing literature, RCTs, meta-analyses, and integrative reviews are significantly less common than in medical or pharmaceutical literature. For many clinical questions in nursing, RCTs may not exist, or they may not even be appropriate. For example, if a nurse is considering how best to prepare a patient for endotracheal suctioning, it would be helpful to inform the patient what suctioning feels like. This type of question does not lend itself to a RCT, but rather to descriptive or qualitative research. In general, qualitative, descriptive, or quasi-experimental studies are much more common methods of inquiry in nursing research than RCTs or meta-analyses. Furthermore, the body of nursing research overall is a newer and less-developed body of research than that of some other health disciplines. So for many clinical questions, nursing research studies may not exist.

Goode and Piedalue (1999) recommend a broader approach and definition for the *evidence* that supports best nursing practices. Goode emphasizes that all types of nursing research, beyond RCTs and meta-analyses, should be considered as potential sources of evidence. She also advocates the use of nine nonresearch sources of evidence:

- pathophysiologic data
- medical record review data
- quality improvement projects
- national and local standards of care
- infection control data, clinical expertise
- benchmarking data
- cost-effectiveness analyses
- patient and family preferences.

Another dilemma for the practicing nurse is the time, access, and expertise needed to search and analyze the research literature to answer clinical questions. In the midst of the current nursing shortage, few practicing nurses have the luxury of leaving their patients to conduct a literature search. Most staff nurses practicing in clinical settings have less than a baccalaureate degree; and therefore, they likely have not been exposed to a formal research course. Findings from research studies are typically very technical, difficult to understand, and even more difficult to translate into applications. Searching, finding, critiquing, and summarizing research findings for applications in practice, are high-level skills that require substantial education and practice.

Discussion Point

If a practicing nurse has no formal education or experience related to research, what strategies should she or he use to find evidence that answers clinical questions and supports best practices?

SUPPORTING BEST PRACTICES

In light of the challenges of providing or implementing best practices, nurses must consider some alternative support mechanisms when searching for the best evidence to support their practice. Six strategies are summarized in Box 3.2.

Garner Administrative Support

The first strategy is to garner administrative support. The implementation of evidence-based best practices should not be an individual, staff nurse-level pursuit. Administrative support is needed to access the resources, provide the support personnel, and sanction the necessary changes in policies, procedures, and practices. Recently, nursing administrators have had increased incentives to support evidence-based best practice, because this approach to care is being recognized as a standard expectation of accrediting bodies,

---

BOX 3.2

Strategies for Finding the Evidence

- Garner administrative support
- Collaborate with a research mentor
- Seek assistance from professional librarians
- Search for sources that have already reviewed or summarized the research
- Access resources from professional organizations
- Benchmark with high-performing teams, units, or institutions

---

such as the Joint Commission on Accreditation of Healthcare Organizations (JCAHO). Evidence-based practice is also one of the expectations associated with the highly regarded Magnet Hospital designation. Most nursing administrators who want their institutions to be recognized for providing high quality care will recognize the value of evidence-based best practice, and therefore, should be willing to provide resources to support it.

Collaborate With a Research Mentor

One way nurse administrators can support the use of best practices is through the provision of nurse experts who can function as research mentors. Advanced practice nurses, nurse researchers, or nursing faculty are examples of nurses who may provide consultation and collaboration to support the process of searching, reviewing, and critiquing research literature and databases to answer clinical questions and identify best practices. Most staff nurses do not have the educational background, research expertise, or time to effectively review and critique extensive research literature in search of the evidence to support best practices. Research mentors can assist with these processes, while staff nurses can often provide the best insight on clinical needs and patient preferences.

Marita Titler and Linda Everett, international experts on evidence-based nursing practice, described their strategies for implementing evidence-based practices for pain management (2001). They recommend the review and adaptation of national practice guidelines for use in local agencies. They use algorithms, charts, and documentation scales as prompts to remind clinicians of the new practices. They also strongly recommend identifying opinion leaders and change champions, experienced and trusted clinicians in the setting, who are willing to lead by example in using the new practices. However, the adoption of evidence-based practice is not limited to expert clinicians. Box 3.3 includes a list of strategies for the new graduate nurse to promote evidence-based best practices.

Seek Assistance From Professional Librarians

Another valuable type of support that is available in academic medical centers, and in some smaller institutions, is a medical librarian. A skilled librarian can save nurses a tremendous amount of time by providing guidance in the most comprehensive and efficient approaches to search the health care literature to find research studies and other resources to support the implementation of best practices.

Search Already Reviewed or Summarized Research

Another strategy nurses can use to expedite the search for evidence and best practice is to specifically seek sources that have already reviewed or summarized the research literature.

Strategies for the New Nurse to Promote Evidence-Based Best Practices

- Keep abreast of the evidence—subscribe to professional journals and read widely
- Use and encourage use of multiple sources of evidence
- Use evidence not only to support clinical interventions, but also for teaching strategies
- Find established sources of evidence in your specialty; don't reinvent the wheel
- Implement and evaluate nationally sanctioned clinical practice guidelines
- Question and challenge nursing traditions, promote a spirit of risk-taking
- Dispel myths and traditions not supported by evidence
- Collaborate with other nurses locally and globally
- Interact with other disciplines to bring nursing evidence to the table

For example, some journals such as *Evidence-Based Nursing* and *WorldViews on Evidence-Based Nursing*, specifically focus on providing summaries, critiques, and practice implications of existing nursing research studies. An example of some topics covered in the July 2004 issue of *Evidence-Based Nursing* include:

- Patient education interventions for adults with diabetes mellitus
- Effects of acetaminophen for postoperative pain
- Elastic compression stockings for prevention of post-thrombotic syndrome

Fall prevention strategies for elders and interventions to decrease alcohol use among college students are two of the topics that were reviewed and summarized in the 2004 issues of the journal *WorldViews on Evidence-Based Nursing*. When conducting a literature search, use of keywords, such as research review or meta-analysis, can assist the nurse in identifying research review articles that have already been published on the topic of interest.

The Cochrane Collaboration is a large international organization comprising several interdisciplinary teams of research scholars that are continuously conducting reviews of research on a wide variety of clinical topics. The Cochrane Collaboration promotes the use of evidence-based practices around the world. Abbreviated (two-page) summaries of such projects are available on the web at *http://www.cochrane.org/index0.htm*. The Cochrane reviews tend to focus heavily on evaluating the effectiveness of medical interventions, for example comparing the effects of different medications for specific conditions. Therefore, many of the Cochrane review summaries are more useful for primary care providers, such as physicians and nurse practitioners, than for staff nurse clinicians. Some of the Cochrane projects of interest to nurses in direct care positions include their reviews of products to prevent pressure ulcers, nursing interventions for smoking cessation, interventions to help patients follow their medication regimens, and interventions to promote collaboration between nurses and physicians.

The Agency for Healthcare Research and Quality (AHRQ) is also a good resource for identifying research reviews and summaries that have already been compiled by national panels of experts. One particularly helpful AHRQ resource is the National Guideline Clearinghouse (NGC) available at *http://www.guideline.gov/*. The mission of the NGC is to "provide physicians and other healthcare providers ... an accessible mechanism for obtaining objective, detailed information on clinical practice guidelines and to further their dissemination, implementation and use" (National Guideline Clearinghouse, 2004).

All of the practice guidelines available through this site are developed through systematic searches and reviews of research literature and scientific evidence by a professional organization, health care specialty association, or government agency. Nursing organizations that have contributed guidelines to the NCG include the Association of Women's Health, Obstetric, and Neonatal Nurses, the Oncology Nursing Society, and the Registered Nurses Association of Ontario. Each guideline includes an abstract summary and a list of recommended practices, strategies, or interventions for a specific clinical condition. The NGC contains more than 1,400 unique practice guidelines.

Access Resources From Professional Organizations

Professional nursing organizations can also provide a wealth of resources to support evidence-based best practices. For example, the American Association of Critical Care Nurses (AACN, 2001) has published several "Protocols for Practice" that are relevant to nursing care in critical care units. These protocols are based on extensive literature reviews conducted by national panels of nurse researchers and advanced practice nurses. A sampling of the topics covered in these protocols is listed in Box 3.4.

Recently, nurse experts from AACN began publishing a new type of resource known as *Practice Alerts*. While the development process is similar to that of the protocols, the product is shorter and more specifically focused on areas where current common practices should change based on the latest research. Some of the topics covered in the Practice Alerts include prevention of ventilator-associated pneumonia, pulmonary artery pressure monitoring, and family presence during resuscitation.

The Association of Women's Health, Obstetric, and Neonatal Nursing (AWHONN) also provides several resources to support evidence-based best practices. The AWHONN Research-Based Practice Program was designed to "advance evidence-based clinical practice using established research utilization procedures, knowledge dissemination methods, and innovative diffusion strategies" (AWHONN, 2004). Through this program, several nationwide, multiyear projects have been completed. Topics addressed through this mechanism have included management of women in second-stage labor, urinary continence for women, neonatal skin care, and cyclic pelvic pain and discomfort management.

BOX 3.4

American Association of Colleges of Nursing's Protocols for Practice

- Care of the Patient With an Arrhythmia
- Continuous Airway Pressure Monitoring
- End-tidal CO_2 Monitoring
- Family Needs and Interventions in Acute Care
- Family Visitation and Partnership
- Noninvasive Blood Pressure Monitoring
- Nutrition Support for the Mechanically Ventilated Patient
- Pain Management in the Acutely Ill
- Promoting Sleep in Acute and Critical Care
- Pulmonary Artery Pressure Monitoring
- Sedation in Patients With Acute Respiratory Failure
- Weaning From Long-Term Mechanical Ventilation
- Weaning From Short-Term Mechanical Ventilation

More recently, AWHONN funded an Evidence-based Clinical Practice Guideline Program. Each of the guidelines includes clinical practice recommendations, referenced rationale statements, quality of evidence ratings for each statement, background information describing the scope of the clinical issue, and a quick care reference guide for clinicians. Breastfeeding support, regional analgesia/anesthesia in labor, promotion of emotional well-being during midlife, and cardiovascular health for women are topics of some of the evidence-based guidelines produced through this program (AWHONN, 2004).

The American Association of Operating Room Nurses (AORN), the Oncology Nursing Society (ONS), and Sigma Theta Tau International also provide web-based resources to facilitate implementation of evidence-based practices. AORN has published Evidence-Based Guidelines for Safe Operating Room Practices, the ONS provides an Evidence-Based Practice Resource Center, and Sigma Theta Tau International publishes web-based continuing education programs and several supportive publications, including *Worldviews on Evidence-Based Nursing*. Web addresses for each of these professional organizations are included in the Web Resources at the end of this chapter, along with other websites that provide helpful resources.

Discussion Point

What institutions, units, teams or individuals in your community can you identify that would be considered regional or national benchmark leaders in the provision of a specialized type of medical or nursing care?

Benchmark With High-Performing Teams, Units, or Institutions

Finally, nurses can use benchmarking strategies to poll nurse experts from high-performing teams, units or institutions to learn more about their best practices for specific clinical problems or patient populations. Leaders of professional nursing organizations, such as Sigma Theta Tau International or the National Association of Clinical Nurse Specialists, can help nurses locate and contact established nurse experts in various areas of specialization. Accrediting organizations, such as the Joint Commission on Accreditation of Healthcare Organizations (JCAHO) can assist in identifying institutions that are known as national leaders in providing specific types of care. The University of Iowa, the University of Rochester, and McMaster University of Ontario are three North American institutions that have established reputations as leaders in evidence-based nursing practice.

Discussion Point

When the investigation reveals a need for an evidence-based change in practice, what strategies are useful for implementing change?

▶ CHALLENGES AND OPPORTUNITIES: STRATEGIES FOR CHANGING PRACTICE

Nurses use several mechanisms for incorporating new research evidence into current practice in the pursuit of promoting best practices. Perhaps the most common mechanism is through the development and refinement of research-based policies and procedures. Fortunately, JCAHO has mandated that healthcare institutions must implement formal processes for reviewing the latest research and assuring that institutional policies and procedures are consistently revised in keeping with current research findings.

Protocols, algorithms, decision trees, standards of care, critical pathways, care maps, and institutional clinical practice guidelines are additional mechanisms used to incorporate new evidence into clinical practice. Each of these formats is used by healthcare teams to guide clinical decision-making and clinical interventions. While nurses often take the lead in developing or revising these devices, participation and buy-in from the interdisciplinary health care team are essential to achieve successful implementation and consistent changes in practice.

In addition to consensus from the interdisciplinary team, support from patients and their families is important. This element of the process is frequently overlooked or not thoroughly considered. As previously mentioned, evidence-based nursing practice involves "...integration of the best evidence available, nursing expertise, and the values and preferences of the individuals, families and communities who are served..." (DiCenso et al., 2004, p. 69). If the review of evidence leads the health care team to recommend an intervention that is inconsistent with the patient or family's values and preferences (such as a specific dietary modification or transfusion of blood products), the recommendation may lead to poor adherence or total disregard by the patient, not to mention a loss of the patient's trust and confidence in the health care team.

Discussion Point

Can you think of situations in which the latest research may be inconsistent with the values of an individual or group of patients?

Challenges to Implementing Evidence-Based Practice

Although evidence-based practices are being discussed and pursued by nurses around the world, several obstacles continue to inhibit the movement. Funk, Champagne, Weiss, and Tornquist (1991) originally studied this problem, and Retsas (2000) used a modification of their survey to poll 400 Australian nurses. He identified several barriers that he grouped into four main factors: accessibility of research findings, anticipated outcomes of using research, support from others, and lack of organizational support, which was perceived to be the most significant limitation. Some of the accessibility problems were lack of clarity or readability of the research reports, confusing statistics, research reports not published fast enough, or not readily available. In the category of anticipated outcomes of using research, nurses expressed concerns about discomfort with change and trying new ideas, no perceived benefits for the nurse, and nurses failing to believe the results or see the value of research. The lack of support from others was primarily related to lack of cooperation from other staff and physicians to support the change. Finally, in relation to

Research Study Fuels the Controversy

Barriers to Evidence-Based Practice

While nurses and physicians around the world agree that the implementation of evidence-based practice is desirable, several barriers often limit progress toward this goal. The purpose of this study was to identify perceived barriers to the implementation of evidence-based practice among general practitioners and nurses working in primary care. This survey was mailed to 356 primary care physicians and 356 primary care nurses in Northern Ireland.

McKenna, H.P., Ashton, S., & Keeney, S. (2004). Barriers to evidence-based practice in primary care. *Journal of Advanced Nursing, 45*(2), 178–189.

Study Findings

The most significant barriers identified by the physicians were the limited relevance of research to practice, difficulty keeping up with constant changes in primary care, and their limited ability to search for evidence-based information. In contrast, the greatest barriers for nurses were poor computer access or resources, poor patient compliance with evidence-based recommendations, and difficulties influencing practice changes in the clinical setting.

lack of organizational support, nurses did not feel they had the authority to change practices, they did not have sufficient time at work to review the research, and the nurses did not feel capable of evaluating or critiquing the research.

McKenna, Ashton, and Keeney (2004) examined barriers to evidence-based practice in the United Kingdom (Box 3.5). They found differences in the barriers identified by nurses and those identified by physicians. Nurses identified barriers associated with poor computer resources, difficulties with changing practices, and poor patient compliance. The physicians in the study were more concerned with the limited relevance of research to the practice setting, difficulties searching for and finding evidence, and difficulty keeping up with all the potential changes in practice.

Omery and Williams (1999) used a qualitative research design to gather perceptions about barriers from clinical nurse researchers across the United States. Of the 20 researchers interviewed, 17 were actively involved in projects directed toward incorporating research evidence into practice. Barriers they identified were lack of resources, such as time, personnel, and funding. The researchers also expressed concerns about the lack of expertise among their nursing staff to read and evaluate research, and problems with institutional cultures that do not value or support the process.

Olade (2004) also found that geography could be a potential barrier. In her study of rural U.S. nurses, only 20.8% of her subjects were involved in evidence-based practice initiatives (Box 3.6). Their perceived barriers were rural isolation and lack of expert research consultants.

Discussion Point

What obstacles would limit your involvement in the process of pursuing evidence-based best practice?

BOX 3.6

Research Study Fuels the Controversy

Evidence-Based Practice Among Rural Nurses

The location and type of practice facilities may have an impact on nurses' use of evidence-based best practices. The purposes of this study were to identify the extent to which rural nurses use evidence-based practice guidelines, to describe their participation in research utilization activities, and to identify the specific barriers they face.

Olade, R. (2004). Evidence-based practice and research utilization activities among rural nurses. *Journal of Nursing Scholarship, 36*(3), 220–225.

Study Findings

Only 20.8% of the participants stated that they were currently involved in research utilization. The two most common areas of research utilization were pain management and pressure ulcer management. Barriers to the use of research included rural isolation and lack of nursing research consultants.

▶ CONCLUSIONS

Many nurses are experiencing success in promoting evidence-based practice. Organizations such as AHRQ and the Cochrane Collaboration provide support to help clinicians overcome some of the barriers, such as the difficulties in obtaining and understanding research reports, and the isolation from colleagues and consultants. The many agencies that support teams of research experts to collect, critique, and summarize the research and other forms of evidence pave the way for frontline clinicians to find and adopt evidence-based best practices.

Yet challenges continue. Too few nurses understand what best practices and evidence-based practice are all about. Organizational cultures may not support the nurse who seeks out and uses research to change long-standing practices rooted in tradition, rather than science. In addition, a stronger connection needs to be established between researchers and academicians studying evidence-based nursing and best practices and staff nurses who must translate those findings into the art of nursing practice. Yet nursing cannot afford to value the art of nursing over the science. Both are critical to making sure that patients receive the highest quality of care possible.

FOR ADDITIONAL DISCUSSION

1. Can decision support tools such as algorithms, decision trees, clinical pathways, and standardized clinical guidelines ever replace clinical judgment?
2. Why does at least some level of disconnect exist between nurse researchers/academics studying best practices and nurses who seek to implement such research into their practice? Is the problem a lack of communication? Do most nurses have access to evidence-based nursing research findings?
3. How static are best practice findings? Can you identify an evidence-based practice that was later found to be ineffective or inappropriate?

4. Are best practices and evidence-based practice more alike or dissimilar?
5. Should best practices be institution-specific or should they always be more generalizable?
6. Is evidence-based nursing research grounded more in quantitative than qualitative research? Are both needed?
7. What can be done to increase the research knowledge base of most practicing registered nurses (RNs), given that almost two thirds of the nursing workforce has been educated at the associate degree level?

REFERENCES

American Association of Critical Care Nurses. (2001). *Protocols for practice*. Aliso Viejo, CA: Author.

Ardery, G., Herr, K., Titler, M., et al. (2003). Assessing and managing acute pain in older adults: a research base to guide practice. *Medsurg Nursing, 12*(1), 7–18.

Association of Women's Health, Obstetric and Neonatal Nurses (AWHONN). (2004). *Research-based practice programs*. Retrieved November 15, 2004 from http://www.awhonn.org/awhonn/?pg=0-874-2190.

Bakken, S., Cimino, J., & Hripcsak, G. (2004). Promoting patient safety and enabling evidence-based practice through informatics. *Medical Care, 42* (2 Suppl), II, 49–56.

Benefield, L.E. (2003). Implementing evidence-based practice in home care. *Home Healthcare Nurse, 21*(12), 804–809.

Bond, A.E., Draeger, C., Mandleco, B., & Donnelly, M. (2003). Needs of family members of patients with severe traumatic brain injury: Implications for evidence-based practice. *Critical Care Nurse, 23*(4), 63–72.

Brazil, K., Royle, J., Montemuro, M., et al. (2004). Moving to evidence-based practice in long-term care. *Journal of Gerontological Nursing, 30*(3) 14–19.

Brent, N.J. (2001). Are ignoring best practice changes putting your agency at legal and financial risk? Case in point: single-lead ECG monitoring in the home. *Home Healthcare Nurse, 19*(11), 721–724.

Buchan, J. (2002). Nursing shortages and evidence-based interventions: A case study from Scotland. *International Nursing Review, 49*(9), 209–218.

Cherry, B. & Jacob, S. (2002). *Contemporary nursing: Issues, trends, & management,* 2nd ed. St. Louis: Mosby.

Civius, D. D. (2003). Forward. In *Best practices: A guide to excellence in nursing care*. Philadelphia: Lippincott Williams & Wilkins.

Craig, J.V. & Smyth, R.L. (2002). *The evidence-based practice manual for nurses*. London: Churchill Livingston.

Devlin, R., Czaus, M., & Santos, J. (2002). Registered Nurses Association of Ontario's best practice guideline as a tool for creating partnerships. *Hospital Quarterly, 5*(3), 62–65.

DiCenso, A., Prevost, S., Benefield, L., et al. (2004). Evidence-based nursing: Rationale and resources. *Worldviews on Evidence-Based Nursing, 1* (1), 69–75.

Driever, M.J. (2002). Are evidenced-based practice and best practice the same? *Western Journal of Nursing Research, 24*(5), 591–597.

Fulbrook, P. & Mooney, S. (2003). Care bundles in critical care: A practical approach to evidence-based practice. *Nursing in Critical Care, 8*(6), 249–255.

Funk, S.G., Champagne, M.T., Weiss, R.A., & Tornquist, E.M. (1991). Barriers to using research findings in practice: The clinician's perspective. *Applied Nursing Research 4*, 90–95.

Geanellos R. (2004). Nursing based evidence: Moving beyond evidence-based practice in mental health nursing. *Journal of Evaluation in Clinical Practice, 10*(2), 177–186.

Gerrish, K. & Clayton, J. (2004). Promoting evidence-based practice: An organizational approach. *Journal of Nursing Management, 12*(2), 114–123.

Goode, C. & Piedalue, F. (1999). Evidence-based clinical practice. *Journal of Nursing Administration, 29*(6), 15–21.

Green, L.W. (2001). From research to "best practices" in other settings and populations. *American Journal of Health Behavior, 25*(3), 165–178.

Hamill, C.T. (2000). Best practices & accreditation extravaganza. *Care Management, 6*(4), 7.

Hinrichs, M., Huseboe, J., Tanq, J.,& Titler, M. (2001). Research-based protocol. Management of constipation. *Journal of Gerontological Nursing, 27*(2), 17–28.

Klardie, K.A., Johnson, J., Mc Naughton, M.A., Meyers W. (2004). Integrating the principles of evidence-based practice into clinical practice. *Journal American Academy of Nurse Practitioners, 16*(3), 98, 100–102, 104–105.

Krugman, M. (2003). Evidence-based practice. The role of staff development. *Journal for Nurses in Staff Development, 19*(6), 279–285.

Larrabee, J. (2004). Advancing quality improvement through using the best evidence to change practice. *Journal of Nursing Care Quality, 19*(1), 10–13.

Ling, C. (2004). *Aim high: Best practices improve patient care*. Retrieved August 28, 2004, from http://www.nurseweek.com/ce/ce120a.html.

Maloni, J., Albrecht, S., Thomas, K., et al. (2003). Implementing evidence-based practice: Reducing risk for low birth weight through pregnancy smoking cessation. *Journal of Obstetric, Gynecologic, and Neonatal Nursing, 32*(5), 676–682.

Maramba, P. J., Richards, S., Myers, A. L., & Larrabee, J. H. (2004). Discharge planning process: Applying a model for evidence-based practice. *Journal of Nursing Care Quality, 19*(2), 123–129.

Mason, D. J. (2002). Who says it's 'best practice'? *American Journal of Nursing, 102*(10), 7.

McKenna, H. P., Ashton, S., & Keeney, S. (2004). Barriers to evidence-based practice in primary care. *Journal of Advanced Nursing, 45*(2), 178–189.

Melnyk, B. (2000). Evidence-based practice: The past, present, and recommendations for the millennium. *Pediatric Nursing, 26*(1), 77–80.

Metheny, N. & Titler, M. (2001). Assessing placement of feeding tubes. *American Journal of Nursing, 101*(5), 36–45.

Mosca, L., Appel, L., Benjamin, E., et al. (2004). Evidence-based guidelines for cardiovascular disease prevention in women. *Circulation, 109*(5), 672–693.

National Guideline Clearinghouse. (2004). *Mission Statement*. Retrieved September 29, 2004 from http://www.guideline.gov/about/mission.aspx.

Olade, R. (2004). Evidence-based practice and research utilization activities among rural nurses. *Journal of Nursing Scholarship, 36*(3),220–225.

Omery, A. & Williams, R. (1999). An appraisal of research utilization across the United States. *Journal of Nursing Administration, 29*(12), 50–56.

Pape, T. (2003). Evidence-based nursing practice: To infinity and beyond. *Journal of Continuing Education in Nursing, 34*(4), 154–161.

Perleth, M., Jakubowski, E., & Busse, R. (2001). What is 'best practice' in health care? State of the art and perspectives in improving the effectiveness and efficiency of the European health care systems. *Health Policy, 56*(3), 235–250.

Ponte, P. R., Branowicki, P., Somerville, J. et al. (2003). Collaboration among nurse executives in complex environments: Fostering administrative best practice. *Journal of Nursing Administration, 33*(11), 596–602.

Retsas, A. (2000). Barriers to using research evidence in nursing practice. *Journal of Advanced Nursing, 31*(3), 599–606.

Rogers, B. (2004). Research utilization—Putting the research evidence into practice. *American Association of Occupational Health Nurses Journal, 52*(1), 14–15.

Sackett, D. L., Strauss, S. E., Richardson, W. S., et al. (2000). *Evidence-based medicine: How to practice and teach EBM* (2nd ed.). London: Churchill Livingston.

Smith, T. T. & Labriola, R. (2001). Developing best practice in arterial sheath removal for registered nurses. *Journal of Nursing Care Quality, 16*(1), 61–67.

Titler, M. & Everett, L. (2001). Translating research into practice. *Critical Care Nursing Clinics of North America, 13*(4), 587–604.

Windle P.E. (2003). Understanding evidence-based practice. *Journal of Perianesthesia Nursing, 18*(5), 360–362.

Zietz, K. & McCutcheon, H. (2003). Evidence-based practice: To be or not to be, this is the question! *International Journal of Nursing Practice, 9*, 272–279.

BIBLIOGRAPHY

Benton, D. (2004). Sharing best practice across the Atlantic. *Nursing Times, 100*(4), 26–27.

Brazil, K. (2004). Moving to evidence-based practice in long-term care: The role of a Best Practice Resource Center in two long-term care settings. *Journal of Geronotology Nursing, 30*(3), 14–19

Caramanica, L., Cousino, J.A., & Petersen, S. (2003). Four elements of a successful quality program. Alignment, collaboration, evidence-based practice, and excellence. *Nursing Adminitration Quarterly, 27*(4), 336–343.

Clarke, L. K. (2003). The 'best practice' approach. *ORL Head and Neck Nursing, 21*(1), 6.

Dawes, M., Davies, P., Gray, A., et al. (1999). *Evidence-based practice: A primer for healthcare professionals*. London: Churchill Livingston.

Dickinson, D., Duffy, A. & Champion, S. (2004). The process of implementing evidence-based practice—the curate's egg. *Journal of Psychiatric Mental Health Nursing, 11*(1), 117–119.

Fulbrook, P. (2003). Developing best practice in critical care nursing: Knowledge, evidence and practice. *Nursing in Critical Care, 8*(3), 96–102.

Gerrish, K., Entwistler, B., Parmakis, G., et al. (2004). Sharing best practice: Developing a web-based database. *British Journal of Nursing, 13*(1), 44–48.

Geyer, S. (2004). Practice, practice. Overcoming barriers to evidence-based nursing. *Materials Management in Health care, 13*(4), 28–29.

Grinspun, D., Virani, T. & Bajnok, I. (2001–2002). Nursing best practice guidelines: The RNAO (Registered Nurses Association of Ontario) project. *Hospital Quarterly, 5*(2), 56–60.

Hancock, H. C. & Easen P. R. (2004). Evidence-based practice—An incomplete model of the relationship between theory and professional work. *Journal of Evaluation in Clinical Practice, 10*(2), 187–196.

Lenfant, C. (2003). Shattuck lecture—Clinical research to clinical practice—Lost in translation? *New England Journal of Medicine, 349*(9), 868–874.

Lewis, P. S. & Latney, C. (2002). Achieve best practice with an evidence-based approach. Create a collaborative environment that improves patient care through consistent outcomes measurement. *Nursing Management, 33*(12), 24, 26–28, 30.

McKenna, H., Ashton, S. & Kenney, S. (2004). Barriers to evidence based practice in primary care: A review of the literature. *International Journal of Nursing Studies, 41*(4), 369–378.

Mohide, E. A. (2003). Building a foundation for evidence-based practice: Experiences in a tertiary hospital. *Evidence-Based Nursing, 6*(4), 100–103.

Nay, R. (2003). Evidence-based practice: Does it benefit older people and gerontic nursing? *Geriatric Nursing, 24*(6), 338–342.

Rycroft-Malone J., Seers, K., Titchen, A., et al. (2004). What counts as evidence in evidence-based practice? *Journal of Advanced Nursing, 47*(1), 81–90.

Sakala, C. (2004). Resources for evidence-based practice. *Journal of Obstetric, Gynecologic, and Neonatal Nursing, 33*(2), 88–91.

Titler, M. G., Cullen, L., & Ardery, G. (2002). Evidence-based practice: An administrative perspective. *Reflections on Nursing Leadership, 28*(2), 26–27, 46, 45.

Titler, M. G.. Kieiber, C., Steelman, V. J., et al. (2001). The Iowa model of evidence-based practice to promote quality care. *Critical Care Nursing Clinics of North America, 13*(4), 497–509.

Wojner, A. W. (2001). *Outcomes management: Applications to clinical practice.* St. Louis: Mosby.

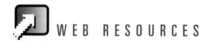 WEB RESOURCES

Agency for Healthcare Research and Quality: Evidence-based Practice	http://www.ahrq.gov/clinic/epcix.htm
Agency for Healthcare Research and Quality: Put Prevention Into Practice	http://www.ahrq.gov/clinic/ppipix.htm
American Association of Critical-Care Nurses	http://www.aacn.org
Appalachian Regional Commission: Best Practices in Healthcare	http://www.arc.gov/index.do?nodeid=1617
Association for Benchmarking Health care	http://www.abhc.org/
Association of peri Operative Registered Nurses	http://www.aorn.org
Association of Women's Health, Obstetric, and Neonatal Nurses	http://www.awhonn.org
Best Practice Initiative, US Department of Health and Human Services	http://www.osophs.dhhs.gov/ophs/bestpractice/default.htm
The Cochrane Collaboration	http://www.cochrane.org/index0.htm
Colorado Department of Public Health, Best Practices Health Topic List	http://www.cdphe.state.co.us/ps/bestpractices/bestpracticeshom.asp
The Joanna Briggs Institute for Promoting and Supporting Best Practice	http://www.joannabriggs.edu.au/about/home.php#
National Guideline Clearinghouse	http://www.guideline.gov/
Oncology Nursing Society	http://www.ons.org
Sigma Theta Tau International—Honor Society of Nursing	http://www.nursingsociety.org
World Health Organization: Best Practices in Health care for Chronic Conditions	http://www.who.int/chronic_conditions/best_practices/en/

4

Socialization and Mentoring

Jeanne Madison

N urses today have many entries and exits from the health care workplace. Nurses change clinical specialties with ease and leave employers for childbirth or childcare, to care for elderly parents, for advanced education, or for international nursing experience. Sometimes they return, often years later, as re-entry or "new" nurses.

Nurses also change from full-time to part-time employment and back again. They enter nursing for the first, second, or third time as young adults, in middle age, or as seniors and they come from diverse ethnic, religious, and social backgrounds. Many are educated in one country but practice in several countries. Given this individual variation as well as diversity in practice patterns, how these nurses are socialized and resocialized in the health care workplace in the 21st century is of profound importance.

▶ SOCIALIZATION: ROLES, SKILLS, VALUES, AND CHANGE

Socialization is the process by which a person acquires the technical skills of his or her society, the knowledge of the kinds of behavior that are understood and acceptable in that society, and the attitudes and values that make conformity with social rules personally meaningful, even gratifying (Hyperdictionary, 2000–2003). Socialization has also been called enculturation.

Resocialization occurs when individuals are forced to learn new values, skills, attitudes, and social rules as a result of changes in the type of work they do, the scope of responsibility they hold, or in the workplace setting itself (Marquis & Huston, 2006). Individuals who frequently need resocialization include experienced nurses who change work settings, either within the same organization or in a new organization, and nurses who undertake new roles. Some nurses adapt easily to resocialization, but most experience some stress with role change.

Before the 1970s, little thought was given to how socialization and resocialization occurred in the health care workplace or how new graduates experienced the transition from student to nurse. It was generally believed that because nurses were educated in the hospital environment, they would not be unduly surprised or alarmed by changes in responsibility and accountability upon graduation from their nursing program. Kramer's work (1974, 1981) on "reality shock" and issues associated with professional socialization led to a renaissance of this thinking, which continues today.

The latest emphasis on socialization research in nursing occurred, coincidentally, at the same time as another sweeping social phenomenon that profoundly changed nursing and the health care workplace forever: the feminist movement. Research about nursing and women's issues expanded significantly against the backdrop of feminism in the Western world.

To nurses in practice and leadership roles, the incongruencies between the subservience of the work world and the professional practice environment expected by college-educated, "enlightened feminist" graduates became abundantly clear. The research spotlight on the female-dominated nursing workplace revealed serious shortcomings and the consequences of maintaining the professional socialization status quo. In addition, an increase in the number of men undertaking nursing education further changed the dynamics within the profession. Clearly, change was needed to meet the expectations of the new professional nurse and to move nursing out from under a medical model and into an accountable and self-governing profession.

During the 1970s, significant, important nursing research focused on analyzing the health care workplace in an effort to understand the long-standing mechanisms that disempowered, denigrated, and marginalized nurses and the nursing profession. It was evident that the oppressive forces in place were entrenched, powerful, and advantageous to those who were in power. Reversing the trajectory of negative nurse socialization was no simple task and could be undertaken only by nurses, individually and collectively.

> ***CONSIDER:** The oppression of nurses has come not only from outside groups, such as medicine and health care administration, but also from within the profession itself.

▶ THE HEALTH CARE WORKPLACE IN THE 21st CENTURY

Negative and positive socialization patterns in the nursing workplace have received wide attention in the literature. The expression used for negative socialization is *horizontal violence*, and it includes manifestations such as bullying, harassment, verbal abuse, and intimidation. Positive socialization is exemplified in the various supportive behaviors associated with mentoring, preceptoring, role modeling, coaching, and guiding. Only recently has significant progress been made for nurses to understand issues associated with the nexus between professional oppression and empowerment.

67

Anger and Hostility

Exactly what is the current experience of new nurses as they are socialized into the health care environment of the 21st century? Thomas (2003) explored the mismanaged and misunderstood issues associated with anger that nurses confront in their workplace (Box 4.1). A disturbing, overarching finding was the presence and extent of nurses' anger with each other. Madison (1997) and Madison and Minichiello (2000) found that for nurses in the workplace, harassers are just as often nurse colleagues as they are members of the medical staff. Thomas (2003), David (2000), Roberts (2000), and Kane and Thomas (2000) identify how hostility is misdirected horizontally between nurses when it seems impossible, unacceptable, or dangerous to direct it at the traditional and long-standing oppressors (e.g., medical staff, supervisors, and administrators). In addition, research by Thomas (2003) suggests that the anger nurses encounter in the health care workplace may vary based on gender differences.

Additionally and unfortunately, not all nurses are altruistic or interested in the development of others and the nursing profession. Many nurses can identify colleagues in the workplace who habitually target entry-level and/or vulnerable staff to undertake responsibilities and tasks that benefit the taskmaster. Often, delegation of tasks in this manner is a pattern or habit and can involve a number of dependent, unacknowledged, and exploited staff. Fawning and groveling behavior is encouraged and expected by the taskmaster. This person can abuse his or her (perceived) authority, position, or experience, and under the guise of a pseudomentoring bond, encourage the development of an inappropriate workplace relationship. Such relationships should not be confused with mentoring and need to be exposed and named.

BOX 4.1

Research Study Fuels the Controversy

Anger and Gender

A recent study into the anger that nurses sometimes encounter in the health care workplace was found to vary based on gender differences:

> Thomas, S. P. (2003). Anger: The mismanaged emotion. *Dermatology Nursing, 15*(4), 351–357.

Study Findings

According to Thomas (2003), the sometimes oppressive, underfunded health care workplace can create justifiable anger among nurses. Taking frustration and anger out on other nurses (or peers) is often seen as "safer" than hostility toward employees or management. Females were described as "anger suppressors" while males were seen as "anger venters." Thomas suggests that women need to learn that relationships do not end when anger is honestly described and men need to consider the consequences of too regular, hostile, aggressive expression.

The study, which outlined alternate strategies for the typical male and female socialization to aggressive and passive communication patterns, suggested that purposeful interpersonal strategies can be effective in reducing and eliminating misdirected anger in the workplace. Setting clear expectations for colleagues in the workplace (e.g., "Don't talk to me that way") is one important way of dealing with misdirected anger. Leaving an abusive situation may also be necessary. Alternately, asking colleagues to stand with you during an abusive situation can be a powerful demotivator for the abuser. The study concluded that nurses need to recognize that recipients of misdirected anger are not responsible for angry abuse and need not accept insulting, aggressive intimidation.

Registered nurses are well placed to recognize and name unacceptable workplace behaviors that they observe. Madison and Minichiello (2004) note that remaining silent or ignoring obviously unhelpful, negative, and discriminatory action in the workplace is no longer an option. Taking action can be intimidating and frightening, but it is necessary and part of a professional's responsibility.

Oppression and Horizontal Violence

The literature is clear that horizontal violence is not unique to nursing; rather, it is found in most oppressed groups and professions. Researchers agree that negative socialization and oppressive behaviors must be eliminated before nurses can assume positive socialization strategies and empower themselves. Understanding typical oppressed-group behavior and horizontal violence is the first step to developing effective change strategies that will reduce and eliminate it.

Oppressed groups typically believe they are oppressed because they are deficient in some way, and most importantly, the oppressor defines these deficiencies (Freire, 1968; Smith, 1995). As this distorted perception is internalized, the oppressed group inadvertently perpetuates the process of oppression. Unsupportive, disempowering, and controlling behaviors *within* the hierarchical nursing structure can easily be identified and demonstrated by horizontal violence. In addition, the oppressive, controlling strategies used by the medical profession and hospital administrators (usually men) are also relatively easy to identify. But the relationship between those behaviors and the self-inflicted, dysfunctional, oppressive behaviors demonstrated within the nursing profession have been exposed and analyzed only recently.

Oppressed group behavior includes a number of widely accepted characteristics: ". . . powerless groups have difficulty taking control of their own destiny because internalized beliefs about their own inferiority lead to a cycle of self-hatred and inability to unite to challenge the inequality of power" (Roberts, 2000, p. 71).

Lee and Saeed (2001, p. 15) assert that "membership in an oppressed group results in reactive behaviors rather than rational, intentional behavior." They describe five characteristics of oppression: "exploitation, marginalization, powerlessness, cultural imperialism, and violence" (Lee and Saeed, 2001, p. 16). They note that historically, nurses have been exploited by the delegation of tasks that were no longer interesting or challenging to medical practitioners. Their salaries and hours of work are unlike any other female-dominated profession.

Just as women are marginalized in society, so nurses continue to be marginalized in the health care workplace. Predominantly male, medical practitioners empowered themselves through their dominance and abuse of power over nurses and women in the workplace. Socially and culturally, physicians have worked hard to maintain their dominance in health care and to control and restrict nurses and other health practitioners. Personal and professional violence against women and nurses from the medical and administrative staff seems to continue in many health care organizations.

Oddly, oppression of nurses often begins early in the educational program when nurses are in their most formative and vulnerable stage. Scarry (1999) describes how the traditional, hierarchical teaching model can continue to perpetuate the oppressive nature of nursing education and thus the health care workplace. Campbell (2003), while exploring ways that nursing school administrators, faculty, and student nurses could cultivate empowerment and positive personal and professional growth, found that nursing students still described a prevailing workplace environment in which nurses treat each other in less than positive ways.

As a nurse academic, Scarry described transforming a nursing curriculum from a passive "student—wise teacher" paradigm to a liberating and empowering model of social action and change agency, and argued that identifying and confronting oppression, as well as developing countermeasures to change the workplace, must start with nursing education.

Discussion Point

What and where are some of the resources nurses can access if they need advice and support when attempting to confront issues of inappropriate, unhelpful, and negative workplace behaviors?

Thomas (2003, p. 356) describes horizontal violence among nurses and the ways that nurses contribute to an oppressive system: "There is no question that nurses have legitimate cause to be angry, given . . . egregious violations of their workplace rights and professional values, but there is abundant evidence that much of their anger is mismanaged." Thomas suggests that nurses do not manage and direct their anger and energy in ways that effect positive change for the future of nurses and nursing. Acknowledging that new graduates are confronted with a challenging and sometimes very negative workplace is critical to progressing the discussion to positive socialization strategies and the ways in which nurses can empower one another.

▶ SOCIALIZATION AND MENTORING: EMPOWERMENT

Mentoring is an intense, positive, discreet, exclusive, one-on-one relationship between an experienced professional and a less experienced novice. Contemporary literature is filled with various definitions and descriptions of mentoring. The mentor relationship is described as similar to the parent-child relationship in that it is usually charged with emotion, and is a serious and mutual, nonsexual loving relationship. The expression "inquisitive teacher" is used when discussing a mentor. From these descriptions, one may assume that mentoring is a high-level human relationship of some significance.

Recently, Roberts (2003) described the characteristics of an effective mentor as a positive attitude, caring toward others, experienced practitioner, good communicator, dedicated to learning, and worthy of trust and admiration. She also noted the importance of appropriate "chemistry" between the mentor and the novice. Clearly, this is different from the more superficial role model or preceptor that is also discussed in the nursing literature. Indeed, a mentor is the highest level of personal and professional relationship. A mentor does everything that a preceptor did . . . and more (Kelly, 1978).

Describing her mentor, Schorr (1979, p. 65) states, "I would have become a nurse without her, but never would I have sought the professionalism, the degree of compassion, the depth of humor, the height of empathy that are set as guidelines for me by the conduct of my mentor."

> *CONSIDER: Mentoring has been identified as one of the most positive interventions to promote socialization for professional and career advancement.

Perhaps most important for nurses is the research from the late 1970s and 1980s that focused on the unique nature of mentoring among women. Sargent (1977) discussed the many positive aspects of the mentor relationship as described in other literature, but emphasized what she considered to be most important. The true value, beyond the teaching, sponsoring, and sharing roles, is the "blessing" in and of itself. To warrant the time and attention ("the blessing") of the mentor is the real worth to the mentee; to have someone believe in one enhances one's belief in oneself.

Business and management literature contains many references and discussions regarding the mentor-mentee phenomenon. Its value to organizational as well as personnel development has been clearly established over the last 30 years. Schein (1978) discusses the obvious situation that exists in organizations when new employees look to more experienced personnel for advice and information. Schein then develops several roles that the willing experienced "mentor" can assume to assist in the development of the new "mentee." The analysis concludes with the observation that the mentor does not necessarily have to be a recognized power figure within the organization, but that experience and willingness to share are important. Other roles common to mentoring are shown in Box 4.2.

Kanter (1977) was one of the earliest businesswomen to identify and use the term *sponsor* to describe the mentor relationship. According to Kanter, the very important

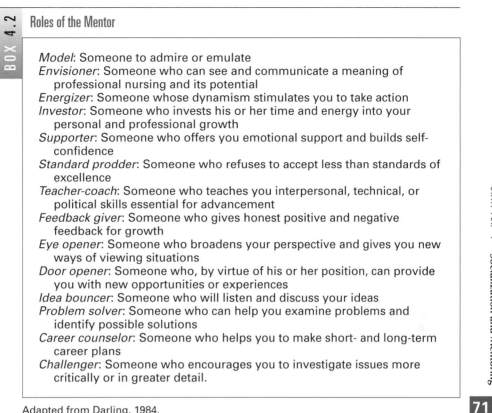

BOX 4.2

Roles of the Mentor

Model: Someone to admire or emulate
Envisioner: Someone who can see and communicate a meaning of professional nursing and its potential
Energizer: Someone whose dynamism stimulates you to take action
Investor: Someone who invests his or her time and energy into your personal and professional growth
Supporter: Someone who offers you emotional support and builds self-confidence
Standard prodder: Someone who refuses to accept less than standards of excellence
Teacher-coach: Someone who teaches you interpersonal, technical, or political skills essential for advancement
Feedback giver: Someone who gives honest positive and negative feedback for growth
Eye opener: Someone who broadens your perspective and gives you new ways of viewing situations
Door opener: Someone who, by virtue of his or her position, can provide you with new opportunities or experiences
Idea bouncer: Someone who will listen and discuss your ideas
Problem solver: Someone who can help you examine problems and identify possible solutions
Career counselor: Someone who helps you to make short- and long-term career plans
Challenger: Someone who encourages you to investigate issues more critically or in greater detail.

Adapted from Darling, 1984.

role that sponsors play in the power struggle at all levels of the organization has three primary characteristics:

- First, the ability to be often in a position to fight for a mentee. The propensity to point out superior performance at important times and promote or support a recommendation from a novice are essential ingredients of the sponsor relationship.
- Second, the ability to bypass the hierarchy and obtain inside information within the organization.
- Last, "reflected power," or support from those with formal or informal power to accelerate the movement of the novice up the organizational ladder.

Stages of the Mentoring Relationship

Hurst et al. (2002) cite four phases in mentoring relationships (Box 4.3). The first phase, *initiation*, occurs when the relationship is established. The second phase, *cultivation*, is characterized by coaching, protection, and sponsorship as well as counseling, acceptance, and the creation of a sense of competence. During this phase, the relationship develops through established meeting times to share and evaluate progress (Pinkerton, 2003). The third phase is *separation* and the fourth is *redefinition*, in which the relationship takes on a new form or ends.

Separation and redefinition are often difficult because the mentor and mentee may share different perceptions about whether it is time to separate and what their new relationship should be. Mentees should outgrow the need for such intense coaching if the

BOX 4.3

Stages of the Mentoring Relationship

1. Initiation
2. Cultivation
3. Separation
4. Redefinition

mentor has done a good job of cultivation. Unfortunately, some mentoring relationships get "stuck" and fail to progress the development of the novice. Personal and workplace circumstances and distractions can cause mentors and protégés to reach a comfort zone that prevents positive and ongoing development of the novice.

Typical mentoring relationships are usually characterized by the participants as intense. Any intense, high-level, interpersonal human relationship that evolves and changes can become a problem and have unfortunate ramifications, particularly in the workplace. As any intense relationship comes to a close, both participants must synchronize the separation or changed relationship. The literature identifies that most mentoring relationships evolve into a warm, lifelong, collegial friendship. Occasionally, either the mentor or protégé is unprepared for the end of a mentoring relationship, or an end is foisted on the participants due to job changes; this can cause serious, unhappy individual and workplace consequences.

D i s c u s s i o n   P o i n t

What strategies can be used when a mentee or protégé remains grateful and connected to the mentor but also begins to feel confined or restricted by a mentoring relationship?

Mentoring Opportunities for Men and Women: Historical Differences

Before the 1970s, the business world functioned on "the good ol' boys" network with mentoring relationships between men—an expected, accepted way to progress up the ladder of opportunity and promotion. The golf course, the locker room, and after-work drinks between workmates all advanced exclusively male mentoring relationships and, in the meantime, excluded women from promotional opportunities. This male-to-male mentoring phenomenon spawned the famous invisible, or "glass," ceiling that reduced career advancement opportunities for women, and thus impacted the predominantly female nursing profession.

Currently, mentoring is recognized as essential for the career development of men and women. This transition, however, has not been without struggle. In the mid-1970s, Henning and Jardin (1977) described the deep and abiding fatherly relationship that existed between 25 women in top management positions in business and industry and the men for whom they worked. All women attributed much of their success and rise to the top to this mentor-like relationship. Epstein (1974) concurred, arguing that for women to succeed, cleverness or professional degrees were simply not enough. Colleagues and seniors had to deem a protégé worthy of "judgment of potential."

Yet the literature suggests that, at least historically, there have not been enough mentors for all the women who want one. Bolton (1980) described four reasons why women do not have enough available mentors. The lack of emphasis on team sports for a girl in childhood could reduce her effectiveness in later life on a business or professional "team." In addition, solitary activities such as cooking and piano lessons are more common to young girls. While the socialization of girls has undoubtedly changed in the past 20 years, at least some of these elements continue to exist.

Boys are still traditionally encouraged to participate in football, baseball, and basketball, developing expertise to use in a team effort. Another reason, according to Bolton, is the potential sexual aspects found in a close personal, albeit business or professional, relationship. Bolton thought that many men fail to perceive talent that merits attention in career women.

> ***CONSIDER:** The socialization of young girls and boys has changed in subtle and not so subtle ways over the past 20 years as research has developed new ways of understanding learning and development. The impact of these changes will gradually change the workplace in expected and sometimes unexpected ways.

In addition, a shortage of mentors for women may be a result of the low number of women in top-level business management who are both willing and available to be mentors to other women. Moreover, the emphasis on the affiliative socialization needs of women could impact the mentoring process. "Belonging" is still associated with feminine socialization; "achieving" is often the focus of socialization for men. Because the purpose of mentoring is achievement, it would seem that mentoring would be inconsistent with feminine socialization; however, the skills of cooperation and collaboration could also support and enhance mentoring.

> ***CONSIDER:** It would be the unusual employer who does not foster women into leadership roles today. Employers are now developing strategies to encourage people from diverse backgrounds (i.e., ethnic, cultural, religious) to achieve promotion and fill leadership roles.

Fortunately, mentoring opportunities for women are increasing. However, the gains are slower for Black women, who report more difficulty finding mentors than their white counterparts. Not having an influential mentor or sponsor was reported in the *Women of Color in Corporate Management Report* (2002) as one of the top barriers to advancement for African American female executives. Of these executives, 46% pointed to "lack of mentoring" as a barrier to their advancement, whereas only 29% of white respondents named that factor. The study also showed that 69% of those with mentors were promoted, compared with 50% of those with no mentors.

Mentoring in Nursing

The presence or absence of mentoring within the nursing profession received attention only in the 1970s when the phenomenon became an important researchable topic. So much societal emphasis had been placed on gaining access to male-dominated professions that the predominantly female service-oriented professions remained underdeveloped until that time. The labeling of "traditional" and "female" apparently had been influential in reducing appropriate attention to the mentoring process in these "traditionally female" occupations. Clearly, mentoring was identified and highly regarded in male-dominated workplaces long before it was noted as having potential for women and later, nurses.

> ***CONSIDER:** Mentoring opportunities for all women, and thus for nurses, have been far more limited than for their male counterparts.

Connie Vance (1977, 1982, 2000) was one of the earliest nurse researchers to explore mentoring in nursing. The mentoring phenomenon and its many permutations is widely acclaimed and largely accepted as an effective strategy for the personal and professional development of nurses in the workplace. It is not an uncommon occurrence to find an editorial or reflective comment in scholarly nursing journals regarding the benefits and positive outcomes associated with mentoring relationships. Mentoring is considered so important that Sigma Theta Tau International (STTI), the honor society of nurses, devoted an entire issue of *Reflections on Nursing Leadership* to the phenomenon (third quarter, 2000). An Internet search via Google uncovered 852 sites for nursing and mentoring.

Discussion Point

What alternatives are available to nurses new to a workplace or feeling that a professional change is on the horizon, if there do not seem to be any available mentors for advice?

Clearly, nurses must actively seek out and perpetuate mentoring relationships. There are an overwhelming number of positive consequences for nurses who find the model that fits their current professional practice and health care workplace. The highly educated professional workforce found in today's health care organizations includes many nurses in powerful positions. Nurses must accept responsibility for individual and collective action to create and maintain an environment that is rewarding and supports positive socialization strategies for themselves and their professional colleagues.

Increasing Opportunities for Mentoring

Not surprisingly, contemporary nursing literature encourages a more assertive, less passive approach to developing a mentoring relationship. Emphasis is placed on the responsibility of leading nurses to bring along, indeed seek out, newer nurses to develop within an area of expertise. Newer nurses are urged to seek out a mentor or mentors to assist them, especially at critical points in their career progress, such as in the beginning or during a change of career direction or promotion. Waiting for a mentor to find a protégé is not always an effective strategy.

As the nursing workforce ages, health care organizations need to identify new ways of valuing mature, older, and experienced nurses and other health care professionals. It is not just the novice in a mentoring relationship who benefits. The mentor also receives many advantages. The recognition as a "chosen one" is evident for many co-workers to see. The gratitude, challenge, and revitalization of acting in a mentoring role are renewing and pleasurable. Participating in and watching a novice develop confidence, assertiveness, and professional skills is a high-level reward for a mentor.

> ***CONSIDER:** In some ancient cultures, older (less productive and dependent) people were placed in canoes and pushed out and away from the shoreline to die. Today, Western cultures are changing the way older people are viewed by placing value and appreciation on the wisdom that comes with experience.*

Before the current nursing shortage, research into the mentoring phenomenon was essentially limited to strategies to assist nurses to gain promotion up and away from the bedside. Encouraging nurses to stay in nursing, and particularly at the bedside, became a new and strategically important goal of mentoring and other supportive behaviors. As the shortage of bedside nurses has spiraled out of control, interest has increased in how mentoring, role modeling, and other supportive behaviors might socialize nurses and improve retention.

Value of Mentoring in Recruitment and Retention

In exploring the value of mentoring in improving recruitment as well as retention, Greene and Puetzer (2002) describe the necessity of "assigning" mentors and mentees when the workplace situation does not allow for spontaneous mentoring relationships to develop. Shapiro et al. (1978) suggest, however, that this is an exercise in futility. Many knowledgeable human relations experts believe that the right interpersonal dynamics must exist. Some believe that it is like falling in love—you cannot force it to happen and "it only works if the chemistry is right" (Williams, 1977). Indeed, much of the available contemporary literature identifies the importance of "chemistry" or the illusive connection that combusts to connect two people in a mentoring relationship. Some have described an "aha" experience as they recognize, on one hand the experience, wisdom, and altruism of a mentor, and on the other, the willingness, potential, and openness of the protégé.

> ***CONSIDER:** Occasionally we meet someone with whom we feel an instant connection. "I really LIKE this person, she/he is on my wave-length. . . . Instinctively, I just trust her. . . . I could talk to him forever." These may be some of the thoughts that precede the development of a mentoring relationship.*

The spontaneous discovery and development of a mentoring relationship within the health care arena would seem the ideal, but there are many examples of successful, planned, and organized mentoring programs. These programs often build on some of the typical mentoring strategies of a coaching or guiding relationship, but at a less intense, more superficial level. Several factors unique to the nursing profession play a role in mentoring and nursing.

- Nurses frequently form informal support groups in an effort to dissipate the high stress of nursing.
- Historically, nurses point to friendships among peers as one of the most satisfying aspects of nursing.
- The intense nature of the mentor relationship is based on heavy personal involvement whereas, historically in nursing, the emphasis has been on serving as a role model, which is a more superficial interpersonal relationship than mentoring.

Owens and Patton (2003) describe their mentoring relationship and note that being too prescriptive about the typical and various roles and characteristics of mentoring can work against the development of such relationships. Human relationships are unique and varied, and there is no reason to expect that all mentoring relationships develop and acquire characteristics according to a formula. Encouraging and celebrating a variety of positive mentoring relationships or one of its derivatives is an important and valuable professional practice.

Farris and Ragan (1981) suggest that concentrating on doing the job well, learning, and self-improvement seem to be the best ways to enable talent. As progress becomes self-evident, many will find that a mentor relationship has naturally developed. Displaying a teachable attitude and an eagerness to learn will also convey a receptive attitude to possible mentors (Williams, 1977).

Mentoring and Developmental Stages

Nurses should be acquainted with adult developmental issues and life transitions as they relate to wellness and illness. Linking this information to the mentoring phenomenon and workplace socialization is important. It will be clear that establishing a mentoring relationship can be enormously important not only to the novice, but also to the mentor.

It was only in the 1970s that Gail Sheehy in *Passages* (Sheehy, 1976) and Daniel Levinson in *The Seasons of Man's Life* (Levinson, 1978) connected mentoring and adult developmental theory. They emphasized that people continue to change throughout their adult life. Levinson found, among other information, that in early adulthood (ages 20 to 40 years), several distinct developmental changes occur in a certain sequence. Young people between 22 and 28 years enter the adult world. From 28 to 33 years they analyze what has occurred so far, and take steps to alter or change what they feel is inappropriate. From 33 years to midlife, they invest in realizing their goals or, as Sheehy describes, "climbing the career ladder."

Near age 40, people stop to take stock of the first half of their life. The compromises that were necessary in the first half of their life and the realization or lack of realization of their goal(s) are crucial components of the infamous midlife transition. At approximately 45 years of age, a pattern is established that modifies a life structure to accommodate the midlife analysis. Both Levinson and Sheehy identified that for many people the last half of their adult life is the fullest and most satisfying. There was evidence that the same transitional periods versus stable periods continue throughout adulthood.

Both works point out clear life stages marked by internal changes not directly related to external changes, such as divorce, death, marriage, births, and the like. Both Sheehy and Levinson refer to the postmidlife analysis period as either fulfilling, renewing, and satisfying or full of resignation and stagnation, depending on how one has dealt with previous transitional periods. This conceptual framework is relevant and pertinent for the nurse in the 21st century.

*CONSIDER: Research indicates that internal (life) changes occur despite external or extrinsic changes. Nurses in today's health care environment frequently encounter workplace transfers and employment changes. It would seem that mentoring relationships would be important strategies to undertake frequently throughout a nursing career and not just upon graduation from an undergraduate nursing program.

The changes and growth, or lack of growth, demonstrated in the different life stages are interconnected. There are always new heights to be climbed "but the next step is not simply another rung on the same ladder. The top of the first ladder turns out to be the bottom rung on a new ladder" (Levinson, 1978, p. 154). During the final thrust toward achievement of success, individuals must necessarily devote themselves to that end at the expense of other important parts of themselves. Many believe that if they become the president of the company or the shop steward or whatever their dream might be, that they will achieve happiness and contentment forever. At midlife an internal mechanism forces most adults to look at the price that has been paid for the place in which they find themselves at midlife.

Levinson and Sheehy both describe the importance of recognizing the costs and gains, and the necessary trade-offs that come to light during midlife analysis. The wisdom that may develop after midlife sets the stage for mentoring. At certain transitional points in life, the mentor relationship has profound and significant value to both participants. Seeing the ladder ahead, one can often see someone ahead who has been climbing.

Schein's (1978) research includes the observation that the midlife analysis exposes a career spent as a leader or a key contributor or dead wood. Levinson states that the mentor functions primarily as a transitional figure. The mentor "is usually older than the protégé by a half-generation, roughly 8 to 15 years" and is experienced as a "responsible, admirable, older sibling" (Levinson, 1978, pp. 177–178). It would appear that the pre-midlife adult would be most susceptible to the protégé role just as the post-midlife adult would be most susceptible to the mentoring role. Welcoming, acquainting, guiding, hosting, and counseling roles would serve both adults well.

Levinson refers to "generativity," or the sense that one feels for the continuity of life and the concern for the future generations. This can be seen at home, at work, in friendships, in government, and by many nurses. Usually, only after midlife does this sense of responsibility for others (development) take an active form. A clear understanding of adult developmental theory lends credence to the significance and importance of mentoring for the mentor as well as the protégé.

▶ CREATING A SUPPORTIVE ENVIRONMENT FOR SOCIALIZATION AND RESOCIALIZATION

The workplace environment is key to nurse satisfaction, retention, and patient care (Pataliah, 2002; Verdejo, 2002; Wright, 2002). Employers and nurse leaders have significant responsibility for creating a workplace that genuinely values supportive behaviors, such as mentoring. Murray (2002) recommends that nurses take advantage of the opportunity to mentor throughout their professional careers.

*CONSIDER: Today's nurses encounter higher workloads and sicker patients than ever before. Energy to combat demeaning and abusive behaviors from workplace colleagues is in short supply, since so much energy must be directed to providing safe and competent patient care. This situation encourages workplace and professional "silence," which is an impediment to individual and professional growth.

Leadership

Highly visible organizational leader(s) must "walk the walk," not merely "talk the talk." All leaders and managers in health care facilities need to demonstrate supportive behaviors themselves and identify and support formal and informal mentoring or other supportive programs at individual as well as departmental levels. For positive socialization, such as mentoring, to flourish and for the nursing profession to reach its greatest potential,

BOX 4.4

Traits of Work Cultures That Promote Positive Socialization

1. Mutual respect is evident in all written and verbal communications.
2. There is appropriate acknowledgment of the ideas and work of others.
3. Superior performance is sought and recognized publicly.
4. Roadblocks to goal achievement or unnecessary bureaucracy in the workplace are identified and addressed promptly.
5. Expectations are clear.
6. Criticism is constructive and given in private.

registered nurses need to be proactive and find ways to facilitate professional and individual growth-producing workplace strategies (Box 4.4).

A workplace culture where mutual respect is evident in all written and verbal communications is an important strategy for organizations to use. One of the favorite pastimes of employees everywhere is to closely observe, and then dissect, each word, behavior, and nuance of their managers, supervisors, and leaders. Appropriate acknowledgment, respectful tones, and public positive reinforcement can have long-term and lasting individual and group consequences. On the other hand, an impatient, poorly expressed personal or professional observation from a high-visibility person in the organization will be described and embellished throughout the organization for far longer than anyone would ever anticipate.

Organizational leaders can use a language that creates a positive and supportive work environment. What is included in the language is as important as what is excluded. Seeking out superior performance, knowing and using people's names, acknowledging the ideas or work of others, and identifying and reducing roadblocks or unnecessary bureaucracy in the workplace need to be everyday occurrences for leaders and managers. On the other hand, "constructive criticism" or even "suggestions" can be unhelpful and more importantly unheeded when presented in front of others. Employing these basic interpersonal and professional communication skills is essential in a workplace that hopes to attract and retain high-quality health care professionals.

Organizations are responsible for the ongoing education and training of all employees including leaders and managers. Poorly trained and performing leaders are the responsibility of the organization's executive and corporate level. Allowing inadequate leaders and leadership to prevail in an organization has long-term serious and negative consequences. Alternatively, an effective, persuasive role model and leader can energize and empower numerous employees and thereby promote a positive, effective workplace. This is particularly important in a health care workplace where highly educated professionals quite clearly know what they expect from their work environment and organizational leadership.

Sponsors, Guides, Preceptors, and Role Models

Organizations can also create work environments supportive of socialization through their use of sponsors, guides, preceptors, and role models. Shapiro, Haseltine, and Rowe (1978) suggested that a continuum exists with mentors and peer pals as endpoints, and sponsors and guides as internal points on the continuum. Mentors are viewed at one end and are the most "intense and paternalistic." Sponsors and then guides are at the two-thirds point; sponsors are less powerful in affecting their charges while guides are invaluable in explaining the system. The peer pal, or today's clinical preceptor, is at the other end of the continuum from a mentor. The peer pal or preceptor encourages a relationship between peers as they help each other succeed and progress.

> ***CONSIDER:** Clinical coordinators or preceptors are commonly assigned to one or more student nurses during their clinical practice placement. Qualities found in the various supportive roles identified here may or may not be readily available to students in today's health care workplace.

Haas et al. (2002) found that a surprising level of camaraderie developed between preceptors and students when preceptored clinical experiences were organized. Haas suggests that attention to the socialization of developing nurses in the real world of evening, night, and weekend shifts promoted a bond between experienced and less experienced nurses. Their experiences did not support the notion that nurses "eat their young."

▶ CONCLUSIONS

Understanding the socialization of novice nurses and the resocialization of nurses in transition or at the peak of their performance is critical to the nursing profession and the health of society. The realization of the full potential of nurses and the nursing profession has a direct impact on patient care and patient outcomes. The history and knowledge that is currently available through the nursing research reviewed here authenticates the importance of understanding and developing a range of strategies that enhance positive, supportive socialization among nurses. The continuing evolution toward professionalization and autonomy that sustains and enhances nurse empowerment is the most effective recruitment and retention strategy available.

Nurses comprise the largest group of health professionals, and most nurses practice nursing within an organization. Considering that hospitals are substantial business enterprises with complicated, multifaceted hierarchies, and that nurses are largely responsible for significant departmental budgets, one cannot help but see that interest and research into professional development and positive socialization, such as mentoring relationships, remain important. Today's health care organizations, administrators, and all health care professionals have a vested interest in recognizing and supporting mentoring programs, relationships, and behaviors.

It is within the hospital organization that most nurses develop or grow as individuals and as professionals. Administrators and medical staff need to consider interdisciplinary mentoring relationships because this cross-fertilization will enhance professional relationships in the health care workplace. Altering the workplace to encourage real partnerships among all health professionals with clear appreciation and acknowledgment of the unique contribution of each discipline remains a challenge. There is much at stake and a way to travel still.

▶ FOR ADDITIONAL DISCUSSION

1. What are some health care workplace behaviors associated with typical oppressed groups?
2. Describe strategies that might be effective in reducing typical oppressed group behavior.

3. Who is advantaged when negative socialization occurs in the health care workplace? Why?
4. Describe five career changes or transitions that might be facilitated by a mentoring relationship.
5. In what ways does a mentoring relationship provide an advantage to the mentor?
6. What are the advantages and disadvantages to a nursing professional of having positive or negative socialization strategies?
7. Will increasing numbers of men in nursing change the frequency or kinds of mentoring relationships that exist in nursing?
8. How can research continue to develop notions associated with positive socialization in the nursing profession?

REFERENCES

Bolton, E. B. (1980). A conceptual analysis of the mentor relationship in the career development of women. *Adult Education, 30*(4), 195–207.

Campbell, S. L. (2003). Cultivating empowerment in nursing today for a strong profession tomorrow. *Journal of Nursing Education, 42*(9), 423–426.

Darling, L. A. (1984). What do nurses want in a mentor? *Journal of Nursing Administration, 14*(10), 42–44.

David, B. A. (2000). Nursing's gender politics: Reformulating the footnotes. *Advanced Nursing Science, 23*(1), 83–93.

Epstein, C. F. (1974). Bringing women in. In R. B. Kundsin, (Ed.), *Women and success.* New York: William Morrow, pp. 13–21.

Farris, R. & Ragan, L. (1981). Importance of mentor-protégé relationships to the upward mobility of the female executive. *Mid-South Business Journal, 1*(4), 24–28.

Freire, P. (1968). *Pedagogy of the oppressed.* New York: Seabury Press.

Greene, M. T. & Puetzer, M. (2002). The value of mentoring: A strategic approach to retention and recruitment. *Journal of Nursing Care Quality, 17*(1), 63–70.

Haas, B. K., Deardorff, K. U., Klotz, L., et al. (2002). Creating a collaborative partnership between academia and service. *Journal of Nursing Education, 41*(12), 518–523.

Henning, M. & Jardin, A. (1977). *The managerial woman.* Garden City, NY: Anchor Press/Doubleday.

Hurst, S., Koplin-Baucum, S., Wilkins, B., et al. (2002). *Mentoring program.* Phoenix, AZ: Good Samaritan Regional Medical Center.

Hyperdictionary. (2000–2003). *Definition of socialization.* Retrieved January 2, 2004, from http://www.hyperdictionary.com/dictionary/socialization.

Kane, D. & Thomas, B. (2000). Nursing and the "F" word. *Nursing Forum 35*(2), 17–24.

Kanter, R. M. (1977). *Men and women of the corporation (pp. 181–184).* New York: Basic Books.

Kelly, L. Y. (1978). Power guide: The mentoring relationship. *Nursing Outlook, 26*(5), 339.

Kramer, M. (1974). *Reality shock: Why nurses leave nursing.* St. Louis: Mosby.

Kramer, M. (January 27—28, 1981). *Coping with reality shock.* Workshop presented at Jackson Memorial Hospital, Miami, FL.

Lee, M. B. & Saeed, I. (2001). Oppression and horizontal violence: The case of nurses in Pakistan. *Nursing Forum, 36*(1), 15–24.

Levinson, D. (1978). *The seasons of man's life (pp. 97–98, 251).* New York: Alfred A. Knopf.

Madison, J. (1997). RN's experiences of sex-based and sexual harassment: An empirical study. *Australian Journal of Advanced Nursing, 14*(4), 29–37.

Madison, J. & Minichiello, V. (2000). Recognizing and labeling sex-based and sexual harassment in the health care workplace. *Journal of Nursing Scholarship, 32*(4), 405–410.

Madison, J. & Minichiello, V. (2004). The contextual issues associated with sexual harassment experiences reported by RNs. *Australian Journal of Advanced Nursing, 22*(2), 8–13.

Marquis, B. & Huston, C. (2006). *Leadership roles and management functions* (4th ed.). Philadelphia: Lippincott Williams & Wilkins.

May, K. M., Meleis, A. I., & Windstead-Fry, P. (1982). Mentorship for scholarliness: Opportunities and dilemmas. *Nursing Outlook, 30*(1), 22–28.

Murray, R. B. (2002). Mentoring: Perceptions of the process and its significance. *Journal of Psychosocial Nursing and Mental Health Services, 40*(4), 44–51.

Owens, J. K. & Patton, J. G. (2003). Take a chance on nursing mentorships: Enhance leadership with this win-win strategy. *Nursing Education Perspectives, 24*(4), 198–204.

Pataliah, B. A. (2002). Mentorship in nursing. *Nursing Journal of India, 93*(6), 125.

Pilette, P. C. (1980). Mentoring: An encounter of the leadership kind. *Nursing Leadership, 3*(2), 22–26.

Pinkerton, S.E. (2003). Mentoring new graduates. *Nursing Economics, 21*(4), 202.

Roberts, D. (2003). Mentoring: The future of nursing. *MedSurg Nursing, 12*(3), 143.

Roberts, S. J. (2000). Development of a professional identity: Liberating oneself from the oppressor within. *Advances in Nursing Science, 22*(4), 71–82.

Sargent, A. G. (1977). *Beyond sex roles*. St. Paul, MN: West.

Scarry, K. D. (1999). Nursing elective: Balancing caregiving in oppressive systems. *Journal of Nursing Education, 38*(9), 423–426.

Schein, E. (1978). *Career dynamics: Matching individual and organizational needs*. Reading, MA: Addison-Wesley, pp. 177–178.

Schorr, T. (1979). Mentor remembered. *American Journal of Nursing, 79*(1), 65.

Shapiro, E. C., Haseltine, F. P., & Rowe, M. P. (1978). Moving up: Role models, mentors and the "patron system." *Sloan Management Review, 19*(3), 51–58.

Sheehy, G. (1974, 1976). *Passages: Predictable crises of adult life*. New York: Bantam.

Smith, S. (1995). *Dancing with conflict: Public health nurses in participatory action-research*. Unpublished doctoral dissertation, University of Calgary, Canada.

Thomas, S. P. (2003). Anger: The mismanaged emotion. *Dermatology Nursing, 15*(4), 351–357.

Vance, C. (1982). The mentor connection. *The Journal of Nursing Administration, 12*(4), 7–13.

Vance, C. (2000). Discovering the riches in mentoring connections. *Reflections on Nursing Leadership, 26*(3), 24–25.

Vance, C. N. (1977). *A group profile of contemporary influentials in American nursing*. Doctoral dissertation, Teachers College, Columbia University.

Verdejo, T. (2002). Mentoring: A model method. *Nursing Management, 33*(8), 15–16.

Williams, M. G. (1977). *The new executive woman*. Radnor, PA: Chilton, pp. 197–198.

Women of color in corporate management. Three years later. (2002). Catalyst. Retrieved April 11 2005, from http://www.catalystwomen.org/knowledge/titles/title.php?page=woc_corpmngt3yrs_01.

Wright, A. (2002). Precepting in 2002. *The Journal of Continuing Education in Nursing, 33*(3), 138–141.

BIBLIOGRAPHY

Bellack, J. (2003). Advice for new (and seasoned) faculty. *Journal of Nursing Education, 42*(9), 383–384.

Bennett, C. (2003). Key to learning: Your mentor and you. *Nursing Standard, 18*(7), 30.

Broome, M. E. (2003). Mentoring: To everything a season. *Nursing Outlook, 51*(6), 249–250.

Cameron, G. (2002). Learning professionalism by celebrating students' work. *Journal of Nursing Education, 41*(9), 425–428.

Christmas, K. (2002). Invest internationally. *Nursing Management, 33*(11), 20–21.

Clark, C. S. (2002). The nursing shortage as a community transformational opportunity. *Advances in Nursing Science, 25*(1), 18–31.

Eifried, S. J. (2003). Bearing witness to suffering: The lived experience of nursing students. *Journal of Nursing Education, 42*(2), 59–67.

Findlay, P. & McKinlay, A., Marks, A., & Thompson, P. (2000). In search of perfect people: Teamwork and team players in the Scottish spirits industry. *Human Relations, 53*(12), 1549–1574.

Grindel, C. G. (2003). Mentoring managers. *Nephrology Nursing Journal, 30*(5), 517–522.

Hagenow, N. & McCrea, M. (1994). A mentoring relationship: Two viewpoints. *Nursing Management, 25*(12), 42–43.

Hand, E. (2002). The preceptor connection. *Nursing Management, 33*(7), 17–18.

Hilgers, J. & Veitch, J. (2002). Guide nursing's next generation. *Nursing Management, 33*(12), 22.

Jackson, M. (2001). A preceptor incentive program. *American Journal of Nursing, 101*(6), 24A–24E.

Juall Carpenito-Moyet, L. (2002). Nurses, it's time to dust off your caps. *Nursing Forum, 37*(3), 3.

Koskinen, L. (2003). Characteristics of intercultural mentoring—A mentor perspective. *Nurse Education Today, 23*(4), 278–285.

Lockerwood-Rayermann, S. (2003). Preceptor leadership style and the nursing practicum. *Journal of Professional Nursing, 19*(1), 32–37.

Madison, J. (1985). *A study to determine nurse administrators' perceptions of the mentoring relationship and its effect on their professional lives*. An unpublished masters thesis, School of Public Health, University of Minnesota.

Mamchur, C. J. & Myrick, F. (2003). Preceptorship and interpersonal conflict: A multidisciplinary study. *Journal of Advanced Nursing, 43*(2), 188–196.

Mentors: One solution to high attrition rates. (June 2003). *Australian Nursing Journal, 10*(11), 37.

Myrick, F. (2002). Preceptorship and critical thinking in nursing education. *Journal of Nursing Education, 41*(4), 154–164.

Poster, E. (2002). The time is now. *Journal of Child and Adolescent Psychiatric Nursing, 13*(3), 95–96.

Oermann, M. H. (2001). One-minute mentor. *Nursing Management, 32*(4), 12–13.

Olson, R. K., Nelson, M., Stuart, C., et al. (2001). Nursing student residency program. *Journal of Nursing Administration, 31*(1), 40–48.

Percival, J. (2002). Manage your mentor. *Nursing Standard, 17*(1), 22.

Pontius, C. (2001). Meant to be a mentor. *Nursing Management, 32*(5), 35–36.

Weber, B. (2002). From bedside to board room: Interviews with nurse COOs and CEOs (Part I). Interview by Alison P. Smith. *Nursing Economics, 20*(3), 109–112.

Working with a mentor or clinical supervisor. (2003). *Nursing Standard, 17*(26), 32–33.

Zungolo, E. (2003). Four years have passed: A public thank you to teachers, mentors, colleagues and friends. *Nursing Education Perspectives, 24*(5), 218.

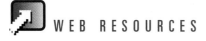

WEB RESOURCES

American Association of Critical-Care Nurses: Education/Training/Mentoring References	http://www.aacn.org/AACN/ICURecog.nsf/ Files/etm/$file/ETM.pdf
AORN *Journal*: Membership Committee Promotes Mentoring	http://www.findarticles.com/cf_dls/m0FSL/ 2_70/55525543/p1/article.jhtml
Computer Mentoring	http://www.nysasn.org/ computer_mentoring.htm
Critical Care Nurse: Make A Difference With Mentoring	http://www.findarticles.com/cf_dls/m0NUC/ 3_22/91111305/p1/article.jhtml
Education: Mentoring Graduate Nurses in Psychiatric Mental Health Settings	http://www.amnhealthcare .com/ featuretopics.asp
Focus on Nursing	http://www.astro.org/publications/ astronews/2003/Jul/FocusNursing.htm
Mentoring Benefits and Issues for Public Health Nurses	http://www.blackwell-synergy.com/links/doi/ 10.1046/j.1525-1446.2001.00101.x/abs/
Mentoring in Health Care	http://www.questia.com
Northwest Public Health Fall/Winter 2003: Mentoring Public Health	http://healthlinks.washington.edu/nwcphp/ nph/f2003/mentoring_phnurses_f2003.html
Nursing Standard: The Professional Home for Nurses on the Net	http://www.nursing-standard.co.uk/ resources/res_levelthree/ RCN-jobsfairseminars03/mentorship-sem.htm
NurseWeek: A Guiding Hand	http://www.nurseweek.com/news/features/ 02-02/mentor.asp
Online Mentoring: The Internet Gives Mentoring Programs a Boost	http://www.nurseweek.com/features/97-3/ mentor.html
Union nurses started a mentoring program to help retain new nurses	http://www.nysut.org/fnhp/amc/ 20010215-amc-agree.html
U.VA Nurse Mentoring Program Ensures High Quality Patient Care	http://www.healthsystem.virginia.edu/ internet/news/Archives00/nurse_ mentoring.cfm

Workforce Issues

2

The Current Nursing Shortage: Causes, Consequences, and Solutions

Carol J. Huston

5

A s government and private insurer reimbursement declined in the 1990s and managed care costs soared, many health care organizations, hospitals in particular, began downsizing to achieve cost containment by eliminating registered nursing jobs or by replacing registered nurses (RNs) with unlicensed assistive personnel. Even hospitals that did not downsize during this period often did little to recruit qualified RNs.

This downsizing and shortsightedness regarding recruitment and retention contributed to the beginning of an acute shortage of RNs in many health care settings by the late 1990s. This shortage, unlike earlier shortages that generally lasted only a few years, is likely to be more severe and lengthier than any nursing shortage experienced thus far (Marquis & Huston, 2006; Perlman, 2004). The shortage is also widespread geographically (indeed worldwide), is likely to worsen before it improves (Upenieks, 2003), and although it exists in all practice settings, is greatest in acute care hospitals. In addition, the causes of the current shortage are numerous and multifaceted, which will make resolution even more difficult.

To assess whether there is a nursing shortage, data must be obtained on both the demand for RNs and the supply. Assessing the demand for RNs is, in many ways, more complicated than assessing the supply, in part because of what some people argue is a lack of clarity in the definition of demand and because of the difficulty in obtaining the data (Brewer & Kovner, 2001). However, from an economic perspective, this shortage is being driven more by the supply side of the supply/demand equation than the demand side. This makes the problem even more difficult to solve because past "quick-fix" economic solutions such as sign-on bonuses, relocation coverage, or new premium packages will only redistribute the inadequate number of nurses, not increase it (Nevidjon & Erickson, 2001). Kimball and O'Neil (2002) concur, suggesting that offering bonuses and recruiting foreign nurses, as hospitals have done during previous shortages, will not be enough to solve the crisis this time. Yet, more than 40% of hospitals continue to offer bonuses of between $1,000 and $5,000 to new hires, with some offering even greater compensation (Hansen, 2002).

*CONSIDER: This nursing shortage is not likely to be fixed by the same solutions that worked in the past.

In addition, solving the current nursing shortage will not be inexpensive. Peter Buerhaus, Senior Associate Dean of Research at Vanderbilt University, said, "The U.S. needs to spend at least $1 billion to make any inroads into the nursing shortage. . . . If we're lucky, we'll get $50 [million] or $60 million" ($1 Billion Needed to Address, 2004).

This chapter will explore factors affecting the current supply of RNs as well as the current and projected demand. In addition, consequences of the shortage will be examined as well as strategies that have been proposed in an effort to confront what is likely one of the greatest threats to quality health care as we enter the 21st century.

▶ THE SUPPLY

Supply refers to the quantity of goods or services that are ready for use or purchase at a given price (Merriam Webster Online Dictionary, n.d.). To evaluate the supply of RNs in the United States, it is necessary to look at both RNs who are currently working and those who are eligible to work, but currently do not. In addition, the current and potential student pool must be part of the supply discussion.

There are currently just over 2.6 million RNs in the United States. Approximately 2.2 million of them are employed, with 1.8 million nurses working primarily in hospitals (Nevidjon & Erickson, 2001). According to a U.S. Department of Health and Human Services, Health Resources and Services Administration (USDHHS-HRSA) report (2002), 1.89 million full-time RNs were working in 2000, whereas approximately 2 million RNs were needed, causing a shortage of 110,000 nurses, or 6%.

Data from the 1980 and 2000 National Sample Survey of Registered Nurses show that although the U.S. population increased 13.7% between 1990 and 2000, the rate of nurses entering the workforce increased just 4.1% between 1996 and 2000, down from 14.2% between 1992 and 1996 (USDHHS-HRSA, 2001). Data from the 2000 survey also showed an estimated 2,696,540 active, licensed RNs in the United States, an increase of only 137,666 nurses from 1996. Although this was a 5.4% increase in the total RN population, the increase was lower than that in any of the previous national surveys. In contrast, the years between 1992 and 1996 showed the highest recorded increase in the RN population: an estimated 14.2%, or 319,058 (U.S. Department of Health and Human Services, 2001).

Declining Enrollment in Nursing Schools

The number of students enrolled or projected to enroll in nursing programs is an important factor in determining RN supply. According to the National Council of State Boards of Nursing, between 1995 and 2001, 28.7% fewer first-time, U.S.-educated nursing school graduates sat for the National Council Licensure Examination for RNs (NCLEX-RN) (VRP Recruitment and Staffing Services, 2003). This translates to 27,729 fewer students in this category (Table 5.1).

Discussion Point

Do you believe that state boards of nursing will be pressured to lower standards for licensure as a result of a reduced number of test takers and an increasing nursing shortage?

TABLE 5.1

Number of Candidates Taking the NCLEX-RN Examination: First-Time, U.S.-Educated Candidates Only

Program	1995	1996	1997	1998	1999	2000	2001
Diploma	7,335	6,346	5,240	3,978	3,161	2,679	2,310
Baccalaureate	31,195	32,278	31,828	30,142	28,107	26,048	24,832
Associate	57,908	55,554	52,396	49,045	45,255	42,665	41,567
Total	96,438	94,178	89,464	83,165	76,523	71,392	68,709

Source: VRP Recruitment Staffing Services (2003).

This decline in NCLEX registrants reflects the 26% decline in nursing school graduates from 1995 to 2000 (USDHHS-HRSA, 2002). Indeed, data from the National League for Nursing indicates declines in enrollments in all types of entry-level nursing programs early this decade, and a study by the American Association of Colleges of Nursing (AACN) found that enrollments in entry-level baccalaureate programs decreased for six consecutive years through fall 2001 (AACN, 1999, 2002c). Enrollments in entry-level nursing programs, however, have increased modestly since fall 2001. In fact, according to survey data released by the AACN in 2005, enrollments in the entry-level baccalaureate programs in nursing increased by 14.1 percent in fall 2004 over the previous year (AACN, 2005). This enrollment increase was even higher than AACN's preliminary data released in December 2004 which showed a 10.6 percent increase (AACN, 2004). Buerhaus (2003) suggests, however, that nursing-school enrollments would have to increase at least 40% annually to put enough new RNs in the pipeline to replace the numbers who are expected to retire in the next 5 to 6 years.

Some of the decline in nursing school enrollment can be attributed to inadequate federal and state funding for nursing education; however, the popularity of nursing as a major field of study has declined as well. The most prominent factor seems to be the expansion of opportunities for capable young women to enter formerly male-dominated professions such as medicine, law, and business. Only half as many women select nursing as a career today as compared with 25 years ago. This represents a decrease of roughly 40% since 1973 in the percentage of college freshmen who indicate that nursing is their top career choice (Staiger, Auerbach, & Buerhaus, 2000). In fact, one study reported that women graduating from high school in the 1990s were 35% less likely to become RNs than women who graduated in the 1970s (Buerhaus, Staiger, & Auerbach, 2000a).

Discussion Point

As the number of women entering nursing continues to decline, should recruitment efforts be directed at bringing more men into the profession?

In addition, Edward O'Neil, professor of family and community medicine and dental public health and director of the Center for the Health Professions at University of California, San Francisco, suggests that declining enrollments in nursing programs may be due, at least in part, to mismatched diversity (Robert Wood Johnson [RWJ] Foundation, 2003).

> *Most nurses are white women, and they do not reflect the diversity of the country. Nursing has not attracted men, and Generation X does not have a value set that makes nursing attractive to them. They [generation X] value anti-institutional, non-hierarchical, flexible environments. Their image of nursing is one of cold, unresponsive institutions lacking, at least in 2002, the high-tech element and flexibility they so value (RWJ, 2003, para 4).*

Some nursing leaders argue that often nurses have little knowledge about what nursing will be like when they choose to enter the field. Joyce Jenkins stated "If they had a little glimpse into what they're getting into, maybe only the people who think they can handle that would do it. That would make room for the people who do have a sincere calling" (McPeck, 2004, p. 19).

Yet, young people know enough about nursing to list working conditions (evening, night, and weekend shifts) and exposure to contagious elements as reasons for not considering nursing a positive career choice (Nevidjon & Erickson, 2001). Heinz (2004) states that work intensity within nursing has dramatically increased as patient lengths of stay have shortened and individual patient acuities have risen. In addition, an increase in patients entering the system has led to frequent admissions, discharges, and transfers. Heinz argues that it is these working conditions, combined with opportunities for limited salary advancement, that have led students to opt out of nursing careers.

Buerhaus states that if schools don't produce the required number of nurses, "the alternative is watching health care facilities turn off their lights. Access will go down and states will have to deal with the issues in a different way" (Perlman, 2004).

Part-Time and Unemployed Nurses: An Untapped Pool?

Some experts have suggested that too much emphasis has been placed on recruiting young people to solve the nursing shortage, and that supply could more easily be increased by bringing unemployed or part-time nurses back to nursing full-time. Indeed, the number of RNs not employed in nursing increased by 28% between 1992 and 2000 (USDHHS-HRSA, 2002).

The reality is, however, that 81.7% or 2,201,813 of active licensed RNs are already employed in nursing (USDHHS-HRSA, 2001). Between 1996 and 2000, the percentage of RNs working either full- or part-time remained unchanged. As of 2000, approximately 71.6% of RNs in the workforce were working full-time and 28.4% were working part-time (U.S. Department of Health and Human Services, 2001).

In addition, the literature on re-entry of RNs into the workplace is pessimistic and suggests that re-entry programs to assist these nurses have not been highly successful (Tone, 2002). "Much of the re-entry literature says that these programs take a lot of effort but do not give much in the way of results. Nurses often think they want to come back, but these days five years is a long time to be away and a lot has changed" (Ecker, as cited in Tone, 2002, para 4).

Yet, Buerhaus, Staiger, and Auerbach (2003) suggest that the current shortage has been alleviated recently, at least in part, by the increased employment of older RNs and the importation of RNs from foreign markets. The authors studied data—collected by the U.S. Bureau of Census's Current Population Survey—on 28,561 nurses ages 21 to 64 employed as RNs between January 1994 and December 2002 to construct and analyze national estimates of annual RN employment and earnings. The authors found substantial growth in foreign-born nurses and nurses older than 50 years of age.

The data show that between 2001 and 2002, the number of employed RNs increased by approximately 100,000, but that RNs older than age 50 and foreign-born RNs accounted for practically all of the increase. Married RNs accounted for 94% of the increase in employment between 2001 and 2002, leading the authors to conclude that the downturn in the U.S. economy in 2002 forced older RNs to return to work. In fact, Buerhaus and colleagues noted that RN employment increased more than 10% in states where unemployment increased the most. In addition, real RN wages increased 5% in 2002—after remaining "essentially flat" from 1994 to 2001—convincing RNs to rejoin the labor market, switch to full-time hours, or work overtime.

Buerhaus (2003) warns, however, that the longer-term outlook for nurse staffing is still grim. This is because the oldest segment of the RN population has demonstrated the most growth in the past 8 years at the same time that the youngest portion of the workforce has declined. The authors believe that unless the United States is able to infuse the workforce with younger RNs or foreign-born workers, there will be a drastic shortage of nurses when the older generation retires. Furthermore, an upswing in the economy could convince older RNs to leave the workforce earlier than expected, hastening the return of a more severe shortage.

▶ THE DEMAND

Demand is defined by Brewer and Kovner (2001) as the amount of a good or service (in this case, an RN) that consumers (in this case, an employer) would be willing to acquire at a given price. A shortage occurs when employers want more employees at the current market wages than they can get. Demand then is derived from the health status of a population and the use of health services.

The National Sample Survey of Registered Nurses projects that by 2005 nearly 2.6 million *full-time* RNs will be needed, a shortfall of 43% (New York State Education Department, 2001). The USDHHS-HRSA (2002) predicts a slow increase in the shortage of nurses between now and 2010, at which time it will have reached 12%. After 2010, the rate will accelerate, due to more nurses leaving the profession than entering. By 2020, the USDHHS-HRSA suggests the shortage will grow to 29%, an estimated 808,400 nurses, or quadruple what it is now.

Statistics from the U.S. Bureau of Labor Statistics are similar and suggest that more than 1 million new nurses will be needed by the year 2010 (Hecker, 2001). In addition, the U.S. Department of Labor projects a 21% increase in the need for nurses nationwide from 1998 to 2008, compared with a 14% increase for all other occupations (Hecker).

A 2002 report by the Joint Commission on Accreditation of Healthcare Organizations shows that in hospitals across the country, 126,000 nursing positions remain unfilled. The same report stated that 90% of long-term care facilities don't even have enough nurses to provide basic care, and some home health care agencies have had to refuse to accept new patients (Sigma Theta Tau International [STTI], 2004).

Causes of Increased Demand

The National Council of State Boards of Nursing (2004) identifies multiple demand factors driving the current shortage. The factors include an 18% increase in the population, a larger percentage of elderly people, medical advances that increase the need for adequately educated nurses, consumerism, the increased acuity of hospitalized patients, and a ballooning health care system.

Mee and Robinson (2003) concur, arguing that a primary cause of increased demand is simply that there are more patients and these patients are older. The population older than age 65 is expected to double between 2000 and 2030, from approximately 35 million to 70 million (U.S. General Accounting Office [GAO], 2001). In addition, people older than age 85 are currently the fastest growing age group (USDHHS-HRSA, 2002). As life expectancy in the United States increases, more nurses are needed to assist the individuals who are surviving serious illnesses and living longer with chronic diseases.

Heinz (2004) agrees, stating that the demand for health care will continue to grow at a staggering rate as the baby-boom generation enters the later stages of their lives. The increased needs of these individuals will require intense health care services, which entail greater hospital bed occupancy and highly skilled nursing care. This is at least part of the reason that average hospital occupancy has increased to the rate of 74.1%. Thus, the demand for health care is expected to steadily increase and the numbers of nurses to care for these patients will lag behind (Heinz).

Geographic Maldistribution of Nurses

Besides shortages of nurses in acute care settings, the nursing workforce is poorly distributed geographically. As this decade began, the greatest concentration of employed nurses was in New England, with 1,075 RNs per 100,000 population. In contrast, the Pacific region had 596 RNs per 100,000 population (Wakefield, 2001).

By 2002, the nursing shortage had been ranked as a "high priority" by 39 states and a "priority" by seven (National Conference of State Legislatures, 2001). These figures were consistent with Perlman's (2004) prediction that 44 states would be grappling with a significant nursing shortage by 2002.

Virtually all states, then, are affected by the current shortage, but the situation in some states is especially dire. For example, California ranks second only to Nevada in the lowest proportion of working RNs per 100,000 population, yet newer figures suggest California will need at least 25,000 more RNs in the next 5 years than will be available (U.S. GAO, 2001) and 60,000 more by 2020 to maintain the current low levels (Case, Mowry & Welebob, 2002). And out-of-state recruitment won't be the answer for California. Half of the RNs currently working in California already are educated in other states or countries (State of California, 1999).

▶ ROOTS OF THE SHORTAGE

Many factors contribute to the current nursing shortage in acute care settings, including an aging workforce, increased employment of nurses in outpatient or ambulatory care settings, high turnover due to worker dissatisfaction, inadequate long-term pay incentives, and an increasing recognition by nurses that they can make more money and act more autonomously as free agents than as full-time employees of a health care organization. These factors and others (Box 5.1) will be discussed in this section.

Nursing as a "Graying" Population

Nursing is a graying population—even more so than the population at large. Data from the USDHHS-HRSA National Sample Survey of Registered Nurses revealed that 52.9% of RNs were younger than the age of 40 in 1980, whereas in 2000 only 31.7% were

---

BOX 5.1

Causes of the Current Nursing Shortage

- ✓ Increasing elderly population (more chronically ill)
- ✓ Increased acuity in acute care settings, requiring higher-level nursing skills
- ✓ Downsizing and restructuring of the late 1990s eliminated many RN positions
- ✓ A relatively healthy economy in the late 1990s and early 2000, which encouraged some nurses to go part-time or quit
- ✓ Aging RN workforce
- ✓ Workplace dissatisfaction
- ✓ Women choosing fields other than nursing for a career
- ✓ Aging faculty for RN programs
- ✓ Inadequate nursing programs to accommodate interested applicants
- ✓ Low ceiling on wages for RNs without advanced degrees
- ✓ Future educator pool for RNs more limited than demand

younger than 40 (USDHHS-HRSA, 2001). Similarly, the number of employed nurses who were 50 years of age or older increased 60% between 1994 and 2000, while the number younger than 35 years of age declined by 17% (Perlman, 2004).

In 2000, Buerhaus, Staiger, and Auerbach (2000b) noted that the average age of the working nurse was 44 years. Berliner and Ginzberg (2002) suggest that the average age of the nurse workforce is 45.2 years, with only 9.1% younger than 30 in 2000. In contrast, in 1980, 25.1% of nurses were younger than 30 (Berliner & Ginzberg).

Wakefield (2001) concurs, stating that over two-thirds of RNs are age 40 and older, and less than 10% are younger than the age of 30. By 2010, more than 40% of RNs will be older than the age of 50 (Buerhaus et al., 2000b), and the average retirement age for nurses is 49 years (New York State Education Department, 2001). This means that there will likely be a vast exodus from the nursing workforce in the next 2 to 10 years, at a time when 43% more nurses are needed.

Discussion Point

What factors have led to the graying of the nursing workforce? Does there appear to be any short-term resolution of these factors?

The Nursing Faculty Are Grayer Yet

To further confound the shortage and efforts to address it, the average age of nursing faculty members in this country continues to increase, narrowing the number of productive years nurse educators can teach. According to the AACN (2003), the mean age for nursing faculty has increased steadily, from 49.7 years in 1993 to 53.3 in 2002 for doctoral faculty, and from 46 years to 48.8 for master's-prepared faculty.

A special survey was conducted by the AACN in 2000 to determine the vacancy rate for faculty. In a national sample of 220 schools, there were 5,132 full-time faculty positions, 379 (7.4%) of which were vacant (AACN, 2003). Full-time educator vacancy rates cited in the literature vary between 3.2% and 9.2%, with vacancies higher in baccalaureate and higher degree programs than in associate degree in nursing programs (California Strategic Planning Committee for Nursing, 2002; Furino, Gott, & Miller, 2000). According to the *Special Survey on Vacant Faculty Positions* released by AACN in June 2003, a total of 614 faculty vacancies were identified at 300 nursing schools across the country (Nurses for a Healthier Tomorrow, Nursing Faculty Shortage, n.d.). The data showed a nurse faculty vacancy rate of 8.6%, an increase from the 7.4% vacancy rate reported by AACN in 2000. Most of the vacancies (59.8%) were faculty positions requiring a doctoral degree. Although vacancy rates of 7% to 8% seem small, any vacant position in a small school can impact the didactic and clinical teaching workload of the remaining faculty, and their effects are cumulative (AACN, 2003).

Even more disturbing are the faculty shortage rates identified by the Southern Regional Educational Board Council on Collegiate Education for Nursing (CEN) (Box 5.2) in its 2002 study. This study clearly demonstrates that an insufficient number of educators are being prepared to replace the resigning and retiring faculty and to fill newly created positions.

Using regression analysis of AACN data between 2000 and 2004 for faculty aged 62 years and younger, Berlin and Sechrist (2002b) found that the mean age for full-time

BOX 5.2

Research Study Fuels the Controversy

Insufficient Faculty Adds to Shortage

The Southern Regional Education Board (SREB) Council on Collegiate Education for Nursing (CEN) conducted a study in July 2002 of 499 academic institutions offering 667 programs in 16 states and the District of Columbia. A total of 6,238 faculty positions were reported for the 2000/2001 academic year with 350 additional positions added in 2001/2002.

Study Findings

A serious shortage of nursing faculty was documented in 16 SREB states and the District of Columbia. Only 28 doctoral graduates were prepared as nurse educators to replace the 72 doctoral faculty who had resigned and the 55 doctoral faculty who had retired. Seven hundred eighty-four additional faculty were expected to retire within the next 5 years. In addition, 971 nurse educators reported not having the minimal academic credential for national accreditation.

The combination of faculty vacancies (432) and newly budgeted positions (350) points to a 12% shortfall in the number of nurse educators needed. The study concluded that unfilled faculty positions, resignations, projected retirements, and the shortage of students being prepared for the faculty role pose a threat to the nursing education workforce over the next 5 years.

doctorally prepared faculty is increasing at almost half a year per year. Retirement projections for individuals who were faculty in 2001 revealed that between 2004 and 2012, 200 to 300 doctorally prepared faculty will be eligible for retirement *each year*, with the modal year of retirement being 2009 (AACN, 2003; Berlin & Sechrist, 2002b).

In addition, the mean age for the 2001 full-time master's faculty cohort is increasing a third of a year per year, and from 2012 through 2018, 220 to 280 master's faculty will be eligible to retire each year, with their modal retirement year being 2015 (Berlin & Sechrist, 2002a). Given that the mean age for nurse faculty retirement is 62.5 years (Berlin & Sechrist, 2002b), faculty will be retiring in record numbers with far too few replacements in the pipeline to keep up with the loss.

*CONSIDER: Even if students can be recruited to become nurses, there may not be enough faculty to teach them.

With less than 1% of nurses holding doctoral degrees and only 10% having master's degrees (Chitty, 2001), the educator pool is already small. In addition, the number of nurses with master's and doctoral degrees prepared for faculty roles has decreased dramatically over the past decade. Only 3.3% of students in master's programs in 1998 were enrolled in education tracks (Chitty). In addition, historical misalignment between practice and education may discourage clinical nursing experts with advanced degrees from pursuing an academic career path.

The latest AACN(2005) data, however, showed a 13.7 % increase in enrollment in master's degree programs in nursing and a 7.3% increase in research focused doctoral programs. Yet, according to AACN, U.S. nursing schools turned away more than 11,000 qualified applicants in 2003 due to insufficient numbers of faculty, clinical sites, and classroom space (AACN, 2005). This is a siginificant increase from the more than 5,000 reported in 2002. Almost 65% of the schools cited faculty shortages as the reason they could not accept all qualified entry-level baccalaureate applicants. Perlman (2004) suggested the numbers were even higher, asserting that schools of nursing turned down at least 15,000 applicants in fall 2003. Indeed, AACN data confirmed that 32,797 qualified applicants were turned way in 2004 due to faculty and resource constraints.

Ada Sue Hinshaw, dean and professor at the University of Michigan School of Nursing, stated "We cannot afford to have colleges and universities deny nurse education to students who want to enter the profession simply because we don't have enough teachers" (AACN, 2002a, para 3). The reality, however, is that not only is this likely to happen, it is almost sure to occur.

The Exodus to Nonacute Care Settings

Another factor compounding the nursing shortage in acute care hospitals is the increasing number of nurses leaving the acute care hospital for employment in community health settings. Just over 18% of RNs are now employed in community health settings (Wakefield, 2001). Although the majority of nurses continue to be employed in hospitals (59.1%), the average national hospital vacancy rate for RNs is between 12% and 15% (Buerhaus et al., 2000a; Case et al., 2002) and is expected to increase to 20% by the year 2020 (Buerhaus et al., 2000a; Heinrich, 2001).

The Free Agent Nurse

An increase in the number of free agent nurses is another aspect that must be examined in assessing supply and demand factors of the current nursing shortage. Full-time employment of nurses is decreasing. Instead, nurses are increasingly assuming the role of *free agent*, a term more common to Generation X than their older counterparts, and this contributes to a shortage in acute care agencies. A free agent nurse is often an independent contractor who sells his or her services to an employer, with the condition that he or she maintains control over the number of hours they are willing to work and working conditions.

Per diem and traveling nurses are two types of free agents. Manion (2002) states that free agents define themselves by what they do, rather than by for whom they do it. In addition, their relationship with the organization is based on a free and open exchange, more of a partnership than an unequal dependency relationship.

Historically, health care organizations have sought to employ full-time workers (employees) so that they could better control the availability of needed human resources. Manion (2002) states, however, that the free agent model of nursing is gaining momentum in health care organizations as they recognize that they need to supplement their full-time employee pool with these skilled workers. Indeed, in a study by the HSM Group (2002), the percentage of facilities using temporary staff or travelers to fill vacancies was 53% in critical care, 34% in the emergency department, 28% in obstetrics, and 24% in operating room/preoperative care. Overall, more than half (54%) of respondents reported using non-permanent RN staff in some capacity.

Similarly, Hansen (2002) reports that nearly 60% of hospitals hire nurses from temporary agencies or traveling nurse companies. With over $7.2 billion spent nationally by hospitals on temporary workers and travelers in 2000 (California Nurses Association, 2001), the impact of the free agent nurse on the current nursing shortage must be examined more carefully.

Workplace Dissatisfaction

Perhaps one of the most significant yet least addressed factors leading to the current RN shortage is workplace dissatisfaction, resulting in high turnover levels and nurses leaving the profession. A study by Strachota, Normandin, O'Brien, et al. (2003) examining why RNs leave or change employment status showed that the most common reason given by respondents was hours worked. Working long shifts, overtime, weekends, nights, and holidays prompted nurses to look for another job. Thirty-seven percent of respondents were unhappy with staffing levels and commented that the workload was too heavy, with no relief in sight. Forty-six percent of the nurses were frustrated with the quality of care they could deliver because of low staffing and increased demands.

Another study by the American Nurses Association (2001) indicated that over half (56%) of the 7,299 nurses surveyed believed that time available for direct patient care had decreased in the past 2 years, and 76% reported an increased patient care load. Seventy-five percent of the nurses indicated that quality of nursing care had declined in their work setting and cited examples of inadequate staffing, delay in providing basic care, and the discharge of patients without adequate information to continue their care. Even more alarming was the finding that 40% of the nurses surveyed would not feel comfortable having a family member or someone close to them cared for in the facility where they worked.

Discussion Point

Why would nurses continue to work in a health care institution where they would not want to have a family member or someone close to them cared for?

Similarly, in a study of over 80,000 staff nurses, 20% of respondents classified the quality of care on their units as fair or poor (Sochalski, 2001). Forty-one percent were moderately or very dissatisfied with their job, citing emotional exhaustion as a leading cause of their dissatisfaction. Study conclusions noted that the frequency of patient adverse incidents increased proportionately with the dissatisfaction and emotional exhaustion of the nurses.

Finally, in a multinational study of 43,000 nurses from more than 700 hospitals in the United States, Canada, England, Scotland, and Germany from 1998 to 1999, Aiken et al. (2001) found that only 34% of surveyed nurses reported that their facility had enough RNs to provide high quality care. Only 43% reported enough support services to get the work done, and 29% reported that their administration listened and responded to their concerns.

*CONSIDER: The nursing shortage cannot be resolved until we address the underlying issues of worker dissatisfaction that caused it in the first place.

Is Pay an Issue?

Salaries also provide mixed incentives for young people to become nurses and for nurse retention. After growing an impressive 3% to 6% annually since the early 1980s, inflation-adjusted hospital RN wages actually *fell* each year between 1994 and 1997, and have risen very little since then (Buerhaus, 2001). As wages fall, holding all else constant, many (but not all) RNs have an economic incentive to reduce the number of hours they work, with some RNs withdrawing from the workplace altogether (Buerhaus). In addition, the economy as we entered the 21st century was fairly strong, with low unemployment and rising consumer confidence. This resulted in some RNs, who were often the second breadwinner in the family unit, reducing their work hours or leaving the workplace entirely (Buerhaus). Many of these same RNs, however, returned to work after the Sept. 11, 2001, attack on the World Trade Center as a result of declining stock market values and lower levels of consumer confidence.

In looking at absolute numbers, a 2003 salary survey showed that the average income for a nurse in 2003 was a respectable $66,020, up $3,230 from 2002 (Steltzer, Woods, & Gasda, 2003). The long-term rise in earnings potential, however, is limited for most nurses. Nurses with more than 20 years of experience had an average annual salary of $70, 270, holding steady with 2002 figures (Steltzer et al.).

Salary is clearly a deterrent for nursing faculty. Graduate students who may have become educators in the past are now opting instead for better-paying positions in clinical and private practice (Huston, 2003; Mee & Robinson, 2003). The average salary of a master's-prepared nurse practitioner working in her or his own private practice was $94,313, according to the 2003 National Salary Survey of Nurse Practitioners (Tumolo & Rollett, 2003). In contrast, AACN reports that full-time nurse faculty with a doctoral degree earned $61,000 in 2002-2003, while faculty with a master's degree earned only $49,000 (Nurses for a Healthier Tomorrow, n.d.).

Discussion Point

Historically, nursing is considered to be an altruistic profession. How critical do you think pay is as a motivator for people to want to become nurses?

Retention: An Undervalued Strategy

An often ignored or at least undervalued aspect of nursing shortages is that highly trained, employable nurses are *voluntarily* leaving the profession because they are dissatisfied with their work. A typical annual turnover rate for hospital nurses in the late 1990s was 15% per year (Advisory Board Company, 2000), although a recent study of RNs' intent to leave their position suggested the situation might be even worse, with 20.5% of the sample stating they were somewhat or very likely to leave their current position (Rambur, Palumbo, McIntosh, & Mongeon, 2003).

Similar turnover rates were found by the HSM Group (2002) in a study commissioned by the American Organization of Nurse Executives in 2000. This study found that the national average turnover rate for RNs in 2000 was 21.3%, although the range was between 10% and 30%. The average RN vacancy rates were highest in critical care (14.6%), medical/surgical care (14.1%), and the emergency department (11.7%).

The western states faced the highest average RN vacancy rate, with 12.2% of budgeted positions unfilled (HSM Group, Ltd., 2002). In addition, the West reported a turnover rate of 22.2%. The Midwest had the lowest average vacancy rate, as compared to other regions (8.9%), and a turnover rate of 20.2%. The South had an average RN vacancy rate of 11% and a higher than average turnover rate of 24% (HSM Group, Ltd.).

> ***CONSIDER:** Retention of precious nurse resources must be a very real part of the solution to the nursing shortage; health care institutions must make a commitment to improve working conditions for nurses.

Clearly, organizations that pay attention to the employee market and understand what people are looking for in the work environment have a better chance to recruit and retain top talent, particularly given the current low unemployment rate (Nevidjon & Erickson, 2001). Jeanna Bozell stated the case for retention articulately with her assertion that:

> *You can recruit till the cows come home. . . . Pull out all the stops, do the sign-on bonuses, basically bribe them in some way to get them in the door. But until you stop the bleeding, they're coming in the front door and leaving out the back door (McPeck, 2004, p. 18).*

▶ THE CONSEQUENCES OF THE SHORTAGE

What are the consequences of a nursing shortage? To answer this question, it is critical first to recognize that patient outcomes are sensitive to nursing interventions and that, as a result, nurse staffing (total hours of care as well as staffing mix) affects patient outcomes. This supposition is certainly supported in a review of the literature, which increasingly suggests that RN staffing affects patient outcomes such as inpatient mortality and other measures of quality of hospital care.

Indeed, numerous studies have been conducted to describe the relationship between nurse staffing levels and clinical outcomes of patients at both the hospital and unit levels; the findings are summarized in Chapter 10. Most studies conclude that there are statistically significant relationships between staffing and patient outcomes; however, researchers agree that more evaluation is necessary (Heinz, 2004).

As such study results are released, collective bargaining agents, the government, policy makers, and special interest groups are taking note and increasingly calling for regulatory oversight of nurse staffing issues (Buerhaus, 2001). And it seems the public is listening. According to a 2002 poll by Vanderbilt University Medical Center's School of Nursing and Center for Health Services Research, most Americans are worried about how the nursing shortage will affect their ability to receive proper medical care (STTI, 2004). The study showed that:

- A total of 81% of Americans recognize there is a nursing shortage; 65% believe it is either a major problem or a crisis.
- A total of 93% agree (and 80% strongly agree) that the nursing shortage jeopardizes the quality of health care in the United States.
- Seniors, aged 55 and older, are particularly sensitive to the shortage's impact on the quality of the health care system.

▶ SOLVING THE SHORTAGE

Just as the issues that caused the current shortage are complex, so too must be the solutions to the problem. Resolution will not be easy. With both demand and supply shortages, creative strategies will need to be implemented in multiple arenas including education, health care delivery systems, policy and regulations, and image brokering (Nevidjon & Erickson, 2001).

This complexity is evident in the following statement by the Tri-Council for Nursing (2003):

> ▶ *There is no simple description of the status of the nursing workforce shortage—present and future. Discussion surrounding this issue is complex and interrelated. It is not possible to isolate single factors or solutions. Rather, a systems perspective review gives the greatest depth and understanding of the relationships between multiple variables. It is critical to include the systematic issues in education, health delivery systems and the work environment. Further, the impact of reimbursement, legislation, regulation and technological advances must also be considered. Failure to consider the relationships among these aspects limits the full appreciation of the nursing workforce shortage complexity.*

This discussion examines only some of the solutions that have been presented to address the current nursing shortage, including redesigning the workplace, increasing the number of nursing students in the pipeline, importing foreign nurses, improving nursing's image, increasing the faculty pool, re-envisioning the profession, and moving toward a self-service approach to patient care. In addition, Box 5.3 includes a list of 11 strategies created by Sigma Theta Tau (2004) for reducing the current shortage.

Redesigning the Workplace

The age of the current nursing workforce is an important factor in the current nursing shortage because nursing can be both physically and mentally taxing, even to the young. We need to redesign patient care delivery models to support the practice of an older workforce, initialize new technology to reduce the physical demands, and offer greater flexibility in scheduling, increased time off, and sabbaticals (Nevidjon & Erickson, 2001).

In addition, RNs must be made to feel valued, and physician-nurse relationships reflecting collegiality and collaboration should be fostered. Additionally, environments of shared governance should be created where nurses actively participate in all decision making related to patient care. Staff nurses should feel empowered, and autonomy should be encouraged. A report by the Joint Commission on Accreditation of Healthcare Organizations (2002) notes that approximately 50 "magnet hospitals" have successfully avoided or overcome shortages (STTI, 2004). Creating positive workplace environments that mirror magnet requirements may go a long way in negating the current shortage.

Support for Nursing Education: Filling the Pipeline

More money is needed in the form of nursing scholarships and loans to encourage young people to enter nursing. Individual nurses and professional organizations must support legislation to improve financial access to nursing education (Albaugh, 2004). The Tri-Council for Nurses urges nurses to advocate for increased nursing education funding under Title VIII of the Public Health Service Act, as well as other publicly funded initiatives, so that there will be the necessary capacity and resources to educate future nurses.

BOX 5.3 Strategies for Addressing the Shortage

- Demonstrate to health care leaders that nurses are the critical difference in America's health system.
- Reposition nursing as a highly versatile profession where young people can learn science and technology, customer service, critical thinking, and decision-making skills.
- Construct practice environments that are interdisciplinary and build on relationships among nurses, physicians, other health care professionals, patients, and communities.
- Create patient care models that encourage professional nurse autonomy and clinical decision making.
- Develop additional evaluation systems that measure the relationship of timely nursing interventions to patient outcomes.
- Establish additional standards and mechanisms for recognition of professional practice environments.
- Develop career enhancement incentives for nurses to pursue professional practice.
- Evaluate the effects of the nursing shortage on the preparation of the next generation of nurse educators, nurse administrators, and nurse researchers and take strategic action.
- Implement and sustain a marketing effort that addresses the image of nursing and the recruitment of qualified students into nursing as a career.
- Promote higher education to nurses of all educational levels.
- Develop and implement strategies to promote the retention of RNs and nurse educators in the workforce.

©2004 Honor Society of Nursing, Sigma Theta Tau International (2004). Reprinted with permission.

99

In 2002, New York passed a health care reform act that provides $1.8 billion over a $3\frac{1}{2}$-year period for health care workforce recruitment, training, and retention in hospitals, nursing homes, and home health care settings (Perlman, 2004). Similarly, California, in 2002, announced a $60 million, 3-year nursing workforce initiative to recruit, train, and retrain nurses for employment in hospitals and other health care facilities (Perlman).

Importation of Foreign Nurses

Given the success hospitals already are having with foreign recruitment and the time required to strengthen the domestic nurse pipeline, Buerhaus et al. (2003) suggest that hospitals may need to continue looking abroad for nurses. They note, however, that such a tactic requires developing a national policy governing nurse quality standards and ensuring the safety of American nurses' jobs. In addition, using foreign labor has complex international implications, creating a drain on some countries' health care systems while shoring up the economies of countries that purposefully export their workers. Because the importation of nurses has such complex ramifications, a separate chapter has been devoted to its discussion (see Chapter 6).

Changing Nursing's Image

More efforts must be made to improve the public's image of nursing. Again, this will not be an easy task given the historical roots of nursing stereotypes and the profession's long history of being unable to effectively change public perceptions regarding professional nursing roles and behaviors (see Chapter 22).

A 2002 poll by Vanderbilt University Medical Center's School of Nursing and Center for Health Services Research confirms that most Americans trust and admire nurses, and would encourage family and friends to consider a nursing career. However, nursing recruitment is hampered by the public's lack of knowledge of the many opportunities available within nursing (STTI, 2004)

Johnson & Johnson, in conjunction with several professional nursing organizations including STTI, launched a multiyear, $20 million national campaign during the Winter Olympics in 2003 to attract more people to the nursing profession (Discover Nursing, 2002; Lindsay, 2002). The "Discover Nursing" campaign includes a website that conveys the benefits of a career in nursing and provides links to nursing schools and scholarship programs. It also profiles nurses in a variety of nursing careers. The campaign also includes a scholarship fund for undergraduate students and nursing faculty. More than 50,000 brochures, posters, and videos have been mailed to high schools, nursing schools, hospitals, and nursing organizations (Lindsay, 2002).

In addition, Nurses for a Healthier Tomorrow (NHT), a coalition of 43 national nursing and health care organizations, has created a website and is running public service announcements and print ads regarding the nursing shortage, in an effort to encourage young people to enter nursing. The campaign has received news coverage across the country (STTI, 2004).

Creating a Nursing Faculty Pool

Solutions must also be directed at the nursing faculty shortage. NHT launched a national advertising campaign titled "Nursing education . . . pass it on" in February 2004 (AACN, 2002a). The faculty recruitment ads depict nurse educators expressing the personal satisfaction and rewards that they receive from their job. The campaign also includes colorful ads depicting nurse educators who encourage teaching careers, an outreach campaign to nursing journals and the mass media, ready-to-run articles in a special edition of the NHT newsletter, and a new career profile on the nurse educator posted on the NHT website.

Re-envisioning the Profession

Perhaps most bold in terms of solutions to the nursing shortage are those presented by Kimball and O'Neil (2002) in their RWJ foundation report *Health Care's Human Crisis-: The American Nursing Shortage*. This report calls for a re-envisioning of the nursing profession itself, so that it can emerge from this crisis stronger and in equal partnership with the profession of medicine. The report suggests that anything less consigns nursing, and the public that depends upon its care, to perpetual cycles of shortage and oversupply.

The report therefore recommends that a national forum to advance nursing be created. An independent body, the forum would draw together a wide range of stakeholders to address the nursing shortage and broader, related health and social issues in four strategic areas (RWJ, 2003). The first would be to support research and pilot programs that would advance the use of breakthrough or "disruptive" strategies within institutions. These strategies would both create new nursing models and study their effects on patient outcomes and satisfaction with care.

Second, to attract and retain a new generation of nurses, and to ensure that the new nursing workforce represents the ethnic and racial diversity of the United States, the forum would focus efforts on reinventing nursing education and work environments to address the needs and values of these new workers. It would foster the creation of new training/educational models and new community-based roles that use nurses' unique skills, while fostering satisfaction and competence. It would develop replicable demonstration projects to attract and retain men, minorities, and special populations, such as single mothers, workers displaced from other professions, and older Americans.

The third strategy proposed for this forum would be to establish a national nursing workforce measurement and data collection system to provide current, consistent, and comparable data that can be aggregated and compared at national, state, and county levels. Such information would be invaluable to health care leaders, nursing educators, and policy makers as they plan for nursing and educational capacity in the future.

Finally, the forum would establish a clearinghouse of effective strategies to advance cultural change within the nursing profession by creating a comprehensive, up-to-date website that is nonterritorial and easy to use and that provides useful information for health care leaders about research, programs, and models that have proven successful in advancing the nursing profession (RWJ, 2003).

> *The National Forum to Advance Nursing is, by any standards, an ambitious proposal, requiring the collective efforts of all stakeholders in the nursing shortage, including communities and consumers. The RWJ Foundation believes that a National Forum to Advance Nursing would provide the necessary structure to bring together all stakeholders in a collective effort to develop meaningful, lasting solutions to the American nursing shortage (RWJ, 2003, para 11–12).*

A Self-service Approach to Patient Care

One must at least consider some fairly radical approaches to the nursing shortage that do not include increasing the number of nurses available. The best known of these is the self-service model.

This model suggests that family members can be used as caregivers to supplement RNs. Mayer (2001) suggests that on a medical-surgical unit, family members would receive education about basic nursing functions (ideally before hospitalization). These family members would then provide most bedside care during the immediate postacute hospital period once the patient has been stabilized. Indeed, self-service nursing is the preferred model of care in many countries.

Critics of this self-service approach suggest that hospitalized patients today are far too ill and their needs are too complex to be cared for by a layperson. Care is too sophisticated and the technology routinely used for care is not known to individuals outside health care. In addition, Nash (2001) suggests that nurses have a responsibility to protect the public from people who do not meet the professional and legal standards of clinical practice.

Nash goes on to say:

> *There is little argument that families are essential to the emotional and social wellbeing of a person in the hospital. They are instrumental in providing familiar and comforting high touch measures of caring. Nurses must find innovative ways to increase the involvement of family in the delivery of care. However, we must be careful not to devalue our professional obligation to the public while we search for better alternatives (2001, p. 459).*

▶ CONCLUSIONS

Many factors have led to the significant professional nursing shortage we face in the early 21st century. Health care providers, the public, and legislators are beginning to recognize that both the problem and the potential consequences are severe. In February 2001, a forum entitled "Hard Numbers, Hard Choices: A Report on the Nation's Nursing Workforce" was held on Capitol Hill and three members of Congress shared their views on the adverse consequences of insufficient numbers and distribution of nurses and also provided a plan to begin addressing these problems (Wakefield, 2001). Today, one would be hard-pressed to find a congressperson or senator who would not identify the current nursing shortage as one of the most serious issues impacting health care today. Yet, efforts to address the shortage have been too few and far between.

Regarding the current shortage, Johnson (2000, p. 402) states: "We have spent lots of time denying, analyzing, and sometimes blaming as well. We have experienced 'analysis paralysis' despite the fact that the demand side of the profession grows higher while the supply side slides further into crisis. We must act collectively, collaboratively, and in concert with a whole host of stakeholders, including all members of the health care team, the community, and Congress as well."

Short-term solutions to the shortage have been attempted, including importing foreign nurses and increasing federal money for nursing education. The recent passage of legislation such as the Nurse Reinvestment Act encourages more students to choose nursing as a career and helps students financially to complete their education. It also encourages graduate students to complete their studies and assume teaching positions in nursing schools.

In addition, many states have introduced or passed legislation designed to improve working conditions or attract more nurses. Four states have passed workforce study bills to study the nursing shortage, and two states have passed bills authorizing funding for nursing education (Williams, 2001). Long-term planning and aggressive intervention, however, will be needed for some time at the national and regional levels to ensure that an adequate, highly qualified nursing workforce will be available in the future to meet the health care needs of the citizens of this country.

Finally, thankfully, the National Council of State Boards of Nursing (NCSBN) (2003) has resisted pressure to lower standards for passing the NCLEX-RN examination as a quick fix to licensing more nurses. Indeed, at their December 2003 meeting, the NCSBN voted to raise the passing standard, effective April 1, 2004, in conjunction with the new 2004 NCLEX-RN test plan. These increases occurred as a result of changes in U.S. health care delivery and nursing practice that increased the acuity of clients cared for by entry-level RNs. "After considering all available information, the Board of Directors determined that safe and effective entry-level RN practice requires a greater level of knowledge, skills, and abilities than was required in 1998, when NCSBN established the current standard" (NCSBN, 2003, para 2).

Yet, more must be done to address the current, mounting nursing shortage, and it is increasingly obvious that multiple solutions to the shortage will be needed. These solutions will require the best thinking of our experts and will likely reshape fundamental core under-pinnings that have been a part of the nursing work world for decades, if not centuries.

Rovin & Formella (2004) argue articulately that the current nursing shortage is not a problem of supply and demand, which is why unbelievable recruitment packages, the importation of foreign nurses, and the active recruitment of RNs across health care institutions haven't really changed anything. "These strategies simply predispose us for another shortage and another" (Rovin & Formella, 2004, p. 163). The only real solution to the nursing shortage is to deal with the causes of the shortage, rather than the symptoms.

Perhaps the Tri-Council for Nursing (2003, para 14) said it best:

> *In order to encourage the development and deployment of nursing personnel with skills appropriate to the health care system, the public, policy makers and the profession must engage in ongoing long-term workforce planning,*

regardless of the perceived or real pressures related to the short-term demand for nursing services. Without measures to reverse the trends discussed above, the nation is in danger of experiencing serious breakdowns in the health care system. Strategies to recruit and retain are costly and must be done with some assurance that these efforts will be accompanied by specific strategies to overcome workforce issues that discourage long-term commitment to a career in nursing.

FOR ADDITIONAL DISCUSSION

1. In what ways do other professions do a better job of attracting younger workers—both men and women?
2. Are salaries a significant driver in the current nursing shortage? At what level would salaries not be a factor?
3. How would increasing the educational level for entry into practice affect the current nursing shortage?
4. Will the demand for RNs in the future be affected by growing technological developments?
5. Why has the nursing workforce historically suffered some degree of a shortage every 10 to 15 years?
6. If magnet hospital criteria were to become the baseline for organizational structure and performance, would nursing shortages exist?
7. Why are starting salaries for nurses with master's and doctoral degrees in academia so low?
8. Why do many health care organizations choose to expend more money on recruitment than on retention strategies? Which is more effective in the short term? In the long term?
9. Is implementation of mandatory minimum staffing ratios in acute care hospitals likely to reduce the nursing shortage in California?

103

REFERENCES

Advisory Board Company. (2000). *Reversing the flight of talent. Executive briefing.* Vol. 1. Washington, DC: Nursing Executive Center.

Aiken, L. H., Clarke, S. P., Sloane, D.M., et al. (2001). Nurses' reports on hospital care in five countries. *Health Affairs, 20*(3), 43–53.

Albaugh, J. A. (2004). Positive ideas and thoughts on the nursing profession: A blueprint to resolving the nursing shortage. *Urologic Nursing, 24*(1), 53–54.

American Association of Colleges of Nursing. (1999). *1998–1999 enrollment and graduations in baccalaureate and graduate programs in nursing.* Washington, DC: Author.

American Association of Colleges of Nursing. (2002a). *Nurses for a Healthier Tomorrow launches campaign to increase number of nurse educators.* Retrieved April 20, 2004, from http://www.aacn.nche.edu/Media/NewsReleases/2004NHTCampaign.htm.

American Association of Colleges of Nursing. (2002b). *Nursing faculty shortage fact sheet.* Retrieved May 18, 2004, from http://www.aacn.nche.edu/Media/Backgrounders/facultyshortage.htm.

American Association of Colleges of Nursing. (2002c). *Nursing school enrollments fall as demand for RNs continues to climb.* Washington, DC: Author. (Last updated March 8, 2004)

American Association of Colleges of Nursing. (May 2003). *AACN white paper. Faculty shortages in baccalaureate and graduate nursing programs: Scope of the problem and strategies for increasing the supply.* Retrieved April 21, 2004, from http://www.aacn.nche.edu/Publications/WhitePapers/FacultyShortages.htm.

American Association of Colleges of Nursing (2005). *New data confirms the shortage of nursing school faculty hinders efforts to address the nation's nursing shortage.* Retrieved April 10, 2005, from http://www.aacn.nche.edu/Media/News-Releases/2005/Enrollments05.htm.

American Nurses Association. (February 6, 2001). *Nurses concerned over working conditions, decline in quality of care, ANA survey reveals.* Retrieved April 20, 2004, from http://nursingworld.org/pressrel/2001/pr0206.htm.

Berlin, L. E. & Sechrist, K. R. (2002a). *Regression analysis of full-time master's prepared faculty in baccalaureate and graduate nursing programs* (unpublished data). Cited in American Association of Colleges of Nursing. (May 2003). *AACN white paper. Faculty shortages in baccalaureate and graduate nursing programs: Scope of the problem and strategies for increasing the supply.* Retrieved April 21, 2004, from http://www.aacn.nche.edu/Publications/WhitePapers/FacultyShortages.htm.

Berlin, L. E. & Sechrist, K. R. (2002b). The shortage of doctorally prepared nursing faculty: A dire situation. *Nursing Outlook, 50*(2), 50–56.

Berliner, H. S. & Ginzberg, E. (2002). Why this hospital shortage is different. *Journal of the American Medical Association, 288*(21), 2742–2744.

Brewer, C. & Kovner, C. T. (2001). Is there another nursing shortage? What the data tell us. *Nursing Outlook, 49*(1), 20–26.

Buerhaus, P. (2001). Expected near and long-term changes in the registered nurse workforce. *Policy, Politics, & Nursing Practice, 2*(4), 264–270.

Buerhaus, P. (November 21, 2003). *Buerhaus study finds influx of foreign, older workers eased RN shortage in 2002, but data portend coming crisis.* Health Care Advisory Board, Nursing Executive Watch. Retrieved April 27, 2004, from http://www.advisoryboardcompany.com.

Buerhaus, P. I., Staiger, D. O., & Auerbach, D. I. (2000a). Implications of an aging registered nurse workforce. *Journal of the American Medical Association, 283*(22), 2948–2954.

Buerhaus, P. I., Staiger, D. O., & Auerbach, D. I. (2000b). Policy responses to an aging registered nurse workforce. *Nursing Economics, 18*(6), 278–284, 303.

Buerhaus, P. I., Staiger, D. O., & Auerbach, D. I. (2003). Is the current shortage of hospital nurses ending? *Health Affairs, 22*(6), 191–198.

California Nurses Association. (July 26, 2001). *CNA blasts study on alleged costs of safe staffing, implementing ratios may be cost neutral, RNs say.* http://66.218.71.225/search/cache?p=CNA+blasts+study+on+alleged+costs+of+safe+staffing,+implementing+ratios+may+be+cost+neutral,+RNs+say.++&u=www.califnurses.org/cna/press/72601.html&w=cna+blasts+study+on+alleged+costs+of+safe+staffing+implementing+ratios+may+be+cost&d=D6DB08845B&c=609&yc=37352&icp=1.

California Strategic Planning Committee for Nursing. (2002). *The California nursing workforce initiative.* Retrieved 10/30/04 from http://www.ucihs.uci.edu/cspcn/TheFinalReport2002.pdf.

Case, J., Mowry, M., & Welebob, E. (June 2002). *The nursing shortage: Can technology help?* Oakland, CA: California Healthcare Foundation.

Cavouras C. (2002). Clinical notebook. Nurse staffing levels in American hospitals: A 2001 report. *Journal of Emergency Nursing, 28*(1), 40–43.

Chitty, K. K. (2001). *Professional nursing. Concepts and challenges* (3rd ed.). Philadelphia: WB Saunders.

Council on College Education for Nursing. (2002). *SREB study indicates serious shortage of nursing faculty.* Atlanta, GA: Southern Regional Education Board.

Discover Nursing. (2002). *The campaign for nursing's future.* Johnson & Johnson HealthCare Systems Inc. Retrieved April 26, 2004, from http://www.discovernursing.com.

Furino, A., Gott, S., & Miller, D. R. (eds.) (2000). *Health and nurses in Texas: The future of nursing: Data for action. A report of the Texas nurse workforce data system.* Austin, TX: Texas Nurses Foundation.

Hansen, B. (2002). Nursing shortage: Are bad working conditions causing deaths? *Congressional Quarterly, Inc. CQ Researcher, 12*(32), 745–768.

Hecker, D. E. (2001). Occupational employment projections to 2010. *Monthly Labor Review, 124*(11), 57–84.

Heinrich, J. (July 2001). *GAO report to health subcommittee on health.* GAO-01-944 Nursing workforce: Emerging nurse shortages due to multiple factors (pp. i–15). Washington, DC: United States General Accounting Office.

Heinz, D. (2004). Hospital nurse staffing and patient outcomes. *Dimensions of Critical Care Nursing, 23*(1), 44–51.

HSM Group, Ltd. (2002). Acute care hospital survey of RN vacancy and turnover rates in 2000. *Journal of Nursing Administration, 32*(9), 437–439.

Huston, C. (2003). Quality health care in an era of diminished resources: Challenges and opportunities. *Journal of Nursing Care Quality, 18*(4), 295–301.

Johnson, J. (2000). The nursing shortage: A difficult conversation. *Journal of Nursing Administration, 30*(9), 401–402.

Joint Commission on Accreditation of Healthcare Organizations. (August 2002). *Healthcare at the crossroads: Strategies for addressing the evolving nursing crisis.* Retrieved 10/30/04 from http://www.bidshift.com/pdf/jhaco_crossroads.pdf

Kimball, B. & O'Neil, E. (2002). *Health care's human crisis: The American nursing shortage.* Alameda, CA: Health Workforce Solutions.

Lindsay, C. (July 10, 2002). A shot in the arm. *Nurseweek.com.* Retrieved April 26, 2004, from http://www.nurseweek.com/news/features/02-07/campaign.asp.

Manion, J. (2002). Emergence of the free agent nurse workforce. *Nursing Administration Quarterly, 26*(5), 68–78.

Marquis, B. & Huston, C. (2006). *Leadership roles and management functions in nursing* (5th ed.). Philadelphia: Lippincott Williams & Wilkins.

Mayer, G. G. (2001). Families as hospital care givers. A self-service approach to the nursing shortage. *Journal of Nursing Administration, 31*(10), 457–458.

McPeck, P. (2004). Can we fix it? *Nurseweek, 17*(5), 17–19.

Mee, C. L. & Robinson, E. (2003). What's different about this nursing shortage? *Nursing 2003, 33*(1), 51–55.

Merriam Webster's Online Dictionary. (n.d.). *Supply.* Retrieved May 18, 2004, from http://www.m-w.com/cgi-bin/dictionary.

Nash, M. G. (2001). Reactions to families as caregivers. *Journal of Nursing Administration, 31*(10), 458–459.

National Conference of State Legislators. (2001). *State health priorities survey.* Washington, DC: Author.

National Council of State Boards of Nursing (NCSBN). (December 11, 2003). *The NCLEX-RN examination passing standard revised for public safety.* Retrieved April 27, 2004, from http://www.ncsbn.org/news/pressreleases_newsnews_press_2003NCLEXPassingStandard.asp.

National Council of State Boards of Nursing (NCSBN). (2004). *Nursing regulation. Education Issues. Education Issue I. Driving the nursing shortage.* Retrieved April 20, 2004, from http://www.ncsbn.org/regulation/nursingeducation_nursing_education_issues1.asp.

Nevidjon, B. & Erickson, J. I. (2001). The nursing shortage: Solutions for the short and long term. *Online Journal of Issues in Nursing, 6*(1). Retrieved March 16, 2004, from http://www.nursingworld.org/ojin/topic14/tpc14_4.htm.

New York State Education Department, Office of the Professions. (April 2001). *The nursing shortage.* Retrieved September 23, 2004, from http://www.op.nysed.gov/nurseshortage.htm.

Nurses for a Healthier Tomorrow. (n.d.). *Nurse educator.* Retrieved April 20, 2004, from http://www.nursesource.org/nurse_educator.html.

Nurses for a Healthier Tomorrow. (n.d.). *Nursing faculty shortage facts and factors.* Retrieved April 20, 2004, from http://www.nursesource.org/04FacultyShortage

$1 billion needed to address U.S. shortage of nurses. (December 2003/January 2004). *Australian Nursing Journal, 11*(6), 21.

Perlman, E. (May 2004). Brother, can you spare an RN? *Governing Magazine. DBA Congressional Quarterly, Inc.* Retrieved May 16, 2004, from http://www.haverstickconsulting.com/pages/%2D1398%2D/.

Rambur, B., Palumbo, M. V., McIntosh, B., & Mongeon, J. (2003). A statewide analysis of RN's intention to leave their position. *Nursing Outlook, 51*(4), 182–188.

Robert Wood Johnson Foundation. (2003). *The American nursing shortage.* Retrieved April 20, 2004, from http://www.rwjf.org/news/special/nursing.jhtml.

Rovin, S. & Formella, N. (2004). Creating a desirable future for nursing. *Journal of Nursing Administration, 34*(4), 163–166.

Sigma Theta Tau International. (2004). *Facts on the nursing shortage in North America.* Retrieved April 26, 2004, from http://www.nursingsociety.org/media/facts_nursingshortage.html.

Sochalski, J. (2001). Quality of care, nurse staffing, and patient outcomes. *Journal of Policy and Politics, 2*(1), 9–18.

Staiger, D. O., Auerbach, D. I., & Buerhaus, P. I. (2000). Expanding career opportunities for women and the declining interest in nursing as a career. *Nursing Economics, 18*(5), 230–236.

State of California, Department of Consumer Affairs, Board of Registered Nursing (BRN). (1999). Unpublished license data.

Steltzer, T. M., Woods, A., & Gasda, K. A. (2003). Salary survey 2003. *Nursing Management, 34*(7), 28–32.

Strachota, E., Normandin, P., O'Brien, N., et al. (2003). Reasons registered nurses leave or change employment status. *Journal of Nursing Administration, 33*(2), 111–117.

Tone, B. (2002). *Re-entry into nursing: Programs woo former nurses.* Nursezone.com. Retrieved May 20, 2004, from http://www.nursezone.com/stories/SpotlightOnNurses.asp?articleID=9782&page=Feature+Stories&profile=Spotlight+on+nurses&headline=Re%2Dentry+into+Nursing%3A+Programs+Woo+Former+Nurses.

Tri-Council for Nursing. (2003). *Policy statement. Strategies to reverse the new nursing shortage.* Retrieved April 27, 2004, from http://nursing.about.com/gi/dynamic/offsite.htm?site=http%3A%2F%2Fwww.nln.org%2Faboutnln%2Fnews_tricouncil2.htm.

Tumolo, J. & Rollett, J. (2003). Gliding higher—NP salaries ascend at a higher pace. *ADVANCE for Nurse Practitioners.* Retrieved April 20, 2004, from http://www.advancefornp.com/common/editorial/editorial.aspx?CC=27756.

2002 SREB Survey highlights. Retrieved May 18, 2004 from http://www.sreb.org/main/Publications/LatestReports/LatestReportsindex.asp

Upenieks, V. (2003). Recruitment and retention strategies: A magnet hospital prevention program. *Nursing Economics, 21*(1), 7–13, 23.

U.S. Department of Health and Human Services Bureau of Health Professions, Division of Nursing. (February 2001). The registered nurse population. National sample survey of registered nurses. *NurseWeek.* Retrieved April 18, 2004, from http://www.nurseweek.com/nursingshortage/rnsurvey.asp.

U.S. Department of Health and Human Services. Health Resources and Services Administration (USDHHS-HRSA). (February 14, 2001). *HRSA national survey cites slowdown in number of registered nurses entering profession.* HRSA News. Retrieved April 28, 2004, from http://newsroom.hrsa.gov/releases/2001%20Releases/nursesurvey.htm.

U.S. Department of Health and Human Services. Health Resources and Services Administration (USDHHS-HRSA). (July 2002). *Projected supply, demand and shortages of registered nurses, 2000–2020.* Retrieved May 18, 2004, from http://bhpr.hrsa.gov/healthworkforce/reports/rnproject/report.htm.

U.S. General Accounting Office (GAO) to the Chairman, Subcommittee on Health, Committee on Ways and Means, House of Representatives. (July 2001). *Nursing workforce: Emerging nurse shortages due to multiple factors.* GAO-01-944. Washington, DC: Author.

VRP Recruitment and Staffing Services. (2003). *Nursing shortage fact sheet.* Retrieved April 26, 2004, from http://www.openmix.com/guideARTICLE2.html.

Wakefield, M. K. (2001). Hard numbers, hard choices: Seeking solutions to the nursing shortage. *Nursing Economics, 19*(2), 80–82.

Williams, B.G. & Hodges, L.C. (2002). SREB Study Indicates Serious Shortage of Nursing Faculty. Retrieved November 1, 2004 from http://www.sreb.org/programs/nursing/publications/02N03-Nursing_Faculty.pdf.

Williams, S. (2001). Common cause: State and federal measures to address shortage find bipartisan support. *NurseWeek, 14*(15), 10–11.

BIBLIOGRAPHY

Advisory Board Company. (2000). *Enfranchising nursing in cost reform.* Washington DC: Author.

An influx of nurses won't solve shortage: Biggest group is older than 50, report says. (2004). *Hospital Employee Health, 23*(2), 23–24.

Anderson, C. A. (2002). A reservoir of talent waiting to be tapped. *Nursing Outlook, 50*(1), 1–2.

Atencio, B. L., Cohen, J., & Gorenberg, B. (2003). Nurse retention: Is it worth it? *Nursing Economics, 21*(6), 262–268.

Berlin, L. E., Stennett, J., & Bednash, G. D. (2002). *2001–2002 salaries of instructional and administrative nursing faculty in baccalaureate and graduate programs in nursing.* Washington, DC: American Association of Colleges of Nursing.

Berlin, L. E., Stennett, J., & Bednash, G. D. (2003a). *2002–2003 enrollment and graduations in baccalaureate and graduate programs in nursing.* Washington, DC: American Association of Colleges of Nursing.

Berlin, L. E., Stennett, J., & Bednash, G. D. (2003b). *2002–2003 salaries of instructional and administrative nursing faculty in baccalaureate and graduate programs in nursing.* Washington, DC: American Association of Colleges of Nursing.

Billings, D. M. (2003). What does it take to be a nurse educator? *Journal of Nursing Education, 42*(3), 99–100.

Bleich, M. R. & Hewlett, P. O. (May 31, 2004). Dissipating the "perfect storm"– Responses from nursing and the health care industry to protect the public's health. *Online Journal of Issues in Nursing, 9*(2). Retrieved June 20, 2004, from www.nursingworld.org/ojin/topic24/tpc24_4.htm.

Bleich, M. R., Hewlett, P. O., Santos, S. R., et al. (2003). Analysis of the nursing workforce crisis: A call to action. *American Journal of Nursing, 103*(4), 66–74.

Boyce, V. J. (2002). Nursing shortage. Everything old is new again. *Policy, Politics, & Nursing Practice, 3*(2), 177–181.

Brewer, C. & Tassone Kovner, C. (2001). Is there another nursing shortage? What the data tell us. *Nursing Outlook, 49*(1), 20–26.

Cline, D., Reilly, C., & Moore, J. F. (2003). What's behind RN turnover? *Nursing Management, 34*(10), 50–53.

Cooksey, J. A., McLaughlin, W., Russinof, H., et al. (2004). Active state-level engagement with the nursing shortage: A study of five Midwestern states. *Policy, Politics & Nursing Practice, 5*(2), 102–112.

Cooper, E. E. (2003). Pieces of the shortage puzzle: Aging and shift work. *Nursing Economics, 21*(2), 75–79.

DeMarco, R. F., Horowitz, J. A., & McLeod, D. (2000). A call to intraprofessional alliances. *Nursing Outlook, 48*(4), 172–178.

Erickson, J. I., Holm, L. J., & Chelminiak, L. (2004). Keeping the nursing shortage from becoming a nursing crisis. *Journal of Nursing Administration, 34*(2), 83–87.

Greipp, M. E. (2003). Salary compression. Its effect on nurse recruitment and retention. *Journal of Nursing Administration, 33*(6), 321–330.

Hinshaw, A. S. (2001). A continuing challenge: The shortage of educationally prepared nursing faculty. *Online Journal of Issues in Nursing, 6*(1). Retrieved September 23, 2004, from http://www.nursingworld.org/ojin/topic14/tpc14_3.htm.

Johnson, J. (2000). The nursing shortage. A difficult conversation. *Journal of Nursing Administration, 30*(9), 401–402.

Kalisch, B. J. (2003). Recruiting nurses. The problem is the process. *Journal of Nursing Administration, 33*(9), 468–477.

Kerfoot, K. (2000). The leader as a retention specialist. *Nursing Economics, 18*(4), 216–218.

Kubar, P. A., Miller, D., & Spear, B. T. (2004). The meaningful retention strategy inventory. *Journal of Nursing Administration, 34*(1), 10–18.

Murray, M. K. (2002). The nursing shortage. Past, present and future. *Journal of Nursing Administration, 32*(2), 79–84.

Needleman, J. & Buerhaus, P. (2001). *Nurse staffing and patient outcomes in hospitals.* Final report, U.S. Department of Health and Human Services, Health Resources and Services Administration Contract. Available http://www.unac-ca.org/pdf/Nurse_Staffing_complete.pdf.

Pinkerton, S. E. (2002). A system approach to retention and recruitment. *Nursing Economics, 20*(6), 296, 299.

Purnell, M. J., Horner, D., Gonzalez, J., & Westman, N. (2001). The nursing shortage. Revisioning the future. *Journal of Nursing Administration, 31*(4), 179–186.

Roark, D. C. (2001). Against the odds: Defining and overcoming the nursing shortage. *Nursing 2001 Career Directory*, 14.

Wagner, C. M. & Huber, D. (2003). Catastrophe and nursing turnover. *Journal of Nursing Administration, 33*(9), 486–492.

White, K. M. (2002). Health care's human crisis: The American nursing shortage. *Policy, Politics & Nursing Practice, 3*(4), 309–312.

Wittmann-Price, R. & Kuplen, C. (2003). A recruitment and retention program that works. *Nursing Economics, 21*(1), 35–38.

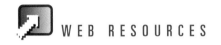

WEB RESOURCES

AACN–Media Relations Nursing Shortage Fact Sheet.	**http://www.aacn.nche.edu/Media/ Backgrounders/shortagefacts.htm**
American Association of Colleges of Nursing	**http://www.aacn.nche.edu**
American Hospital Association	**http://www.aha.org**
American Nurses Association	**http://www.ana.org**
Bureau of Labor Statistics	**http://www.bls.gov/**
Discover Nursing campaign. Johnson & Johnson Healthcare Systems, Inc.	**http://www.discovernursing.com**
Fagin, C. (February 2001). *When Care Becomes a Burden. Diminishing Access to Adequate Nursing.* Milbank Memorial Fund.	**http://www.milbank.org/010216fagin.html**
National Council of State Boards of Nursing	**http://www.ncsbn.org**
National League for Nursing	**http://www.nln.org**
National Student Nurses Association	**http://www.nsna.org**
Nevidjon, B.& Erickson, J. (2001). The Nursing Shortage: Solutions for the Short and Long Term. *Online Journal of Issues in Nursing*, 6(1).	**http://www.nursingworld.org/ojin/ topic14/tpc14_4.htm**
Nurse.com	**http://nurse.com/NurseContent/**
Nurses for a Healthier Tomorrow. *Facts About the Nursing Shortage.* (Sigma Theta Tau International, 2001)	**http://www.nursesource.org/ facts_shortage.html**
Nurses for a Healthier Tomorrow. Nurse Educator Recruitment Campaign.	**http://www.nursesource.org/ campaign_news.html**
Office of the Professions. New York State Education Department. (2001). *The Nursing Shortage*	**http://www.op.nysed.gov/ nurseshortage.htm**

Importing Foreign Nurses

Carol J. Huston

M
any countries have had cyclical shortages of nurses, but they were usually caused by increasing demand outstripping a static or slowly growing supply of nurses (Buchan, 2001b, p. 203). Currently, the situation is more serious. Demand continues to grow while supply decreases as a result of an aging workforce, a projected dramatic increase in nursing retirements in the coming decade, and a smaller pool of individuals entering nursing, particularly young women, who have chosen formerly male-dominated professions such as medicine, law, and business instead of nursing. Indeed, the majority of member states of the World Health Organization, including Australia, Canada, the United States, France, Germany, Ireland, and the United Kingdom, report shortages, maldistribution, and the inappropriate utilization of nurses (Kingma, 2001; Kline, 2003).

One increasingly common means of alleviating current nursing shortages has been to recruit foreign nurses. International recruitment and *nurse migration*—moving from one country to another in search of employment—has been viewed as a relatively cheap, "quick fix" solution to rapidly increasing shortages.

In the past, nurse migration was mostly opportunistic or based on individual motivation and contacts (Buchan, 2001b). "What is occurring now is the active planning of international recruitment on a large scale – an employer or agency targets one country, aiming to recruit 20, 50, or 100 nurses at a time and developed countries are jumping on the merry-go-round and trying to recruit nurses from each other, but some are also targeting developing countries" (Buchan, p. 203). In addition, developing countries are recruiting from each other, even within the same geographic region (e.g., Caribbean nations and South Africa) (International Council of Nurses [ICN], 2002). Table 6.1 summarizes the current dynamic nature of nurse migration in select countries around the world.

▶ GLOBAL MIGRATION OF NURSES: "PUSH" AND "PULL" FACTORS

To understand what is driving the global migration of nurses, it is first necessary to examine what are known as the "push" and "pull" factors of nursing migration. *Push factors* are those things that push or drive nurses to want to leave their countries to go to another. *Pull factors* are those things that draw the nurse toward a different country. Low pay, poor career structures, lack of educational opportunities, the continued devaluation of nursing because it is "women's work," and violence at the workplace or in wider society are common push factors for nurses (Buchan, 2001b).

Pull factors typically include higher pay, better career structures, more opportunities for further education, and in some cases, safety from the threat of violence (more prevalent in less developed countries). In addition, shared language, common educational curriculum, and postcolonial ties between countries influence which developing countries are targeted as sources of nurses (Buchan, 2001b).

Similarly, Kingma (2001) suggests that the three primary driving forces or pull factors for nurse migration are the search for professional development, better quality of life, and personal safety. Pay and learning opportunities are the most frequently reported incentives for nursing migration. Career opportunities are considered key incentives for nurses emigrating from high income countries.

TABLE 6.1 Impact of Push–Pull Migration on Select Countries

Australia	Has called for a national workforce plan. Primarily recruits from the United Kingdom and New Zealand.
China	Has second largest nursing workforce in the world (surpassed only by the United States). Currently has oversupply of nurses, especially from secondary nursing schools. Actively seeking to prepare nurses for CGFNS certification in hopes of exportation to the United States (Xu, 2003).
Canada	Lost a significant number of nurses to the United States during health care cutbacks levied by the Canadian government during the 1990s (Bryant, 2001). Now doing foreign recruiting themselves and lobbying for a loosening of nurse migration restrictions (Bryant, 2001).
Ireland	As little as 20 years ago, Ireland was inviting U.S. hospitals over, setting up job fairs for their abundant pool of nurses (Bryant, 2001). Now they are competing for business and recruiting nurses primarily from South Africa, the Philippines, the United Kingdom, Australia, and India (Buchan et al., 2003). Thus, Ireland has moved from being a traditional "exporter" of nurses to an importer. In 1990, three-fourths of new nurses on the Irish nursing register were "home grown"; in the first 6 months of 2000, more than half the additions were from nonIrish sources (Buchan, 2001b). Many of these nurses came from the United Kingdom—a reverse migration.
Norway	The main inflow of nurses has been from other Scandinavian countries. There has been some additional recent recruitment from the Philippines and Poland, but all recruitment is controlled by a state recruitment agency, with a cap on numbers (Buchan et al., 2003).
The Philippines	Since the late 1960s, the Philippines has been the world's leading exporter of nurses and has also sent more professional immigrants to the United States than any other country in the world (University of Minnesota, n.d.). This is actively endorsed by the Philippine government because these nurses send money home on a regular basis, thereby contributing to the homeland economy (Gamble, 2002).
South Africa	Buckling under a massive HIV/AIDS epidemic, South Africa is desperate to retain nurses and doctors that are easily seduced by the promise of better pay and better living and working conditions (Bryant, 2001). Currently recruiting nurses from Jamaica and the Caribbean, the South African government proposed to the Commonwealth (an association of 53 countries, representing 1.8 billion people, e.g., New Zealanders, South Africans, Zambians, Kenyans, Canadians, Australians and more; see *http://www.thecommonwealth.org/Templates/Internal.asp?NodeID=20596*) that recruitment of health professionals from developing countries take place only within formal bilateral agreements between richer and poorer nations (Kline, 2003).
Saudi Arabia	Now gets most of its nurses from the Philippines—the very same place where most countries, including the United States, are doing the majority of their recruiting (Bryant, 2001).
United Kingdom	In 1999/2000, internationally recruited nurses accounted for one in three new admissions to the U.K. nursing professional register (Buchan, 2001b). In 2001/2002, approximately 40% of the "new" nurses on the U.K. nursing register came from nonU.K. sources (Buchan, 2001b). The three most important source countries were South Africa, Australia, and the Philippines (Buchan, 2001b). The Department of Health in the United Kingdom has established practice guidelines in international recruitment for National Health service employers (Kline, 2003).
United States	Recruiting heavily from the Philippines, Canada, and South Africa. Proposed the Rural and Urban Health Care Act of 2001 to expand the existing H-1C visas to ease the immigration of foreign nurses, although this has been resisted by the American Nurses Association (Kline, 2003).

TABLE 6.2   Push and Pull Factors for Nurse Migration

Push Factors	Pull Factors
Low pay (absolute and/or relative)	Higher pay (and opportunities for remittances)
Poor working conditions	Better working conditions
Lack of resources to work effectively	Better resourced health systems
Limited career opportunities	Career opportunities
Limited educational opportunities	Provision of postbasic education
Impact of human immunodeficiency virus and acquired immunodeficiency disease	Political stability
Unstable/dangerous work environment	Travel opportunities
Economic instability	Aid work

Source: Buchan, J., Parkin, T., & Sochalski, J. (2003). *International nurse mobility: Trends and policy implications.* Retrieved February 10, 2004, from *http://www.icn.ch/Int_Nurse_mobility%20final.pdf.*

> *CONSIDER: Nurse migration is often a symptom of deep-seated problems in a country's nursing labor markets relating to long-term relative underinvestment in the profession and its career structure (Buchan, 2001b).

"To an extent, there is a 'mirror image' of push and pull, related to the relative level of pay, career prospects, working conditions and environment available in the source country and in the destination country. Where the relative gap (or perceived gap) is significant, then the 'pull' of the destination country will be felt" (Buchan, Parkin, & Sochalski, 2003 para 11). However, other factors that act as push factors in some countries include the impact of human immunodeficiency virus and acquired immunodeficiency disease on health system workers; concerns about personal security in areas of conflict; and economic instability. Other pull factors, such as the opportunity to travel or to participate in foreign aid work, also influence some nurses (Buchan et al., 2003).

It is important to remember that developed countries, such as Australia, the United Kingdom, and the United States, are the primary destinations of most migrant nurses (Kline, 2003). These destination countries are able to recruit nurses as a result of a large number of pull factors. Many internationally recruited nurses report they would have preferred to remain in their home country, with family and friends, in a familiar culture and environment (ICN, 2002), but that push and pull factors were overwhelming in their decision to migrate. A summary of push and pull factors for nurse migration are shown in Table 6.2. In addition, Box 6.1 displays the findings from Buchan and colleagues's (2003) study of push and pull factors leading to nurse migration in nine countries.

▶ THE IMPACT OF GLOBAL MIGRATION ON DEVELOPING COUNTRIES

A review of the literature suggests that different countries have experienced different impacts as a result of the push–pull of international nurse migration. Some national governments and government agencies have encouraged the outflow of nurses from their country. For example, for many years, "the Philippines government has endorsed and facilitated initiatives aimed at educating, recruiting, training, and placing its Filipino

BOX 6.1

Research Study Fuels the Controversy

Why Do Nurses Emigrate?

This study draws upon case studies from Australia, the Caribbean, Ghana, Ireland, Norway, the Philippines, South Africa, the United Kingdom, and the United States and examines factors that lead to nurse migration, both from developing to developed countries and between developed countries.

Buchan, J., Parkin, T., & Sochalski, J. (2003). International nurse mobility: Trends and policy implications. Retrieved February 10, 2004, from http://www.icn.ch/Int_Nurse_mobility%20final.pdf

Study Findings

This study suggests that although a number of factors stimulated the mobility of nurses, the fundamental problems that stimulated the nurses' desire to work in another country—such as poor pay, excessive workloads, and violence in the workplace— have not been adequately addressed. As a result, developed countries with nursing shortages have been able to turn to a "quick fix" of international recruitment by offering better salaries, career opportunities, professional development, and improved conditions of employment.

The authors conclude that it is inadequate policy responses by governments to the fundamental causes of nursing shortages that have been driving the dynamics of aggressive and sometimes exploitive international recruitment. They argue that recruiting nurses into a dysfunctional health system is at best a short-term solution, with ethical implications.

Three options were identified for national and international governments to change these dynamics.

- Support for improvements in pay, working conditions, and the prestige of nurses in their own countries.
- Encouragement and bilateral facilitation of "country-to-country" managed or regulated flows of nurses.
- Exploration of the feasibility and implementation of a plan to flow compensation from the recruiting country back to the source country. This compensation could be directly or indirectly monetary, as part of a donor package, or it could be in the form of a return flow of better-trained staff.

---

expatriates in jobs all over the world" (Gamble, 2002, p. 176). This is likely the result of a financial imperative, to encourage the generation of remittance income, or a response to labor market oversupply. Or it may be an attempt to develop a long-term improvement in the skills base of the nursing workforce by encouraging short-term outflow to other countries where training is available (Buchan et al., 2003).

The reality is that in countries like the Philippines, "becoming a nurse is often marketed as a path to success in a western country and a way to send money home to support the family" (Shepard, 2003). More than 5 million Filipinos work overseas, for example, and send home more than $6 billion a year, 60% of it from the United States and Canada. Remittances are the country's single largest source of foreign trade (Shepard, 2003).

China, another country that continues to report a significant surplus of nurses, especially those prepared at the secondary school level, is also actively seeking to export nurses (Xu, 2003). Yet recent reports from South Africa, Ghana, the Caribbean, and even the Philippines highlight that the outflow of nurses has had several major negative impacts linked to the effect on remaining staff, to reductions in the level and quality of services, and to loss of specialist skills (Buchan et al., 2003).

One of the most commonly cited impacts associated with global migration today, particularly from developing countries, is the "brain drain" of nursing resources. Brain drain refers to the loss of skilled personnel and the loss of investment in education (Kline, 2003) that is experienced when those human resources migrate elsewhere. Xu (2003) defines it as the migration of professionals and technical personnel to other countries, resulting in perceived loss of real or potential human capital to their homelands.

In some cases, aggressive recruitment, by which large numbers of recruits are sought, may significantly deplete a single health facility or contract an important number of newly graduated nurses from a single educational institute. This has significant local and regional implications (ICN, 2002). Complaints of brain drain are increasingly heard from donor countries such as India, the Philippines, South Africa, and Zimbabwe. These nations argue that their human health care resources are being extracted at a time when they are most needed (Record Overseas Numbers, 2002). In addition, many of the countries that are exporting nurses are also experiencing a nursing shortage.

* **CONSIDER:** The majority of countries importing foreign nurses are primarily white and donor nations are typically exporting nurses of color. The issue of race and the global economics of nursing should be examined in terms of impact on both supplier and donor countries.

Kingma (2001) suggests that the negative effects of international migration on "supplier" countries are beginning to be recognized, but that they have not been effectively addressed. The problems caused for some developing countries by nurse migration are severe. "They are losing scarce, and relatively expensive-to-train resources. Levels and quality of care in their countries are suffering. In addition, many of the nurse recruits are relatively young, and these countries may be losing out on future leaders in the profession" (Buchan, 2001b, p. 204).

* **CONSIDER:** The positive global economic/social/professional development resulting from international migration needs to be weighed against a substantial brain and skills drain experienced by supplier countries (Kingma, 2001).

Brain drain is not just occurring in nursing. Despite Europe's efforts to stop its scientific brain drain, more and more of the continent's brightest young researchers are choosing to pursue careers abroad. In a study released by the European Commission, 75% of European graduate students studying in the United States said they would prefer to stay after finishing their doctoral work because they feel the United States offers better career and employment opportunities for scientists (Bosch, 2003). The majority of an estimated 400,000 European researchers now working in the United States—the equivalent of 4% of Europe's total pool of research and development resources—will end up staying (Bosch, 2003).

Just because the brain drain that occurs in nursing resources also occurs in other disciplines does not make it acceptable. It does, however, suggest that the individual's right to choose cannot be easily negated simply because the donor country does not want to lose its intellectual resources.

Finally, one must consider whether recruiting foreign nurses to solve acute staffing shortages is simply a poorly thought out, quick fix to a much greater problem, and whether in doing so, not only are donor nations harmed, but the issues that led to the shortage in the first place are never addressed. Certainly, one must at least question whether wholesale foreign nurse recruitment would even be necessary if importer nations made a more concerted effort to improve the working conditions, salaries, empowerment, and recognition of the native nurses they already employ. Indeed, one must question whether importation occurs in an effort to avoid the costs of doing so.

> ***CONSIDER:** Importing foreign nurses to solve America's nursing shortage only puts a Band-Aid on the problem. The factors that led to the nursing shortage in the first place still need to be resolved.

Controversy regarding the ethics of international recruitment of nurses is not new. In 1948, the ICN wrote to the Chief Nurse in England complaining that English employers were "poaching" nurses from Sweden and the Netherlands to help combat a postwar nursing shortage (Buchan, 2001a, 2001b).

Whenever resources are limited, ethical issues regarding their allocation are likely to arise. In the case of global nurse recruitment and migration, the ethical principles of autonomy, utility, and justice seem most relevant. Certainly, there must be some sort of a balance between the right of individual nurses to choose to migrate (autonomy), particularly when push factors are overwhelming, and the more utilitarian concern for the donor nations' health as a result of losing scarce nursing resources.

Discussion Point

Should the right for the individual nurse to migrate (autonomy) override what is best for the donor nation (utilitarianism)?

Justice, or fairness, is another ethical principle that seems appropriate to this discussion because it examines how social and material goods are distributed to or withheld from members of a group or society (Haddad, 2002). Does global recruitment violate the principle of justice, particularly if a shortage is not being solved, and is merely being shunted to a country less well equipped to deal with the shortage (Kingma, 2001)?

Buchan (2001b) argues that importer countries have an obligation first to ensure that their own houses are in order, investing in attractive career structures and improving retention and the return of their own nurses. He also argues that importer countries need to incorporate an ethical dimension to international recruitment activity, by identifying which developing countries can least afford to lose nurses and by steering recruiters away from these countries.

Buchan argues further that there is a clear need for international agencies to better monitor the international flows of nurses, to highlight where problems are occurring and to identify which importer countries are being aggressive and unethical in their recruitment activities. "In an era of globalization, with free mobility of labour, no country can anticipate being totally self-sufficient in its nursing resources. But those developed countries that have the resources should work harder to be self-reliant" (Buchan, 2001b, p. 204).

International Council of Nurses' Position on Recruitment and Importation

One international agency, the ICN, has issued a position statement arguing for ethics and good employment practices in international recruitment (Box 6.2). The ICN, a federation of more than 124 national nurses' associations, represents millions of nurses worldwide (ICN, 2002). The ICN position statement confirms the right of nurses to migrate, as well as the potential beneficial outcomes of multicultural practice and learning opportunities supported by migration, but acknowledges potential adverse impacts on the quality of health care in donor countries.

BOX 6.2

ICN Position Statement on Nurse Retention, Transfer and Migration (1999)

ICN and its member associations firmly believe that quality health care is directly dependent on an adequate supply of qualified nursing personnel.

ICN recognizes the right of individual nurses to migrate, while acknowledging the possible adverse effect that international migration may have on health care quality.

ICN condemns the practice of recruiting nurses to countries where authorities have failed to address human resource planning and problems that cause nurses to leave the profession and discourage them from returning to nursing.

In support of the above ICN :

- Disseminates information on nursing personnel needs and resources and on the development of fulfilling nursing career structures.
- Provides training opportunities in negotiation and socioeconomic welfare-related issues.
- Disseminates data on nursing employment worldwide.
- Takes action to help reduce the serious effects of any shortage, maldistribution and misutilization of nursing personnel.
- Advocates adherence nationally to international labor standards.
- Condemns the recruitment of nurses as a strike-breaking mechanism.
- Advocates for open and transparent migration systems (recognizing that some appropriate screening is necessary to ensure public safety).
- Supports a transcultural approach to nursing practice.
- Promotes the introduction of transferable benefits, e.g., pension.

National nurses' associations are urged to:

- Encourage relevant authorities to ensure sound human resources planning for nursing.

- Participate in the development of sound national policies on immigration and emigration of nurses.
- Promote the revision of nursing curriculum for basic and postbasic education in nursing and administration to emphasize effective nursing leadership.
- Disseminate information on the working conditions of nurses.
- Discourage nurses from working in other countries where salaries and conditions are not acceptable to nurses and professional associations in those countries.
- Ensure that foreign nurses have conditions of employment equal to those of local nurses in posts requiring the same level of competency, and involving the same duties and responsibilities.
- Ensure that there are no distinctions made among foreign nurses from different countries.
- Monitor the activities of recruiting agencies.
- Provide an advisory service to help nurses interpret contracts and assist foreign nurses with personal and work-related problems, such as institutional racism, violence, sexual harassment.
- Provide orientation for foreign nurses on the local cultural, social and political values and on the health system and national language.
- Alert nurses to the fact that some diplomas, qualifications or degrees earned in one country may not be recognized in another.
- Assist nurses with their problems related to international migration and repatriation.

The ICN also condemns the practice of recruiting nurses to countries where authorities have failed to implement sound human resource planning and to seriously address problems that cause nurses to leave the profession and discourage them from returning to nursing. The position statement also denounces unethical recruitment practices that exploit nurses or mislead them into accepting job responsibilities and working conditions that are incompatible with their qualifications, skills, and experience. The ICN and its member national nurses' associations call for a regulated recruitment process, based on ethical principles that guide informed decision making and reinforce sound employment policies on the part of governments, employers, and nurses, thereby supporting fair and cost-effective recruitment and retention practices.

Mistreatment of Foreign Nurses

Shepard (2003) states it can cost a U.S. hospital $10,000 to find and bring in a foreign nurse. Despite the cost and the additional investment of time and energy that goes into recruiting foreign nurses, some of these hospitals reportedly treat the imported nurses poorly, once they arrive. These nurses may receive substandard jobs or wages or be subjected to illegal practices by their employers. Such was the case in 2001, when the media reported the poor treatment of Indian and Filipino nurses recruited to United Kingdom private sector nursing homes (Buchan, 2001b). This occurred despite good practice guidelines being issued to all National Health Service employers in 1999 by the Department of Health.

Similarly, Tabone (2000) reported that Filipino nurses were actively recruited for work in the United States (Texas) in 2000, but were offered wages significantly below the prevailing wage rate in Texas ($13.85 per hour for a nurse with 4 years of experience including cardiology and emergency department experience). These nurses were locked into the low wages for years. Prevailing domestic wages for a nurse with that experience, according to the Texas Workforce Commission and the U.S. Department of Labor, was around $19 per hour. The Texas Nurses Association sent a formal complaint to the Immigration and Naturalization Service (INS) and requested that INS investigate the situation, since it was likely happening in other states as well.

> *CONSIDER: Due to the lack of regulatory oversight of global nurse migration contracting, foreign nurses are at increased risk for employment under false pretenses and may be misled as to the conditions of work, remuneration, and benefits.

There are also reports that overzealous recruiters have made false promises to foreign nurses regarding job opportunities and wages, charged exorbitant migration fees to bring the nurses to the new country, and virtually forced the now migrated registered nurse (RN) to work long hours in substandard working conditions. Part of the reason for this is that private for-profit agencies have increasingly become involved in the search for nursing personnel and there is generally no designated body that regulates or monitors the content of contracts offered. Internationally recruited nurses may be particularly at risk of exploitation or abuse due to the difficulty of verifying the terms of employment as a result of distance, language barriers, cost, and naiveté.

Discussion Point

Should there be regulatory oversight of foreign nurse recruitment?

Haddad (2002) also voices her concern that foreign nurses may not receive the respect they deserve in the workplace as a result of negative bias by their peers, who regard them as outsiders. Socializing foreign nurses, which is addressed later in this chapter, appears to be an ethical imperative as well as a management issue.

▶ THE INTERNATIONAL COMMUNITY ADDRESSES THE PROBLEM

The nursing shortage and resulting global migration issues have led several national governments to intervene, and as a result, some countries have made progress in tackling the ethical issues associated with global recruitment and migration of nurses. It is likely only through cooperation at organizational and governmental levels that a win-win solution to nurse migration will be found (Buchan 2001b).

Some Governments Respond

Within the last few years, England, Ireland, and Canada have published national nursing strategies for dealing with staff shortages (Buchan, 2001a). Like professional nursing organizations in the United States, Norway has issued a policy statement on the ethics of international recruitment. The Netherlands, Ireland, and the Scandinavian countries also have good practice guidelines on international recruitment, or are looking at developing guidelines. Some countries have initiated or examined various policy responses to reduce outflow–such as "bonding" nurses to home employment for a specified time after completion of training or negotiating a compensation fee, from either the emigrating nurses or the importing country (Buchan et al., 2003). "This may not be effective if compliance is not monitored or if there is scope to 'buy out' of the bond. The scope for compensation claims continues to be raised in international fora [forums], but there is little evidence that such schemes have been effective in the past" (Buchan et al., p. 3).

Another response has been to recognize that outflow cannot be halted if principles of individual freedom are to be upheld, but the outflow that does occur must be managed and moderated. The "managed migration" initiative being undertaken in the Caribbean is one example of a coordinated intervention to minimize the negative impacts of outflow while realizing at least some benefit from the process (Buchan et al., 2003).

The Department of Health in England funded advertising campaigns to attract recruits and "returners'" to nursing. It also admitted more nursing students to nursing programs, supported an increase in pay for newly qualified nurses, and made a concerted effort to make working lives in the National Health Service more attractive and rewarding (Buchan, 2001a). Although this campaign is having a positive effect on nursing numbers, the National Health Service Plan in England makes it explicit that England will continue to be an active recruiter in international nursing labor markets. In addition, Spain and England have created a formal agreement for Spanish nurses to work in the National Health Service in England for defined periods, which may lay a groundwork for other countries to follow (Buchan, 2001b).

Professional Organizations Take A Stand

But it is the ICN that has created the most comprehensive plan for addressing ethical global nurse recruitment and migration. The ICN (2002) has identified 13 principles necessary to create a foundation for ethical recruitment, whether international or intranational contexts are being considered. The ICN suggests that all health sector

BOX 6.3 Principles of Ethical Global Nurse Recruitment and Migration

1. Effective planning and development strategies must be introduced, regularly reviewed, and maintained to ensure a balance between supply and demand of nurse human resources.
2. Nursing legislation must authorize regulatory bodies to determine nurses' standards of education, competencies, and standards of practice and to ensure that only individuals meeting these standards are allowed to practice as a nurse.
3. Because the provision of quality care relies on the availability of nurses to meet staffing demand, nurses in a recruiting region/country and seeking employment should be made aware of job opportunities.
4. Nurses should have the right to migrate if they comply with the recruiting country's immigration/work policies (e.g., work permit) and meet obligations in their home country (e.g., bonding responsibilities, tax payment).
5. Nurses have the right to expect fair treatment (e.g., working conditions, promotion, and continuing education).
6. Nurses and employers are to be protected from false information, withholding relevant information, misleading claims and exploitation (e.g., accurate job descriptions, benefits/allocations/bonuses specified in writing, authentic educational records).
7. There should be no discrimination between occupations/professions with the same level of responsibility, educational qualification, work experience, skill

requirement, and hardship (e.g., pay, grading).
8. When nurses' or employers' contracted or acquired rights or benefits are threatened or violated, suitable machinery must be in place to hear grievances in a timely manner and at reasonable cost.
9. Nurses must be protected from occupational injury and health hazards, including violence (e.g., sexual harassment) and made aware of existing workplace hazards.
10. The provision of quality care in the current highly complex and often stressful health care environment depends on a supportive formal and informal supervisory infrastructure.
11. Employment contracts must specify a trial period when the signing parties are free to express dissatisfaction and cancel the contract with no penalty. In the case of international migration, the responsibility for covering the cost of repatriation needs to be clearly stated.
12. Nurses have the right to affiliate to and be represented by a professional association and/or union to safeguard their rights as health professionals and workers.
13. Recruitment agencies (public and private) should be regulated and effective monitoring mechanisms such as cost-effectiveness, volume, success rate over time, retention rates, equalities criteria, and client satisfaction should be introduced.

Source: Adapted from ICN, 2001.

stakeholders—patients, governments, employers, and nurses—will benefit if this ethical recruitment framework is systematically applied. These principles are shown in Box 6.3. In addition, policy questions and subsidiary research questions related to international nurse recruitment are shown in Box 6.4.

The U.S. Role in Nurse Migration: Issuing Visas

By the end of the year, Tenet Healthcare Corp. hopes to recruit at least 100 registered nurses from Northern Ireland to hospitals in the Southeast through a special visa program passed last year by Congress (cited by Bryant, 2001).

This type of press release is increasingly commonplace, and highlights the role that the U.S. government plays in the nurse migration issue: issuing visas. Xu, Xu, and Zhang (1999) state that under normal circumstances, the Department of Labor is

BOX 6.4

International Nurse Mobility: Questions on Policy and Subsidiary Research

Source Countries

Policy

- Should outflow be supported or encouraged? (to stimulate remittance income or to end oversupply)
- Should outflow be constrained or reduced? (e.g., to reduce "brain drain"; if so, how—what is effective and ethical?)
- Should recruitment agencies be regulated?

Research

- What are the destination countries for outflow?
- How much of outflow is permanent or temporary? (short- or long-term?)
- How much of outflow is going to health sector–related employment/education in other countries; what proportion to non–health-related destinations?
- What is the size of outflow to other countries compared to the outflow to other sectors within the country?
- What is the impact of outflow?
- Why are nurses leaving?
- How should flows be monitored?

Destination Countries

Policy

- Is inflow sustainable?
- Is inflow a cost-effective way of solving skills shortages?
- Is inflow ethically justifiable?
- Should recruitment agencies be regulated?

Research

- What are the source countries for inflow?
- How much of inflow is permanent or temporary?
- How much of inflow is going to health sector–related employment/ education in the country; what proportion to non–health-related destinations?
- Is inflow effectively managed?
- Why are nurses coming?
- How should flows be monitored?

International Agencies

- How should international flows of nurses be monitored?
- In the context of the working relationship with the country's government, what is the appropriate role/response of the agency to the issue of international nurse mobility?
- Should it [international agency] intervene in the process (e.g., developing ethical framework, supporting government-to-government contracts, introducing regulatory compliance)?

Source: Buchan, J., Parkin, T., & Sochalski, J. (2003). *International nurse mobility: Trends and policy implications.* Retrieved February 10, 2004, from *http://www.icn.ch/Int_Nurse_mobility%20final.pdf.* Reprinted with permission.

required by law to certify to the Department of State and the INS when an alien is hired that: 1) no U.S. citizens and permanent residents are available or qualified for a given job, and 2) the employment of an alien will not adversely affect the wages of the concerned profession. This has come to be known as *labor certification* (Xu et al., 1999).

The main purpose of this legal provision has been to protect the domestic labor market; however, the immigration laws have provided preferential provisions for members of certain professions in the national interest of the United States, and created a list of occupations and professions, including nursing, that do not require labor certification. Because nursing has been classified as one of the shortage areas in the U.S. economy, a so-called blanket waiver of the labor certification is in place.

Indeed, since the U.S. Immigration Act of 1965, skilled labor, and in particular, individuals from countries of the Asia-Pacific Triangle, were no longer selectively denied access to immigration (Brush & Berger, 2002). In addition, from 1962 to 1989, foreign nurses were regarded as "professionals" under U.S. immigration laws and could therefore seek an H-1 temporary work visa in the United States. As a result, the influx of nurses from other countries, especially the Philippines, Korea, and Thailand, increased dramatically.

In 1989, the Immigration Nursing Relief Act (INRA) was created as a 5-year pilot program (Xu, 2003). The INRA stipulated that only health care facilities with "attestations" approved by the Department of Health could obtain H-1A occupation visas to employ nurses on a temporary basis. Consequently, other occupations that formerly fell into the H-1 category became part of the new H-1B category (Xu, 2003).

In 1990, Congress passed the Immigration and Nationality Act, which is the legal foundation for current immigration policies. In this act, nursing continued to be listed as a shortage area. In 1999, the Nursing Relief for Disadvantaged Areas Act created H-1C occupational visas, which were perceived largely as an effort to renew the INRA of 1989, but with more restrictions (Xu, 2003). These temporary visas were created for foreign nurse graduates seeking employment in designated U.S. facilities (serving primarily poor patients in inner cities and some rural areas) (Brush & Berger, 2002). The *Federal Register* mandated that the total number of H-1C visas be limited to 500 each year, be valid for years without extension, and be capped at 25 nurses in states with a population of fewer than 9 million and 50 nurses in states with a population over 9 million (Murthy, 2004).

In addition, some foreign nurses applied for work in the United States via the H-1B visa. This nonimmigrant visa status allows recruiting of shortage professionals into jobs that require a 4-year university degree (Tabone, 2000). Of particular interest is the fact that unlike the scientists and computer professionals currently being brought into the United States under H-1B status, registered nurses no longer qualify, because the Fifth Circuit Court ruled in February 2000 that RN hospital jobs do not currently require a bachelor's degree in nursing credential, regardless of recruiter requirements.

Shepard (2003) states that the H-1B status does have a quota limit, but some nurses can apply if they have a specialized skill, particularly in intensive care, management, and specialty nursing areas. Xu (2003) concurs, stating that foreign nurses can get work under the H-1B visa but that U.S. employers must convince immigration officials that specific jobs do meet the H-1B requirement on a case-by-case basis. According to Thibodeau (2003), only 79,100 H-1B visas were issued during the 2001–2002 fiscal year, down sharply from the 163,600 issued in the previous year, and far below the 195,000 cap set by Congress.

Another way nurses get work visas in the United States has been under the immigrant E3 to I-140 status ("greencard" or permanent resident). In this case, RNs can be brought into the country and become permanent residents through petition to the INS (Tabone, 2000). A problem with this visa status is that it does not require labor certification, so the Department of Labor does not have to certify that the wage offered to the nurse is the prevailing wage. However, the law does state that foreign nurses entering under I-140 cannot have a negative impact on domestic wages (Tabone, 2000).

D i s c u s s i o n   P o i n t

Does the increased importation of foreign nurses directly or indirectly impact the prevailing wages of domestic RNs?

Still other foreign nurses have sought employment in the United States in accordance with the North American Free-Trade Agreement (NAFTA), enacted in December 1993. NAFTA established a reciprocal trading relationship between the United States, Canada, and Mexico and allowed for a nonimmigrant class of admission exclusively for business and service trade individuals entering the United States (Brush & Berger, 2002). Thus, under NAFTA's auspices, Mexican and Canadian nurses can work in the United States under a specially created Trade NAFTA (TN) visa.

On July 26, 2003, the U.S. Bureau of Citizenship and Immigration Services ruled that foreign-educated health care professionals, including nurses who are seeking temporary or permanent occupational visas, as well as those who are seeking NAFTA status, must successfully complete a screening program before receiving an occupational visa or permanent (green card) visa (Commission on Graduates of Foreign Nursing Schools, 2003). This screening, completed by the Commission on Graduates of Foreign Nursing Schools (CGFNS), includes an assessment of an applicant's education to ensure that it is comparable to a nursing graduate in the United States, verification that licenses are valid and unencumbered, successful completion of an English-language proficiency examination, and verification that the nurse has either earned certification by the CGFNS or passed the National Council Licensure Examination for Registered Nurses (NCLEX-RN) (Bola et al., 2003; Xu et al., 1999). Steefel (2004) argued that border cities such as Detroit, Buffalo, and Seattle would be hardest hit by the new certification rules.

Nurses who entered the United States after the ruling on July 26, 2003, had one year from entry to produce a visa certificate from a U.S. Department of Homeland Security (DHS)–approved agency such as CGFNS. Nurses in the United States before July 26, 2003, had until July 26, 2004, to produce the certificate (Steefel, 2004).

The National Council of State Boards of Nursing and the Organization of Nurse Executives, however, asked the DHS to delay implementation of certification rules for certain health care workers, including nurses, for at least 18 months, citing that 10,000 to 15,000 nurses currently licensed by their state nursing boards and practicing in the United States might not be able to continue to work if they could not obtain certification (RNews Capsules, 2004; Steefel, 2004). The American Nurses Association (ANA), however, opposed such a delay, noting that the new rules were originally passed in 1996 and suggesting that the one-year transition period should have been adequate for foreign nurses to start the certification process (Steefel, 2004). Yet on Monday, July 19, 2004, the U.S. Citizenship and Immigration Services (USCIS) announced that Canadian and Mexican health care workers who entered the United States on a TN (Trade NAFTA) visa and were employed in the United States and held a valid U.S. license before September 23, 2003, would continue to be exempt from the prescreening requirements for one additional year (USCIS Extends Deadline, 2004).

Discussion Point

Should implementation of the new certification rules be delayed until the immediate nursing shortage is resolved? Should manpower issues take precedence over concerns regarding patient safety?

ENSURING COMPETENCY OF FOREIGN NURSES: COMMISSION ON GRADUATES OF FOREIGN NURSING SCHOOLS

Nursing is one of the most highly regulated health professions in the United States, and a license is required to practice in all 50 states and U.S. territories. Before 1977, endorsement and taking the State Board Test Pool Examination (SBTPE) were the two ways for foreign nurses to obtain a license (Xu et al., 1999). SBTPE tested the foreign graduate's English language proficiency and knowledge of U.S. nursing practice, but alarmingly, only 15% to 20% of foreign RNs typically passed the NCLEX-RN (CGFNS, 2004). Indeed, between 1969 and 1978, as many as 85% (70,000) of the 82,000 foreign nurse graduates taking the SBTPE failed, compared to 17% of U.S. nurses (Maroun & Serota, 1988).

As a result of this high failure rate and a concern for patient safety, the ANA and the National League of Nursing (NLN), with collaboration from the Department of Labor and INS, established CGFNS in 1977 as an independent, nonprofit organization (Xu et al., 1999). CGFNS was intended to protect foreign nurse graduates and the American public by "establishing order out of confusion, bringing fairness and equity to an often chaotic situation, protecting foreign educated nurses against exploitation, and contributing to safe nursing practice in the United States" (CGFNS, as cited by Brush & Berger, 2002, p. 110). CGFNS was to accomplish this by evaluating and testing foreign graduates via a certification program, before they left their home countries, to ensure that there was a reasonable chance for them to pass the NCLEX-RN in the United States. Such a certification examination minimized the foreign nurses' potential economic loss and emotional suffering should they not be able to be licensed in the United States, and helped to protect the welfare of the American public (Xu et al., 1999).

> *__CONSIDER:__ Recruiting internationally may be a quick-fix solution, but it is far from clear that it is a cost-effective solution.

However, the examination was not intended to be a substitute for the state board licensing examination. Through a contract with NLN, which had designed the NCLEX-RN, a CGFNS qualifying examination was developed. The examination consists of two parts to test the applicant's knowledge of nursing and the English language (both written and oral) (Xu et al., 1999). The nursing section was modeled after the NCLEX-RN and covers the basic five areas of nursing: medical, surgical, pediatric, maternal, and psychiatric. The presumption of the examination was that the applicant had adequate preparation in the five content areas and the English language. To avoid any apparent conflict of interest,

CGFNS does not offer any preparatory courses or publish remedial materials concerning the examination (Xu et al., 1999).

Today, the CGFNS qualifying examination is offered in six cities in the continental United States and in over 30 countries around the world (Xu et al., 1999). Since its inception, the CGFNS has boosted the licensure rate for foreign graduates from the 15% to 20% range up into the 85% to 90% range (CGFNS, 2004). However, 58 Mexican nurses took the test for U.S. licensure in 2002, and only 16 were successful, far below the licensure rate of nurses from the Philippines, India, South Korea, and Nigeria, where schools actually train nurses for work in the United States (Recruiters Help Mexican, 2004).

More than 23,000 foreign nurses took the NCLEX-RN in 2002, up from approximately 20,000 the year before (Freiss, 2003). Of those, more than half were from the Philippines. Until 2005, the NCLEX-RN was offered only in the United States and its territories; however, in June 2004, the National Council of State Boards of Nursing (2004) announced that NCLEX-RN testing would begin in January 2005 in Seoul, South Korea; London, England; and Hong Kong, China.

Neither the National Council of State Boards of Nursing nor the U. S. government keeps a tally of how many foreign-educated nurses are licensed and working in the United States, but anecdotal accounts abound of health care companies spending as much as $10,000 per hire in recruiting efforts and immigration costs to fill their vacancies (Freiss, 2003).

Discussion Point

If the money that is currently being spent on recruitment and immigration of foreign nurses was instead spent on resolving the domestic nursing issues that led to a shortage in the first place, would international nurse recruitment even be necessary?

▶ ASSIMILATING THE FOREIGN NURSE THROUGH SOCIALIZATION

The ethical obligation to the foreign nurse does not end with his or her arrival in a new country. The sponsoring country must do whatever it can to see that the migrant nurse is assimilated into the new work environment as well as the new culture. Ryan (2003) suggests that socialization to the professional nursing role is one of four basic needs that must be addressed if foreign nurses are to adapt successfully to American workplaces. Ryan suggests that initially, foreign nurses must be introduced to American jargon and variations in nursing practice delivery because language is reported to be a significant barrier (Kingma, 2001). Then many must be supported through a period of cultural, professional, and psychological dissonance that is associated with anxiety, homesickness, and isolation. Finally, these nurses must be integrated within the institution so that they develop a sense of community life on the nursing unit.

Bola et al. (2003) state that international nurses also frequently experience culture shock regarding nonverbal communication, which may interfere with their assimilation. "Patients or staff with limited cultural competence may interpret nonverbal communication, such as eye contact or smiling, as disrespectful" (Bola et al., p. 41).

Ryan (2003) suggests that using a cultural diversity enhancement group (CDEG) and a "buddy program" may help socialize these international nurses. The CDEG includes staff nurses and management personnel from varied ethnic backgrounds who agree to buddy with the international nurses to make them feel welcomed in the organizational culture and to assist them regarding basic services, places, or necessary items they need to know about or have. Bolla et al. (2003) concurs, suggesting that without a support system, international nurses may question their ability to solve problems and function successfully because the values and behaviors helpful in solving problems in their home country may not be helpful here.

Many migrant nurses are afraid to express dissatisfaction or to ask for help, for fear they will no longer have a job or because they fear being sent home. In addition, many of the families left behind in donor countries count on the migrant RN sending money home to improve their living standard. All of these factors place migrated nurses at increased risk for abuse and failure to assimilate.

▶ CONCLUSIONS

Nurse migration and its associated ethical dilemmas is one of the most serious issues facing the nursing profession today. Clearly, developed countries have an advantage in terms of pull factors to recruit migrant nurses from less developed countries, and less developed countries are the ones most likely to suffer the devastating effects of "brain drain." One must ask, however, whether this quick fix solution to the nursing shortage has become too commonplace and too easy. Does it keep recruiter countries from dealing with the issues that led to their shortage in the first place? Does it negatively impact prevailing domestic wages and artificially alter what should be normal supply/demand curves in the health care marketplace? Of even greater concern is the lack of regulatory oversight of contracting with foreign nurses, placing them at risk for unethical, if not illegal, employment practices in their host country.

Clearly, some countries and professional nursing organizations are beginning to address these issues. So, too, are national governments and regulatory agencies, in an effort to protect both the migrant nurses and the public those nurses will serve. Yet, in the meantime, what may be hundreds of thousands of nurses are migrating internationally, and the potentially negative impacts of this increasing trend, on both the migrant nurse and the donor nation, are only now becoming apparent.

Brush and Berger (2002, p. 113) state that it remains to be seen whether new renditions of old solutions will revitalize and sustain nursing in the long run or simply have short-term effects. They go on to say, that "if the latter is true, foreign nurse graduates will remain a vital local response to the imbalance in nurse supply and demand in years ahead."

FOR ADDITIONAL DISCUSSION

1. Are the requirements for foreign nurses to get visas in the United States adequate?
2. Does CGFNS certification and passage of the NCLEX-RN examination in the United States assure competency of the foreign nurse graduate?
3. As long as international nurse recruitment is a viable option, will the problems that have led to a nursing shortage in the first place be addressed?

4. Should donor countries develop nurse migration policy efforts that limit human resource exports?
5. How can government and professional nursing organizations work together to ensure that recruitment practices of foreign nurses are both ethical and appropriate?
6. How does the ethical principle of veracity (truth-telling) apply to the zealous recruiting efforts seen, particularly in developing countries?
7. Is government regulatory oversight of foreign nurse recruitment efforts in conflict with America's value of capitalistic, free enterprise?

REFERENCES

Bola, T. V., Driggers, K., Dunlap, C., & Ebersole, M. (2003). Foreign-educated nurses. Strangers in a strange land. *Nursing Management, 34*(7), 39–42.

Bosch, X. (2003). Brain drain robbing Europe of its brightest young scientists. *Lancet, 361*(9376), 2210–2212.

Brush, B. L., & Berger, A. M. (2002). Sending for nurses: Foreign nurse migration, 1965–2002. *Nursing Health and Policy Review, 1*(2), 103–115.

Bryant, J. (May 4, 2001). Hospitals go overseas for nurses. *Atlanta Business Chronicle.* Retrieved February 10, 2004, from http://atlanta.bizjournals.com/atlanta/stories/2001/05/07/story1.html.

Buchan, J. (2001a). Guest editorial. *International Nursing Review, 48*(2), 65–68.

Buchan J. (2001b). Nurse migration and international recruitment. *Nursing Inquiry, 8*(4), 203–204.

Buchan, J., Parkin, T., & Sochalski, J. (2003). *International nurse mobility: Trends and policy implications.* Retrieved February 10, 2004, from http://www.icn.ch/Int_Nurse_mobility%20final.pdf.

Commission on Graduates of Foreign Nursing Schools (CGFNS). (August 26, 2003). *Bureau of Citizenship and Immigration Services issues final rule on health care professionals seeking occupational visas.* Accessed June 16, 2005, from http://www.cgfns.org/prog-cert.shtml.

Commission on Graduates of Foreign Nursing Schools (CGFNS). (2004). *Certification program.* Retrieved April 29, 2004, from http://www.cgfns.org/prog-cert.shtml.

Freiss, S. (2003). *U.S. looks abroad for nurses.* VRP Recruitment and Staffing Services, LLC. Retrieved April 29, 2004, from http://www.openmix.com/guideARTICLE.html.

Gamble, D. A. (2002). Filipino nurse recruitment as a staffing strategy. *Journal of Nursing Administration, 32*(4), 175–177.

Haddad, A. (2002). Ethics in action. *RN, 65*(79), 25–26, 28.

International Council of Nurses. (1999). *Position statement: Nurse retention, transfer, and migration.* Retrieved February 10, 2004, from http://www.icn.ch/psretention.htm.

International Council of Nurses. (2001). *Ethical nurse recruitment.* Retrieved May 16, 2004, from http://www.icn.ch/psrecruit01.htm.

International Council of Nurses. (2002). *Career moves and migration: Critical questions.* Retrieved May 24, 2004, from http://www.icn.ch/CareerMovesMigangl.pdf.

Kingma, M. (2001). Nursing migration: Global treasure hunt or disaster-in-the-making? *Nursing Inquiry, 8*(4), 205–212.

Kline, D. S. (2003). Push and pull factors in international nurse migration. *Journal of Nursing Scholarship, 35*(2), 107–111.

Maroun, V. M., & Serota, C. (1988). Demanding quality when foreign nurses are in demand. *Nursing and Health care 9*(7), 360–363.

Murthy, S. (2004). *United States immigration. Overview: H1C visas for registered nurses.* Retrieved July 24, 2004, from http://www.murthy.com/news/UDh1covr.html.

National Council of State Boards of Nursing. (June 1, 2004). *NCSBN selects first three countries to offer NCLEX abroad.* Retrieved June 20, 2004, from http://www.ncsbn.org/news/pressreleases_18AE335B87C947939F012B4542B6AEAD.htm

Record overseas numbers join UK nurse register. (2002). *Australian Nursing Journal, 10*(1), 16.

Recruiters help Mexican nurses attain U.A. licensure. (July 12, 2004). *Nurseweek* (California), p. 28.

RNews capsules. Delay sought for implementing certification rules. (2004). *Reflections on Nursing Leadership, 30*(2), 11.

Ryan, M. (2003). A buddy program for international nurses. *Journal of Nursing Administration, 33*(6), 350–352.

Shepard, S. (February 7, 2003). Recruitment process of foreign nurses gets a boost from INS. *Memphis Business Journal.* Retrieved February 10, 2004, from http://www.visalaw.com/news/02102003mbj.htm.

Steefel, L. (July 12, 2004). Bridges or barriers. *Nurseweek* (California). pp. 11–13.

Tabone, S. (2000). 2000 update: Foreign nurse recruitment. *Texas Nursing, 74*(8), 9, 15.

Thibodeau, P. (January 28, 2003). H-1B visa awards drop in '02. *Computer World.* Retrieved May 25, 2004, from http://www.computerworld.com/careertopics/careers/story/0,10801,77949,00.html.

University of Minnesota. (n.d.). *Around the U. A mixed message.* Retrieved February 10, 2004, from http://www1.umn.edu/urelate/kiosk/12.99text/legacy.html.

USCIS extends deadline for prescreening requirement for some Canadian and Mexican nurses. (July 21, 2004). *Nursing World.* Retrieved July 22, 2004, from http://www.nursingworld.org/inc/prtnewsarchive.htm.

Xu, Y. (2003). Are Chinese nurses a viable source to relieve the U.S. nurse shortage? *Nursing Economics, 21*(6), 269–274.

Xu, Y., Xu, Z, & Zhang, J. (1999). International credentialing and immigration of nurses: CGFNS. *Nursing Economics, 17*(6), 325–331.

BIBLIOGRAPHY

Davis, C. R. & Nichols, B. L. (2002). Foreign-educated nurses and the changing U.S. nursing workforce. *Nursing Administration Quarterly, 26*(2), 43–51.

Davis, C. (2003). How to help international nurses adjust: Use these practical tips to help international nurses make an effective transition to U.S. practice. *Nursing 2003 Career Directory, 33,* 28–29.

Davis, C. (2004). Crossing borders: International nurses in the U.S. workforce. *Imprint, 51*(2), 49–51.

Davis, C. R. (2004). International nurses: Adapting to U.S. nursing practice. *Nursing 2004 Career Directory, 34 226,* 26–28, 30.

DiCicco-Bloom, B. (2004). The racial and gendered experiences of immigrant nurses from Kerala, India. *Journal of Transcultural Nursing, 15*(1), 26–33.

Dixon, M. E. (September 3, 2003). Nurses move for better working conditions. *Advance Online Editions for Nurses.* Retrieved June 20, 2004, from http://nursing.advanceweb.com/common/EditorialSearch/AViewer.aspx? cc = 21456.

Flynn, L. J. & Aiken, L. H. (2003). Does international nurse recruitment influence practice values in U.S. hospitals? *Journal of Nursing Scholarship, 34*(1), 67–73.

Gerrish, K. & Griffith, V. (2004). Integration of overseas registered nurses: Evaluation of an adaptation programme. *Journal of Advanced Nursing, 45*(6), 579–587.

Global nursing partnerships: Strategies for a sustainable nursing workforce. (2001). Atlanta: Emory University. Available from www.nursing.emory.edu.

NMC barred from EU talks on nurse migration. (2002). *Nursing Times, 98*(41), 6.

Ollier, C. (2004). As global nurse migration accelerates, WHO study warns of unintended consequences. *Patient Care Staffing Report, 4*(2), 4–5.

Ondeck, D. M. (2001). Credentialing corner. Offsetting the nursing shortage with international nurses. *Home Health Care Management Practice, 13*(3), 236–238.

Stone, P. W., Tourangeau, A. E., Duffield, C. M., Hughes, F., Jones, C. B., O'Brien-Pallas, L., et al. (2003). Evidence of nurse working conditions: A global perspective. *Policy, Politics, & Nursing Practice, 4*(2), 120–130.

Wessling, S. (Winter 2003). Does the NCLEX-RN® pass the test for cultural sensitivity? *Minority Nurse,* 46–50.

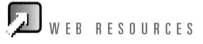

WEB RESOURCES

American Organization of Nurse Executives (AONE): Policy Statement on Foreign Nurse Recruitment	http://www.hospitalconnect.com/aone/advocacy/ps_foreign_recruitment.html
Commission on Graduates of Foreign Nursing Schools	http://www.cgfns.org/
Commonwealth Code of Practice for the International Recruitment of Health Workers.	http://www.thecommonwealth.org/shared_asp_files/uploadedfiles/%7B7BDD970B-53AE-441D-81DB-1B64C37E992A%7D_CommonwealthCodeofPractice.pdf
International Council of Nurses: International Forum Discusses Alternatives to Nurse Migration	http://www.icn.ch/sewapr-sept03.htm#2
International Nurse Mobility Trends and Policy Implications. (World Health Organization, International Council of Nurses, & Royal College of Nursing)	http://www.nursingspectrum.com/InternationalNursing/Resources/IntNurseMobility.pdf
Immigrant and Non-Immigrant Visas for Nurses	http://www.jamaicans.com/articles/immigration/im_0203.htm
National Council Licensure Examination for Registered Nurses (NCLEX-RN) (providing information on the NCLEX examination)	http://www.ncsbn.org/
Nursing Migration: Global Treasure Hunt or Disaster-in-the Making?	http://www.blackwell-synergy.com/links/doi/10.1046/j.1440-1800.2001.00116.x

Distance Learning: One Strategy for Furthering Nursing Education and Easing the Nursing Shortage

7

Catherine Wilde McPhee

The depth and complexity of the current nursing shortage are well documented in Chapter 5. So, too, were multiple strategies to speed its resolution. One such strategy was to increase the funding for nursing education (scholarships, loans, grants) so that more young people could be recruited into the profession. Although this funding and the improved financial access it offers certainly are an important part of recruiting more students into nursing, offering more nontraditional pathways to a nursing education must also be explored. This chapter, therefore, explores the use of distance education as a means of both advancing nursing education and alleviating the nursing shortage.

Distance education, also known as *distributed learning*, uses a wide range of computing and communications technologies to provide learning opportunities beyond the time and place constraints of the traditional classroom (The CSU Center for Distributed Learning, 2004). Educators say that distance education, by its nature, draws in students who wouldn't otherwise be able to pursue coursework because of lack of access to a campus or because work, family, or economic considerations preclude full-time, on-site education (American Association of Colleges of Nursing [AACN] (2000). Indeed, most students who take online courses do so for the convenience of balancing work schedules and course availability (Leasure, Davis, & Thievon, 2000). Online distance education also meets the needs of students who prefer more independence in their learning.

Yet distance education is not without its critics. Like most major change, distance education has encountered resistance levels ranging from eager anticipation to absolute refusal to consider accepting anything to be an educational modality that does not include a traditional classroom, students, and faculty.

To complicate the issue, distance education also consists of more than just taking the same courses that are offered in the traditional classroom and offering them online. Technology-mediated teaching strategies change the way teaching and learning occur. In addition, distance education challenges the traditional relationships between students and faculty and between students and academic institutions. These changes require new ways of assessing the quality of education and new strategies regarding how to best support student learning (AACN, 1999). Distance education, then, is not for everyone.

To better understand the complexities of these issues, this chapter begins by looking at the history of distance education and then explores the use of distance education for educating the nursing professional. Next, the chapter compares distance learner outcomes with learner outcomes in traditional delivery systems and also examines the "quiet concerns" about quality in distance education programs and the need for quality regulation. The chapter concludes by examining what distance education offers the nursing profession, both in terms of reducing the current shortage and in terms of advancing the educational preparation of practicing nurses.

▶ DISTANCE LEARNING: HISTORICAL PERSPECTIVES

Although not new, distance education is certainly a change in the approach to education delivery. Initially, "distance learning" referred merely to education being offered at a geographic location other than the campus where one was enrolled. However, when looking at distance learning from a historical perspective, one notes that it comes in multiple formats and is distributed in multiple ways (Table 7.1).

TABLE 7.1 Historical Milestones in Distance Education

1873	Print medium and correspondence studies
1920s	Radio: the "first distance education technology"
1950s	Telephone; audio conferencing; first nursing audio conference; psychiatric course offered by the University of Nebraska
1960s–1980s	Television; video-based systems including cable, microwave, and satellite; provide more of a "classroom feeling"
1966	First successful group of computer-assisted instruction (CAI) for continuing nursing education: Programmed Logic for Automatic Teaching Operations (PLATO)
1972	Ohio State University initiates first CAI course
1980s	CAI expands with availability of asynchronous and synchronous technology
1990s	Internet access proliferates

Source: Armstrong, Gessner, Cooper, 2000.

Distance education began with print medium and correspondence studies in the 1870s as the postal service began distributing correspondence studies to students across the United States. Radio programs of the 1920s, however, could be described as the first "distance education technology." In the early 1950s, telephone and audio conferencing became available. Next, television and video-based systems were able to provide a more classroom-like setting. Although moving slowly for approximately 30 years, computer technology for distance education jumped to the forefront and computer-assisted instruction then developed quickly (Armstrong, Gessner, & Cooper, 2000).

More recently, distance education has changed significantly due to the increased use of computer-mediated learning, the Internet, and other related technologies. In response to these advancements in technology, distance education now refers to any course being offered at any time and any place other than in a classroom on the campus where one is enrolled. It is not bound by time or place. According to Reinert and Fryback, it is a set of teaching and/or learning strategies that meet the learning needs of students separate from the traditional classroom setting and sometimes from the traditional roles of faculty (Care & Scanlon, 2000). Distance education requires that teachers and learners are separate from each other. It does not include activities in which the teacher travels to an alternative site to deliver a traditional course or class (AACN, 1999).

Distance education has experienced many changes in the past years, and will continue to evolve with the phenomenal growth of telecommunications technologies. McGonigle and Mastrian suggested almost 10 years ago that "Nurses will need to become adept users and information connoisseurs . . . discriminating users of the

Discussion Point

Are younger learners today better prepared for distance learning as a result of life-long exposure to computer technology? Do you believe most nurses are adept users of computer technologies?

cyberspacial arena that spans the informational gambit from junkyard to goldmine" (Armstrong et al., 2000, p. 68). Note that these authors suggested that nurses should not only be able to use the technology, but also be discriminatory in gathering information.

ACCESS TO CONTEMPORARY FORMS OF DISTANCE LEARNING

Currently, a variety of methods are used for distance learning. Courses are now referred to as *Internet-enabled*, *Web-based*, *computer-mediated*, *online*, *synchronous*, and *asynchronous*. The differences among these terms have to do with the amount the computer is required to complete course requirements, whether students will be required to use the Internet to access the course or course materials, and how much flexibility students will have in completing course requirements according to their personal schedules.

For example, online programs can be entirely Web-based or have some required on-campus requirements or clinical experiences. Students may also be allowed to complete 100% of their course requirements at a time of their choosing (asynchronous) or students may be required to meet at predetermined times, in person or in virtual environments (synchronous), to speak in chat rooms, create presentations, or hear video-streamed lecture interaction.

*CONSIDER: A high school graduate in New Jersey attends nursing school at the university of her dreams in California . . . without leaving her home or support system.

When distance learning is described as "more accessible" or "more available," it can mean several things. It may mean that courses are available in geographic areas where institutions of higher learning don't exist. And, for the most part, distance education course requirements are amenable to the schedule of the learner, rather than the individual teacher or institution. In addition, "more accessible" or "more available" distance education may simply mean that more courses can be offered, not because they take less time to teach, but because the availability of educators is increased as a result of faculty members being given the flexibility to teach according to their schedules.

However, a policy by the Institute for Higher Education [IHE] (1999) challenges the public to carefully scrutinize the notion of "easy access" to education that has been suggested by some distance education advocates. Computer-mediated learning requires special skills of students and more sophisticated technical support if students are to interact fully. In addition, the IHE encourages potential students to question the quality of the access. For example, although courses are available, does the student have the skills and technical support to access the course as planned?

D i s c u s s i o n   P o i n t

Does the general public perceive that distance education courses are "easier" than those offered in a traditional classroom?

The IHE also advocates that more research be done to determine if the advantage of easier access is overshadowed by difficulties not normally encountered by students in on-campus programs. Much research has been done in this area, yet many studies have not answered this question empirically. Research must continue at a pace consistent with advancements in technology (IHE, 1999).

WHY DISTANCE EDUCATION IN NURSING?

Nurses have many different motivations for attaining or furthering their education using distance education modalities. Nurses identified traveling long distances to a campus-based course as a major barrier to further education (White, Roberts, & Brannan, 2003). Precious time spent en route to campus, coupled with high fuel and automotive costs, could also easily be perceived as a deterrent. In addition, geographic barriers to nursing education continue to exist. Many rural areas continue to be underserved by institutions of higher learning. Even now, many students and nurses drive, and even fly, hours to a university to meet their educational needs. In addition, work and family obligations necessitate a more flexible learning environment (Dixon, Hordern, & Borland, 2001). These factors clearly make distance education an excellent solution for the student who wants to begin or advance his or her educational preparation in nursing.

Today's nurses need increased education and training to deliver complex patient care. Distance technology makes it cost effective to run smaller, more specialized classes, which enhance the quality of learning. Specialty courses can be tailored to address geographic shortages in nursing specialties and meet specific community health needs. It is not just the inadequate number of nurses, but also the distribution and lack of preparation that are contributing to the current nursing shortage.

Fortunately, the advent of technology has expanded the capacity of educational institutions to reach far beyond their geographic areas. Educators point out that distance education courses may fight "brain drain" from rural communities because adult students who learn within their communities are more likely to practice there, and working nurses taking distance education courses can continue to serve their patients while continuing their education (AACN, 2000).

The financial burden of an education in nursing is also prohibitive to many students, particularly minorities. Although distance education is likely no cheaper in terms of tuition than on-campus courses, it allows learners greater flexibility in terms of maintaining jobs (income) while they go to school, reduces travel time, and may reduce costs that would have to be spent on child care.

Compensation by employers and increased funding by private and governmental agencies for all education, including distance education, encourages people to enter nursing and to continue their nursing education. The increased use of technology in education may increase access to and ultimately lower the cost of education (AACN, 1999).

*CONSIDER: Distance education may cost a student less as a result of decreased travel costs and time and less time missed from work.

FINANCIAL AID FOR DISTANCE EDUCATION

The Nurse Reinvestment Act, signed by President George W. Bush in August 2002, directs that grants be awarded to schools of nursing and health care providers to develop programs aimed at recruiting students to enter nursing, promoting re-entry into the profession, and providing specialty training. Organizations can receive funding from grants to implement programs with the purpose of advancing nursing practice through career ladders, clinical best practices, and other retention strategies (Smith, 2002).

Unfortunately, a law known as the "50% rule" bars colleges from participating in federal financial aid programs if at least half of their students study online or if more than half of the institution's courses are offered at a distance. As demand for distance education increases, this law, originally intended to prevent fraudulent distant learning institutions from exploiting federal aid programs, may deny a significant number of distance education students access to federal aid.

Discussion Point

Is the 50% rule fair? What do you believe are the driving forces behind this law?

A recent report by the General Accounting Office (GAO) disclosed that institutions are already being affected by the law—or may be soon. The GAO recommends that the Department of Education continue to grant colleges waivers from the 50% rule while monitoring the performance of distance education and developing an alternative way to detect fraud. Changes in this law will allow equal access to federal aid by distance education students as well as the institutions that develop these programs to meet the ever-expanding needs of their populations, some of whom are nurses or future nurses (Foster, 2004).

▶ SCOPE OF DISTANCE EDUCATION IN NURSING

Online degree programs in nursing have multiplied rapidly in recent years, and the new reality is that distance education for nursing now exists for associate- through doctorate-level degrees. The choice of which educational program is offered frequently depends upon school preferences and culture (AACN, 2000).

In a 1998 survey conducted by the American Association of Colleges of Nursing (AACN, 1999), 51% of nursing schools reported they were engaged in some form of distance education. In addition, registered nurse (RN) to bachelor of science in nursing (BSN), RN to master of science in nursing (MSN), and MSN in many advanced practice majors are available online today (Stokowski, 2004). Numerous online doctoral programs also exist including complete or partial online Doctor of Philosophy (PhD) programs at respected universities such as Duquesne, the University of Arizona, and the University of Colorado.

In a distance learning survey conducted by the National Council of State Boards of Nursing (NCSBN, 2004), a large majority of state boards responded that distance learning is being used in basic RN, RN to BSN, and advanced practice programs. Most of the programs are postlicensure programs such as RN to BSN, MSN, or postmaster's certification programs. Only three of the boards (New York, Wisconsin, and Illinois) reported an entry-level RN program that offered most of its coursework through distance education, although many boards reported such programs were in development. Almost half (45%) of the states reported that they have programs that offer the majority of the coursework through distance education (NCSBN, 2004).

D i s c u s s i o n   P o i n t

Is distance education more appropriate for one educational level than another (e.g., graduate-level education more so than undergraduate education? RN to BSN more than RN entry?) Why or why not?

STUDENT NEEDS IN DISTANCE LEARNING

Historically, much of the literature on distance learning has been directed at preparing faculty members to teach online or looking at special needs that faculty teaching distance courses might have. This was reinforced by Hara and King (2000), who reported that the current literature inadequately addresses distance students' needs. More recently, however, there is greater awareness that distance students do indeed have unique needs.

Palloff and Pratt (2003) propose that what the virtual student needs is very clear: communication and feedback, interactivity and a sense of community, and adequate direction and empowerment to carry out the tasks required of the course. The National Center for Education Statistics reports, however, that it may be more complex than that, because online learners range in age from late adolescence to late adulthood. To meet student needs, distance education faculty are challenged to move beyond traditional pedagogical teaching strategies that work well in a classroom setting. To present courses that are not only technologically effective, but also meaningful from the virtual learner's standpoint, distance education faculty need to use adult learning theory (andragogy) (Fidishun, 2000).

In addition, distance students frequently need clarification regarding how they are to engage with the instructor, the material, or one another. Unlike the traditional classroom, where a student often has a choice of whether to participate in a discussion, online learners generally do not have this option. For this reason, online learning needs to be learner-centered and learner-focused (Palloff & Pratt, 2003).

Palloff & Pratt (2003) also state that the virtual student:

- Needs to have access to a computer and modem or high-speed connection and the skills to use them
- Must be open-minded about sharing personal details about his or her life, work, or other educational experiences
- Cannot be hindered by the absence of visual cues in the communication process
- Should be willing to commit a significant amount of time to his or her studies weekly and should not see the course as the "softer, easier way"
- Is or can be developed into a critical thinker
- Has the critical ability to reflect
- Most importantly, holds a belief that high-quality learning can happen anywhere and anytime

Meeting these student needs does not mean that all students will be satisfied with their distance education experience. Some students report dissatisfaction with online courses. Points of distress that occur are often related to the technology in use, course content, and communication (Hara & King, 2000). Indeed, Huston, Shovein, Damazo, and Fox (2001) suggest that a student's computer skill levels are often predictive of his or her satisfaction with distance learning.

Discussion Point

What technology hardware and skills are typically needed by the distance learner to be successful in completing distance education courses?

Communication, however, is another critical aspect of student satisfaction with distance learning. Hara and King's (2000) qualitative study identified periodic distressing experiences by students related to communication breakdown and technical difficulties between themselves and faculty or other students. Sometimes this occurs because the faculty members teaching these online courses have had little or no training in distance education. Hara and King suggest that these issues have not been adequately addressed and need further exploration.

Other students express frustration with not being given the independence and freedom they need to complete online course requirements. Most students who choose distance education as a learning modality are self-motivated and disciplined and certainly these two characteristics should be predictive of success.

▶ CONTROVERSIES REGARDING DISTANCE EDUCATION IN NURSING

Can Nursing Be Taught Online?

Using distance education to teach nurses is not without controversy. When first introduced, there were concerns, which are still voiced today, that Internet education for a practice- and competency-based profession, such as nursing, would fail to produce nurses who were equally competent to those from traditional programs.

Common questions about the appropriateness of distance education for nurses include whether there is adequate clinical experience and adequate opportunity to develop necessary skills such as professional socialization and critical thought. The inherent nature of nursing as a clinical profession requires that all students have the opportunity to develop professional practices through collaboration with faculty, peers, mentors, and experts (Billings, 2000). Clinical practice experiences are essential to the socialization and development of this professional role. Nursing is a practice-and competency-based profession, which makes the opportunity for clinical experience an issue of great concern.

Accrediting bodies require all distance education courses in nursing to have the same clinical requirements as those in the traditional setting. Each accreditation and program-review entity incorporates its review of distance education programs as a component of site visit—evaluator training (AACN, 2002). The school providing the distance program must deem clinical sites and preceptors competent. Various accrediting bodies, including the Joint Commission on Accreditation of Healthcare Organizations and state departments of health service, document that established standards are met at the facilities. According to AACN (2000), experienced deans report that developing quality clinical preceptorships for students in remote settings is challenging, but doable. They agree with the opinion that preceptorships should be conducted completely independent of one's professional work.

Discussion Point

Should faculty be required to make onsite visits for students completing preceptorships in distance education programs?

Can Distance Education Nursing Students Be Socialized to the Professional Nursing Role?

Professional socialization has long been identified as a crucial aspect of nursing students' development. One's first response to distance education might be that such socialization is likely very difficult without the face-to-face interaction of traditional education. However, the literature actually suggests that both socialization and student interactions can be enhanced by using distance education technologies (Huston et al., 2001) (Box 7.1).

Box 7.1

Research Study Fuels the Controversy

Successes of RN-to-BSN Bridge Course

One strategy used to ease the transition of the RN student into BSN education is the RN-to-BSN bridge course. This article detailed course objectives, course content, course implementation, and preliminary outcomes of a primarily distance learning RN-to-BSN bridge course at a northern California University.

The 6-week, two-unit course summarized in this article introduced RN-to-BSN learners to the university and to professional roles assumed by baccalaureate-prepared nurses. Adult learning theory was presented and personal learning styles and critical thinking skills were assessed for program and career planning. Learning strategies to promote critical thinking were emphasized. Values clarification was utilized as a tool to improve decision making. In addition, time management was emphasized as a tool for personal and organizational management. This course also introduced tools for distance learning such as WEB CT, electronic mail, and computerized database searches.

Huston, C., Shovein, J., Damazo, B., & Fox, S. (2001). The RN-BSN bridge course: Transitioning the re-entry learner. *Journal of Continuing Education in Nursing, 32*(6), 1–4.

Study Findings

Preliminary learner outcomes suggested greater than expected increases in role and campus socialization as well as computer literacy as a result of RN-to-BSN bridge course implementation. Notably, students quickly created their own support groups online to discuss common challenges and issues associated with their return to school. The authors concluded that an RN-to-BSN bridge course can be used successfully to ease the transition of students re-entering the academic environment, and may be the link that allows RN-to-BSN students to effectively face the concurrent challenges of role socialization and computer literacy while mastering course content and course objectives.

Distance education students have been found to communicate openly with each other and with their faculty and to form close bonds. More reflection before interaction often leads to more logical and coherent viewpoints than those expressed by classroom-based students. Many faculty members say they get to know students better in online programs than in face-to-face classes. This results, they say, from students being required to participate actively in every class and/or from students feeling more comfortable expressing themselves from a distance (Snow, 2003).

Online, no one dominates the conversation. The shy student has an equal chance of being heard. Because it is a faceless environment, the distance learning environment tends to facilitate participants sharing more of themselves (Loftus, 2001; Nesler, Hanner, Melburg, & McGowan, 2001). Picture a dozen nurses at the same hospital participating in the same distance education program. Would they not tend to develop their own group, resulting in more social support through increased interaction?

> *****CONSIDER:** A quantitative study comparing professional socialization of senior BSN students enrolled at campus-based programs, senior BSN students at distance programs, and nonnursing students reported that although students in both nursing programs scored higher than nonnursing students, the students in the distance programs demonstrated even more professional socialization than students in the campus-based programs (Nesler et al., 2001).

Nesler's finding that senior BSN students in distance programs demonstrated more professional socialization than those students in campus-based programs is important to distance education given the current focus on student outcomes by accreditors and other evaluators of higher education (2001). Nesler and colleagues concluded that students enrolled in distance programs achieve professional socialization through alternative means. For example, most students enter distance programs with significant health care experience and continue to work at least part-time while in school, often forming preceptor relationships. The authors caution that the effect of the distance-learning environment on professional socialization should be reassessed as more distance programs become available to nurses earlier in their careers and to students seeking original licensure as a registered nurse.

Can Students in Distance Learning Programs Achieve the Desired Outcomes?

Although outcomes achieved with traditional classroom learning have been viewed as the gold standard of quality education, experts suggest that online education is as effective as classroom learning. Perhaps this is because the learner-centered environment compensates for the lack of face-to-face interaction.

Potempa (2001) explains that data gathered since 1912 show no significant difference in learning outcomes between distance education and traditional classroom education. Similarly, a 1999 review by researcher T. L. Russell, conducted from 1928 to 1997, found no significant differences in the competencies of students taught by the traditional classroom methods versus distance education. This study showed that distance education methods do not negatively affect quality of outcomes (AACN, 2000).

Armstrong and colleagues (2000) also found that students learn via distance education as well as they do via traditional formats, such as classrooms, conferences, or seminars. Leasure and colleagues (2000) found the same in their study comparing student outcomes in an undergraduate research course taught using both web-based learning technology and traditional pedagogy.

Another descriptive comparative study by Buckley (2003) of classroom-based, web-enhanced, and web-based nutrition courses for undergraduate nursing students found no differences in student learning outcomes. Students in this study were able to grasp the content at comparable levels regardless of how they received the materials. Zucker and Asselin (2003) also found little difference between online and traditional classroom students' nursing course grades and ratings of satisfaction.

According to AACN (2000), Rebecca Jones, Director of the School of Nursing and Health Sciences at Texas A&M University-Corpus Christi, reported that students in distance programs tended to perform as well as other students, with greater education rates over time.

Some researchers have even suggested that distance education learners have better outcomes than traditional learners do. Distance students benefit when the role of faculty changes to facilitator or guide, rather than a provider of information. For example, Leasure and colleagues' (2000) study proposed that critical thought is developed more quickly for the distance student in response, partly, to the asynchronous and collaborative nature of the experience. Leasure's study showed that students tended to default to the course faculty in the traditional classroom setting whereas students in the web-based learning environment more readily demonstrated synthesis of information provided by others and themselves. In addition, some proponents of online education argue that its ability to foster thoughtful discussion—through e-mail, chat rooms, and discussion boards—may be the technology's greatest strength (Shea & Boser, 2001).

Another advantage identified in the Leasure study (2000) was that, rather than being given data, students in online courses can be directed to use evidence-based practice sources. The development of this skill, to easily navigate and discover these resources, will make empirical data more easily available for use in practice. Distance learning, then, allows students to develop certain skills, such as critical thought and retrieval of empirical evidence, both required outcomes for the nursing graduate.

How Do Faculty Roles Differ in Distance Education From Traditional Settings?

As technology becomes more integrated into distance education and the role of the student evolves, so too must the role of the distance faculty educator. Distance students need to recognize that often, with the introduction of distance education, faculty must become learners, too. The learning curve for faculty to master new technology can be huge, and the time invested can be enormous. The AACN (1999) reports that superior distance education programs require substantial institutional financial investment in equipment, infrastructure, and faculty development.

According to Watts (2003), distance education faculty need to use the new technologies along *with* students in an exploration and analysis of the world and its meaning. In addition to preparing and posting materials, faculty must be able to respond to students' email and review online activity in chat rooms in a timely manner.

---

*CONSIDER: "The transition from a traditional classroom to online learning and emancipatory teaching often requires faculty to transition to new teaching and learning paradigms and no intrapersonal conflict is likely during the transition" (Shovein, Huston, Fox, & Damazo, in press).

Because of the uniqueness of distance faculty and student interactions, students would be wise to evaluate certain characteristics of their instructor. Distance learning can be disquieting for faculty as they frequently lose familiar landmarks when their reliance on visual and embodied cues is challenged (Diekelmann, 2000). Care and Scanlan (2000) explain that online faculty must be more than the content expert; they also must be the encourager, motivator, interpreter, and mentor. Students can evaluate several key characteristics that increase the likelihood that an instructor will be successful in facilitating an online course:

▸ Flexibility
▸ A willingness to learn from one's students
▸ A willingness to give up control to the learners in both course design and the learning process
▸ A willingness to collaborate
▸ A willingness to move away from the traditional faculty role (Palloff & Pratt, 2002).

*CONSIDER: As competition for students extends beyond traditional boundaries with distance education, the notion that both students and faculty are aligned with one academic institution is changing (AACN, 1999). As innovation threatens to transform the fundamental nature of education, as it is now, angst and anxiety are on the rise (Potempa, 2001).

Discussion Point

Given that there are inadequate numbers of nursing faculty to teach the nurses that will be needed to solve the current nursing shortage—and that nursing faculty are even "grayer" than nurses in general—does distance education offer new opportunities for retired faculty to reenter the workforce and teach part-time without the commitment of being onsite?

How Can Quality in Distance Education Programs Be Assured?

The number of distance education programs in nursing has increased dramatically, and this increase can be expected to continue. Yet, it is not always easy to discern the quality of these programs. Thus, in addition to identifying one's ability to be successful with teaching online, the distance education process itself must be evaluated.

The *Seven Principles of Good Practice in Undergraduate Education*, originally reported by the American Association for Higher Education in 1987, but further developed by Chickering and Ehrman in 1996, often serves as a gold standard for traditional undergraduate education. Graham, Kursat, Byung-Ro, Craner, and Duffy (2001) applied these seven principles of good practice to online education (Box 7.2), along with corresponding lessons for online instruction. Faculty using these principles can accomplish learner-focused online education to meet the needs and wants of the virtual student (Palloff & Pratt, 2003).

BOX 7.2

Seven Principles of Best Practice and Corresponding Lessons for Online Education

Principle 1: Good practice encourages student–faculty contact.
Lesson for online instruction: Instructors should provide clear guidelines for interaction with students.
Principle 2: Good practice encourages cooperation among students.
Lesson for online instruction: Well-designed discussion assignments facilitate meaningful cooperation among students.
Principle 3: Good practice encourages use of active learning techniques.
Lesson for online instruction: Students should present course projects.
Principle 4: Good practice gives prompt feedback.
Lesson for online instruction: Instructors need to provide two types of feedback: information feedback and acknowledgment feedback.
Principle 5: Good practice emphasizes time on task.
Lesson for online instruction: Online courses need deadlines.
Principle 6: Good practice communicates high expectations.
Lesson for online instruction: Challenging tasks, sample cases, and praise for quality work communicate high expectations.
Principle 7: Good practice respects diverse talents and ways of learning.
Lesson for online instruction: Allowing students to choose project topics allows diverse views to emerge.

Source: Graham, Kursat, Byung-Ro, Craner, & Duffy, 2001.

In a white paper, *Distance Technology in Nursing Education*, the AACN (1999) recognizes recent technological advances as opportunities to improve "dramatically" the quality of and access to nursing education. This statement proposes that careful use of technology in education may well enhance the profession's ability to educate nurses for practice, prepare future nurse educators, and advance nursing science at a time when there is an insufficient number of professional nurses, qualified nurse faculty, and nurse researchers.

Despite the research already presented on distance learner outcomes, questions continue regarding the quality of distance education curricula, clinical standards, accreditation, and jurisdiction issues (Discenza, Howard, & Schenk, 2002). Scientifically based knowledge about outcomes, what teaching and learning practices contribute to positive outcomes, what support needs to be in place for students and faculty, or how web technology and its tools contribute to teaching and learning are still being discovered through research.

The continuing question of quality outcomes in distance learning programs for nursing has, however, been addressed by various professional nursing organizations. These identified standards should be used in assessing any distance program for nursing. For students who choose to pursue distance education, it is imperative that they choose a program approved by a regional accrediting body, the professional association of a specific field of study, and/or a state agency (Shea & Boser, 2001).

For example, through its Council of Regional Accrediting Commissions, the eight regional accrediting commissions developed a *Statement of Commitment and Best Practices for Electronically Offered Degree and Certificate Programs in 2000* (Western Interstate Commission for Higher Education [WICHE], 2001a, 2001b). In addition, the Alliance for Nursing Accreditation, composed of 14 national and specialty nursing organizations and accrediting/certification bodies, developed a *Statement on Distance Education Policies* (AACN, 2002) to assure the public that nursing education programs maintain a high standard of quality. This statement directed that distance learning programs must meet the same academic program and support standards and accreditation criteria as programs provided in face-to-face formats. Other standards for distance education nursing programs (AACN, 2002) identified by the Alliance for Nursing Accreditation are shown in Box 7.3.

BOX 7.3

Standards for Distance Education Nursing Programs

1. Student outcomes are consistent with the stated mission, goals, and objectives of the program.
2. The institution assumes the responsibility for establishing a means to assess student outcomes, including both program and specific course outcomes, and that results are used for continuous program improvement.
3. Mechanisms for ongoing faculty development and involvement in the area of distance learning and the use of technology in the teaching–learning process are established.
4. Appropriate technical support for faculty and students is provided.
5. The program provides learning opportunities that facilitate development of students' clinical competence and professional role socialization and measures these student outcomes.
6. The program provides or makes available resources for the student's successful attainment of all program objectives.
7. Each accreditation and program review entity incorporates the review of distance education programs as a component of site visitor/evaluator training.

Source: AACN, 2002.

The National Council of State Boards of Nursing also addressed distance learning issues for educators during an Educational Network telephone conference in 1999. Dr. Maria Connolly, Dean of the College of Nursing and Allied Health at the University of St. Francis in Joliet, Illinois, nationally and internationally renowned for her work in distance learning, shared her expertise. Five components to be used for evaluating web-based courses were presented. These are listed in Box 7.4. Dr. Connolly (NCSBN, 2003) also suggested three publications to be used when evaluating distance-learning courses:

▶ *Distance Education Guidelines for Good Practice:* Higher Education Program and Policy Council, May 2000. This can be purchased from the American Federation of Teachers Higher Education Department, 555 New Jersey Ave. NW, Washington, DC 20001.
▶ *Best Practices for Electronically Offered Degree and Certificate Programs:* Western Cooperative for Educational Telecommunications. Available at *www.wiche.edu/telecom.*
▶ *AACN White Paper on Distance Technology in Nursing Education:* From July 1999. Available at *www.aacn.nche.edu/publications/positions/whitepaper.htm*

BOX 7.4

Five Components for Evaluating Web-Based Courses

1. Text with syllabi: weekly agenda; classes developed with PowerPoint (or other graphics that convey the message being taught); reading assignments
2. Live chat sessions (synchronous)
3. Postdiscussion questions (asynchronous)
4. Online testing and grade book
5. Broadcast emailing

Source: NCSBN, 2003.

Finally, a study by Billings (2000) proposed a framework to assess the interaction of technology used to offer web-based courses in nursing, the teaching/learning practices in these courses, and the outcomes enabled by the technology. Concepts from her model include outcomes, educational practices, faculty support, learner support, and use of technology. This model, adapted from several others, is unique in that it specifies the associated operational variables and their relationship to each concept. These variables can be particularly helpful in assessing specific courses. According to the author, questions about these concepts in web-based courses for nursing students should be answered by faculty. Using a theory-driven framework such as that of Billings will guide inquiry and thereby provide evidence to establish best practices for both learning and teaching in web-based nursing courses.

▶ DISTANCE LEARNING AND SPECIFIC STUDENT POPULATIONS

RN to BSN Students

In 1996, the National Advisory Council on Nurse Education and Practice recommended that a federal policy be adopted to achieve a basic nurse workforce in which at least two-thirds hold baccalaureate or higher degrees in nursing by the year 2010 (AACN, 1999). Currently only 32% of RNs are prepared at the baccalaureate level, and only 43% of the RN workforce possesses baccalaureate, master's, or doctoral degrees (Tri-Council for Nursing, 2001).

The recent study by Aiken, Clarke, Cheung, Sloane & Silber (2003) has been a motivating factor for facilities and government to increase opportunities, funding, and compensation for those wanting to attain a BSN or advanced degree. In this study, Aiken and colleagues found that surgical patients have a substantial survival advantage if treated in hospitals with a higher proportion of nurses educated at the baccalaureate or higher level. Astonishingly, the study's key findings concluded that at least 1,700 preventable deaths could have been realized in Pennsylvania hospitals alone if the nursing staff comprised 60% of BSN-prepared nurses and the nurse-to-patient ratio had been 1:4.

Dr. Kathleen Ann Long, President of AACN, states, "Dr. Aiken's research clearly shows that baccalaureate nursing education has a direct impact on patient outcomes and on saving lives" (AACN, 2003, para 2). Perhaps these data can be used to encourage more nurses with associate degrees to continue their education toward a BSN. Only 16% of associate degree–prepared nurses go on to obtain post-RN nursing or nursing-related degrees (AACN, 2003). The accessibility and flexibility of distance RN-to-BSN programs could clearly meet the needs of a workforce that desperately needs to respond to such compelling findings.

One finding from the Aiken (2003) study that was not so publicized was that a nurse's years of experience had no impact on mortality or failure-to-rescue rates. This is important information when considering that the nurse workforce is aging. It is contrary to the long-held belief that the nurse expert can compensate for advanced education with experience. Presented correctly, these data could stimulate the experienced nurse to obtain a baccalaureate degree and stimulate a career that has, perhaps, become less fulfilling. If this goal becomes easier to achieve, through a distance RN-to-BSN program, the chances that a nurse would pursue this route may increase.

Refresher Course Students

Approximately a half million nurses in the United States are not actively employed in nursing. Nurses not presently employed in nursing may be enticed back into the workforce because of distance education refresher courses. Refresher courses, usually provided by schools of nursing or hospital-based continuing education departments, generally offer these courses in the traditional approach of classroom didactic followed by clinical practice. The cost of such programs and their dependence on class size to be cost-effective require them to pull from a large geographic area.

Nurses returning to work after an absence from the clinical setting may not possess current knowledge and skills, and they may face unfamiliar advances in workplace technology. Deterrents to their return could be lack of availability or accessibility of refresher courses.

Also, according to Quant (2001), adults who participate in refresher courses are voluntary learners with diverse life and work experiences. Unlike undergraduate study, the purpose of a refresher course and clinical component is to provide feedback and correct errors. Although this group may prefer the independent online format, they require motivation and reassurance so that they can be successful returning to an academic environment.

*CONSIDER: Nurses who participate in refresher courses may experience uncertainty and lack of confidence in their own abilities to cope with new information and practice.

In the fall of 2000, an online refresher course was begun at Kennesaw State University in Georgia. This was in response to the university's inability to meet the demand for refresher courses for nurses in faraway rural areas. The course was developed using an interactive distance education model designed at the University of Wisconsin, Madison (White et al., 2003). The course included four components deemed necessary to bridge the distance between the instructor and the learner without the assistance of nonverbal cues: humanizing or creating a good learning environment; getting the learner to participate; using the right message so that it is received, understood, and remembered; and eliciting feedback from the learner (Armstrong et al., 2000).

Several educational issues were identified and addressed as this online refresher course evolved. These included technical support including computer availability and competence, testing issues related to participants not needing a course grade or to sit for the state licensing examination, and the need for additional faculty development before teaching.

◗ CONCLUSIONS

Is distance learning appropriate for nursing education? Can it produce nurses competent in the social, behavioral, and clinical skills needed for the humanistic, practice-oriented discipline of nursing? Those in favor of distance education say there is no excuse for not using new and available tools. They believe that intelligent use of technology will extend both reach and results (Watts, 2003).

Yet, despite numerous research studies suggesting that distance education is an effective method of providing education to nurses, controversy continues and "quiet concerns" about quality perpetuate. For those unsure that distance education methods can produce desired learner outcomes, regulatory bodies are in place to evaluate these programs, and the current standards emphasize the same academic rigor as those used in evaluating on-campus programs.

Each student must determine if distance learning is right for him or her. Similarly, each teacher will need to determine individually if he or she wants to use distance education technologies to connect with students.

The contributions of distance education to the nursing shortage could not have come at a better time. The nursing profession needs distance education to attract nurses who cannot access traditional school settings. Distance education can also help retain and attract nurses to practice by providing advanced degrees, which correspond with higher levels of job satisfaction.

In addition, given the aging of nursing educators, the incentives of distance education may be significant to faculty retention and recruitment. Working from a "virtual classroom" in one's home might be tempting to faculty, especially those thinking of retirement. Master's-prepared nurses also could pursue careers in education more easily via online doctoral courses while remaining in the workforce.

Despite the quality safeguards and the obvious benefits of increasing the number of entry modes into nursing education, there are skeptics who will be slow to embrace any nontraditional learning method. Hutchinson, the first editor for *The Journal of Continuing Education in Nursing*, stated:

> ◗ *The decision [for using distance education] is ours—either lift the anchor or maintain the status quo. If you decide to take the plunge . . . Study all alternative methods. Chart your course, but don't expect smooth sailing. Batten down the hatches. Use all relevant navigational guides. Steady at the helm . . . Damn the torpedoes . . . And full speed ahead. (Armstrong et al., 2000, p. 68)*

Perhaps the most noteworthy thing about this quote is that it was authored in 1976. Thirty years later, it still holds true. The bottom line is that distance education in nursing is here to stay and is, in fact, gaining momentum. The increasing number of quality distance education programs will only assist in advancing nursing education and alleviating the nursing shortage.

Shovein et al. (in press) states:

> ◗ *The reaction to computer technology will probably follow patterns of the past, which consist of those who fearlessly embrace it, those who are prudently cautious, and those who will fight it to the end. Eventually, it will come down to the balance and the way in which the technology is applied and the purpose for which it is used. The formidable task remains what it has always been for a nursing educator, to design learning paradigms that awaken the awareness of another to a nursing consciousness.*

1. Can online learning using an interactive, community-based approach be used effectively across disciplines, specifically, nursing?

2. Using the standards identified in this chapter, how would one go about evaluating the quality of a distance education program in nursing?

3. Should national standards be set for distance education courses in nursing?

4. Can students learn to relate well in a multidisciplinary environment when their dominant educational experiences have been technology based?

5. How can faculty effectively oversee and assess clinical competence in distance modalities, particularly in prelicensure programs?

6. What noncurricular supports are necessary for students enrolled in distance education programs?

7. What are the findings of the research on the effectiveness of distance education? Are they valid? Are there gaps in the research that require further investigation?

REFERENCES

Aiken, L., Clarke, S. P., Cheung, R. B., Sloane, D. M., & Silber, J. H. (2003). Educational levels of hospital nurse and surgical patient mortality. *Journal of the American Medical Association, 290*(12), 1617–1623.

American Association of Colleges of Nursing (AACN). (July 1999). *White paper: Distance technology in nursing education.* Retrieved July 27, 2004, from http://www.aacn.nche.edu/publications/positions/whitepaper.htm.

American Association of Colleges of Nursing (AACN). (January 2000). *Issue bulletin: Distance learning is changing and challenging nursing education.* Retrieved April 18, 2005, from http://www.aacn.nche.edu/publications/issues/jan2000.htm.

American Association of Colleges of Nursing (AACN). (March 2002). *Alliance for nursing accreditation statement on distance education policies.* Retrieved April 18, 2005, from http://www.aacn.nche.edu/Education/disstate.htm.

American Association of Colleges of Nursing (AACN). (September 23, 2003). *AACN applauds new study that confirms link between nursing education and patient mortality.* Retrieved April 18, 2005, from http://www.aacn.nche.edu/Media/NewsReleases/2003AikenStudy.htm.

Armstrong, M., Gessner, B., & Cooper, S. (2000). POTS, PANS, and PEARLS: The nursing profession's rich history with distance education for a new century of nursing. *The Journal of Continuing Education in Nursing, 31*(2), 63–70.

Billings, D. (2000). A framework for assessing outcomes and practices in web-based courses in nursing. *Journal of Nursing Education, 39*(2), 60–67.

Buckley, K. (2003). Evaluation of classroom-based, Web-enhanced, and Web-based distance learning nutrition courses for undergraduate nursing. *Journal of Nursing Education, 42*(8), 367–370.

Care, W. & Scanlon, J. (2000). Meeting the challenge of developing courses for distance delivery: Two different models for course development. *The Journal of Continuing Education for Nursing, 31*(3), 121–128.

The CSU Center for Distributed Learning. (2004). *Welcome to the CSU Center for Distributed Learning.* Retrieved April 18, 2005, from http://www.cdl.edu.

Diekelmann, N. (2000). Technology based distance education and the absence of physical presence. *Journal of Nursing Education, 39*(2), 51–52.

Discenza, R., Howard, C., & Schenk, K. (2002). *The design and management of effective distance learning programs.* Hershey, PA: Idea Group.

Dixon, H., Hordern, A., & Borland, R. (2001). The breast cancer distance education program: Development of a course for specialized breast cancer nurses. *Cancer Nursing, 24*(1), 44–52.

Fidishun, D. (2000). *Andragogy and technology: Integrating adult learning theory as we teach with technology.* Retrieved April 18, 2005, from http://www.mtsu.edu/~itconf/proceed00/fidishun.htm.

Foster, A. (2004). Limit on aid for distance students may do more harm than good, congressional report says. *The Chronicle of Higher Education.* Retrieved April 18, 2005, from www.chronicle.com/daily/2004/02/2004022703n.htm.

Graham, C., Caglitay, K., Byung-Ro, L., Craner, J., & Duffy, T.M. (March/April 2001). Seven principles of effective teaching: A practical lens for evaluating online courses. The Technology Source. Suny Network. Retrieved May 5, 2005 from http://sln.suny.edu/sln/public/original.nsf/dd93a8da0b7ccce0852567b00054e2b6/b495223246cabd6b88256a090058ab98?OpenDocument.

Hara, N. & King, B. (2000). *Students' distress with a Web-based distance-learning course: An ethnographic study of participants' experiences.* Retrieved May 1, 2004, from http://www.slis.indiana.edu/CSI/WP/wp00-01B.html.

Huston, C., Shovein, J., Damazo, B., & Fox, S. (2001). The RN-BSN bridge course: Transitioning the re-entry learner. *Journal of Continuing Education in Nursing, 32*(6), 250–253.

Institute for Higher Education (IHE). (1999). *Policy: What's the difference? A review of contemporary research of the effectiveness of distance learning in higher education.* Retrieved April 18, 2005, from http://www.ihep.com/difference.pdf.

Leasure, A., Davis, L., & Thievon, S. (2000). Comparison of student outcomes and preferences in a traditional vs. World Wide Web based baccalaureate nursing research course. *Journal of Nursing Education, 39*(4), 149–154.

Loftus, M. (2001). But what's it like? *U.S. News and World Report, 131*(15), 56–57.

National Council of State Boards of Nursing (NCSBN). (2003). Distance learning issues for educators. *Council Connector, 3*(1), 4. Retrieved April 18, 2005 from http://www.ncsbn.org.

National Council of State Boards of Nursing (NCSBN). (2004). *2002–2003 NCSBN distance learning survey results.* Retrieved April 18, 2005, from http://www.ncsbn.org/regulation/nursingeducation_nursing_education_distance_learning_survey_results.asp.

Nesler, M., Hanner, M., Melburg, V., & McGowan, S. (2001). Professional socialization of baccalaureate nursing students: Can students in distance nursing programs become socialized? *Journal of Nursing Education, 40*(7), 293–302.

Palloff, R. & Pratt, K. (2002). Beyond the looking glass: What faculty and students need to be successful online. In K. E. Rudestam & J. Schoenholtz-Read (Eds.). *Handbook of online learning* (pp. 171–184). Thousand Oaks, CA: Sage.

Palloff, R. & Pratt, K. (2003). *The virtual student: A profile and guide to working with online learners.* San Francisco: John Wiley & Son.

Potempa, K. (2001). Guest editorial: Where winds the road of distance education in nursing? *Journal of Nursing Education, 40*(7), 291–292.

Quant, T. (2001). Education for nurses returning to practice. *Nursing Standard, 15*(17), 39–41.

Shea, R. & Boser, U. (2001). So where's the beef? *U.S. News and World Report, 131*(15), 44–54.

Shovein, J., Huston, C., Fox, S., & Damazo, B. (2005-in press). Challenging traditional teaching and learning paradigms: Online learning and emancipatory teaching. *Nursing Education Perspectives.*

Smith, A. (2002). Responses to the nursing shortage: Policy, press, pipeline, and perks. *Nursing Economics, 20*(6), 287–290.

Snow, S. (April 18, 2003). Virtual learning: Hot and happening or cold and distant? *Tampa Bay Business Journal.* Retrieved April 18, 2005, from http://tampabay.bizjournals.com/tampabay/stories/2003/04/21/focus1.html.

Stokowski, L. (2004). Trends in nursing: 2004 and beyond. *Topics in Advanced Practice Nursing eJournal, 4*(1). Retrieved April 18, 2005, from http://medscape.com/viewarticle/466711.

Tri-Council for Nursing. (2001). *Policy statement: Strategies to reduce the new nursing shortage.* Retrieved March 5, 2004, from http://www.nursingworld.org/pressrel/2001/sta0205.htm.

Watts, M. (2003). *Technology: Taking the distance out of learning.* San Francisco: Jossey-Bass.

Western Interstate Commission for Higher Education (WICHE).(2001a). *Best practices for electronically offered degree and certificate programs.* Retrieved November 12, 2004, from http://www.wcet.info/resources/accreditation/Accrediting%20-%20Best%20Practices.pdf.

Western Interstate Commission for Higher Education (WICHE). (2001b). *Statement of commitment by the regional accrediting commissions for the evaluation of electronically offered degree and certificate programs.* Retrieved November 12, 2004, from http://www.wcet.info/resources/accreditation/Accrediting%20-%20Commitment.pdf.

White, A., Roberts, V., & Brannan, J. (2003). Returning nursing to the workforce: Developing an online refresher course. *The Journal of Continuing Education in Nursing, 34*(2), 59–63.

Zucker, D. & Asselin, M. (2003). Migrating to the Web: The transformation of a traditional RN to BS program. *The Journal of Continuing Education in Nursing, 34*(2), 86–89.

BIBLIOGRAPHY

American Association of Colleges of Nursing (AACN). (October 9, 2003). *Fact sheet: The impact of education on nursing practice.* Retrieved November 12, 2004, from http://www.aacn.nche.edu/edimpact.

Billings, D. (1999). Program assessment and distance education in nursing. *Journal of Nursing Education, 38*(7), 292–293.

Chickerling, A. & Ehrmann, S. (1996). *Implementing the seven principles: Technology as lever.* Retrieved April 18, 2005, from http://www.tltgroup.org/programs/seven.html.

Donald, J. (2002). *Learning to think: Disciplinary perspectives.* San Francisco: Jossey-Bass.

Fest, G. & Leighty, J. M. (August 23, 2004). Direct flight. *Nurseweek.* Retrieved April 18, 2005, from http://www.nurseweek.com/news/Features/04-08/bsn.asp.

Heinrich, J. (2001). *Nursing workforce: Emerging nurse shortages due to multiple factors.* GAO report number 01-944. Washington, DC: U.S. General Accounting Office, pp. i–15 .

Mannix, M. (2001). Buyer, be wary. *U.S. News & World Report, 131*(15), 68–71.

Moore, M. & Kearsley, G. (1996). *Distance education: A systems view*. Belmont, CA: Wadsworth.

National Council of State Boards of Nursing (NCSBN). (1996). *Distance learning/Web definitions: A resource for the model education rules.* Retrieved April 18, 2005, from http://www.ncsbn.org/regulation/nursingeducation_nursing_education_distance_learning_definitions.asp.

Peterson, D. S. (2004). Education anytime, anywhere. *Advance for Nurses, 1*(5), 35–36.

Potempa, K., Stanley, J., Davis, B., Miller, K., Hassett, M., & Pepicello, S. (2001). Survey of distance technology use in AACN member schools. *Journal of Professional Nursing, 17*(1), 7–13.

Wills, C. & Stommel, M. (2002). Graduate nursing students' precourse and postcourse perceptions and preferences concerning completely Web-based courses. *Journal of Nursing Education, 41*(55), 193–201.

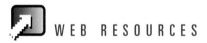 WEB RESOURCES

American Association of Colleges of Nursing (AACN)	http://www.aacn.nche.edu/
American Association for Higher Education (AAHE)	http://www.aahe.org
American Nurses Association	http://www.nursingworld.org
Institute for Higher Education	http://www.ihep.com
Multimedia Educational Resource for Learning and Online Teaching (MERLOT)—free membership site with links to online learning materials along with annotations and peer reviews	www.merlot.org
National Council of State Boards of Nursing (NCSBN)	http://www.ncsbn.org
Sigma Theta Tau International (STTI)	http://www.stti.iupui.edu
University of Chicago Student Counseling and Resource Service	http://counseling.uchicago.edu/vpc/virtulets.html
Western Cooperative for Educational Telecommunications (WCET)	http://www.wcet.info
Western Interstate Commission for Higher Education (WICHE)	http://www.wiche.edu

Unlicensed Assistive Personnel and the Registered Nurse

Carol J. Huston

8

In an effort to contain spiraling health care costs, many health care providers in the 1990s restructured their organizations by eliminating registered nurse (RN) positions and/or by replacing licensed professional nurses with unlicensed assistive personnel (UAP). The American Nurses Association (ANA) defines UAP as "unlicensed individuals who are trained to function in an assistive role to the licensed registered nurse in the provision of patient/client care activities as delegated by the nurse. The term includes, but is not limited to nurses aides, orderlies, assistants, attendants, or technicians" (1997, para 13). More contemporary titles include partners in care, nurse extenders, patient care technicians, patient care assistants and health care assistants. In fact, UAP are represented by almost 65 different job titles (Zimmerman, 2004).

Fifty-seven percent of hospital chief executive officers reported their hospitals were restructured in the 1990s, with personnel being reduced in approximately 90% of these restructured hospitals (Aiken, Clarke, Sloane, & Sochalski, 2001). In addition, skill mix reductions (i.e., declines in the proportions of RNs on unit staffs) occurred in approximately 70% of these hospitals (Aiken et al).

By the late 1990s, hospitals were actively recruiting the RNs who had been let go just a few years before. RNs who lost their jobs, however, were slow to return to the acute care setting, despite a widespread, worsening nursing shortage. As a result, hospitals again increased their use of UAP early in the 21st century, in an effort to supplement their licensed nursing staff.

Both as a result of the restructuring of the 1990s and the current serious nursing shortage, the skill mix in many hospitals today has proportionately more UAP than RNs (Seago, 2000). Indeed, almost all RNs in acute-care institutions and long-term care facilities today are currently involved in some way with the assignment, delegation, and supervision of UAP.

Several reasons are commonly cited for increasing the use of UAP. The primary argument for using UAP in acute care settings is usually cost, although the current professional nursing shortage is a contributing factor (Marquis & Huston, 2006). Another widely recognized benefit of using UAP is that they can free professional nurses from tasks and assignments (specifically, nonnursing functions) that can be completed by less well-trained personnel at a lower cost (Huston, 1996).

So why has the increased use of UAP created so much controversy? The answer is that in many institutions, UAP are not supplements to, but replacements of, professional RN staff. This is of concern because limited empirical research exists regarding what percentage of the staffing mix can safely be represented by UAP without negatively impacting patient outcomes. In addition, minimum national educational and training requirements have not been established for UAP and their scope of practice varies from institution to institution. All of these issues raise serious questions as to whether greater use of UAP represents an effective solution to dwindling health care resources or whether it is an economically driven, short-term response that could lead to the apocalypse of registered nursing (Huston, 1996) and compromised patient outcomes.

This chapter, however, does not intend to advocate for the elimination of UAP. Instead, this chapter will address what safeguards must be incorporated in the use of UAP so that safe, accessible, and affordable nursing care is possible.

MOTIVATION TO USE UNLICENSED ASSISTIVE PERSONNEL

The primary arguments for using UAP are maximizing human resources and cost reduction. UAP can maximize human resources because they free professional nurses from tasks and assignments that do not require independent thinking and professional judgment. This is significant because much of a typical nurse's time is spent on nonnursing tasks and functions.

Glazer (2000) defines nonnursing tasks and functions as activities that do not require a great deal of judgment or decision making based on nursing knowledge or expertise and that do not change based on the individual client or situation. Sample nonnursing activities that fit this definition include bandaging a cut, making a bed, taking a temperature, feeding a client, measuring intakes and outputs, and obtaining a weight or height (Glazer).

In Hayes's study of 118 RNs in a large medical center, 100% of respondents reported doing nonnursing functions "usually" or "almost always." This occurred despite 87% of respondents "disagreeing" or "strongly disagreeing" that RNs should perform such tasks. This performance of nonnursing functions by RNs did not change despite expansion of the UAP job description, the assistance of head nurses in identifying and prioritizing nonnursing functions for staff nurses, and the provision of an educational program for nurses on delegation. The study did not speculate as to why nurses continued to perform such functions despite an increasing perception that these were tasks they should not be doing (Hayes, 1994).

In a more recent study by Aiken et al., nurses across five different countries still reported spending a significant amount of time on nonnursing tasks (such as transporting patients, delivering or retrieving food trays, and housekeeping activities), while care requiring their professional skills (such as pain control, oral hygiene, skin care, or teaching patients and family) was left undone (Aiken et al., 2001).

In addition, *Keeping Patients Safe: Transforming the Work Environment of Nurses*, the third in a series of reports on health care quality issued by the Institute of Medicine (2003), stated that documentation of patient information and care given consumed an estimated 13% to 28% of a hospital nurse's time and that the time required for home care nurses was estimated to be even greater.

Discussion Point

Why are professional registered nurses still completing so many nonnursing tasks? Are they reluctant to delegate them to ancillary personnel or are there inadequate support personnel to take on these tasks?

Cost savings associated with UAP use, the second argument for increased UAP use, are unclear. Morgan, DeRose, and Vallance (2003) described the implementation of a staffing mix change at Southwest Florida Regional Medical Center, which added one UAP per 10 patients on dayshift, and one UAP per 15 patients on evening and night shifts. The plan's overall proposed cost totaled $722,733 annually, but reduced the average hourly rate by $0.22 per hour across all units combined.

Buerhaus and Staiger (1999), however, report that UAP use failed to produce anticipated cost savings in some hospitals. Many of these hospitals resumed reliance on RNs, due to the greater flexibility associated with a larger cadre of RNs. Research by McClung (2000) also found mixed results in a decade of studies addressing financial benefits of UAP use. Some studies reported cost savings, others reported neutral effects on the budget; still others reported cost increases.

► EDUCATIONAL REQUIREMENTS FOR UNLICENSED ASSISTIVE PERSONNEL

Some monitoring of the regulation, education, and use of UAP has been ongoing since the early 1950s (Kido, 2001); however, most of this has been for *certified nurse's aides*. The Omnibus Budget Reconciliation Act (OBRA) of 1987 established regulations for the education and certification of *nurse's aides* (minimum of 75 hours of theory and practice and successful completion of an examination in both areas). Yet no federal or community standards have been established for training the more broadly defined UAP (Huston, 1996).

Indeed, a study by Ventura (1999) found that the training for most UAP varied from less than 1 week to 4 or more weeks and Case (2004) suggests that the training is usually completed by the employing facility and occurs without formal certification. Formal training programs that do exist are completed at vocational schools and community colleges. They typically focus on long-term care, and provide certifications only as necessary to meet state requirements.

*CONSIDER: A high school diploma is not required to work as UAP in acute care settings.

Some agencies argue that the work experience reported by their UAP is a substitute for formal education and training. Research done by Anthony, Casey, Chau, and Brennan (2000) suggests, however, that while work experience for licensed nurses is associated with positive outcomes for patients, overall experience for UAP was not associated with differences in patient outcomes. Potter and Grant (2004) did report, however, that experienced UAP shared stories of "knowing their patients." This level of knowing did not involve scientific principles or a detailed knowledge base such as that possessed by an RN, but was a practical level of knowing that allowed them to contribute to the patient care process.

Discussion Point

Is it possible for RNs to assess individual UAP's "knowing" of patients and if so, should this influence their task assignment to that UAP?

Thomas, Barter, and McLaughlin (2000) state that some standards and guidelines are now required for the preparation and use of UAP in certified home health agencies and skilled nursing facilities. Still, this formal training is often inadequate. In 2002, the Office of the

Inspector General of the Department of Health and Human Services issued a report on *Nurse Aide Training* (Texas Nurses Association [TNA], 2004). This report, which looked at the training of nurse aides for nursing homes, concluded that nurse aide training had not kept pace with the changes in long-term care settings and that teaching methods for nurse aides were ineffective and teaching sessions too brief to provide the didactic and hands-on experience that was necessary to achieve competence. The report urged improvement of competency evaluation program requirements for nurse aides.

Of even more concern is the fact that nurse aides are used even more widely today than in 1998 when TNA convened its first task force on the subject. Today, nurse aides are being used in many settings other than long-term care. Extended utilization and reports on the need to set specific competency-based training make it inappropriate for nurse aides to continue to be trained to deliver care only in long-term care settings (TNA). For efficiency and safety, it is clear that a standardized curriculum that addresses the skill sets needed in the many settings where nurse aides are utilized should be implemented. TNA argues that since aides support the care delivered by RNs and licensed vocational nurses, it is logical that the aides' education should be under the purview of the nursing board (TNA, 2004).

Similar to long-term care, the education and training of UAP in acute-care settings is inadequate. In fact, there are no required educational standards or guidelines, that cross state lines and jurisdictions, for the use of UAP in acute-care settings (Thomas et al., 2000). Instead, UAP educational and training requirements for acute-care settings are generally facility based and the UAP is often trained only in the skill sets needed for that particular facility (Case, 2004). This is important to remember when UAP transfer from one facility to another because no assumption should be made about UAP competency levels to perform certain tasks, despite their work experience.

The increased use of UAP, called by some the "de-skilling of the nursing workforce," raises concern among consumers and legislators alike. The result is the introduction of legislation at the state level. In 1998, 20 states introduced legislation to regulate UAP practice through registration and certification. A few states proposed direct regulation of UAP by passing legislation that required UAP to be certified by meeting education and competency requirements (Kido, 2001). Legislation introduced in five states required the state boards of nursing to register or certify UAP and four other states introduced legislation that requires the Department of Health to regulate UAP (Kido).

Discussion Point

Why has the movement to regulate UAP education and training occurred only at the state level? Why has there been no national movement to do the same?

The need for state legislation to regulate UAP education and training should not imply, however, that all UAP are undereducated and unprepared for the roles they have been asked to fill. Indeed UAP educational levels vary from less than that of a high school graduate to those holding advanced degrees (Case, 2004). It merely suggests that RNs, in delegating to UAP, must make no assumptions about the educational preparation or training of that UAP. Instead, the RN must carefully assess what skills and knowledge each UAP has, or risk increased personal liability for the failure to do so.

UNLICENSED ASSISTIVE PERSONNEL SCOPE OF PRACTICE

In addition to existing state regulations regarding UAP education and training as well as required competencies, many professional nursing organizations have studied the use and impact of UAP and are adopting position statements regarding their use. In the early 1990s, the ANA took the position that the control and monitoring of assistive personnel in clinical settings should be performed through the use of existing mechanisms that regulate nursing practice. Typically, this includes the state board of nursing, institutional policies, and external agency standards (ANA, 1992).

In follow-up, many state boards of nursing issued recommendations regarding scope of practice for UAP or attempted to delineate the relationship between RNs and UAP. In a 1998 survey of 53 state and territorial boards of nursing, a majority of states reported that they had regulations/guidelines for RNs who supervised UAP and regulations that protected the use of the RN title (Thomas et al., 2000). Few states, however, used the ANA or National Council of State Boards of Nursing (NCSBN) definitions for delegation, supervision, or assignment. Most states also reported that there was no standardized curriculum in place for UAP employed in acute-care hospitals, and more than half the states reported that no plans existed for developing such a curriculum (Thomas et al., 2000). The end result, then, is that there is no universally accepted scope of practice for UAP (Kupperschmidt, 2002).

Some state boards of nursing have issued task lists for UAP (lists of activities considered to be within the scope of practice for UAP). However, the NCSBN warns that by creating task lists for UAP, an unofficial scope of practice is created and the training of UAP should not include the notion that such individuals will be performing activities independently (Simpkins, 1997). Task lists also suggest there is no need for delegation, as the UAP already has a list of nursing activities he or she may perform without waiting for the delegation process (Marquis & Huston, 2006).

Discussion Point

What happens when the condition of a patient changes? Is the training of UAP adequate to recognize changes in clients' conditions that warrant seeking intervention from the licensed nurse?

One major national effort to define the scope of practice for UAP was undertaken by the ANA in their delineation of tasks appropriate for UAP practice. These tasks, divided into direct and indirect patient care activities are shown in Box 8.1. Still, despite efforts by the ANA and state boards of nursing, the reality is that at the institutional level, most health care organizations interpret regulations broadly, allowing UAP a broader scope of practice than that advocated by professional nursing associations or state boards of nursing. In addition, while some institutions limit the scope of practice for UAP to nonnursing functions, many organizations allow the UAP to perform skills traditionally reserved for the licensed nurse (Huston, 1997).

Gordon (1997) concurs, stating that UAP usually have little background in health care and only rudimentary training. "Yet they may insert catheters, read EKGs [electrocardiographs], suction tracheotomy tubes, change sterile dressings, and perform

Direct and Indirect Patient Care Activities Appropriate to Unlicensed Assistive Personnel Scope of Practice

Direct patient care activities assist the patient/client in meeting basic human needs within the institution, at home, or in other health care settings. This includes activities such as assisting the patient with feeding, drinking, ambulating, grooming, toileting, dressing, and socializing, and direct patient care activities may involve collecting, reporting, and documenting data related to these activities. These data are reported to the RN who uses the information to make a clinical judgment about patient care.

Activities delegated to the UAP do not include health counseling or teaching or do delegated activities require independent, specialized nursing knowledge, skill, or judgment.*

Indirect patient care activities are necessary to support the patient and the patient's environment, and only incidentally involve direct patient contact. These activities assist in providing a clean, efficient, and safe patient care milieu and typically encompass help with chores; companion care; housekeeping; transporting; clerical, stocking, and maintenance tasks.

*_Judgment_ is defined as the intellectual process that a nurse exercises in forming an opinion and reaching a clinical decision based on an analysis of the evidence or data.
Source: ANA, 1997.

other traditional nursing functions. To keep patients from becoming unduly alarmed, some hospitals now prohibit nurses from wearing name badges that identify them as RNs. Thus everyone at the bedside is some kind of 'patient care technician'—regardless of how little training or experience she or he has" (p. 86).

*CONSIDER: Given the lack of national regulatory standards regarding the scope of practice for UAP, many health care institutions allow UAP to complete tasks traditionally reserved for licensed practitioners.

Kido concurs, arguing that a number of acute-care hospitals have expanded the UAP role to include catheter insertion and care, tracheal care and suctioning, phlebotomy, blood glucose monitoring, observation of skin integrity, and measurements such as intake and output, calorie count, and height and weight (Kido, 2001).

In some cases, UAP known as _unlicensed medication administration personnel_ (UMAP) also administer medications. Indeed, in the summer of 2001, draft legislation was circulated in Ohio to allow medication technicians to dispense medications in all long-term care facilities in that state (Trossman, 2002). There was no preset curriculum to train them and it was up to the facility to provide the training. In addition, the UMAP were to work under the direction of the nurse—so the responsibility and accountability for medication administration would still have belonged to the nurse. The nursing home industry dropped the legislative proposal after becoming sidetracked by a bill designed to reduce their liability insurance costs (Trossman, 2002), although the Ohio Nurses Association has worked diligently since that time to assure that such a proposal never resurfaces.

*CONSIDER: As of 2002, a total of 22 states were using UMAP (Trossman, 2002).

153

A similarly expanded scope of practice for UAP was reported by Young, who stated that emergency department assistants (EDAs) in her hospital, in England, after an 8-week induction period, are allowed to perform certain clinical duties "once thought of as requiring traditional nursing skills" (Young, 2004, para 2). These include cardiopulmonary resuscitation, taking observations, assisting in 'theatre,' attending to personal hygiene needs, and applying dressings. Young even predicts that in the future, EDAs may be allowed to carry out venipuncture and cannulation.

School nurses are also waging a battle to stop expansion of UAP practice in terms of the drugs they are allowed to administer (i.e., currently only licensed school nurses can administer insulin). It is the position of the National Association of School Nurses (2002) that the use of assistive personnel may be appropriate to supplement professional school nursing services in certain situations, but they should never supplant school nurses or be permitted to practice nursing without a license.

Indeed, a University of Iowa study conducted by McCarthy, Kelly, and Reed (2000) reported that nearly half of the school nurses surveyed reported medication errors in their schools during the previous year. A major factor in medication errors was the use of "unlicensed assistive personnel" such as school secretaries, health aides, teachers, parents, and even students, to administer medications. Only 25% of the nurses said they administered all the medication in their schools. The other 75% said that unlicensed personnel routinely dispense medications to students.

The reality then is that in many settings, UAP are inappropriately performing functions that are within the legal practice of nursing. This is likely a violation of the state nursing practice act and poses a threat to public safety. Auckenthaler (2002, para 7) articulately states:

> *"Those who hold the purse strings and who are held accountable by regulation and having a responsibility to comply with State and Federal rules for reimbursement have taken matters into their own hands. By using some creative muscle they have collectively empowered the hospital industry (themselves) to enhance the scope of care practices of the UAP thus avoiding additional regulatory oversight."*
>
> *There are no rules governing care delivered by an unlicensed employee of the hospital who conveniently falls under policy guidelines having set protocols established or condoned by a medical director. What this means is that fewer, costly, RNs will be necessary for direct patient care.*
>
> *Any direct care given is the purview of nursing practice and falls under nursing governance. The public should not be duped into believing they are the recipients of care from a qualified and highly educated RN when instead they are the recipients of a moderately paid, undereducated, poorly prepared hospital employee who may have no prior background or experience in health care (Auckenthaler).*

*CONSIDER: Many patients given direct care by UAP assume that UAP are licensed nurses. This confusion is promulgated when health care professionals do not include their credentials on their nametags or introduce themselves to patients according to their actual job title.

Barter (2002) echoes Auckenthaler's concern, stating that certain professional responsibilities related to nursing care must never be delegated. These professional responsibilities include patient assessment, nursing diagnosis, care planning, patient teaching and patient outcome evaluation. Similarly, the ANA argues that the underlying principles shown in Box 8.2 should be used by RNs and health care institutions to assure that the UAP scope of practice is appropriate.

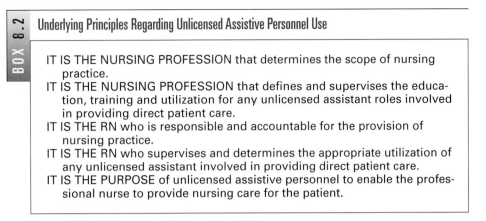

BOX 8.2   Underlying Principles Regarding Unlicensed Assistive Personnel Use

IT IS THE NURSING PROFESSION that determines the scope of nursing practice.

IT IS THE NURSING PROFESSION that defines and supervises the education, training and utilization for any unlicensed assistant roles involved in providing direct patient care.

IT IS THE RN who is responsible and accountable for the provision of nursing practice.

IT IS THE RN who supervises and determines the appropriate utilization of any unlicensed assistant involved in providing direct patient care.

IT IS THE PURPOSE of unlicensed assistive personnel to enable the professional nurse to provide nursing care for the patient.

Source: 1992 ANA Position Statement on UAP.

It is critical then that the RN never lose sight of his or her ultimate responsibility for ensuring that patients receive appropriate, high-quality care. This means that while the UAP may complete nonnursing functions such as bathing, vital signs, and the measurement and recording of intake and output, it is the RN who must analyze that information using highly developed critical thinking skills and then use the nursing process to see that desired patient outcomes are achieved. Only RNs have the formal authority to practice nursing, and activities that rely on the nursing process or require specialized skill, expert knowledge, or professional judgment should never be delegated (Zimmerman, 2004).

▶ UNLICENSED ASSISTIVE PERSONNEL AND PATIENT OUTCOMES

The outcomes associated with the increased use of UAP are not fully known; however, an increasing number of studies clearly demonstrate a direct link between decreased RN staffing and declines in patient outcomes. Some of these declines in patient outcomes include an increased incidence of patient falls, nosocomial infections, and medication errors (Blegen, Goode, & Reed, 1998; Huston, 1997, 2001; Lichtig, Knauf, & Milholland, 1999).

A benchmark study by Kovner and Gergen (1998) showed that patients who had surgery in hospitals with fewer registered nurses per patient than other hospitals ran a higher risk of avoidable complications following their operations. The study found hospitals that provided 1 additional hour of nursing care per patient day than the average nursing care hours per patient day had almost 10% fewer patients with urinary tract infections and 8% fewer patients with pneumonia.

Hall, Doran, and Pink (2004) reported similar findings in their descriptive correlational study of 19 teaching hospitals in Ontario, Canada. The researchers found that the lower the proportion of professional nursing staff employed on a unit, the higher the number of medication errors and wound infections. Similarly, Dunton, Gajewski, Taunton, and Moore (2004) reported higher fall rates were associated with fewer nursing hours per patient day and a lower percentage of registered nurses, although the relationship varied by unit type.

In addition, a benchmark study by Needleman, Buerhaus, Mattke, Stewart, and Zelevinsky (2002) of 799 hospitals in 11 states (covering 5,075,969 discharges of medical patients and 1,104,659 discharges of surgical patients) showed that lower levels of RN staffing in hospitals were associated with an increased risk of potentially fatal complications in patients. Among medical patients, a higher proportion of hours of care per day provided by RNs and a greater absolute number of hours of care per day provided by RNs were associated with a shorter length of stay and lower rates of both urinary tract infections and upper gastrointestinal bleeding. A higher proportion of hours of care provided by RNs was also associated with lower rates of pneumonia, shock or cardiac arrest and "failure to rescue," which was defined as death from pneumonia, shock or cardiac arrest, upper gastrointestinal bleeding, sepsis, or deep venous thrombosis.

A more complete review of the literature on the relationship between nurse staffing, staffing mix, and patient outcomes is included in Chapter 5, The Current Nursing Shortage.

▶ REGISTERED NURSES AND UNLICENSED ASSISTIVE PERSONNEL: THEIR WORKING RELATIONSHIP

The nursing literature is filled with reports about ways in which RNs and UAP work together to meet patient goals. Some models appear to be more successful than others and Potter and Grant (2004) argue that how an RN and UAP partner has implications for care delivery, and ultimately patient outcomes.

In a study of the organizational culture of acute care nursing units, Seago (2000) found that UAP frequently assume a thinking and behavior style of dependence and opposition. This suggests that UAP may believe it is necessary to be critical, resistant to authority, or to demonstrate an increased need for recognition when interacting in the work environment. Seago also found that UAP demonstrate a positive concern for the people they care for and have a need to do well in the caregiver role and concluded that the culture of the workgroup was critical to understanding the relationship between RNs and UAP.

One model that has been proposed to describe a positive relationship between RNs and UAP was developed by the National Council of State Boards of Nursing (1998). This model suggests that unlicensed personnel may be used across the continuum of care but suggests that more supervision is required by the RN of the UAP as client dependence increases and client competence decreases. The model also delineates care situations that are client directed from those where the activities must be delegated by the nurse. The purpose of developing this model was to assist nurses in identifying where greater supervision and delegation are needed in working with UAP.

▶ REGISTERED NURSE LIABILITY FOR SUPERVISION AND DELEGATION OF UNLICENSED ASSISTIVE PERSONNEL

Delegation has long been a function of registered nursing, although the scope of delegation and the tasks being delegated have changed dramatically the past two decades. In their classic 1995 position paper, the National Council of State Boards of Nursing (1995, para 6) defined *delegation* as "transferring to a competent individual the authority to perform selected tasks in selected situations. The nurse retains the accountability for the delegation."

In the 1990s, some health care institutions began assigning social workers, housekeeping personnel, dietary workers, respiratory therapists, and clinical laboratory staff to nursing departments under the supervision of a nurse manager (Hood & Leddy, 2003). As a result, the professional nurse (RN) role changed in many acute care institutions from one of direct care provider to one requiring delegation of patient care to others. Instead of spending time with patients, the RN supervised the care given by the other health care professionals on the team as well as the UAP (Hood & Leddy).

This role of delegator and supervisor increased the scope of legal liability for the RN. Although there is limited case law involving nursing delegation and supervision, it is generally accepted that the RN is responsible for adequate supervision of the person to whom an assignment has been delegated (Huston, 1996). Although nurses are not automatically held liable for all acts of negligence on the part of those they supervise, they may be held liable if they were negligent in the supervision of those employees at the time they committed the negligent acts (Marquis & Huston, 2006).

Liability is based on a supervisor's failure to determine which patient needs could safely be assigned to a subordinate or for failing to closely monitor a subordinate who requires such supervision. Experienced nurses have traditionally been expected to work with minimal supervision. The RN who delegates care to another competent RN does not have the same legal obligation to closely supervise that person's work as when the care is delegated to UAP. In assigning tasks to UAP, then, the RN must be aware of the job description, knowledge base, and demonstrated skills of each person.

> *__CONSIDER:__ The UAP has no license to lose for "exceeding scope of practice" and nationally established standards to state what the limits should be for UAP in terms of scope of practice, do not exist. It is the RN who bears the legal liability for allowing UAP to perform tasks that should be accomplished only by a licensed health care professional.

Hood and Leddy (2003) suggest, however, that delegating to UAP is not that different from the past, wherein RNs delegated work to licensed practical nurses (LPNs) or nurse aides. RNs, who are always accountable for the care given, continue to be responsible for instructing UAP as to who needs care and when. Hood and Leddy argue, however, that UAP should also be accountable for knowing how to properly perform their segment of assigned care and for knowing when other workers should be called in for tasks beyond the limits of their knowledge and training. As such, despite the legal doctrine of *respondeat superior* (the employer can be held legally liable for the conduct of employees whose actions he or she has a right to direct or control), UAP do carry some accountability of their own and always have (Hood & Leddy).

Case (2004) agrees, arguing that although *respondeat superior* applies only to the employer, an RN, LPN, UAP and other employees are nonetheless responsible for their own actions. The RN then may be sued individually for delegation, only if it is inappropriate according to the state's nurse practice act and the policies of the facility (Case).

Discussion Point

Do most UAP believe they can be held legally liable and accountable for their actions if they are delegated to do something by an RN, that is beyond their scope of practice or training?

Regardless of liability issues, the need for nurses to have highly developed delegation skills has never been greater than it is today. The ability to use delegation skills appropriately will help to reduce the personal liability associated with supervising and delegating to UAP. It will also ensure that clients' needs are met and their safety is not jeopardized.

CREATING A SAFE WORK ENVIRONMENT

Huston (1996) suggests that there are things health care organizations can do to increase the likelihood that UAP are used both effectively and appropriate as members of the health care team.

First, the organization must have a clearly defined organization structure in which RNs are recognized as leaders of the health care team. This organization structure must facilitate RN evaluation of UAP job performance and encourage UAP accountability to the RN. In addition, UAP should be assigned to a specific nurse, not to patients or to tasks, as they are to be under the direct supervision of an RN (Palmier, 1998) (Box 8.3).

Job descriptions must also be developed by health care agencies that clearly define the roles and responsibilities of all categories of care givers. These descriptions should be consistent with that state's Nurse Practice Act as well as community standards of care and should reflect differences between the roles of licensed and unlicensed personnel. Policies should facilitate adequate supervision of UAP by RNs and restrict UAP to simple tasks that can be performed safely. In addition, worker credentials should be readily apparent on the nametags worn by nursing health care personnel.

Second, uniform training and orientation programs for UAP must be established to ensure that preparation is adequate to provide at least minimum standards of safe patient care. These training and orientation programs should be based on clearly defined job descriptions for UAP. Additionally, organizational education programs must be developed for all personnel to learn the roles and responsibilities of different categories of care givers. "Nurses who understand UAP's clinical capabilities and work ethic are more likely to delegate appropriate tasks, freeing the nurse to spend time on activities that require professional judgment and expertise" (Kupperschmidt, 2002, p. 280). In addition, to protect their patients and their professional license, RNs must continue to seek current information regarding national efforts to standardize scope of practice for UAP and professional guidelines regarding what can be safely delegated to UAP.

Additionally, there must be adequate program development in leadership and delegation skills for RNs before UAP are introduced. Delegation is a learned skill and much can be done to better prepare RNs for this role. Educational programs that produce graduate nurses must explore the nature of the RN role, with a focus on professional nurse leadership roles, to better prepare them to meet the challenges of working in restructured health care settings. Practicing RNs should have opportunities for continuing education in the principles of delegation and supervision. This will allow them not only to recognize the limitations of UAP scope of practice, but also to gain confidence in differentiating between skills requiring licensure and those that do not.

Finally, before enlisting the assistance of a UAP, Sheehan (2001) states that nurses should consider the following:

▶ How does this task affect the patient's safety and potential for harm?
▶ What is the stability and acuity of the patient's condition?
▶ What is the nature and complexity of the task?
▶ What type of technology does the task involve?
▶ Will the task effect infection control and safety issues on the unit?

> ## Box 8.3
>
> ### Research Study Fuels the Controversy
>
> **Registered Nurses, Unlicensed Assistive Personnel, and Patient Care**
> To better understand the working relationships between RNs and UAP and the influence this has on patient care delivery, the authors' organization conducted a qualitative investigation involving focus sessions with separate groups of RNs and UAP. Twenty-two staff (13 RN and 9 UAP), representing 22 of 32 patient care units, participated in the study. Subjects were asked to tell their stories of "good" and "difficult" working relationships and the care delivery practices on their units.
>
> > Potter, P., & Grant, E. (January 2004). Understanding RN and unlicensed assistive personnel working relationships in designing care delivery strategies. *Journal of Nursing Administration, 34*(1), 19–25.
>
> ### Study Findings
> Trust was found to be central for effective RN and UAP relationships. Such trust was fostered when UAP were assigned to work with only one RN on a given shift. UAP reported that when they were assigned to work with multiple RNs on a single shift, that it was difficult to partner or work together in ways that built trust or familiarity with one another's work habits. Other qualities that contributed to positive working relationships between RNs and UAP were initiative, good communication, showing an appreciation for each other's contributions, and demonstrating a willingness to help each other with tasks.
>
> The study also found inconsistencies in how UAP orientation was conducted. Some patient care units required UAP to only work with UAP preceptors while others had UAP undergo orientation with RN preceptors for various periods. UAP who did not have an RN mentor found it difficult to understand the RN's role.
>
> The study also revealed that there was no standardized approach used by RNs in providing a beginning shift report to the UAP. UAP did not attend the change-of-shift report. RNs typically provided a report at some point after the change of shift, but times when this occurred varied across units, with delays of 1 to 2 hours being common. The study's authors concluded that joint patient rounds would allow RNs and UAP to share a common plan of care for their assigned patients.
>
> The study concluded that successful RN and UAP partnering allows staff to share a common patient care focus, have ready access to one another during the course of a shift, and have a means to maintain ongoing and timely communication regarding patient conditions and response to treatment. The result is successful working relationships, improved care delivery, and improved patient care outcomes.

▶ THE UNLICENSED ASSISTIVE PERSONNEL SHORTAGE

Finally, if all the issues related to the education, training, scope of practice, and delegation to UAP are resolved, there may be an even greater problem. There may not be enough UAP to meet the need that has been established. High turnover rates and severe shortages of direct-care workers have been the reality the past several years irrespective of care setting (Harmuth, 2002).

There are currently 2.3 million UAP, which comprise almost 25% of all health care workers in health care delivery settings (Rainer, 2004), and a Bureau of Labor Statistics report estimates that by 2008, the demand for nonprofessional direct care staff, such as UAP, will increase by more than 80% from the 1998 level (Kupperschmidt, 2002).

Indeed, currently there is a nationwide shortage of well-trained UAP in all settings and while a majority of states responding to a state-level interagency task force reported recruitment and retention of support personnel as a major area of concern, only 31% were actively addressing the situation (Kovner, 2002). Similarly, a study in 2002 by The Center for Health Workforce Studies in New York, found that 64% of states reported a shortage of certified nurses assistants and 62% reported shortages of home health aides.

One problem contributing to this shortage is the 80% to 100% nationwide annual turnover rate for nursing assistants (Kupperschmidt, 2002). A survey by the University of North Carolina at Chapel Hill's Institute on Aging showed 100% annual turnover rates in North Carolina nursing homes, 119% in adult care homes, and 53% in home care agencies (Harmuth, 2002).

The reasons for this high turnover rate are varied, but low pay and the physical and emotional demands of the job are certainly a part of it. Harmuth (2002) suggests that direct care workers in long-term care often care for persons with cognitive impairments and/or dementia that can result in difficult communications and disruptive behaviors. In addition, many persons being cared for have chronic illnesses that lead to declining health and death.

In addition, some employers provide UAP few, if any, employer-paid benefits such as health insurance coverage, retirement benefits, or child care. Also, there are few career paths for aides who do not want to achieve a licensed job category (e.g. LPN, RN), and some direct care workers complain about the lack of exposure to "real-life" job demands during training (Harmuth, 2002). "Further, even though nurse aides and other direct care workers provide much of the hands-on care, they lack opportunity for meaningful input into patient care planning or health services provision, and they receive inadequate recognition and appreciation by families, residents, or employers" (Harmuth, p. 89).

Working conditions are also often less than ideal. Because of UAP turnover and absenteeism, those UAP who do work, must often work short-handed, which leads to greater stress. A study released by the California HealthCare Foundation in December 2004 showed that only one in 10 of California's skilled nursing facilities fully comply with all federal care standards for minimum nursing staff requirements, and that requirement is only 3.2 hours of nursing care per patient per day (Nursing Homes Fall Short, 2004). To add to all this, UAP have high injury rates—ranking third, in fact, behind truck drivers and laborers for the largest number of work-related injuries and illnesses resulting in time away from work (U.S. Department of Labor, 1999).

> ***CONSIDER:** "The number of staff on duty (in nursing homes) varies according to the three shifts of the day, but the brunt of work falls on the certified nursing aides. They perform the hands-on tasks needed by residents for an average of less than $10 an hour, and the way those direct-care workers approach their jobs makes all the difference in the satisfaction of patients and families" (Rotstein, 2002, para 65).

Overcoming both the current and future UAP shortage will not be easy. The pool of younger females, who traditionally comprise UAP (particularly in long-term care settings), is stagnant (Rotstein, 2002). Rotstein states this lack of manpower—or more accurately, womanpower—is already used often by the long-term care industry to defend its shortcomings. Indeed, a government study found that fewer than one in 10 nursing homes employs the optimum number of nurses and aides. Few facilities are ever cited for understaffing, however, because minimum government standards are set far below the levels needed to help assure high quality care (Rotstein).

Indeed, Rainer (2004) suggests that a variance in minimum staffing levels exists across hospitals and nursing homes and, according to the *Keeping Patients Safe* report, minimum standards for staffing in nursing homes need to be updated. Federal regulations are out of date and do not reflect new knowledge on safe staffing levels. Minimum standards for RNs require only one licensed nurse in a nursing home regardless of its size.

In addition, research by Anthony, Standing, and Hertz (2000), who examined the congruence between RN and UAP perceptions of nursing practice, found significant differences in philosophy of patient care and perceived accountability for team and patients between RNs and UAP. This finding suggests that assumptions about the interchangeability of RNs and UAP in the staffing mix must be examined carefully.

The bottom line, then, is that "the demand for these workers (UAP) is growing rapidly and the difficulty of meeting future demand is exacerbated by the fact that the population of persons who have traditionally filled these jobs is declining. In the absence of timely and successful action to strengthen recruitment and reduce turnover rates, we will not have the sheer numbers of direct care workers needed, much less will we succeed in attracting—and keeping—the caring and dedicated workers that family members and society expect and deserve" (Harmuth, 2002, p.93).

▶ CONCLUSIONS

The increased use of UAP presents both opportunities and challenges for the American health care system. UAP play an increasingly integral role in care delivery today. Indeed, they provide most of the paid long-term care needed in this country (Harmuth, 2002). Harmuth goes so far as to say that UAP are essential to achieving quality care and to preserving, to the greatest extent possible, the dignity and independence of persons who must rely on others for help with care needs. Kupperschmidt (2002, p. 280) agrees, stating that UAP who are "competent, satisfied with their work situation, and have relatively stable work histories can be a major benefit to their organizations."

Yet, the challenge continues to be using UAP only to provide personal care needs or nursing tasks that do not require the skill and judgment of the RN. With increasing patient loads and the current nursing shortage, many health care organizations and the RNs who work within them, are tempted to allow UAP to perform tasks that should be limited to professional nursing practice. Nurses must remember, however, that the responsibility for assuring that patients are protected and that UAP do not exceed their scope of practice, ultimately falls to the RN. The American Association of Nurse Attorneys [AANA] (n.d.) concurs, arguing that "patients must be protected so that only those unlicensed assistive personnel who have been screened, trained and periodically evaluated, are assisting in care." When UAP are allowed to encroach into professional nursing care, patients are placed at risk.

Stepanek (2003, para 21) states: "UAP were brought into health care ostensibly to assist the RN in the provision of care: The lines defining the practice between these nonlicensed 'helpers' and highly-educated RNs have blurred to the point where patients no longer routinely know the qualifications of the person providing their care. Name badges that previously read, 'Registered Nurse' now read 'nursing services staff,' leaving patients uninformed and less than confident. This 'removing of the guardrails' that once ensured patients with quality nursing should be every bit as terrifying as a rocky mountain drive is to a committed acrophobic... if not more so."

When patients approach health care, they too assume that the guardrails are in place; however, for patients, the blurring of the lines between the practice of RNs and UAP makes it nearly impossible to make an informed decision about continuing their journey.

Certainly at some point, given the increasing complexity of health care and the increasing acuity of patient illnesses, there is a maximum representation of UAP in the staffing mix that should not be breached (Huston, 1996). Those levels have not yet been determined. Nor have states been able to reach a consensus regarding the education, training, and scope of practice needed for UAP to safely practice. Until these answers are found, the likelihood is that UAP will continue to constitute a significant portion of the nursing workforce and the boundary between UAP and RN practice will continue to be blurred.

FOR ADDITIONAL DISCUSSION

1. Is cost or the nursing shortage the greater driving force in increased UAP use in acute care hospitals today?
2. Is institutional training and certification of UAP a precursor to future initiatives for institutional licensure of registered nurses?
3. Are the cost savings associated with increased UAP use offset by the need for greater supervision by RNs and potential declines in patient outcomes?
4. Should UAP be allowed to administer medications? Perform intravenous cannulation? Change sterile dressings?
5. Do you believe that patients typically are aware whether it is the UAP or licensed nurse that is caring for them?
6. How comfortable do you believe most RNs are in the role of delegator to UAP? Do you believe most RNs feel clarity regarding role differentiation between the RN and the UAP?
7. Should the training and certification of UAP fall under the purview of state boards of registered nursing?

REFERENCES

Aiken, L. H., Clarke, S. P., Sloane, D. M., & Sochalski, J. (May 2001). Cause for concern: Nurses' reports of hospital care in five countries. LDI Issue Brief. *Leonard Davis Institute of Health Economics, 6*(8), 1–4. Retrieved April 18, 2005, from http://www.upenn.edu/ldi/issuebrief6_8.pdf.

American Association of Nurse Attorneys. (n.d.). *The American Association of Nurse Attorneys Recommendations regarding unlicensed assistive personnel.* Retrieved April 18, 2005, from http://www.taana.org/shownews.asp?newsid = 50.

American Nurses Association (1992) Position statement. *Registered nurse utilization of unlicensed assistive personnel.* Retrieved April 18, 2005, from http://www.nursingworld.org/readroom/position/uap/uapuse.htm.

American Nurses Association (1997). *Attachment I: Definitions related to ANA 1992 position statements on unlicensed assistive personnel.* Retrieved April 18, 2005, from http://www.ana.org/readroom/position/uap/uapuse.htm.

Anthony, M. K., Standing, T., & Hertz, J. E. (October 2000). Factors influencing outcomes after delegation to unlicensed assistive personnel. *Journal of Nursing Administration, 30*(10), 474–481.

Anthony, M. K., Casey, D., Chau, T., & Brennan, P. F. (2000). Congruence between registered nurses' and unlicensed assistive personnel perception of nursing practice. *Nursing Economics, 18*(6), 285–293.

Auckenthaler, L. (November 2002). President's message. Opportunities. *Nevada RNFormation, 11*(4), 3.

Barter, M (2002). Follow the team leader. *Nursing Management, 33*(10), 54–57.

Blegen, M. A., Goode, C. J., & Reed, L. (1998). Nurse staffing and patient outcomes. *Nursing Research, 47*(1), 43–50.

Buerhaus, P. & Staiger, D. (1999). Trouble in the nurse labor market? Recent trends and future outlook for nurse earnings and employment. *Health Affairs, 18*(1), 214–222.

Case, B. (July 19, 2004). Delegation skills. *Advance for Nurses, 1*(3), 20–26.

Center for Health Workforce Studies (November 2002). *State responses to health workers shortages: Results of 2002 survey of states.* School of Public Health. University of Albany–SUNY. Retrieved April 18, 2005, from http://www.phppo.cdc.gov/owpp/docs/library/2002/State%20Responses%20to%20Health%20Workforce%20Shortages.pdf.

Dunton, N., Gajewski, B., Taunton, R. L. & Moore, J. (2004). Nurse staffing and patient falls on acute care hospital units. *Nursing Outlook, 52*(1), 53–59.

Glazer, G. (June 23, 2000). *What makes something a nursing activity or task? Online Journal of Issues in Nursing.* Retrieved April 18, 2005, from http://www.nursingworld.org/ojin/tpclg/leg_9.htm.

Gordon, S. (1997). What nurses stand for. *The Atlantic Monthly, 279*(2), 80–88.

Hall, L. M., Doran, D., & Pink, G. H. (January 2004). Nurse staffing models, nursing hours, and patient safety outcomes. *Journal of Nursing Administration, 34*(1), 41–45.

Harmuth, S. (2002). *The direct care workforce crisis in long-term care. North Carolina Medical Journal, 63*(2), 87–94. Retrieved April 18, 2005, from http://www.ncmedicaljournal.com/mar-apr-02/ar030205.pdf.

Hayes, P. M. (1994). Non-nursing functions: Time for them to go. *Nursing Economics, 12* (3), 120–125.

Hood, L. J. & Leddy, S. K. (2003). *Conceptual bases of professional nursing* (5th ed.). Philadelphia: Lippincott Williams & Wilkins.

Huston, C. (1996). Unlicensed assistive personnel: A solution to dwindling health care resources or the precursor to the apocalypse of registered nursing? *Nursing Outlook, 44*(2), 67–73.

Huston, C. (1997). *The replacement of registered nurses by unlicensed personnel: The impact on three process/outcome indicators of quality.* Unpublished doctoral dissertation, University of Southern California.

Huston, C. (June 2001). Contemporary staffing mix changes: Impact on postoperative pain management. *Pain Management Nursing, 2*(2), 65–72.

Institute of Medicine. (2003). *Keeping patients safe: Transforming the work environment of nurses.* Washington DC. National Academies Press. Available online at www.nap.edu.

Kido, V. (November 2001). The UAP dilemma. *Nursing Management, 32*(11), 27–29.

Kovner, C. (2002). Nursing care providers in home care: A shortage of nonprofessional, direct care staff. *American Journal of Nursing, 102*(1), 91.

Kovner, C. & Gergen P. (1998). Nurse staffing levels and adverse events following surgery in U.S. hospitals. *Image: Journal of Nursing Scholarship, 30*(4), 315–321.

Kupperschmidt, B. R. (2002). Unlicensed assistive personnel retention and realistic job previews. *Nursing Economics, 20*(6), 279–283.

Lichtig, L. K., Knauf, R. A., & Milholland, D. K. (1999). Some impacts of nursing on acute care hospital outcomes. *Journal of Nursing Administration, 29*(2), 25–33.

Marquis, B., & Huston, C. (2006). *Leadership roles and management functions in nursing* (5th ed.). Philadelphia: Lippincott Williams & Wilkins.

McCarthy, A., Kelly, M. W., & Reed, D. (November 2000). Medication administration practices of school nurses. *Journal of School Health, 70*(9), 371–376.

McClung, T. (2000). Assessing the reported financial benefits of unlicensed assistive personnel in nursing. *Journal of Nursing Administration, 30*(11), 530–534.

Morgan, S. P., DeRose, C., & Vallance, J. (Nov. 1, 2003). Reduce workload intensity with PCTs. *Nursing Management, 34*(11), 9.

National Association of School Nurses (June 2002). Position statement. *Using assistive personnel in school health services programs.* Retrieved April 18, 2005, from http://www.nasn.org/positions/2002assistive.htm.

National Council of State Boards of Nursing. (1995). *Delegation: Concepts and decision making process.* National Council of State Boards of Nursing Position Paper. Chicago. Retrieved April 18, 2005, from http://www.ncsbn.org/regulation/uap_delegation_documents_delegation.asp#Introduction.

National Council of State Boards of Nursing (April 1998). *Diagram to illustrate roles of nurses and AP at different points of client competence/self care continuum.* Retrieved April 18, 2005, from http://www.ncsbn.org/regulation/uap_delegation_documents_nurseroles.asp.

Needleman, J., Buerhaus, P., Mattke, S., Stewart, M., & Zelevinsky, K. (May 30, 2002). Nurse staffing levels and the quality of care in hospitals. *New England Journal of Medicine, 346*(22), 1715–1722.

Nursing homes fall short, study finds. (December 1, 2004). *The Sacramento Bee,* p. A3, column 1–3.

Palmier, D. (1998). How can the bedside nurse take a leadership role to affect change for the future? *Concern, 27*(1), 16–17.

Potter, P. & Grant, E. (January 2004). Understanding RN and unlicensed assistive personnel working relationships in designing care delivery strategies. *Journal of Nursing Administration, 34*(1), 19–25.

Rainer, S. (2004). Nurses work environments require changes for the safety of patients. Originally printed in the November-December 2003 issue of *Texas Nursing.* Retrieved August 9, 2004 from http://www.njsna.org/Rainer's%20Report/march_5_2004.htm.

Rotstein, G. (September 22, 2002). No place like home: Nursing homes struggle with too few nurses, aides for growing elderly population. post-gazette.com. *Health and Science.* Retrieved April 18, 2005, from http://www.post-gazette.com/healthscience/20020922nursinghomes0922p1.asp.

Seago, J. (2000). Registered nurses, unlicensed assistive personnel, and organizational cultures in hospitals. *Journal of Nursing Administration, 30*(5), 278–286.

Sheehan, J. P. (April 2001). Legal checkpoints. UAP delegation: A step-by-step process. *Nursing Management, 32*(4), 22.

Simpkins, R. W. (1997). Using task lists with unlicensed assistive personnel. *Insight, 6*(2), 1–5.

Stepanek, C. (December 1, 2003). Executive director's column. Removing the guardrails. *Nebraska Nurse*, 36 (4), 2, 4. Retrieved August 9, 2004 from Ebsco Host.

Texas Nurses Association (2004). *Nursing issues*. Retrieved April 18, 2005, from http://www.texasnurses.org/nursingissues/proposedres_04.htm.

Thomas, S. A., Barter, M., & McLaughlin, F. E. (March 2000). State and territorial boards of nursing approaches to the use of unlicensed assistive personnel. *Journal of Nursing Administration's Healthcare Law, Ethics, and Regulation, 2*(1), 13–21.

Trossman, S. (2002). No shortage of excuses: Nurses worry that health care industry will use staffing crisis to replace RNs. *American Nurse, 34*(6). Retrieved from Academic Search Elite.

Ventura, M. (1999). Staffing issues. *RN, 62* (2), 26–30.

Young, A. (2004). The developing role of EDAs. *Emergency Nurse, 11* (10), 10–11. Retrieved August 9, 2004 from Academic Search Elite.

Zimmermann, P. (2004). Delegating to unlicensed assistive personnel. *Nursing Spectrum*. Education/CE. Self-study modules. Retrieved April 18, 2005, from http://www.medi-smart.com/delegation-ce1.htm.

BIBLIOGRAPHY

Bernreuter, M., and Cardona, M. (1997). Survey and critique of studies related to unlicensed assistive personnel from 1975 to 1997, Part 2. *Journal of Nursing Administration, 27*(7/8), 49–55.

Cady, R. (2001). Focus on the law. Legal issues surrounding the use of unlicensed assistive personnel. *The American Journal of Maternal Child Nursing, 26*(1), 49.

Cardinale, A. (2003). 2-week training not enough.... "Medication administration by unlicensed caregivers: A model program"... June 2003 issue (vol. 29, no. 6). *Journal of Gerontological Nursing, 29* (11), 8.

Conant, S. M. (2004). Viewpoint. Is 'skilled nursing home' a misnomer? Least educated providers constitute largest proportion of workforce. *American Journal of Nursing, 104*(6), 11.

Flores, K. (2000). Board approves task force revisions to Rule 218, Delegation of Selected Nursing Tasks by Registered Professional Nurses to Unlicensed Personnel for public comment. *RN Update, 31*(2), 4.

Fowler, V. (2003). Health care assistants: Developing their role to include nursing tasks. *Nursing Times, 99*(36), 34–37.

Hansten, R. (2001). Continuing education. Delegating to UAPs: Making it work... Unlicensed assistive personnel. *Nurseweek California, 14*(3), 16–18.

Higginbotham, E. (2003). Advice of counsel. Should an unlicensed technical handle invasive tasks? *RN, 66*(9), 77.

Host, P. (2004). *School medication administration*. About Inc. Retrieved April 18, 2005, from http://www.bipolar.about.com/cs/kids_parents/a/0207_schoolmeds.htm.

Kaiser, C. (2002). The UAP dilemma. *Nursing Management, 33*(3), 6.

Kopishke, L. R. (2002). Unlicensed assistive personnel: A dilemma for nurses. *Journal of Legal Nurse Consulting, 13*(1), 3–7.

Kupperschmidt, B. R., (2001). UAPs: To have and to hold. *Nursing Management, 32*(3), 33–35.

Lange, J. W. (2002). Patient identification of caregivers' titles: Do they know who you are? *Applied Nursing Research, 15*(1), 11–18.

McCarthy, A.M. (2000). Medication administration practices of school nurses. *Journal of School Health, 70*(9), 371–376.

Registered nurse utilization of unlicensed assistive personnel. (2000). *Prairie Rose, 69*(3), 5a.

Rhom, L. R. (2002). Delegation of authority. *Journal of Undergraduate Nursing Scholarship, 4*(1). Retrieved April 18, 2005, from http://juns.nursing.arizona.edu/articles/Fall%202002/Rohm.htm.

Spellbring, A. M. (2003). Medication administration by unlicensed caregivers: A model program. *Journal of Gerontological Nursing, 29* (6), 48–54.

Spencer, S. A. (2001). Education, training, and use of unlicensed assistive personnel in critical care. *Critical Care Nursing Clinics of North America, 13*(1), 105–118.

Standing, T. (2001). Nurses' narratives of outcomes after delegation to unlicensed assistive personnel. *Outcomes Management for Nursing Practice, 5*(1), 18–23.

Suchanek, M. K. (2000). Surgical technologists... "health policy issues" article regarding unlicensed assistive personnel (UAP) (2000). *Association of Perioperative Registered Nurses Journal, 72*(2), 179–180.

Sullivan, G. J. (2004). Advice of counsel. Protecting patients from an aide who is careless. *RN, 67*(1), 68.

Sullivan, G. J. (2003). Advice of counsel. How to manage unlicensed staffers to reduce risk. *RN, 66*(11), 76.

Thomas, S. A. (2000). State and territorial boards of nursing approaches to the use of unlicensed assistive personnel. *Journal of Nursing Administration's Healthcare Law, Ethics and Regulation, 2*(1), 13–21.

Tuttas, C.A. (2003). Decreasing nurse staffing costs in a hospital setting. *Journal of Nursing Care Quality, 18*(3), 226–240.

Workplace restructuring may include certified medication aides. (2004). *Arizona Nurse, 57*(1), 6.

Zimmermann, P. G. (2000). The use of unlicensed assistive personnel: An update and skeptical look at a role that may present more problems than solutions. *Journal of Emergency Nursing, 26*(4), 312–317.

WEB RESOURCES

American Association of Colleges of Nursing. Tri Council for Nursing. Statement on Assistive Personnel to the Registered Nurse.

http://www.aacn.nche.edu/Publications/positions/tricounc.htm

AORN Official Statement on Unlicensed Assistive Personnel (Sunset Review 10/2004)

http://www.aorn.org/about/positions/unlicensed.htm

Commonwealth of Massachusetts. Principles for Appropriate Utilization of Unlicensed Assistive Personnel in Acute Care Hospitals.

http://www.mass.gov/dph/dhcq/cicletter/princip2.htm

National Association of School Nurses (NASN). Position Statement. Using Assistive Personnel in School Health Services Programs. (2002)

http://www.nasn.org/positions/2002ps/assistive.htm

1992 ANA Position Statement- Registered Nurse Utilization of Unlicensed Assistive Personnel. Updated 1997.

http://www.nursingworld.org/readroom/position/uap/uapuse.htm

New Jersey State Nurses Association Position Statement on Unlicensed Assistive Personnel (Revised 9/99)

http://www.njsna.org/Position_Statements/Unlicensed_Assistive_Personnel.html

Oncology Nursing Society. Position statement on the use of assistive personnel in cancer care. Revised September 2002.

http://www.ons.org/publications/positions/AssistivePersonnel.shtml

The Role of Unlicensed Assistive Personnel in The Nursing Care for Women and Newborns. Association of Women's Health, Obstetric, and Neonatal Nurses (AWOHNN) position statement.

http://www.awhonn.org/awhonn/?pg=875-4730-5400-7330

U.S. Department of Labor. Bureau of Health Statistics. Nursing, Psychiatric, and Home Health Aides. (Modified March 24, 2004)

http://stats.bls.gov/oco/ocos165.htm

Diversity in the Nursing Workforce

Carol J. Huston

9

Diversity has been defined as the differences among groups or between individuals. Many definitions of diversity include the acknowledgment that not everyone is alike and that these differences must be acknowledged for understanding and growth to occur (Cook, 2003).

Diversity in any given population comes in the form of age, gender, religion, customs, sexual orientation, physical size, physical and mental capabilities, beliefs, culture, ethnicity, and skin color; it also encompasses opportunity and representation (Waters, 2004). Yet, despite increasing diversity (particularly ethnic and cultural) in this country, the nursing workforce is homogenous, at least in terms of ethnicity and gender. For decades, the overwhelming majority of nurses in the United States have been White, female, and middle-aged (Newell-Withrow & Slusher, 2001).

This lack of ethnic, gender, and generational diversity is a concern not only for the nursing profession, but also for the clients who are served. A review of the literature reveals a clamor for greater diversity as a profession. Raymond Grady, Board Chairperson of the Institute for Diversity in Health Management, stated:

> *There is irrefutable evidence that the demographics of our society are changing. The patients and families who come to our hospitals for care will reflect these demographic shifts. If we are to assure the delivery of high quality, culturally sensitive, and proficient health care, then the physicians, nurses, technicians, and executives responsible for delivering that care must reflect the communities they serve (Catholic Health Association, 2004, para 3).*

Indeed, Gould (2003) argues that it is only through a diverse provider community that racial and ethnic minorities can receive the highest quality of care.

Historically, despite this stated need for and appreciation of the benefits of a diverse health care workforce, efforts to increase the number of minority professionals have not been highly successful. The reasons for this are many, but Bowen and Bok (1998) argue that the roots are found in racism, lack of sustained funding for the programs, and lack of institutional commitment.

Discussion Point

For nursing care to be culturally and ethnically sensitive, must it be provided by a culturally and ethnically diverse nursing population?

This chapter focuses primarily on three aspects of diversity in the nursing workforce: ethnicity, gender, and generational. Factors leading to the lack of ethnic and gender diversity in nursing are explored, as are individual and organizational strategies to address the problem. (The importation of foreign nurses as a factor in workforce diversity is discussed in Chapter 6.) In addition, the efforts of current professional nursing organizations to increase diversity in the profession are examined. Finally, the impact of generational diversity on workers and workplace functioning is presented.

▶ ETHNIC DIVERSITY

Ethnic Diversity in the United States

Demographic data from the 2000 U.S. Census showed that the U.S. population has continued to diversify over the past 30 years, with minority populations increasing at a faster rate than the White, non-Hispanic population (U.S. Census Bureau, 2000). The seven ethnic categories in the 2000 census were:

1. White
2. Black or African American
3. Hispanic
4. Asian
5. American Indian and Alaska Native
6. Native Hawaiian and other Pacific Islanders
7. Some other race

In interpreting U.S. Census Bureau data for 2000, the question on race was different from the race question on the 1990 census in several ways. Most significantly, respondents were given the option of selecting one or more race categories to indicate their racial identities; however, minorities who reported their race as White, either alone or in combination with one or more other races, were included in the numbers for Whites in 2000.

Census 2000 data showed that the White, non-Hispanic population was still the largest racial and ethnic group in the United States, comprising approximately 69% of the population. This was down from about 83% in 1970, but in total numbers, at approximately 196.8 million in 2002, it was the highest it has ever been (U.S. Census, 2003).

U.S. Census Bureau data also revealed that in 2002, the Hispanic population became the largest minority in the United States, comprising approximately 13.5% of the U.S. population (U.S. Census, 2003). This was up from approximately 4.5% in 1970, the first census in which Hispanic origin was identified. The Black population comprised approximately 13% of the total population, while Asians and Pacific Islanders comprised approximately 4% of the population. American Indians and Alaska Natives comprised only 1% of the population. And for the first time in the history of the census, approximately 2.4% of the population chose to identify themselves as belonging to more than one race. Predictions are that ethnic minorities will comprise an estimated 37% of the population in the United States by 2025 (U.S. Census Bureau, 1999).

Ethnic Diversity in Nursing

There were significant differences between the ethnic and gender demographics of the U.S. population and those of the nursing workforce in the United States in the year 2000 (Table 9.1). The 2000 National Sample Survey of Registered Nurses showed that 12.3 %, or 333,368, of all registered nurses (RNs) in the United States reported being from one or more racial or ethnic minority backgrounds (News from NINR, 2001). This is higher than the 246,364 minority nurses (9.7%) reported in 1997 (Buerhaus & Auerbach, 1999), yet considerably lower than the 31% minority representation found in the general population.

Male nurses are a bit more diverse than their female counterparts; however, the differences are small. Eighty-six percent of male nurses are White (non-Hispanic), 6% are Asian–Pacific Islander, 4% are Hispanic, 3% are Black (non-Hispanic), and 1% are American Indian/Alaskan Native (Chung, 2003).

TABLE 9.1

Comparison of U.S. Population and Registered Nurse Workforce in Terms of Ethnicity and Gender

Characteristic	Year 2000 U.S. Census Data (% representation)	Year 2000 Registered Nurse Workforce (% representation)
Gender: men	49	5.4
Gender: women	51	94.6
White (non-Hispanic)	69	86.6
Black/African American	13	4.9
Asian	4.2	3.5
Native Hawaiian/Pacific Islander		
American Indian/Alaskan native	1	0.5
Hispanic/Latino	13.5	2.0
Two or more races	2.4	1.2

Source: The Registered Nurse Population, 2000; U.S. Census Bureau, 2003.

Clearly, increasing diversity in the nursing profession must begin with the aggressive recruitment and retention of minority students. Staiger, Auerbach, and Buerhaus (2003) note that the number of racial and ethnic minorities enrolled in nursing schools during the 2000–2001 academic year increased slightly from the previous year, according to the annual survey by the American Association of Colleges of Nursing (AACN). Minorities graduating from nursing programs with a bachelor of arts or an advanced degree (e.g., master of science in nursing, master of arts in nursing, doctorate, or Nursing Doctorate) also showed slight increases compared with the previous year. However, this growth was not experienced by all racial/ethnic minorities or for all degrees, and there were fewer White graduates as well.

Recruiting Minority Students Into Nursing

Carol (2001) suggests that the nursing profession has failed to tap into underrecruited, diverse cultural groups such as African Americans, Hispanic Americans, Latino Americans, and Native Americans. Many experts suggest this is because many diverse groups of women and men are economically disadvantaged and are the product of inferior education systems that are not open to or accepting of diversity (Newell-Withrow & Slusher, 2001). Often this has led to an underdevelopment of basic learning skills such as reading, writing, and critical thinking (Parker, 1998); thus, some diverse students are unable to achieve the grades and test scores required to enter nursing schools. Newell-Withrow and Slusher concur, arguing that although academic achievement is an important predictor of success in nursing, inadequate recognition has been given to commitment, dedication, and a strong sense of caring.

The AACN (2002, para 6) also agrees, arguing that "increasing diversity implies expanding the traditional pool of qualified applicants for the academic experience and employment by appropriately defining variables reflecting the value and worth of the human experience." It should require an admissions and employment process that fully encompasses the principles of equal opportunity, and qualified applicants should represent the cultural, racial, ethnic, economic, gender, and social diversity of the broader population. The goal, then, "should be to create a community of culturally competent scholars, including faculty, students, staff, and practitioners, who support a world view of interconnectivity and community" (AACN, 2002, para 6).

*CONSIDER: Retention of minority nursing students should improve if these students are given solid academic preparation and if the environment in which they are educated is accepting of and hospitable to students from diverse backgrounds.

Progress, however, is slow. Price (2001) reports that there is a correlation between professionals' acceptance of diversity and increases in the numbers of diverse groups in the nursing workforce. The same is likely true for nursing education. Newell-Withrow and Slusher (2001) suggest that when diversity is conceptualized, there is a need to think in broader terms that lead to new models for learning, such as integration of students' lived experiences into nursing curriculums and incorporation of paradigms that build on the wealth of experiences that the students bring to nursing and nursing education, while enhancing basic learning skills.

Discussion Point

Should more resources (time, energy, money) be devoted to recruitment or retention of minority students? Is a two-pronged approach (emphasizing both recruitment and retention) necessary?

170 Retaining Minority Students in Nursing

Despite the challenges inherent in recruiting minority students, recruiting them is often easier than retaining them. The literature overwhelmingly suggests that minority students face more barriers than their White counterparts. Some of these barriers are shown in Box 9.1.

Inadequate preparation at the high school level (poor study habits as well as inadequate writing, reading, and communication skills) is a major contributor to the attrition rate of minority students (Abriam-Yago, 2002; Feist-Price, 2001; Villarruel, Canales, & Torres, 2001). In addition, because many minority students are the first in their families to attend college, it is difficult for family members to provide adequate support due to their lack of information about college and the rigors of higher education (Abriam-Yago, 2002; Feist-Price, 2001).

Finances are also often a barrier to minority students, who must work at least part time to subsidize the cost of their college education. In addition, when faced with the decision of whether to continue their education, many minority students' decisions are heavily influenced by their financial situation (Nugent, Childs, Jones, & Cook, 2004).

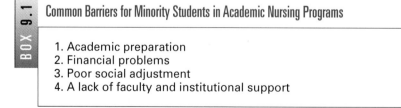

BOX 9.1

Common Barriers for Minority Students in Academic Nursing Programs

1. Academic preparation
2. Financial problems
3. Poor social adjustment
4. A lack of faculty and institutional support

Source: Nugent, Childs, Jones, & Cook, 2004.

Minority students also tend to experience more difficulty with social adjustment in the college environment, particularly when they are attending a predominantly White institution. Feelings of isolation, not belonging, and not being understood are common among minority students (Furr & Elling, 2002; Steffan Dickerson, Neary, & Hyche-Johnson, 2000). This is especially true when there are small numbers of minority faculty and administrators.

Nugent et al. (2004) suggest that to improve the retention and graduation rates of minority students in nursing, an educational environment supporting the needs of all students, regardless of cultural, ethnic, or gender background, must exist. This environment must include academic support, financial support, self-development and professional/leadership development, faculty mentoring, and institutional awareness.

The Health Resources and Services Administration (HRSA) is currently addressing the need for financial support by offering the Health Careers Opportunity Program, Centers of Excellence and Minority Faculty Fellowship grants to schools and health professions training programs to increase diversity within the health fields. The grants provide disadvantaged and underrepresented minority students and faculty opportunities to enhance their academic skills and obtain the support needed to graduate from health professions schools or faculty development programs. HRSA also provides grants to health professions training programs to create scholarships, loans, and loan repayments for disadvantaged students and faculty (HRSA National Survey, 2001).

Wenzel and Utz (2002) suggest that another strategy to promote minority student retention and graduation from schools of nursing is to create a success-oriented milieu and to provide supplementary opportunities to enhance student learning. These strategies will transmit the joy of learning to minority students and promote a thirst for new knowledge while enhancing student socialization.

Perhaps one of the most articulate and well-organized documents for helping nurse educators develop strategies to assist culturally diverse students in being successful, regardless of their educational level, has been created by the AACN. This document, *Effective Strategies for Increasing Diversity in Nursing Programs* (AACN, 2001), highlights numerous successful campaigns undertaken by nursing schools to increase diversity in their nursing programs. Examples of strategies in the seven key areas identified in the document are shown in Box 9.2.

> *CONSIDER: Nugent et al. (2004) suggest that although much emphasis has traditionally been placed on recruitment strategies targeting minority students, it is the retention and graduation of minority students that will begin to change the cultural face of nursing.

BOX 9.2   Seven Key Strategy Areas Identified in AACN's Effective Strategies for Increasing Diversity in Nursing Programs (2001)

1. Presenting an inclusive image
2. Reaching out to diverse student populations
3. Making connections at the middle/high school level
4. Supporting students through the application process
5. Mentoring as the key to retention
6. Facilitating student success
7. Launching a coordinated outreach campaign

Ethnic Diversity in Education and Health Care Administration

The exact number of minority nurses in leadership positions has not been determined; however, data from the AACN 2000–2001 Salaries of Instructional and Administrative Nursing Faculty in Baccalaureate and Graduate Programs in Nursing survey suggests that only 9.2% of all full-time instructional faculty members in baccalaureate and graduate programs are members of racial/ethnic minority groups. There was no significant increase over the previous year (Staiger, Auerbach, & Buerhaus, 2003).

In addition, when compared to the previous year's figures, there was very little change in the number of minority faculty members who held full professorships (9.9% in 1999–2000 vs. 9.3% in 2000–2001), but the number of associate and assistant minority professors declined (22% vs. 24% and 42% vs. 44.2%, respectively). Additionally, there was a decrease in the number of tenured or tenure track minority nurse faculty between the two academic years, but the number of non–tenure track minority faculty was up by approximately 5% (35.4% vs. 30%) (Staiger et al., 2003).

Research suggests that although minority percentages are increasing in nursing, a significant divide exists between Black and White health care executives, especially at the senior decision-making levels. According to research conducted by the National Association of Health Services Executives (NAHSE), the American College of Healthcare Executives (ACHE), and the Institute for Diversity in Health Management, 62% of White male respondents hold top executive positions, while only 44% of Black male respondents are in the same job (Gould, 2003). The numbers are even worse for women, with 44% of White female respondents holding top jobs, and just 26% of Black women (Box 9.3).

Similarly, reports heard at the first national London Black and Minority National (LBMN) Health Service Network conference in 2003 suggested that the United Kingdom's Black and ethnic minority nurses are being denied senior nursing roles in favor of White co-workers (Minority Nurses Denied, 2003). Despite 38.2% of the workforce at London's King's College Hospital being Black or of ethnic minority origin, only 22.4% of these nurses held senior roles. Spokesperson Wendy Gay, head of human resources at the hospital, affirmed that minority nurses were applying for senior nursing positions, but fewer were being short listed for the posts than White applicants, and they were being appointed in even fewer numbers (Minority Nurses Denied, 2003).

Burda (2003, para 1) goes so far as to say that "the field of health care management continues to be an old boy's network and it's getting even Whiter despite efforts to promote racial and gender diversity in the ranks of the industry leadership." This comment followed the release of an ACHE study conducted in collaboration with the Association of Hispanic Healthcare Executives, the Executive Leadership Development Program of the Indian Health Services, the Institute for Diversity in Health Management, and the NAHSE. This study of 1,621 health care executives in 2002 showed that 62% of the White males in the sample held senior management positions (chief executive officer, chief operating officer, and senior vice-president), up from 51% in 1997, and that the percentage point gap between White male and female senior health care executives had increased from 16 percentage points to 22 in the same time period (Burda).

In addition, more than half of the RNs in racial/ethnic minority groups who are in the workforce hold less than a baccalaureate education (National Advisory Council on Nurse Education and Practice, 2000), which likely limits their opportunities for advancement into leadership positions. Racial and ethnic minorities are also underrepresented as nurse researchers (Ezenwa, 2003). As a result, the National Institutes of Health funds the

BOX 9.3

Research Study Fuels the Controversy

Executive Health Care Positions and Race

The National Association of Health Services Executives (NAHSE), the American College of Healthcare Executives (ACHE), and the Institute for Diversity in Health Management attempted to document the representation of Blacks, Hispanics, and other minorities in senior health care executive leadership with three rounds of studies in 1992, 1997, and 2002.

> Gould, S. (2003). A long road ahead: Diversity studies show progress but minority, women execs still lack opportunities. *Modern Healthcare, 33*(34), 37.

Study Findings

The studies document that although the positive percentages are rising, a significant divide continues to exist between Black and White health care executives, especially at the senior decision-making levels. Sixty-two percent of White male respondents hold top executive positions, while only 44% of Black male respondents are in such jobs. The numbers are worse for women. Forty percent of White female respondents hold the top jobs, while just 26% of Black females do.

Although minorities are faring better in raw percentage terms since 1992, a closer review reveals that Whites tend to be running hospitals, agencies, and systems, while minorities are making strides mostly at the level of departmental, clinical, and association management.

Gould speculates that the "glass ceiling" is still in existence as a result of discrimination, and that when controlled for experience, one must acknowledge that the longevity of Blacks in top executive positions is much less than that of their White counterparts. Black executives leave these positions more frequently than Whites because of lack of salary increases, discrimination and disparity in the boardroom, and the presence of long-serving Whites in more senior positions. Only half of the White respondents said they thought something needed to be done to change the situation.

173

Stipends for Training Aspiring Researchers program to enhance recruitment of minority students into research careers.

Ethnic Professional Associations in Nursing

There is a professional association for almost every ethnic group in nursing, including the National Black Nurses Association, established in 1971; the National Association of Hispanic Nurses, founded in 1975; the Philippine Nurses Association of America, formed in 1979; and the National Alaska Native American Indian Nurses Association. See Box 9.4 for more information on these groups.

Discussion Point

If our goal is to better appreciate and merge cultural and ethnic diversity in nursing, why do culturally and ethnically diverse nurses separate themselves with their own professional nursing organizations?

BOX 9.4

Ethnic Professional Associations in Nursing

Support groups and professional associations abound among nurses in the United States. Some of the groups formed to address specific issues related to ethnic diversity in nursing include the following:

National Black Nurses Association

The National Black Nurses Association (NBNA), founded in 1971, represents approximately 150,000 Black nurses from the United States (with 76 chartered chapters nationwide), the Eastern Caribbean nations, and Africa, (NBNA, n.d.). The mission of the NBNA is to provide a forum for collective action by Black nurses to "investigate, define and determine what the health care needs of African Americans are and to implement change to make health care available to African Americans and other minorities that is commensurate with that [health care] of the larger society."(NBNA)

National Association of Hispanic Nurses

The National Association of Hispanic Nurses (NAHN), founded in 1975, strives to serve the nursing and health care delivery needs of the Hispanic community and the professional needs of Hispanic nurses (NAHN, n.d.). NAHN is committed to improve the quality of health and nursing care for Hispanic consumers and to provide equal access to educational, professional, and economic opportunities for Hispanic nurses.

Philippine Nurses Association of America

The Philippine Nurses Association of America (PNAA) was formed in 1979 in an effort to address the issues and concerns of Filipino nurses in the United States. Its mission is to widen the Filipino nurses' global perspective by providing a link through which they can communicate and promote fellowship with nurses from the mainland United States, the Philippines, and other places, and if called for, to join forces in enhancing and uplifting the well-being of Filipino nurses (PNAA, n.d.).

National Alaska Native American Indian Nurses Association

The National Alaska Native American Indian Nurses Association (NANAINA) was founded upon its predecessor organization, the American Indian Nurses Association and later, the American Indian Alaska Native Nurses Association. The NANAINA is dedicated to supporting Alaska Native and American Indian students, nurses, and allied health professionals through the development of leadership skills and continuing education. It also advocates for the improvement of health care provided to American Indian and Alaska Native consumers and culturally competent health care (NANAINA, 2004). Similar goals exist for the Asian and Pacific Islander population as described by the Asian and Pacific Islander Nurses Association.

▶ GENDER DIVERSITY

Gender Diversity in Nursing

Diversity goals in nursing are not just directed at ethnicity—they also frequently include increasing the number of men in nursing. Just 5.9% of the nation's 2.7 million RNs are men (up from 5.4% in 1996), according to the March 2000 National Sample Survey of Registered Nurses. Males also account for approximately 8% of students enrolled in 4-year college nursing programs (Doheny, 2004; HRSA National Survey, 2001). These are the highest percentages since the 1900s.

Despite a call to increase the number of men in nursing, progress in this regard has been slow for many reasons. Stereotypes of male nurses as being different or gay due to their close working relationship with women abound, and there are few male faculty role models in nursing. Many nursing textbooks refer to the comforting caregiver nurse as "she," and make no mention of the male gender, except as sickly, demanding patients.

[*CONSIDER: Caregiving is not just a feminine trait.]

These stereotypes suggest that male nurses are incapable of, or at least less capable of, caring, compassion, and nurturing than female nurses. Clearly, this is not the case, yet it does pose socialization and acceptance challenges for male nurses. In Milligan's (2001) qualitative study of male nurses working in acute care hospital settings, male nurses emphasized meeting patient needs, effective communication, and information giving as core components of their practice. Yet they were sensitive to the male stereotype that they would be less capable in completing these tasks.

Negative stereotypes also emerged in Evans's (2002) study of male nurses who reported being cast in stereotypes of being either a sexual aggressor or gay. Study participants suggested that these stereotypes sexualize the touch of male nurses and create complex and contradictory situations of acceptance, rejection, and suspicion of men as nurturers and caregivers. They also situated male nurses in highly stigmatized roles in which they were subject to accusations of inappropriate behavior. Evans reported that for male nurses, this situation creates a heightened sense of vulnerability and the continual need to be cautious while touching and caring for patients. Ultimately, this situation impacts on the ability of male nurses to do the caring work they came into nursing to do. This difficulty of socializing into what has long been perceived as a woman's occupation is depicted in Figure 9.1.

At least partly as a result of these stereotypes, some patients have gender preferences (more commonly female) for their caregivers. In a longitudinal study of gender, age, and experience on preferences for female or male nurses, Chur-Hansen (2002) found that younger females prefer young female nurses. Experience with male nurses was limited, but was not highly predictive of preferences or attitudes. In-depth, qualitative research was recommended to understand better the reasons for preferences and attitudes in both male and female patients.

In addition, Whittock and Leonard (2003) note that male nurses experience exclusion from gender-specific areas of care, and that these exclusions come primarily from female nursing colleagues rather than female patients. McCrae (2003) appropriately questions this strong bias against male obstetric nurses because obstetricians are traditionally male.

In addition, two court cases have confused the issue further. In one case, the courts ruled that female gender is a legitimate qualification for labor and delivery nurses yet the Equal Employment Opportunity Commission determined these qualifications to be discriminatory (Boughn, 1994; Cude, 2004).

Russell Tranbarger, President of the American Assembly for Men in Nursing (AAMN), suggests that the challenges men face in nursing are the same ones they have faced for many years—a need to degender nursing and to overcome the concept that nursing is a woman's job (LeMaire, 2003). Tranbarger goes on to say:

> Look in our nursing journals and we see an awful lot of women. Two of the men on the Vietnam Wall are male nurses, yet we don't hear of them. Three thousand men were drafted into the Army in 1965 as nurses, yet they tell you they never needed to draft nurses because a ready supply of women volunteered. That's just not the case. There were many male nurses working at the World Trade Center site, and it was good to see some interviewed by the news media. That provided a positive visibility for men in nursing (LeMaire, 2003, para 11).

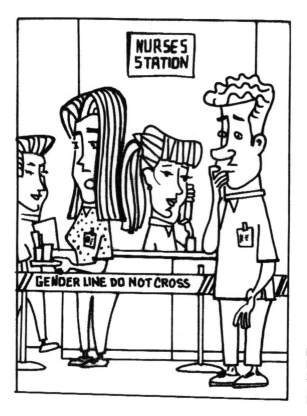

FIGURE 9.1 Challenges faced by men in nursing. Copyright 2002, MedZilla, Inc. *http://www.medzilla.com.* Reprinted with permission.

According to AACN, nursing schools are spearheading the national campaign to increase gender diversity in the profession. But many experts feel that simply getting more male bodies into classroom seats is not enough. Nursing programs, they argue, must also make significant changes in their curricula and teaching styles to create a more positive and nondiscriminatory learning environment for nursing students who happen to be men (Williams, 2003).

Is There a Male Advantage in Nursing?

In contrast to these arguments, Kleinman (2004) suggests that the minority status of men in nursing often results in advantages, including hiring and promotion, that help rather than hinder their careers, unlike women in male-dominated professions. Indeed, research undertaken by Whittock, Edwards, McLaren, and Robinson (2002) suggested that working part-time and taking career breaks, more common to female nurses, results in female nurses falling behind male colleagues in terms of career development and promotion prospects. In addition, managers tended to select men over women (particularly those who work part-time) for advancement roles in the hospital setting.

Additionally, although sex role stereotyping may limit recruitment of men into nursing, Kleinman (2004) suggests these obstacles to entry into practice are superseded by a quest for personal and professional power among men that facilitates professional career advancement in nursing. Kleinman suggests this occurs because traditional health care organizations were organized and managed along the lines of patriarchal family structures that favor male dominance. Under this system, men have been socialized to issue orders, assign tasks, and provide a sense of direction, whereas women suggest, support, and carry out orders (Cunningham, 1999). Similarly, Boughn (2001) states that although male and female nursing students seek empowerment, female students want to empower others whereas male students want to empower themselves.

Men in nursing also appear to have an economic advantage. In a study of 28,955 nurses from the 1992 and 1996 National Sample Survey of Registered Nurses, Kalist (2002) reported that male nurses averaged approximately 12% more in earnings than their female counterparts, approximately $48,833 as compared to $43,472. Approximately 90% of the female–male earnings differential could not be explained by variables in the regression model.

Similarly, a salary survey of more than 1,000 nurses in 2003 demonstrated salary gaps for nurses based on gender, but suggested that the disparity is decreasing (Steltzer, Woods, & Gasda, 2003). In 2003, the difference between male and female nurse salaries was $1,700, much narrower than the $5,361 deficit reported in 2002 by Kalist.

> *CONSIDER: Many experts suggest that the power of the profession would be elevated if more men were to become nurses. Yet, men in nursing hold a disproportionately large share of the high-income jobs in nursing and have higher salaries than their female counterparts.

Why Are Men Leaving Nursing?

In an analysis of RNs' intentions to leave their position, Rambur, Palumbo, McIntosh, and Mongeon (2003) found that 23% of male nurses intended to leave their positions, as compared to 20% of the female nurses. Of those intending to leave, however, 75% of the males were intending to leave for reasons of job dissatisfaction, in comparison to 50% of the females. Furthermore, males were more likely to be intending to leave as a result of dissatisfaction with salary, with 53% of males citing this reason as compared to 26% of females.

> *CONSIDER: Recent graduates of the nation's nursing schools are leaving the profession more quickly than their predecessors, with male nurses leaving at a much higher rate than their female counterparts.

The study also found that the dropout rate for new graduates of both genders is accelerating—increasing from 2% of men in 1992 to 7.5% of men in 2000, and from 2.7% of women in 1992 to 4.1% of women in 2000. Approximately 7.5% of new male nurses left the profession within 4 years of graduating from nursing school, compared to 4.1% of new female nurses (Is There a Male Nurse?, 2002). Some experts argue that this is because nursing still lacks status and therefore nurses are often demeaned by other health professionals. Male nurses may be less willing to tolerate this kind of treatment.

Job satisfaction also differs by gender, with 75% of new female nurses reporting they were satisfied with their jobs compared with only 67% of male nurses. Among nurses established in their careers, 69% of women and 60% of men reported being satisfied with their jobs (Is There a Male Nurse?, 2002).

Recruiting Men Into Nursing: Is Affirmative Action Required?

Dr. Luther Christman points to the mysterious lack of affirmative action in nursing as one of the major reasons for the shortage of men in nursing (Medzilla Asks: Is There a Need?,

2002). He says that affirmative action worked in medicine, paving the way for women to become doctors, and engineering, where women were once shunned.

Today, according to 2002/2003 and prior editions of the *Physician Characteristics and Distribution in the U.S.*, representation of female physicians in medicine continues to show steady increases (Medzilla Asks: Is There a Need?, 2002). In 1980, women comprised 11.6% of the physician workforce, but by 2000 they accounted for 24% of the total physician population. In the academic year 2000–2001, of the students enrolled in U.S. medical schools 44.6% were women, according to the American Medical Association.

D i s c u s s i o n   P o i n t

Affirmative action has been used successfully to increase the presence of some underrepresented minorities in health care. Should the same be done to increase the number of men in nursing?

According to Dr. Christman, although the least expensive and easiest way to increase men in nursing would be affirmative action, legislators are slow to support the concept. According to Dr. Christman:

> *There were two studies done years ago—one was done at the University of Pennsylvania in the early '60s and that showed that only 23% of women worked full time from the time they graduated until they retired in nursing. But 97% of men worked full time; the same as men do in all the professions. Some 20 years later the University of Illinois replicated the study and found there was a change. Now 32% of women were working full time but the men's record was the same. When I bring this up at nurse meetings, I get nothing but a cold stare. No one wants to break the grip of White women on nursing. It's a built in construct (Christman, as cited in Medzilla Asks: Is There a Need?, 2002, para 8).*

Heasley says that to attract men into nursing there will have to be a paradigm shift, starting with a new name and image (Medzilla Asks: Why Are There So Few Male Nurses?, 2002). He questions whether nurses should be called *medics*, because this is a term that could be positive for both men and women.

▶ GENERATIONAL DIVERSITY IN NURSING

The average age of an RN in this country is somewhere between 44 and 46 years of age (Berliner & Ginzberg, 2002; Buerhaus, Staiger, & Auerbach, 2000). In addition, over two-thirds of registered nurses are age 40 and older, and less than 10% are under the age of 30 (Wakefield, 2001). Clearly, if one believes that ethnically and gender diverse providers are needed to appropriately care for diverse populations, then attention must be paid to generational diversity as well.

Age: The Latest Issue

"During the last six or seven years, the whole idea of age has become the latest diversity issue, taking its place up there beside gender, race, color and creed," said Carolyn Martin,

PhD, dean of faculty at Rainmaker Thinking Inc., Connecticut, at the journal *Nursing Management*'s Recruitment & Retention Conference in Orlando, Florida. "As long as there have been human people on this planet, there has been generational conflict" (Wood, 2003, para 2).

The problem, then, is not that the nursing workforce lacks generational diversity, but that typically, four generations have not cohabitated together, at the same time, in a profession. Given the current nursing shortage and the need both to retain and recruit older nurses and to bring new, young nurses into the field, generational issues must be examined further.

Defining the Generations

The research increasingly suggests that the different generations represented in nursing today have different value systems, which greatly impacts the settings in which they work. Hill (2004) describes the "veteran generation" as those nurses born between 1925 and 1942. Having lived through several international military conflicts (World War II, the Korean War, and Vietnam), they're often averse to risk (particularly in regard to personal finances), respectful of authority, supportive of hierarchy, and disciplined (Hill). These nurses are less likely to question organizational practices and more likely to seek employment in structured settings (Marquis & Huston, 2006).

McNeese-Smith and Crook (2003) posit that the "boom generation" (born 1943–1960) and the "silent [or veteran] generation" (born 1925–1942) have more traditional work values and ethics; however, the boom nurses are more materialistic and are willing to work long hours at their jobs. Hill (2004) points out, however, that many nurses in this age group have been taught to think as individuals from a young age and to express themselves creatively. These nurses then may be best suited for work that requires flexibility, independent thinking, and creativity.

"Generation Xers" (born between 1961 and 1981), in contrast, may lack the interest in lifetime employment at one place that prior generations have valued, instead valuing greater work hour flexibility (McNeese-Smith & Crook, 2003). Hill (2004) argues that this is because family structure changed during this generation's formative years. Many were raised as latchkey children because both parents worked outside the home. Many of this generation became disillusioned with the values of corporate America. Thus, this generation, while no less interested in success than the generations preceding them, typically chooses to define success in their own terms (Hill).

"Generation Y" (born 1978–1986) represents the first cohort of truly global citizens; these nurses frequently seek roles that will push their limits (Martin, 2003). They are also optimistic, upbeat, self-confident, volunteer-minded, and socially conscious, all of which have staffing implications.

Hill (2004) suggests that although generational diversity poses new management challenges, it also provides a variety of perspectives and outlooks that enhance workplace balance and productivity. Hill goes on to say that recognizing and integrating the different generations will increase understanding among peers and will help peers feel more positive about themselves, their peers, their jobs, and the efforts of management. In addition, patients should benefit from the optimal outcomes that occur as a result of a higher-performing team.

Gerke (2001) concurs, arguing that generational diversity is not new, but that four generations working side by side has not occurred before. This climate offers challenges and opportunities for leaders, and also provides opportunities to further diversify a workforce to more closely resemble the clients they serve and to identify the best thinking of so many perspectives.

▶ PROFESSIONAL ORGANIZATIONS SPEAK OUT

Many professional nursing organizations have issued position statements or recommendations on diversity in the past decade. In 1997, AACN, the national voice for baccalaureate and higher degree education programs, drafted a position statement that suggests that diversity and inclusion have emerged as central issues for organizations and institutions and that leadership in nursing must respond to these issues by finding ways to accelerate the inclusion of groups, cultures, and ideas that traditionally have been underrepresented in higher education (AACN, 2002). Moreover, the position statement argues that health care providers and the nursing profession should reflect and value the diversity of the populations and communities they serve.

The American Nurses Association (ANA) (1998) issued a position statement on discrimination and racism in health care in1998 and stated its commitment to working toward the eradication of discrimination and racism in the profession of nursing, in the education of nurses, in the practice of nursing, and in the organizations in which nurses work. Certainly, the ANA Code of Ethics for Nurses (2001) advocates diversity in its assertion that "the nurse, in all professional relationships, practices with compassion and respect for the inherent dignity, worth and uniqueness of every individual, unrestricted by considerations of social or economic status, personal attributes, or the nature of health problems."

In November 2003, Sigma Theta Tau, the international honor society of nursing, published a white paper entitled *Community Through Diversity: A Diversity Statement for Sigma Theta Tau International*. It stated that diversity creates an opportunity to support a mosaic of cultural distinctiveness and nursing excellence through inclusiveness, personal and professional development, and the stimulation to think in different ways (Wilson, Sanner, & McAllister, 2003).

In contrast, the International Council of Nurses (ICN) does not have a diversity statement, but rather has embedded *diversity* in its policy and practice (Wilson et al., 2003). One example comes from the ICN Code of Ethics for Nurses, "Nursing care is unrestricted by considerations of age, colour, creed, culture, disability or illness, gender, nationality, politics, race or social status" (ICN, 2000).

Some professional organizations have gone beyond simply arguing the need for diversity, and have instead given monies to advance the cause. The American Association of Critical Care Nurses announced that it would award $1,500 scholarships, funded by the nursing website *www.RN.com*, to attend the 2003 National Teaching Institute & Critical Care Exposition. These scholarships were open to nurses from groups that are underrepresented in nursing, particularly ethnic minorities and those who have developed successful programs to serve ethnic minority patients and families and/or increase involvement of underrepresented groups in nursing (Applications for AACN Minority, n.d.).

Despite the backlash in the late 1990s over the practice of affirmative action in helping racial and ethnic minorities enter the health professions, the Bureau of Health Professions within the HRSA, U.S. Department of Health and Human Services, has held steadfast to its goal of ensuring representation of underrepresented minorities in the health professions by prioritizing this goal in funding opportunities (Montes, 2000).

▶ CONCLUSIONS

Projections suggest that current ethnic minorities are likely, in the not too distant future, to become the majority of the U.S. population. This diversity, however, is not reflected in the nursing workforce or in schools of nursing. Similarly, men are underrepresented in nursing, and efforts to increase the number of men in the nursing profession are even fewer than those directed at increasing ethnic diversity. Finally, generational diversity is occurring in all health care organizations; however, few organizations have directly confronted the implications of how to deal with this diversity or examined the impact it has on the quality of care provided.

Diversity, equity, and parity are business imperatives but should also be moral imperatives. "Although vanishing from the national leadership agenda, the health care industry must see equal opportunity as a priority" (Gould, 2003, p. 37). Using "change by drift" strategies to address the lack of ethnic and gender diversity in nursing has been ineffective. It has become increasingly clear that proactive, well thought out strategies at multiple levels and by multiple parties will be needed before diversity in the nursing profession will mirror that of the public it serves.

FOR ADDITIONAL DISCUSSION

1. What are the strongest driving and restraining forces for increasing ethnic diversity in nursing? For increasing gender diversity in nursing? For having a multigenerational nursing workforce?
2. Should funding for diversity initiatives come from federal or state governments?
3. Should the institutions that reap the benefits of a diverse workforce share the costs to make that happen?
4. Should there be different nursing school entry requirements for minority students than for their White counterparts?
5. Will having more men in nursing raise the status of the profession?
6. Why have women been better able to overcome stereotypes in medicine than men have in nursing?
7. How does the use of mentors assist in both the recruitment and the retention of minority (ethnic and gender) nurses?
8. Does a multigenerational nursing workforce improve patient care? If so, how?

REFERENCES

Abriam-Yago, K. (2002). Degrees of success: Academic forum. Mentoring to empower: An unusual mentoring program in California helps minority students master the "three Cs" of academic success—communication, comfort level and confidence. *Minority Nurse*, 64–65.

American Association of Colleges of Nursing. (2001). Effective strategies for increasing diversity in nursing programs. Retrieved April 21, 2005, from http://www.aacn.nche.edu/Publications/issues/dec01.htm.

American Association of Colleges of Nursing. (2002). A position statement. Diversity and equality of opportunity. Retrieved April 21, 2005, from http://www.aacn.nche.edu/publications/positions/diverse.htm.

American Nurses Association. (1998). Position statement. Discrimination and racism in health care. Retrieved April 21, 2005, from http://www.nursingworld.org/readroom/position/ethics/etdisrac.htm.

American Nurses Association. (2001). Code of ethics for nurses with interpretive statements. Retrieved April 21, 2005, from http://www.nursingworld.org/ethics/code/ethicscode150.htm.

Applications for AACN minority continuing education scholarships due Feb. 1. (n.d.). Retrieved April 21, 2005, from http://www.nursezone.com/student_nurse_center/default.asp?articleID=9943.

Berliner, H. S. & Ginzberg, E. (2002). Why this hospital shortage is different. *Journal of the American Medical Association, 288*(21), 2742–2744.

Boughn, S. (1994). Why do men choose nursing? *Nursing & Health Care, 15*(8), 406–411.

Boughn, S. (2001). Why women and men choose nursing. *Nursing Health Care Perspectives, 22*(1), 14–19.

Bowen, W. G. & Bok, D. (1998). *The Shape of the River.* Princeton, NJ: Princeton University Press.

Buerhaus, P. & Auerbach, D. (1999). Slow growth in the United States of the number of minorities in the RN workforce. *Image: Journal of Nursing Scholarship, 32*(2), 179–183.

Buerhaus, P., Staiger, D., & Auerbach, I. (2000). Policy responses to an aging registered nurse workforce. *Nursing Economics, 18*(6), 278–284, 303.

Burda, D. (2003). A melting pot it's not: ACHE study finds health care management still dominated by Whites, men despite efforts to promote greater diversity. *Modern Healthcare, 33*(32), 6–7, 14–15.

Carol, R. (Summer 2001). Closing the gap. *Minority Nurse, 18*–22, 24.

Catholic Health Association. (June 6–9, 2004). 89th Catholic health assembly. Retrieved April 21, 2005, from http://www.chausa.org/04ASSEMB/MONDAY_M5.ASP.

Chung, V. (2003). *Men in nursing.* Retrieved April 21, 2005, from http://www.minoritynurse.com/features/nurse_emp/08-30-00c.html.

Chur-Hansen, A. (2002). Preferences for female and male nurses: The role of age, gender and previous experience—year 2000 compared with 1984. *Journal of Advanced Nursing, 37*(2), 192–198.

Cook, C. (2003). The many faces of diversity: Overview and summary. *Online Journal of Issues in Nursing, 8*(1). April 21, 2005, from http://www.nursingworld.org/ojin/topic20/tpc20ntr.htm.

Cude, G. (2004). Do men have a role in maternal-newborn nursing? *AWHONN Lifelines, 8* (4), 343–347.

Cunningham, A. (1999). Nursing stereotypes. *Nursing Standard, 13*(45), 46–47.

Doheny, K. (2004). *Men in nursing.* Retrieved April 21, 2005, from http://www.healthscout.com/news/68/516423/main.html.

Evans, J. A. (2002). Cautious caregivers: Gender stereotypes and the sexualization of men nurses' touch. *Journal of Advanced Nursing, 40*(4), 441–448.

Ezenwa, M. (2003). *Degrees of success: Mentorship in black and white.* Retrieved April 21, 2005, from http://www.minoritynurse.com/features/undergraduate/11-01-03f.html.

Feist-Price, S. (2001). African American faculty mentoring relationships at predominantly White institutions. *Rehabilitation Education, 15,* 47–53.

Furr, S. R. & Elling, T. W. (2002). African American students in a predominantly White university: Factors associated with retention. *College Student Journal, 36,* 188–203.

Gerke, M. L. (2001). Understanding and leading the Quad Matrix: Four generations in the workplace: The traditional generation, Boomers, Gen-X, Nexters. *Seminars for Nurse Managers, 9*(3), 173–181.

Gould, S. (2003). A long road ahead: Diversity studies show progress but minority, women execs still lack opportunities. *Modern Healthcare, 33*(34), 37.

Health Resources and Services Administration. (2004). *Diversity.* Retrieved April 21, 2005, from http://bhpr.hrsa.gov/diversity/default.htm.

Hill, K. S. (2004). Defy the decades with multigenerational teams. *Nursing Management, 35*(1), 32–35.

HRSA national survey cites slowdown in number of registered nurses entering profession. (2001). *HRSA News.* Retrieved April 21, 2005, from http://newsroom.hrsa.gov/releases/2001%20Releases/nursesurvey.htm.

International Council of Nurses (ICN). (2000). *The ICN code of ethics for nurses.* Retrieved April 21, 2005, from http://www.icn.ch/icncode.pdf.

Is there a male nurse in the house? (2002). Retrieved April 21, 2005, from http://www.cbsnews.com/stories/2002/09/06/health/printable521057.shtml.

Kalist, D. E. (2002). The gender earnings gap in the RN labor market. *Nursing Economics, 20*(4), 155–162.

Kleinman, C. S. (2004). Understanding and capitalizing on men's advantages in nursing. *Journal of Nursing Administration, 34*(2), 78–82.

LeMaire, B. (2003). *5 minutes with Gene Tranbarger, on men in nursing.* Retrieved April 21, 2005, from http://www.nurseweek.com/5min/tranbarger.asp.

Marquis, B. & Huston, C. (2006). *Leadership roles and management functions in nursing* (5th ed.). Philadelphia: Lippincott Williams and Wilkins.

Martin, C. A. (2003). Transcend generational timelines. *Nursing Management, 34*(4), 25–26, 28.

McCrae, M. J. (2003). Men in obstetrical nursing: Perceptions of the role. *MCN, The American Journal of Maternal Child Nursing , 28*(3), 167–173.

McNeese-Smith, D. K. & Crook, M. (2003). Nursing values and a changing nurse workforce: Values, age, and, job stages. *Journal of Nursing Administration, 33*(5), 260–270.

Medzilla asks "is there a need for affirmative action in the nursing field"? (2002). Retrieved April 21, 2005, from http://www.medzilla.com/press62502.html.

Medzilla asks "why are there so few male nurses"? Retrieved April 21, 2005, from http://www.medzilla.com/press61102.html.

Milligan, F. (2001). The concept of care in male nurse work: An ontological hermeneutic study in acute hospitals. *Journal of Advanced Nursing, 35*(1), 7–16.

Minority nurses denied senior roles. (2003). *Australian Nursing Journal, 10*(9), 16.

Montes, H. (2000). Recruitment challenges being met by HRSA Bureau of Health Professions. Retrieved April 21, 2005, from http://apha.confex.com/apha/128am/techprogram/paper_10291.htm.

National Advisory Council on Nurse Education and Practice. (2000). *Report to the Secretary of Health and Human Services and Congress. A national agenda for workforce racial/ethnic diversity.* Washington, DC: U.S. Department of Health and Human Services, Health Resources and Services Administration, Bureau of Health Professions, Division of Nursing.

National Alaska Native American Indian Nurses Association. (2004). *About us—NANAINA. History.* Retrieved April 21, 2005, from http://www.nanaina.com/about_us/main.html.

National Association of Hispanic Nurses. (n.d.). Home page. Retrieved April 21, 2005, from http://www.thehispanicnurses.org.

National Black Nurses Association. (n.d.). Home page. Retrieved April 21, 2005, from http://www.nbna.org.

Newell-Withrow, C. & Slusher, I. L. (2001). Diversity: An answer to the nursing shortage. *Nursing Outlook, 49*(6), 270–271.

News from NINR. Nursing shortage. (2001). Retrieved April 21, 2005, from http://ninr.nih.gov/ninr/news-info/pubs/outlookmay01.html.

Nugent, K. E., Childs, G., Jones, R., & Cook, P. (2004). A mentorship model for the retention of minority students. *Nursing Outlook, 52*(2), 89–94.

Palmer, P. (1998). The courage to teach. San Francisco: Jossey-Bass.

Philippine Nurses Association of America. (n.d.) *About us. Brief history.* Retrieved April 21, 2005, from http://www.geocities.com/pna_hawaii/history.html.

Price, C. (2001). Short staffing watch. *American Nurse, 33*(3), 20.

Rambur, B., Palumbo, M. V., McIntosh, B., & Mongeon, J. (2003). A statewide analysis of RN's intention to leave their position. *Nursing Outlook, 51*(4), 182–188.

The registered nurse population. National sample survey data. Registered nurse population gender and racial/ethnic background March 2000. (March 2000). Retrieved April 21, 2005, from http://bhpr.hrsa.gov/healthworkforce/reports/rnsurvey/rnss1.htm#T1.

Staiger, D. O., Auerbach, D. I., & Buerhaus, P. I. (2003). Minority enrollments up, but not minority faculty. Retrieved April 21, 2005, from http://www.minoritynurse.com/features/faculty/07-09-01c.html.

Steffan Dickerson, S., Neary, M. A., & Hyche-Johnson, M. (2000). Native American graduate nursing students' learning experiences. *Journal of Nursing Scholarship, 32*(2), 189–196.

Steltzer, T. M., Woods, A., & Gasda, K. A. (2003). Salary survey 2003. *Nursing Management, 34*(7), 28–32.

U.S. Census Bureau. (1999). *Resident population of the United States: Middle series projections, 2015–2030, by sex, race, and Hispanic origin, with median age.* Retrieved April 21, 2005, from http://www.census.gov.

U.S. Census Bureau. (2000). *The White population: 2000. Census 2000 brief.* Retrieved April 21, 2005, from http://www.census.gov/prod/2001pubs/c2kbr01-4.pdf.

U.S. Census Bureau. (2003). *Diversity continues to grow in the U.S.* Retrieved April 21, 2005, from http://www.factfinder.census.gov/jsp/saff/SAFFInfo.jsp?geo_id=01000US&_geo Context=&_street=&_county=&_cityTown=&_state=&_zip=&_content=tp9_race_ethnicity.html&_water-mark=people_watermark.gif&_gnId=0&_gtId=0&_title=Race+and+Ethnicity&_lang=en&_sse=on.

Villarruel, A. M., Canales, M., & Torres, S. (2001). Bridges and barriers: Educational mobility of Hispanic nurses. *Journal of Nursing Education, 40*(6), 245–251.

Wakefield, M. K. (2001). Hard numbers, hard choices: Seeking solutions to the nursing shortage. *Nursing Economics, 19*(2), 80–82.

Waters, V. L. (2004). Cultivate corporate culture and diversity. *Nursing Management, 35*(1), 36–37.

Wenzel, J. & Utz, S.W. (2002). Male and minority nurses: Solutions to current problems confronting our profession. *Virginia Nurses Today, 10*(3). Retrieved February 23, 2004, from EBSCO HOST database.

Whittock, M., Edwards, C., McLaren, S., & Robinson, O. (2002). The tender trap: Gender, part-time nursing and the effects of "family friendly" policies on career advancement. *Sociology of Health and Illness, 24*(3), 305–326.

Whittock, M. & Leonard, L. (2003). Stepping outside the stereotype. A pilot study of the motivations and experiences of males in the nursing profession. *Journal of Nursing Management, 11*, 242–249.

Williams, D. (2003). *Looking for a few good men.* Retrieved April 21, 2005, from http://www.minoritynurse.com/features/nurse_emp/05-03-02a.html.

Wilson, A. H., Sanner, S. J., & McAllister, L. E. (2003). The honor society of nursing, Sigma Theta Tau International diversity white paper. Retrieved April 21, 2005, from http://www.nursingsociety.org/about/Diversity_white_paper.pdf.

Wood, C. (2003). Managing to bridge the generation gaps. Retrieved April 21, 2005, from http://www.nursezone.com/stories/SpotlightOnNurses.asp?articleID=10976&page=Feature+Stories&profile=Spotlight+on+nurses&headline=Managing+to+Bridge+the+Generation+Gaps.

BIBLIOGRAPHY

Alexis, O. (2002). Diversity and equality: Recruiting and retaining overseas ethnic minority nurses in the NHS. *Nursing Management, 9*(5), 22–25.

American Assembly for Men in Nursing. (n.d.) Home page. Retrieved April 21, 2005, from http://aamn.org/.

Ballestas, H. C. (2002). Cultural barriers: Recruiting minority nurses. Viewpoint. *American Journal of Nursing, 102*(8), 14.

Bessent, H. & Fleming, J. W. (2003). The Leadership Enhancement and Development (LEAD) project for minority nurses (in the new millennium model). *Nursing Outlook, 51*(6), 255–260.

Blecher, M. B. (2001–2004). What color is your whistle? Reporting incidents of wrongdoing in your workplace is always a risky business–but for minority nurses who blow the whistle, the stakes are even higher. *Minority Nurse.* Retrieved April 21, 2005, from http://www.minoritynurse.com/features/nurse_emp/05-03-02c.html.

Boyd, T. (2002). Male nurses give a real sense of balance. *Australian Nursing Journal, 10*(1), 3.

Campinha-Bacote, J. (2003) Many faces: Addressing diversity in health care. *Online Journal of Issues in Nursing, 8*(1), 3. Retrieved April 21, 2005, from http://nursingworld.org/ojin/topic20/tpc20_2.htm.

Chwedyk, P. (2003). Vital signs. Diversity leadership initiative aims to develop more minority health care executives. Retrieved April 21, 2005, from http://www.minoritynurse.com/vitalsigns/dec03-6.html

Clausing, S. L. (2003). Generational diversity: the Nexters. *AORN Journal, 78*(3), 373–379.

Cooper, K. (2003). Surge in recruits follows push for diverse workforce. *Nursing Standard, 18*(3), 7.

Drone, C. (2002). More nurses speak out: We need male nurses! . . . "A male RN warns other men to avoid the nursing profession." *RN, 65*(7), 14.

Foti, S. (2003). Nurses with borders. Retrieved April 21, 2005, from http://www.minoritynurse.com/features/nurse_emp/04-17-03.html.

Frusti, D. K., Niesen, K. M., & Campion, J. K. (2003). Creating a culturally competent organization. *Journal of Nursing Administration, 33*(1), 31–38.

Harding, T. (2003). Male nurses: the struggle for acceptance. *Kai Tiaki Nursing New Zealand, 9*(4), 17–19.

Harringan, R. C., Gollin, L. X., & Casken, J. (2003). Barriers to increasing native Hawaiian, Samoan, and Filipino nursing students: Perceptions of students and their families. *Nursing Outlook, 51*(1), 25–30.

Hilton, L. (May 14, 2001). A few good men. Retrieved April 21, 2005, from http://www.nurseweek.com/news/features/01-05/men.html.

Kalist, D. E. (2002). The gender earnings gap in the RN labor market. *Nursing Economics, 20*(4), 155–162.

Leeman, J., Goeppinger, J., Funk, S., & Roland, E. J. (2003). An enriched research experience for minority undergraduates: A step toward increasing the number of minority nurse researchers. *Nursing Outlook, 51*(1), 20–24.

Marquand, B. (2003). On the front lines of diversity. Retrieved April 21, 2005, from http://www.minoritynurse.com/features/nurse_emp/11-01-01c.html.

Meadus, R. J. (2000). Men in nursing: Barriers to recruitment. *Nursing Forum, 35*, 5–12.

Rudan, V. T. (2003). The best of both worlds: A consideration of gender in team building. *Journal of Nursing Administration, 33*(3), 179–186.

Schmeiding, N. J. (2000). Minority nurses in leadership positions: A call for action. *Nursing Outlook, 48*(3), 120–127.

Tucker-Allen, S. (2003). Increasing minority nurses means increasing minority nursing faculty members. *Association of Black Nursing Faculty (ABNF) Journal, 14*(1), 3.

Van Dyke, M. (Fall 2003). Management plan: Meet five minority nurses in health care management positions whose ability to defy the odds, break through the barriers and take courageous risks helped them rise to the top of their field. *Minority Nurse,* 20–26.

Villarruel, A. M. (2002). Viewpoint. Recruiting minority nurses: We're asking ourselves the wrong questions. *American Journal of Nursing, 102*(5), 11.

Wenzel, J. (2002). Male and minority nurses: Solutions to current problems confronting our profession. *VA Nurses Today, 10*(3), 1, 4–5

Westphal, R. J. (2003). Historical perspectives. Remember the Maine! Remember the men! The first male nurses held military rank and served in the Spanish-American war. *American Journal of Nursing, 103*(5), 77.

Williams, D. (Summer 2002). Honoring diversity: Under the leadership of one of the nation's most distinguished minority nurses, Sigma Theta Tau International launches a bold initiative to increase the racial, cultural and gender diversity of its membership. *Minority Nurse,* 40–45.

Williams, D. (Fall 2002). A world of opportunities: Working in foreign countries is a great way for minority nurses to learn new skills, experience other cultures and make a real difference in improving global health. *Minority Nurse,* 20–24.

Williams, D. (Winter 2003). Degrees of success. Welcome to the real world: Surviving the transition from nursing school to your first job as an RN can make the difference between a successful career and early burnout—especially for new minority and male nurses. *Minority Nurse,* 55–60.

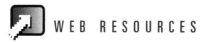 WEB RESOURCES

American Assembly for Men in Nursing	http://AAMN.org
American Medical Student Association, Diversity in Medicine	www.amsa.org/div
Asian & Pacific Islander Nurses Association	http://www.aapina.org
Diversity Rx	http://www.diversityrx.org
The Center for Cross-Cultural Health	http://www.crosshealth.com
Center for Healthy Families and Cultural Diversity, Department of Family Medicine/UMDNJ, Robert Wood Johnson Medical School	www2.umdnj.edu/fmedweb/chfcd/INDEX.HTM
Commission on Graduates of Foreign Nursing Schools	http://www.cgfns.org
Equal Employment Opportunities Commission (EEOC)	http://www.eeoc.gov
Men in Nursing (historical information)	http://www.nurses.info/history_men.htm
Minority Nurse	http://www.minoritynurse.com

National Alaska Native American Indian Nurses Association	www.nanaina.com
National Association of Hispanic Nurses	http://www.thehispanicnurses.org
National Black Nurses Association	http://www.nbna.org
National Coalition of Ethnic Minority Nurse Associations	http://www.ncemna.org/officers.html
The Office of Minority Health, Department of Health and Human Services	http://www.omhrc.gov
Philippine Nursing Association—Hawaii	http://www.geocities.com/pna_hawaii/ history.html
Southern Regional Education Board: Racial/Ethnic and Gender Diversity in Nursing Education	http://www.sreb.org/programs/Nursing/ publications/Diversity_in_Nursing.asp

Workplace Issues

3

Mandatory Staffing Ratios: Are They Working?

10

Carol J. Huston

F or some time now, economics has been the primary driver in dictating changes in the registered nurse (RN) skill mix in hospitals. As a result, the trend for at least the past decade has been to reduce RNs in the staffing mix and to replace them with less expensive alternatives. Empirical research increasingly concludes, however, that the number of RNs in the staffing mix has a direct impact on quality care and in particular, patient outcomes. In response, legislators, health care providers, and the public are increasingly demanding adequate staffing ratios of RNs in acute care settings.

Indeed, this movement has already begun. At least 28 states, with the backing of some nursing organizations, have moved toward imposing mandatory licensed staffing requirements (Leighty, 2004), and one state (California) has already enacted legislation requiring mandatory staffing ratios that affect hospitals and long-term care facilities. Massachusetts, New York, Florida, Michigan, and Oregon are close behind (Leighty), although similar bills have failed in Virginia, New Jersey, Hawaii, and Missouri (Hopkins, 2000).

This chapter explores factors driving legislative mandates for minimum RN representation in the staffing mix. California's experience, as the first state to implement minimum staffing ratios, will be detailed, as will its struggle to define appropriate ratios and the challenges of implementing staffing ratios in an era of limited fiscal and human resources. The chapter concludes by looking at the movement of other states toward adopting minimum staffing ratios and examining strategies that have been suggested as alternatives to staffing ratios.

*CONSIDER: The literature continues to suggest that increasing the number of RNs in the staffing mix leads to safer workplaces for nurses and a higher quality of care for patients.

▶ STAFFING RATIOS AND PATIENT OUTCOMES

Numerous studies in the past decade examined the link between staffing mix and patient outcomes (Table 10.1). Most have suggested a link between the increased representation of RNs in the staffing mix and improved patient outcomes.

*CONSIDER: A recent study by Blakeman Hodge, Romano, Harvey, Samuels, Olson, Saure et al. (2004) suggests that variations in skill mix were identified in their study of California acute care hospitals, and that the proportion of RNs in the staffing mix ranged from 30% to 84%, depending on the unit type surveyed.

Few studies, however, have had as much impact on determining safe staffing ratios as the research done by Aiken et al. (2002). This study of over 10,000 nurses and 230,000 patients in 168 hospitals concluded that in hospitals with higher patient-to-nurse ratios, surgical patients had a greater likelihood of dying within 30 days of admission as well as increased odds of failure-to-rescue (mortality following complications). This occurred because the time nurses have for surveillance, early detection, and timely intervention—particularly with patients who are not at high risk, but who are vulnerable to other unfavorable outcomes—has a direct impact on patient outcomes.

TABLE 10.1

Selected Research on Nurse Staffing Levels and Patient Clinical Outcomes

Citation	Description
Blegen, M. A., Goode, C. J., & Reed, L. (1998). Nurse staffing and patient outcomes. *Nursing Research, 47*(1), 43–50.	The proportion of hours of care delivered by RNs was inversely related to the unit rates of medication errors, pressure ulcer rates, and patient/family complaints.
Lichtig, L. K., Knauf, R. A., & Milholland, D. K. (1999). Some impacts on nursing on acute care hospitals outcomes. *Journal of Nursing Administration, 29* (2), 25–33.	Both higher nurse staffing and a higher proportion of RNs were significantly related to shorter lengths of stay. Lower adverse outcome rates were more consistently related to a higher proportion of RNs.
Needleman, J., Buerhaus, P., Mattke, S., Stewart, M., & Zelevinsky, K. (February 28, 2001). Nurse staffing and patient outcomes in hospitals. (Health Resources Services Administration Contract No. 230-99-0021). Available at http://bhpr.hrsa.gov/dn/staffstudy.htm.	A strong and consistent relationship was found between nurse staffing levels and mix of personnel, particularly RNs, and five patient outcomes in medical patients and one outcome in surgical patients.
Aiken, L. H., Clarke, S., Sloane, D., Sochalski, J., Reinhard, B., Clarke, H., et al. (2001). Nurses report on hospital care in five countries. *Health Affairs, 20*(3), 43– 52.	Only 30%–40% of nurses reported that there were enough RNs to provide quality care and enough staff to get the work done.
Sochalski, J. (2001). Quality of care, nurse staffing, and patient outcomes. *Policy, Politics, & Nursing Practice, 2*(1), 9–18.	One out of every five nurses reported that the quality of care on their unit was fair or poor. Workload played a role in these quality assessments, but it was the consequences of the workload that played a more prominent role.
Joint Commission on Accreditation of Healthcare Organizations. (August 2002). Healthcare at the crossroads: Strategies for addressing the nursing crisis. Retrieved December 8, 2003 from http://www.jcaho.org/about+us/public+policy+initiatives/health+at+the+crossroads.pdf.	Inadequate nurse staffing has been a factor in 24% of the 1,609 cases involving patient death, injury, or permanent loss of function that were reported between 1997 and 2002.
Aiken, L., Clarke, S. P., Sloane, D. M., Sochalski, J., & Silber, J. H. (2002). Hospital nurse staffing and patient mortality, nurse burnout, and job dissatisfaction. *Journal of the American Medical Association, 288* (16), 1987–1993.	For each additional patient over four in a nurse's workload, the risk of death increases by 7% for surgical patients. Patients in hospitals with the highest patient-to-nurse ratio (eight patients per nurse) have a 31% greater risk of dying than those in hospitals with four patients per nurse. On a national scale, staffing differences of this magnitude may result in as many as 20,000 unnecessary deaths each year.
Potter, P., Barr, N., McSweeney, M., & Sledge, J. (2003). Identifying nurse staffing and patient outcome relationships: A guide for change in care delivery. *Nursing Economics, 21*(4), 158–166.	Negative correlation between percentage of RN hours and patient's perception of pain. Positive correlation between percentage of RN hours and patient satisfaction.
McGillis Hall, L., Doran, D., & Pink, G. H. (2004). Nurse staffing models, nursing hours, and patient safety outcomes. *Journal of Nursing Administration, 34*(1), 41–45.	The lower the proportion of professional nursing staff employed on a unit, the higher the number of medication errors and wound infections. The less experienced the nurse, the higher the number of wound infections.

The study found that staffing at six patients per nurse, rather than four, would result in an additional 2.3 deaths per 1,000 patients and 8.7 additional deaths per 1,000 patients with complications. Staffing at eight patients per nurse, rather than six, would incur an additional 2.6 deaths per 1,000 patients and 9.5 deaths per 1,000 patients with complications. Uniformly staffing at eight patients per nurse, rather than four, was expected to entail five excess deaths per 1,000 patients and 18.2 complications per 1,000 patients. In addition, patients had a 31% higher chance of dying within 30 days of admission (Aiken et al., 2002; Bonifazi, 2002; Center for Nursing Advocacy, 2002).

Within days of the study's release, an editorial entitled "Dying for Lack of Nurses" (2002) appeared in the *New York Times*, commenting on the research by Aiken et al. A similar opinion piece was published in the *Philadelphia Inquirer* on the same day (Daily Health Policy Report, 2002). Others quickly followed, such as a *New York Times* editorial entitled "Cases; Prescription, Quite Simply, Was a Nurse" (Zuger, 2002). In fact, over the next few weeks and months, Aiken's study results were summarized, repeated, and analyzed in detail in almost all public forums and by most professional health care organizations. The message was clear: there is a direct link between nurse-to-patient ratios and mortality rates from preventable complications, and the inadequate numbers of RNs places the public is at risk.

Discussion Point

Why did the study by Aiken et al. (2002) garner so much national attention in so many public forums? Were the findings significantly different than earlier studies? Was it timing? Was it how "the message" was managed?

ARE MANDATORY STAFFING RATIOS REALLY NEEDED?

It is little surprise, then, that one proposed solution to Aiken's (2002) research findings was the implementation of minimum mandatory RN-patient staffing ratios in acute care hospitals. Numerous articles have appeared in the media attesting to grossly inadequate staffing in hospitals and nursing homes, and professional nursing organizations, such as the American Nurses Association (ANA), have expressed concern about the effect poor staffing has both on nurses' health and safety and on patient outcomes (Kovner, 2000).

The Institute for Health and Socioeconomic Policy (IHSP) analyzed 18.2 million California hospital discharge records and other data collected from state agencies and the hospital industry between 1994 and 1997. They found that there was an 8.8% increase in the average number of patients for which an RN cared for, a 7.2% decrease in the number of RNs employed, and a 7.7% jump in the number of patients per staffed bed between 1995 and 1998 (Gordon, 2000).

Kathleen Dracup, Dean of the University of California, San Francisco, School of Nursing, stated:

> We have anecdotal reports of 10 patients per 1 nurse on surgical/medical floors. Years ago, that might have been safe because patients weren't as sick and stayed for longer times. Now, the patient population is older, sicker, more vulnerable, and needs to be assured that enough nurses are available (Leighty, 2004, p. 15).

Similar comments were reported by the New York State Nurses Association in their study of the state's RNs. Twenty-two percent of the nurse respondents stated that they were responsible for 10 or more patients; hospital surgical nurses reported an average patient load of 9.4 patients and critical care nurses, 3.14 patients (Gordon, 2000). Forty-six percent of the nurses reported that they could not provide the level of care that patients needed.

Adequate staffing, then, is needed to assure that care provided is at least safe and, hopefully, of high quality. Proponents of state regulation of RN-to-patient ratios suggest that such ratios protect the most basic elements of the public health care we take for granted, and argue that the government must take on this responsibility to ensure that safe health care is provided to all Americans (Kovner, 2000).

CONSIDER: The bottom line is that minimum staffing ratios would not have been proposed if staffing abuses and the resultant decline in the quality of patient care had not occurred in the past.

Hopkins (2000) suggests, however, that there are three arguments against staffing ratios. The first is that the current nursing shortage will make it difficult to fill the slots when the ratios appear; the second is that the ratios may merely serve as a Band-Aid to the greater problems of quality of care; and third, that numbers alone do not ensure improved patient care, because not all RNs have equivalent clinical experience and skill levels.

Indeed, conclusions from the Aiken study clearly state that "results do not directly indicate how many nurses are needed to care for patients or whether there is some maximum ratio of patients per nurse above which hospitals should not venture" (Aiken et el., 2002, p. 1990). In addition, Peter Buerhaus, a leading researcher who has studied the relationship between nurse staffing and patient outcomes, suggests that legislation to mandate fixed ratios carries a high potential of leading to the economic and political devaluation of the nursing profession and fails to effectively deal with the issues surrounding nurse staffing (American Organization of Nurse Executives [AONE], 2003).

Similarly, Graf et al. suggest that the current focus on staffing ratios as a means to assure appropriate care for patients ignores the very real differences among patients in their needs for nursing care. They argue that patients and patient days are not equal and that the need for nursing care varies significantly among patients and over the length of stay for individual patients. As the intensity of patient care needs increases and length of stay decreases, staffing ratios generate inadequate estimates of nursing resource requirements (Graf et al., 2003).

Other critics argue that staffing may actually decline with ratios because they might be used as the ceiling or as ironclad criteria if institutions are not willing to make adjustments for patient acuity or RN skill level. Vessey, Andres, Fountain, and Wheeler (2002) also suggest that mandatory staffing ratios create significant opportunity costs that may restrict employers and payors from responding to market forces; subsequently, they may not be able to take advantage of improved technological support or respond to changes in patient acuity.

Other critics of minimum staffing ratios have argued that mandated ratios will divert resources away from patient care and into compliance. Still others argue that it is health care professionals—not legislators or regulators—who understand health care and are best qualified to determine staffing needs. This may be the case, but given that hospitals are no longer exempt from "big business," profit-driven motives, one must question whether what is best for patients can be separated from what is best financially for the institution.

Finally, critics of staffing ratios claim that mandating specific staffing ratios in an environment already experiencing a shortage of nurses will lead to a reduction in hospital services, increased emergency room diversions, increased unit closures, and increased expenses as hospitals pay additional labor costs for overtime and temporary agency nurses (AONE, 2003). Indeed, it is the position of the AONE that "mandatory nurse staffing ratios will only serve to increase stress on a health care system that is overburdened by an escalating national and international shortage of registered professional nurses and that such ratios have the potential to create a greater risk to public safety" (AONE, Para 5).

Yet, proponents of legislated minimum staffing ratios argue that the implementation of staffing ratios will actually improve nurse satisfaction and thus, retention. This improvement in the work environment should subsequently attract new nurses as well as part-time and nonemployed nurses back into the full-time nursing workforce, thus actually alleviating the nursing shortage, not making it worse.

▶ CALIFORNIA AS THE PROTOTYPE FOR MANDATORY STAFFING RATIOS

Passing the Legislation

California has had a minimum licensed nurse-to-patient ratio requirement (Title 22 of the California Code of Regulations) for intensive care and coronary care units for over two decades; however, no minimums were established for other types of acute care units. Given increasing pressure from nursing unions in the state, increasing bad press about poor quality care, the increased use of unlicensed assistive personnel as direct care providers, and skyrocketing patient loads for licensed nurses in acute care, California stepped forward as the first state in the nation to implement mandatory minimum staffing ratios.

Under Assembly Bill (A.B.) 394 ("Safe Staffing Law"), passed in 1999 and crafted by the California Nurses Association (CNA), all hospitals in California were to comply with the minimum staffing ratios shown in Table 10.2 by January 1, 2004 (CNA,

TABLE 10.2 Minimum Registered Nurse Staffing Ratios for Hospitals in California Effective January 2004

Unit	Registered Nurse–Patient Ratio
Critical Care/ICU	1:2
Neonatal ICU	1:2
Operating Room	1:1
Labor and Delivery	1:2
Antepartum	1:4
Postpartum couplets	1:4
Postpartum women only	1:6
Pediatrics	1:4
Step-down (initial)	1:4
Step-down (in 2008)	1:3
Medical/Surgical (initial)	1:6
Medical/Surgical (in 2005)	1:5
Oncology (initial)	1:5
Oncology (in 2008)	1:4
Psychiatry	1:6
Emergency Room	1:4

Source: California Nurses Association, (2003b).

2003c). These ratios, developed by the California Department of Health Services (CDHS) with assistance from the University of California, Davis, represented the maximum number of patients an RN could be assigned to care for, under any circumstance. In addition, this legislation prohibited unlicensed personnel from performing certain procedures such as medication administration, venipuncture, parenteral or tube feedings, inserting nasogastric tubes, inserting catheters, tracheal suctioning, assessment of patient conditions, patient education, and moderately complex laboratory tests (Spetz, 2001).

The Struggle to Determine Appropriate Ratios

Developing draft regulations for minimum staffing ratios was challenging for the CDHS because data was not readily accessible regarding the distribution of nurse staffing in California hospitals, the number of hospitals likely to be affected by the minimum staffing requirements, or the expected costs of this legislation (Spetz, 2001). In addition, the ratios were meant to supplement valid and reliable patient classification systems (PCS), which had been required in California hospitals since 1996. The problem was that although California hospitals had been required to submit their PCS data to the state, there was no standardization and little guidance about what characterized a valid PCS or what criteria should be used in determining the PCS (Seago, 2002). Therefore PCS data yielded little if any, helpful information to the CDHS in determining appropriate ratios.

Discussion Point

The California Healthcare Association advocated the use of PCS as the gold standard for staffing decisions rather than staffing ratios. The CNA argued for the reverse. What motives may have been driving these positions?

Cost was also an unknown. Projections by the Public Policy Institute of California (PPIC) in July 2001 suggested that many hospitals in California could see their expenditures for RNs increase between 5% and 41%, depending on the staffing ratios eventually adopted by the state (California Healthcare Association [CHA], 2001). PPIC research fellow Joanne Spetz publicly lamented how little information the CDHS really had to draw up recommended staffing ratios and suggested that putting a price tag on various staffing options was a very important start, but that more information was needed about the potential benefits of higher ratios on the quality of care (CHA, 2001). (Aiken et al.'s 2002 study had yet to be published.) Spetz continued "It's important that we get this right: The rest of the nation is watching California closely" (CHA, 2001, para 4).

At least in part as a result of limited empirical data, proposals received by CDHS suggested a wide range of minimum staffing ratios and even more widely differing estimates of cost. The CHA, a hospital trade group representing the interests of nearly 500 hospital and health system members in California, called for a minimum staffing ratio of one nurse to 10 patients on medical-surgical units, whereas the University of California, Davis recommended a ratio of one to six (Seago, 2002). The Service Employees International Union (SEIU), the United Nurses Association (UNA) of California, and Kaiser Permanente argued for minimum ratios in medical-surgical units of one to four, and the CNA recommended one to three (Seago, 2002).

Not surprisingly, the proposal by CHA, which represented the interests of hospitals, recommended more patients per nurse than any of the other proposals and produced the smallest increase in costs (an estimated average annual increase of nearly $200,000 per hospital) (CHA, 2001). The SEIU proposal, which was endorsed by Kaiser Permanente, was estimated by the PPIC to cost over $1.3 million per hospital annually, and the CNA proposal was estimated to cost hospitals up to $2.3 million yearly (CHA, 2001).

To complicate the picture further, a study by Berliner, Kovner, and Zhu (2002) suggested that instead of the $1.1 billion cost projected by the U.C. Davis Center for Health Services Research in Primary Care and the Center for Nursing Research to implement a ratio of four patients to one nurse in medical-surgical units (the standard approved by the SEIU, UNA, and Kaiser), that true costs were likely to be about half of that (close to $500 million annually). They further argued that the revenues of hospitals in California were approximately $40 billion in 2000, and even if the billion-dollar figure was accurate, the increase would be very small in terms of total revenue—only a 2.5% increase in overall costs.

Following months of waiting and almost 2 years of wrangling, the final minimum staffing ratios were announced in January 2002.

Then California Governor Gray Davis, in a press conference at St. Vincent's Medical Center in Los Angeles, announced that his administration supported a ratio of one nurse to every six patients in medical-surgical units—twice the number of patients supported by the CNA and four fewer than that favored by the CHA, which represented the state's 470 hospitals (Tieman, 2002). Actual regulations were released later that spring with 45 days allocated for public comment. Hospitals in California were also required to continue to keep a PCS in place and to staff according to the PCS if it called for a larger number of nurses than the minimum ratios set by the CDHS.

Kay McVay, president of the CNA, stated "No other state or governor in the U.S. has taken such a profound and courageous step in the face of the heated opposition of the powerful health care industry. These ratios will help us bring *nurses* back to the bedside" (California Patients and Nurses Win Minimum Staffing Ratios, 2002, Para 3).

Delays in Implementation

Implementing the ratio legislation proved to be just as difficult as determining what the ratios should be. The first challenge that arose was interpreting the meaning and intent of the legislation's language in regard to what constituted "licensed nurses." Almost immediately, questions were raised about whether the minimum mandatory ratios had to reflect RN representation in the staffing mix or whether licensed vocational/practical nurses (LVNs) would meet the requirement.

CNA argued that the intent of the law was to regulate minimum RN staffing. The SEIU argued, however, that limiting ratio compliance to RNs was "rewriting history" because both RNs and LVNs were licensed by state boards (Russell, 2002). This set up an adversarial relationship between CNA—a group of 45,000 RNs—and SEIU, which included 30,000 California RNs and 5,000 LVNs as well as hospital orderlies (Russell).

The issues were aired at a public hearing before the state Department of Health Services in San Francisco and a determination was provided that the ratios referred to RNs only and that LVNs would be authorized to practice only under the direction of an RN or licensed physician.

Questions were then raised as to whether hospitals could eliminate/reduce their nonlicensed staff in an effort to save costs, since the number of RNs would be increased. The CNA argued that the ratios were based on CDHS surveys of existing hospital staffing patterns, including the percentage of LVNs and other nursing staff, and it was their position that any hospitals that cut nonRN nursing staff must hire additional RNs, beyond the minimum staffing ratios, to assure safe patient care (CNA, 2003c). Yet, the state chose not to weigh in, arguing that their position was to regulate minimum RN–patient ratios; as a result, many hospitals immediately began reducing the number of support personnel to offset the increased cost of RN staff.

Finally, the CHA, with the help of Senator Aanestad, introduced new legislation (A.B. 847) to the California State Senate Health and Human Services committee in April 2003, attempting to delay implementation of the 1:5 minimum nurse–patient staffing ratio on medical–surgical units. Authors of the bill argued that such a delay was necessary until additional data could be gathered regarding implementation costs and to ascertain whether an adequate number of RNs were available to meet the required ratios (Hospital Industry Attempt to Delay Staffing Ratio, 2003).

Opponents of the delay argued that the manner in which the proposal was being formulated would push implementation far into the future, and possibly preclude it altogether. The end result was that "the committee was not swayed by the hospital industry's arguments and the bill was voted down, with only two Republicans in favor, with little debate" (Hospital Industry Attempt to Delay Staffing Ratio, 2003, para 5).

Still, resistance to staffing ratio implementation continued. CNA alleges that the California hospital industry held seminars across the state to advise hospital administrators how to undermine and avoid compliance with the new RN staffing ratios. CNA (2003a) argues that the advice included:

▶ Voluntarily closing or downsizing beds or units, citing an inability to "find" sufficient RNs to meet the ratios. The goal here was to fan hysteria in hopes of softening public support for the ratios, winning regulatory exemptions to compliance, and generating political support for legislation to repeal or suspend the ratios.
▶ Delaying elective surgeries due to health care "emergencies," both to force RNs on staff to work more hours and to engage in a public relations war to subvert the ratios.
▶ Distorting the use of acuity systems or other tools to reduce staffing.
▶ Discharging patients more quickly so that staffing could be reduced.
▶ Laying off nonRN staff thereby increasing the RN workload and violating the intent of A.B. 394.
▶ Challenging or ignoring RN efforts to monitor and protest violations.
▶ Continuing to use existing, even expired, "program flexibility" waivers from the Department of Health Services (DHS) to avoid compliance with the ratios and hope that no one noticed.
▶ Pressuring or cajoling the DHS not to enforce the law.
▶ Reintroducing A.B. 847 that would have required indefinite delays in implementation of ratios until studies proved there were sufficient numbers of RNs and that ratios improve patient outcomes.

The Struggle to Implement the Ratios

Despite these efforts and a pervasive, ongoing resistance to staffing ratio implementation, the staffing ratio mandate did become effective January 1, 2004. But were hospitals ready and willing to implement these changes?

Leighty (2004, p. 15) suggests that although many large hospital systems in California were prepared to meet the minimum staffing ratios when the mandate took effect, many other acute care facilities "have scrambled to comply in the face of a statewide nursing shortage." Many smaller hospitals, with budget deficits, had to seek waivers from the CDHS because of their difficulty in meeting ratios. Waivers are allowed; however, hospitals must be rural and meet very strict conditions. In the first three weeks of the mandate, the CDHS received 67 requests for flexibility and waivers from hospitals. Nine were denied, two were found to be in compliance, and one was approved (Leighty, 2004). The other cases are pending. Only one hospital reported closing as a result of staffing ratios in the first five months after implementation of the law (Wood, 2004).

D i s c u s s i o n   P o i n t

Should small, rural hospitals be given waivers for the mandatory staffing ratios? Is this justified by the patient population characteristics or is it simply an economic incentive to keep these hospitals viable?

The "At All Times" Clause

Almost immediately after implementation, clarification was needed regarding interpretation of the law in regards to ratio coverage "at all times." A ruling by the CDHS blindsided many hospitals in its strict interpretation that ratios had to be maintained at all times, including breaks and lunches. For many hospitals, this meant hiring additional rotating staff to fill in for nurses when they leave the bedside for short periods (breaks, lunch, transporting patients, etc.) or face being noncompliant.

As a result, the CHA filed a lawsuit December 30, 2003, challenging the ruling and arguing that the nation's second worst nursing shortage makes compliance with the "at-all-times" ruling impossible (Leighty, 2004; Nurse, Hospital Showdown Goes to Judge, 2004). Jan Emerson, CHA spokesperson, asked "What happens if a nurse needs to go to the bathroom? You have to get another nurse to come stand there" (CA Ratios Become Law, 2004, pp. 5–6).

The court heard the case in a Sacramento courthouse May 14, 2004, while CNA held a rally in the city. CNA director Rose Ann DeMoro warned that "there would be a mass revolt if the judge reversed the rules that took effect in January" (Nurse, Hospital Showdown Goes to Judge, 2004, para 3).

In a 10-page ruling, issued May 26, 2004, the judge dismissed the hospital association lawsuit, saying that not adhering to the "at all times" clause would make the nurse-to-patient ratios meaningless, a sentiment echoed by the CNA. CHA vice president Dorel Harms called the ruling a disservice to patients, and an industry spokeswoman said the association was considering an appeal (Judge Rejects Hospital Challenge, 2004).

D i s c u s s i o n   P o i n t

Is an "at all times" ruling necessary to assure quality health care?

Assuring Compliance: The Role of the California Department of Health Services

The CDHS is charged with compliance oversight of minimum staffing ratios in acute care hospitals and is enforcing these regulations in the same general manner in which they have enforced intensive care and critical care unit staffing regulations for the past 28 years.

Compliance with the regulations may be verified during a periodic survey or by investigating a complaint that is specific to staffing or staffing ratios (California's Nurse to Patient Staffing Ratios, 2004).

Although there is no statutory timeframe within which CDHS must initiate an on-site investigation in response to a complaint against an acute care hospital, by existing policy, CDHS will initiate an investigation within 48 hours if a credible allegation of serious and immediate jeopardy to patients is received. If the allegation does not constitute serious and immediate jeopardy, the complaint will be investigated during the next periodic survey or along with the next "serious" complaint (California's Nurse to Patient Staffing Ratios, 2004).

If a violation of the ratio requirements occurs, CDHS will issue a deficiency notice to the hospital and require an acceptable plan of correction. CDHS may verify that the plan of correction has been implemented and the deficiency corrected during any subsequent complaint investigation or periodic survey.

There is no penalty or monetary fine for a violation of the ratio regulations. However, if the CDHS concludes that the violation of the ratios is so severe that it poses an immediate and substantial hazard to the health or safety of patients, CDHS may order the hospital to reduce the number of patients or close a unit until additional staffing is obtained (California's Nurse to Patient Staffing Ratios, 2004).

> ***CONSIDER:** If there are no monetary fines from the CDHS for noncompliance, what will motivate California hospitals to continue to comply with mandated staffing ratios?

The reality, however, is that few hospitals in California have been inspected for compliance with nurse–patient ratios, and resources have not allowed for random checks on nurse–patient ratios (Few Hospitals Checked, 2004). Indeed, the CDHS had inspected only 28 of the 451 acute-care hospitals by November 2004 and 15 of these hospitals did not meet mandated staffing levels (Few Hospitals Checked). All 15 of these hospitals were required to develop a plan for compliance.

The Bottom Line: Has Registered Nurse Staffing Improved in California Hospitals?

Both the CNA and the CHA are actively tracking compliance of staffing ratios. A study by CNA, 1 month after implementation of mandatory staffing ratios (February 2004), suggests that staffing ratios have improved staffing in 68% of California's acute care hospitals (Staffing Improved at Nearly 70%, 2004) (Box 10.1). Yet, many hospitals are still struggling. As of January 21, 2004, 86 hospitals had self-reported that they were not complying with the ratios on some units (Leighty, 2004).

The CHA tracks compliance more formally, surveying 300 of its 450 member hospitals weekly. The CHA reports that 4 months after implementation (April 5–12, 2004), 87% of responding hospitals reported they were unable to meet the "at-all-times" requirement for staffing (Wood, 2004). Jan Emerson, vice president of external affairs for the CHA, stated that "the majority of hospitals were meeting the ratios at the beginning of the shift, but the at-all-times compliance requirement is the real problem" (Wood, 2004, para 7).

In a survey by the Governance Institute, a membership organization that focuses on board education for approximately 450 hospitals and health systems across the country, California chief executive officers (CEOs) reported spending an average of $5.34 million

BOX 10.1

Research Study Fuels the Controversy

Implications of Mandatory Staffing Ratios

A study was completed by the California Nurses Association of 114 hospitals (30% of the general acute care hospitals in the state), 1 month after mandatory staffing ratios took effect in January 1, 2004. The results were based on interviews with RNs in the hospitals.

> Staffing improved at nearly 70% of California hospitals. (February 2004). *California Nurse, 10* (2), 13.

Study Findings

Some large hospital systems in California, such as Kaiser Permanente and the University of California Medical Centers, used the 4-year lag time between passage of AB 394 and its implementation both to hire additional RNs and to begin meeting the ratios in most clinical areas. This was generally not the case, however, for hospitals in smaller, rural areas.

Overall, this study found that 68% of surveyed hospitals had improved their staffing conditions as a result of mandatory staffing ratio implementation. Approximately 58% of the hospitals were generally in compliance with the requirements of the law. Hospitals represented by the California Nurses Association as their bargaining agent, had the greatest compliance rates, with 74% improving staffing conditions and 62% in general compliance.

The study did, however, find two ongoing issues: 1) the inappropriate use of LVNs, and 2) the efforts of some hospitals to reduce support staff, thus increasing RN's workloads and decreasing time spent with patients.

in fiscal 2004 to implement the ratios (Phillips, 2004). The median cost estimate for implementing staffing ratios was $3 million, with a range of $225,000 for smaller hospitals to $40 million for large systems with as many as 20 hospitals. Yet 73% of those California CEOs said they didn't have enough RNs to meet the requirements, and one-third said they may need to occasionally close units or cut services to meet the law. Nearly 87% of California respondents said they anticipated controversy over the law's interpretation (Phillips, 2004).

The most recent state data available suggest that 78 complaints had been filed with the CDHS November 2004 (Few Hospitals Checked, 2004). These complaints were followed up by the CDHS to assure that patients were not in immediate jeopardy of health or safety. Yet, the overwhelming majority of hospitals in California will not be inspected until their regularly scheduled inspection every 3 years. As a result, it remains unclear how many are complying with the ratios (Few Hospitals Checked, 2004).

Some of these implementation struggles may be related to the normal issues that arise whenever a new law takes effect; however, the reality may be that California lacks the nursing resources needed to implement its own law. And to further cloud the picture, minimum ratios were to get tougher in 2005, with the minimum nurse-patient ratio in medical–surgical units dropping from 1:6 to 1:5 (CA Ratios Become Law, 2004). However, California Governor Arnold Schwarzenegger announced in November 2004 that this ruling would be delayed to 2008. The CNA argued that the governor was bowing to special interests in the health care industry while the CHA maintained the new ratios were impossible to implement due to the current severe nursing shortage

(Nurse Ratio Delay Blasted, 2004). In March 2005, a state Superior Court judge sided with the CNA and ruled that the governor had overstepped his authority in delaying the further reduction in the number of nurses to patients on medical–surgical units. The judge argued that the financial state of hospitals did not give the state the right to delay implementing the law, because the law's intent was to improve patient safety. Hospitals were told to comply immediately. Both the hospital industry and the state vowed to appeal the court decision.

▶ SIMILAR INITIATIVES IN OTHER STATES

It appears that other states are likely to soon follow California's lead. According to the Governance Institute survey, 52% of hospital CEOs reported that they expect their state legislature to consider mandated ratios in the next 2 years. Of those who expect the issue to come up, 25% thought their state would pass it. Many of those respondents were from New York, New Jersey, Pennsylvania, Florida, Illinois, Kentucky, Michigan, Oregon, and Texas. Asked whether they thought mandated ratios would help with recruitment and retention, 93% of respondents said no, saying the problem is supply and that ratios don't account for acuity, among other reasons (Phillips, 2004).

Some states, however, are actively pursuing minimum staffing ratio legislation. The Massachusetts Nursing Association, with support from more than 200 advocacy groups, is backing a state legislative bill, B.H. 182, to mandate staffing ratios in that state (Leighty, 2004). This bill, although similar to California's, would require no more than a 1:4 nurse–patient ratio on medical–surgical units, where California currently requires no more than a 1:5 ratio. The bill would also ask for a 1:1 and up to a 1:3 ratio for emergency departments, a 1:1 ratio in labor units, and a 1:2 ratio in intensive care units.

The New York State Nurses Association (NYSNA) is also furthering legislation that calls for mandatory nurse–patient ratios in that state. Although New York state law currently requires "sufficient nurse staffing to meet patients' needs," there are few specific requirements that define safe staffing (NYSNA Calls for Expanded . . . , 2004). The newly proposed legislation, which has been introduced in both the Senate and the Assembly, would require the state to establish RN-to-patient ratios in hospitals and health care facilities to disclose staffing ratios and patient outcomes.

On August 15, 2003, Michigan Nurses Association members went to the Capitol and attended a press conference to introduce the Patient Protection Act (H.B. 5049). This act is a three-bill package of legislation designed to support and strengthen the nursing profession (Leading the Charge Toward . . . , 2003). One key part of the act mandates an acuity system and annual staffing plan that includes minimum nurse-to-patient ratios. The bill has been referred to the Committee on Health Policy for review.

Similarly, Representative Joni Jenkins introduced H.B. 91, the Patients' Bill of Rights, in the Kentucky House of Representatives in 2002. The bill seeks to assure safer staffing and protect patients and nurses against forced overtime. H.B. 91 is now with the House Health and Welfare Committee (State Staffing Legislation, 2002).

An assembly bill (A.B.313) was also introduced into the Nevada legislature on March 13, 2003, requiring certain health care facilities employing nurses to establish a staffing plan and to provide adequate staffing. It also provides certain minimum ratios for nurse staffing and establishes maximum limits on work hours (Nevada Organization of Nurse Leaders, 2004). The bill remains in the Legislative Committee on Health Care, awaiting an interim subcommittee study of system staffing for delivery of health care in Nevada.

◗ OTHER ALTERNATIVES

Efforts are also under way, in both California and the rest of the nation, to explore alternatives to improve nurse staffing that do not require legislated minimum staffing ratios. California Congresswoman Lois Capps, in partnership with the ANA, introduced the "Quality Nursing Care Act of 2004" into the House of Representatives on December 8, 2003. If enacted, this bill will "mandate the development of staffing systems in hospitals aimed at ending the wide-spread practice of health care facilities stretching their nursing staff with unsafe patient loads, mandatory overtime, 'floating' to specialty units without training and orientation, and other practices that would undermine the delivery of safe, quality care" (Safe Staffing Initiatives, 2004, pp. 1, 3). Specifically, it mandates the development of staffing systems that require the input of direct-care RNs and it provides whistleblower protection for RNs who speak out about patient care issues, including levels of nurse staffing. It also requires public reporting of staffing information.

The bill also establishes a requirement for minimum staffing ratios incorporating *ANA's Principles of Nursing Staffing*. Thus, rather than establishing a specific numeric ratio, it requires a staffing system be developed that "ensures a number of RNs on each shift and in each unit of the hospital to ensure appropriate staffing levels for patient care" (Safe Staffing Initiatives, 2004, p. 3). A summary of the proposed staffing requirements presented in this bill are shown in Box 10.2.

Seago (2002) also suggests alternatives to minimum staffing ratios in her discussion of innovative staffing formulas and her initial attempts to conceptualize nurse workload beyond staffing ratios, nursing care hours per patient day, and PCS scores. The Joint Commission on Accreditation of Healthcare Organizations (JCAHO) also unveiled an alternative to mandatory staffing ratios in 2002, suggesting that staffing ratios "miss the point" because they only measure staffing and not patient outcomes (FNA Report, 2002). As a result, JCAHO implemented staffing standards, which became effective January 1, 2003, requiring health care organizations to monitor a minimum of four outcome indicators of the 21 that have been developed by JCAHO. Two must be human resource indicators, such as overtime use, and two must be clinical or service indicators, such as patient complaints or patient falls (FNA Report). Health care organizations are expected to analyze the collected data with regard to staffing effectiveness and adjust staffing levels accordingly.

BOX 10.2   Components of the Proposed "Quality Nursing Care Act of 2004"

Requires acute care staffing systems to:

1. Be created with input from direct-care RNs or their designated representative
2. Be based on the number of patients and level and intensity of care to be provided, with consideration given to patient admissions, discharges, and transfers on each shift
3. Account for architecture and geography of the environment and available technology
4. Reflect the level of preparation and experience of those providing care
5. Reflect staffing levels recommended by specialty nursing organizations
6. Provide that an RN not be forced to work in a particular unit without having first established that she or he is able to provide professional care in such a unit

Source: Safe Staffing Initiatives, (2004).

▶ CONCLUSIONS

The literature is clear that increasing RN representation in the staffing mix improves patient outcomes. What is not clear is what the optimal staffing levels are for various patient populations and when costs associated with staffing mix become unreasonable in terms of attempting to improve patient outcomes. In addition, given the lessons that have already been learned with the "RN/LVN debate" and the "at-all times" requirement, more thought must be given as to how strictly staffing ratio regulations are to be interpreted and how enforcement can be effective when there are no monetary consequences for breaking rules. In addition, the intermingling roles of state government as a legislator of minimum staffing ratios, compliance officer, disciplinary enforcer, and potential funding source to assist with mandated ratio implementation needs further examination and clarification.

The implementation and subsequent evaluation of mandatory staffing ratios in California in 2004 should provide some insight into these ongoing issues that will be helpful to other states that choose to follow in California's footsteps. Clearly the enactment of California's nurse-to-patient ratio law is undergoing some "birthing pains" (Leighty, 2004, p. 14) and concerns continue about whether hospitals can find enough nurses, whether they can afford the cost of hiring additional staff in times of financial uncertainty, and whether they can come up with creative solutions to meet staffing ratios "at all times," including breaks and lunches (Leighty).

It is not clear yet whether California has the resources (both human and fiscal) that it will need to make successful staffing ratio implementation a reality. The implementation struggles thus far have been significant. The fact that it took 5 years from passage of the legislation to mandated implementation is telling. What is even more telling are the number of hospitals in California that currently report difficulty in meeting staffing ratio requirements and the pervasive resistance that continues to be a part of its implementation.

DeMoro (2002) argues, however, that California, the birthplace of managed care and many restructuring programs that eroded patient-care standards and created the worst hospital nursing shortage in years, now offers a new model and the first genuine hope for ending that shortage and rebuilding a tattered nursing infrastructure.

Mary Foley, past president of the ANA, agrees and stated:

▶ *Government intervention is necessary when the marketplace is not protecting patients, and we commend the governor (of California) both for putting patient care concerns first and for addressing a nurse staffing crisis that is fast reaching crisis proportions, not just in California, but across the nation (Hashing Out California's Staffing Ratios, 2002, para 4).*

⏩ FOR ADDITIONAL DISCUSSION

1. If California is struggling to meet the mandatory staffing ratios implemented in 2004, how will they cope with increased requirements effective in the years to come?
2. In an effort to cut the costs associated with implementing minimum RN staffing ratios, many hospitals have eliminated their support staff. Have RNs gained anything?
3. Should LVNs be counted to meet minimum mandatory staffing ratio requirements?
4. Is allowing hospitals to determine their own staffing needs a little like having the "fox guard the chicken coop"?
5. Does the implementation of mandatory staffing ratios in the midst of a severe national nursing shortage make sense? Why or why not?

6. At what point does cost related to staffing mix become so prohibitive that society will be willing to accept some increase in patient morbidity and mortality?

7. What critical lessons should other states learn from California's experience thus far in implementing mandatory staffing ratios?

REFERENCES

Aiken, L. H., Clarke, S. P., Sloane, D., Sochalski, J., & Silber, J. (2002). Effects of nurse-staffing on nurse burnout and job-dissatisfaction and patient deaths. *Journal of the American Medical Association (JAMA), 288,* 1987–1993.

American Organization of Nurse Executives (AONE). (2003). AONE policy statement on mandated staffing ratios. Retrieved April 25, 2005, from http://www.hospitalconnect.com/aone/advocacy/ps_ratios.html.

Berliner, H., Kovner, C., & Zhu. C. (2002). *Nurse staffing ratios in California hospitals: A critique of the final report on hospital nursing staff ratios and quality of care.* Retrieved April 25, 2005, from http://www.nursealliance.org/patients/BerlinerKovneretal.pdf.

Blakeman Hodge, M., Romano, P. S., Harvey, D., Samuels, S. J., Olson, V. A., Sauve, M. J., et al. (2004). Licensed caregiver characteristics and staffing in California acute care hospital units. *Journal of Nursing Administration, 34*(3), 123–133.

Bonifazi, W. L. (2002). JAMA study reports critical consequences of staffing ratios. *Nursing Spectrum.* Retrieved April 25, 2005, from http://community.nursingspectrum.com/MagazineArticles/article.cfm?AID=8035.

CA ratios become law. (2004). *The American Nurse, 36*(1), 5–6.

California Healthcare Association. (2001). *Minimum nurse staffing requirements could cost California hospitals between $200,000 and $2.3 million annually.* Retrieved April 25, 2005, from http://www.calhealth.org/calanswers/nurstaf_costs.htm.

California Nurses Association. (2003a). *Hospital industry seminars advise administrators how to evade RN ratios.* Retrieved from http://www.calnurse.org/102103/hospindustry.html.

California Nurses Association. (2003b). *RN alert. Final ratios approved. CNA wins protection for RNs.* Retrieved from http://www.calnurse.org/finalrat/finratrn7103.pdf.

California Nurses Association. (2003c). *RN staffing ratios: It's the law.* Retrieved, from http://www.calnurse.org/102103/safestaffqa.html

California patients and nurses win minimum staffing ratios. Retrieved April 25, 2005, from http://users.rcn.com/wbumpus/sandy/seachange80.htm.

California's nurse-to-patient staffing ratios for general acute care hospitals: Frequently asked questions and responses from the California State Agency that regulates hospital licensing requirements. (2004). *Nevada RNformation, 13*(1), 6–7.

Center for Nursing Advocacy. (2002). *Groundbreaking study shows that nurse short-staffing increases patient mortality, nursing dissatisfaction and nursing burnout.* Retrieved April 25, 2005, from http://www.nursingadvocacy.org/news/2002oct23_jama.html.

Daily Health Policy Report. (2002). Retrieved April 25, 2005, from http://www.kaisernetwork.org/daily_reports/rep_index.cfm?DR_ID=14258.

DeMoro, R. A. (2002). What California has started. *Modern Healthcare, 32*(13), 26.

Dying for lack of nurses. (2002). *New York Times. Late Edition-Final.* p. A34.

Few hospitals checked for nurse-patient ratios. (2004). *Enterprise Record.* Column 5/6. p. 4A.

FNA Report: JCAHO on Nurse Staffing. (2002). *Florida State Association of Rehabilitation Nurses (FSARN) Newsletter, 10*(3), 5. Retrieved April 25, 2005, from http://www.fsarn.org/newsletters/dec2002.pdf.

Gordon, S. (2000). Nurse, interrupted. *The American Prospect, 11*(7), 26–30.

Graf, C. M., Millar, S., Feilteau, C., Coakley, P. J., & Erickson, J. I. (2003). Patients' needs for nursing care. *Journal of Nursing Administration, 33*(2), 76–81.

Hashing out California's staffing ratios. (2002). *The American Nurse, 34*(2), 1, 16–17.

Hopkins, M. E. (2000). Tip of the iceberg: Amid a sea of hot button issues, staffing ratios rise to the surface. *Nurseweek.* Retrieved April 25, 2005, from http://www.nurseweek.com/news/features/00-10/wages.asp.

Hospital industry attempt to delay staffing ratios. (2003). *California Nurse, 99*(3), 5.

Judge rejects hospital challenge to nurse staffing law. (2004). *Chico Enterprise Record,* p. 6A.

Kovner, C. T. (2000). State regulation of RN-to-patient ratios. *American Journal of Nursing, 100*(11), 61–63.

Leading the charge toward legislated staffing ratios. (2003). *Michigan Nurse, 76*(9), 9.

Leighty, J. (2004). Uncharted waters. *Nurseweek, 17*(5), 14–16.

Nevada Organization of Nurse Leaders. (2004). *Legislative issues that are important to NONL.* Bill name AB313. Retrieved April 25, 2005, from http://www.nonl.org/pages/news/legislature/AB313/.

Nurse, hospital showdown goes to judge. (2004). *Chico Enterprise Record,* p. 6A.

Nurse ratio delay blasted. (2004). *The Sacramento Bee.* p. A3, column 6.

NYSNA calls for expanded nurse-patient ratios. (January/February 2004). *The American Nurse, 36*(1), 6.

Phillips, K. (2004). *Some CEOs see mandated ratios as growing idea.* NurseZone.com. Retrieved April 25, 2005, from http://www.nursezone.com/job/MedicalNewsAlerts.asp?articleID=12012.

Russell, S. (2002). Does 'licensed' in 2004 law mean only RNs? Unions debate nurse-patient ratios ahead. SFGate.com. Retrieved April 25, 2005, from http://www.sfgate.com/cgi-bin/article.cgi?file=/chronicle/archive/2002/11/20/BA31607.DTL&type=printable.

Safe staffing initiatives get another boost in Congress. (2004). *The American Nurse, 36*(1), 1, 3.

Seago, J. A. (2002).The California experiment: Alternatives for minimum nurse-to-patient ratios. *Journal of Nursing Administration, 32*(1), 48–58.

Spetz, J. (2001). What should we expect from California's minimum nurse staffing legislation? *Journal of Nursing Administration, 31*(3), 132–140.

Staffing improved at nearly 70% of California hospitals. (2004). *California Nurse, 10*(2), 13.

State staffing legislation (as of April 26, 2002). SEIU District 1199 NW. Retrieved April 25, 2005, from http://www.seiu1199nw.com/appResources/scPages/mandatoryovertime.cfm.

Tieman, J. (2002). Absolute minimum. *Modern Healthcare, 32*(4), 8–10.

Vessey, J. A., Andres, S., Fountain, M., & Wheeler, A. (August 2002). Rx for the nursing crisis? The economic impact of mandatory RN staffing to patient ratios. *Policy, Politics & Nursing Practice, 3*(3), 220–227.

Wood, D. (2004). *Nursing news. California staffing ratios head to the courts.* NurseZone.com. Retrieved April 25, 2005, from http://www.nursezone.com/job/MedicalNewsAlerts.asp?articleID=12360.

Zuger, A. (2002). Cases; Prescription, quite simply, was a nurse. *New York Times* Late Edition-Final, p. F5.

BIBLIOGRAPHY

Blakeman Hodge, M., Asch, S. M., Olson, V. A., Kravitz, R. L., & Sauve, M. J. (2002). Developing indicators of nursing quality to evaluate nurse staffing ratios. *Journal of Nursing Administration, 32*(6), 338–345.

Bolton, L. B., Jones, D., Aydin, C. E., Donaldson, N., Storer Brown, D. (2001). A response to California's mandated nursing ratios. *Journal of Nursing Scholarship, 32*(2), 179–184.

Board on Health Care Services (HCS) and Institute of Medicine. *Keeping patients safe: Transforming the work environment of nurses* (2004). National Academies Press. Retrieved December 8, 2004 from http://www.nap.edu/books/0309090679/html/162.html.

Buerhaus, P. I. & Needleman, J. (2000). Policy implications of research on nurse staffing and quality of patient care. *Policy, Politics & Nursing Practice, 1*(1), 5–16.

Clarke, S. P. (2003). Balancing staffing and safety. *Nursing Management, 34*(6), 44–48.

Clarke, S. P. & Aiken, L. H. (2003). Failure to rescue. *American Journal of Nursing, 103*(1), 42–47.

De Moro, R. A. (2002). What California has started . . . staffing ratios, union activism are national solutions to the nursing shortage. *Modern Healthcare, 32*(13), 26.

Gonzales-Torre, P. L., Adenso-Diaz, B., & Sanchez- Molero, O. (2002). Capacity planning in hospital nursing: A model for minimum staff calculation. *Nursing Economics, 20*(1), 28–36.

Kovner, C. T., Jones, C. B., & Gergen, P. J. (2000). Nurse staffing in acute care hospitals, 1990–1996. *Policy, Politics, & Nursing Practice, 1*(3), 194–204.

Leading the charge toward legislated staffing ratios. (2003). *Michigan Nurse, 76*(9), 9.

Leighty, J. (2004). Safety in numbers. *Nurseweek* (California), 25–27.

Lester, D. (2002). Staffing ratios. *Nursing, 32*(6), 12.

Malloch, K., Davenport, S., & Hatler, C. (2003). Nursing workforce management. Using benchmarking for planning and outcomes monitoring. *Journal of Nursing Administration, 33*(10), 538–543.

Manthey, M. (2001). A core incremental staffing plan. *Journal of Nursing Administration, 31*(9), 424–425.

Mason, D. J. (2003). How many patients are too many? Legislating staffing ratios is good for nursing. *American Journal of Nursing, 103*(11), 7.

McGillis, L., Doran, D., & Pink, G. H. (2004). Nurse staffing models, nursing hours, and patient safety outcomes. *Journal of Nursing Administration, 34*(1), 41–45.

McVay, K. & DeMoro, D. (2002). Point/counterpoint. Regulated staffing ratios: Not "if " but "how." *Nursing Leadership Forum, 6*(4), 92, 95–99.

Mercer, A. L., Kehl, S., & McDonald, G. V. (2004). Viewpoints on nurse/patient ratios. Mandatory nurse/patient ratios: A good idea or not? *Nursing 2004, 34*(1), 8, 10.

Michigan Nurses Association. (2004). The business case for reducing patient-to-nursing staff ratios and eliminating mandatory overtime for nurses. Retrieved April 25, 2005, from http://www.minurses.org/spc/MNA%20Report%200607.pdf.

Seago, J., Spetz, J., Coffman, J., Rosenoff, E., & O'Neil, E. (2003). Minimum staffing ratios: The California workforce initiative survey. *Nursing Economics, 21*(2), 65–70.

Staffing standards are part of the solution. (2004). *California Nurse, 100*(2), 10–12.

Stone, P. W., Tourangeau, A. E., Duffield, C. M., Hughes, F., Jones, C. B., O'Brien-Pallas, L., et al. (2003). Evidence of nurse working conditions: A global perspective. *Policy, Politics, & Nursing Practice, 4*(2), 120–130.

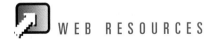

WEB RESOURCES

American Federation of Teachers (AFT) AFL-CIO. Policy Statement on Safe Staffing.   **http://www.aft.org/topics/ healthcare-staffing/policy.htm**

American Medical Directors Association: Position on Direct Care Staffing in Nursing Homes   **http://www.amda.com/library/governance/ resolutions/h02.htm**

American Nurses Association: Government Affairs. Background Info and Legislative Maps. Nurse Staffing Plans and Ratios

American Nurses Association Supports Legislative Proposal to Improve Staffing in Nursing Homes

AONE Policy Statement on Mandated Staffing Ratios (Dec. 2003)

Borgatti, C. (July 28, 2003). Are safe staffing ratios the solution? *Nursing Spectrum*. (Debate over HB 1282 to establish minimum staffing ratios in the state of Massachusetts)

California Department of Health Services

California Healthcare Association

California Nurses Association Position Statement on RN Staffing Ratio

California Nurses Association. Q & A on the Ratios

Society of Gastroenterology Nurses and Associates. Position Statement on Minimal RN Staffing for Patient Care in the Gastrointestinal Endoscopy Unit

Staffing and Productivity in the Emergency Care Setting (2003)

http://www.nursingworld.org/GOVA/STATE/2003/ratio1203.pdf

http://www.nursingworld.org/pressrel/2002/pr0509.htm
http://www.hospitalconnect.com/aone/advocacy/ps_ratios.html

http://community.nursingspectrum.com/MagazineArticles/article.cfm?AID=10182

http://www.dhs.ca.gov
http://www.calhealth.org
http://www.calnurse.org/?Action=content&id=198
http://www.calnurse.org/?Action=content&id=179
http://www.sgna.org/resources/statement14.cfm

http://www.ena.org/about/position/PDFs staffing-productivity.PDF

Mandatory Overtime in Nursing: How Much? How Often?

11

Carol J. Huston

One short-term means of dealing with the current nursing shortage has been to require nurses to work extra shifts, often under threat of "patient abandonment" or punitive measures. *Mandatory overtime*, also called *compulsory* or *forced* overtime, occurs when employees are required to work more hours than are standard (generally 40 hours per week) or risk employer reprisals such as job loss, demotion, or threat of assignment to unattractive tasks or shifts (Golden & Jorgensen, 2002).

Mandatory overtime often results from unanticipated events such as unplanned leave, unexpected vacancies, or sudden changes in patient care requirements (Report to Congress, 2002). However, it also is used by some hospital administrators simply as a way to save money by limiting recruitment and benefit expenses.

Mandatory overtime is not new, nor is it restricted to nursing. Fandray (2000) states that the globalization of the world's economy, abetted by a revolution in computer technology, has made the notion of a 40-hour work week increasingly anachronistic. Indeed, Golden and Jorgensen (2002) report that almost one-third of the American workforce regularly works more than the standard 40-hour work week, and one-fifth work more than 50 hours per week. This occurs because in the United States (unlike most European countries) employment is *at will*, meaning that employers can dismiss employees for any reason—except for gender, race, age, or disability—or for no reason at all (Golden & Jorgensen). Thus, employees who refuse to work overtime can lose their jobs or face other reprisals.

Indeed, the last known attempt to directly measure the extent of mandatory overtime in the United States with specific survey questions in a nationally representative sample was the 1977 Quality Employment Sample of the University of Michigan. Approximately 45% of respondents stated that overtime work was "mostly up to their employers," 44% said "it was up to them," and the remainder said it was up to both of them. Approximately 19% reported they would have suffered a penalty if they had refused to work required overtime (Golden & Jorgensen, 2002).

Yet, nurses argue that mandatory overtime in nursing is not comparable to mandatory overtime in other fields, because the consequences of being overly fatigued for the nurse may literally have life-and-death consequences. Proponents of mandatory overtime argue that it is an economic reality given how limited labor health care resources are. The problem is that both positions are correct.

This chapter will define overtime, examine the extent of the use of mandatory overtime in nursing, discuss the consequences of mandatory overtime in nursing as identified in the literature, and look at staffing alternatives that might alleviate the problem.

▶ LEGISLATING MANDATORY OVERTIME

The Fair Labor Standards Act

The definition of what constitutes overtime or how it should be calculated has historically varied from state to state or from industry to industry. There are, however, national standards in terms of the Fair Labor Standards Act (FLSA) of 1938. This act, which regulates overtime, currently imposes no limits on overtime hours, nor does it prohibit dismissal or any other sanction for declining overtime work (Golden & Jorgensen, 2002).

The FLSA requires that payroll employees (those who are not "exempt" from the overtime requirements of the FLSA) be paid an overtime premium of at least one and one-half times the regular rate of pay for each hour worked over 40 in a week.

> ***CONSIDER:** Labor laws such as the FLSA need to be amended to protect workers against excessive work hours and mandatory overtime and to protect the public from the dangers of an overburdened, stressed workforce (Golden & Jorgensen, 2002).

Recent Changes to Federal Overtime Rules

There have, however, been recent changes to the federal overtime rules. These new changes, which became effective August 23, 2004, define exemptions from the FLSA for what were traditionally called "white-collar" employees. The new rules increased the amount of money employees could earn before they were no longer eligible to receive overtime pay from $65,000 a year to $100,000 a year (Phillips, 2004).

Almost immediately, some nursing leaders expressed concern that the lack of clear language in the new rules opened the door for employer attempts to reclassify nurses as exempt from overtime protections historically given to workers under the FLSA (Trossman, 2004b). This occurred because under the new regulations, employees who are "learned professionals" and who earn a salary of at least $455 a week cannot earn overtime pay. Nurses meet the criteria of learned professional, which is defined in part as employees who perform work that requires advanced knowledge in the sciences and that this may make them ineligible for overtime pay (Trossman, 2004b). Some nurses, however, could still be eligible for overtime pay if they were classified by employers as hourly—not salaried—employees. In fact, the most recent Department of Labor Fact Sheet for nurses states that RNs paid on an hourly basis should receive overtime pay (Phillips, 2004).

The new rules also appear to make it easier to classify registered nurses (RNs) as salaried employees, and salaried employees are not eligible for overtime. As of November 2004, RNs from two constituent member organizations had reported plans by their employers to reclassify nurses as salaried employees to avoid having to pay overtime (Efforts Continue, 2004). In addition, the new rules include employees fulfilling the role of "team leader" within the administrative exemption (Trossman, 2004b). Team leaders are employees who lead a team of other employees in completing a major project. This ruling would mean that team leaders do not have to have direct supervisory responsibility to be exempt from overtime pay. Trossman suggests that although it is unlikely that the administrative exemption will apply to many RNs, this change is likely to cause confusion.

The final rule also indicates that state laws and collective bargaining agreements can require greater protections beyond those outlined in the FLSA. However, the *Coalition to Preserve Overtime Rights for Registered Nurses* questions whether unionized workers ultimately will lose overtime protections or other benefits when they negotiate contracts under the new federal rules, because some unions link their contract language on overtime to the FLSA standards (Trossman, 2004b).

As a result of these concerns, Iowa Senator Tom Harkin introduced a bill in May 2004 to the U.S. Senate that provided that no category of workers eligible for overtime under the old rules—including hourly paid RNs—would lose that right (Efforts Continue, 2004). Rep. Obey of Wisconsin introduced a similar amendment to the bill in the House of

CHAPTER 11   Mandatory Overtime in Nursing: How Much? How Often?

209

Representatives that was approved on September 9, 2004. The American Nurses Association (ANA), however, suggests that threats remain to passage of the final version of the bill and that President George W. Bush has threatened to veto it (Efforts Continue, 2004).

Legislating Limits on Nursing Overtime

In March 2001, a bill entitled the Registered Nurses and Patients Protection Act was introduced to the House of Representatives (H.R. 1289). This bill would prohibit employers from requiring licensed health care employees to work more than 8 hours in a single workday or 80 hours in any 14-day work period—except in the case of a natural disaster or declaration of emergency by federal, state, or local government officials (Battle Brews over Bill, 2001). H.R. 1289 was referred to the House Committee on Education and the Workforce on March 29, 2001.

In addition, in summer 2002, the Safe Nursing and Patient Act of 2003 (H.R. 745/S. 373) was introduced. This bill seeks to amend title XVIII of the Social Security Act by limiting the number of mandatory overtime hours a nurse may be required to work. The act would prohibit health care facilities that receive Medicare funding from requiring a RN or licensed practical nurse (LPN) to work beyond an agreed-to, predetermined, regularly scheduled shift (ANA, July 8, 2004). In no instance could a nurse be required to work more than 12 hours in a 24-hour period or for more than 80 hours in a 2-week period—a provision that would prevent an institution from altering shift schedules in a way that would undermine the law.

The bill also includes nondiscrimination protections for nurses who refuse overtime and for nurses who provide information and/or cooperate with investigations about the use of overtime. Exceptions would include cases of declared national, state, or local emergency (ANA, July 8, 2004).

State Legislation

States are increasingly taking a role in both defining mandatory overtime and putting delimiters around its use. In 2000, California's Industrial Welfare Commission issued a ruling that barred forced overtime, but it only covered health care workers in the private sector who worked 12-hour shifts and were not represented by a contract (Vernarec, 2000). The ruling did, however, state that nurses could be required to work an additional 4 hours in an emergency.

Legislation to restrict mandatory overtime by nurses has passed in states such as Maine, Oregon, and New Jersey (American Association of Critical Care Nurses Public Policy, 2002). In addition, in May 2004, Connecticut became the 10th state—and the second in 2004—to place limits on overtime for nurses in hospitals (Dixon, 2004). The Connecticut legislation prohibits hospitals from requiring nurses to work longer than their scheduled shifts except in defined circumstances such as participating in a surgical procedure until the procedure is completed or a public health emergency. The state senator who wrote the bill predicted that it would protect the health and well-being of health care workers and their patients; in contrast, a hospital executive said the bill ignored the impact on patients of too-few available nurses (Dixon).

In 2004, West Virginia also enacted legislation prohibiting a hospital from mandating a nurse to accept an assignment of overtime (Dixon, 2004), after having similar bills die in the state Senate as a result of opposition from state hospitals (Nurses Progress Further, 2003). Similar legislation was introduced in 2004 in Florida, Georgia, Hawaii, Illinois, Iowa, Massachusetts, Michigan, Missouri, New York, Ohio, Pennsylvania, Rhode Island, Tennessee, Vermont, Washington, and Wyoming (Allabaugh, 2004; Dixon, 2004).

In addition, boards of nursing in several states, including Michigan, Alabama, California, Oregon, and Ohio, have developed clear statements differentiating patient abandonment and employee abandonment (Kany, 2001). These statements define *employment abandonment* as nurses leaving their places of work to avoid injury to patients or to themselves. (See "Patient Abandonment" later in this chapter for more on this issue.)

▶ MANDATORY OVERTIME IN NURSING

A review of the literature suggests that the use of mandatory overtime varies greatly from institution to institution and from state to state. Some of the lowest reported mandatory overtime rates were reported by veterans hospitals, with less than 3.5% of overtime hours in 2001 being reported as mandatory (Report to Congress, 2002; see Box 11.1 for more information). Even with these low rates, the Veterans Administration states that it is unable to totally eliminate mandatory overtime and that any legislative restrictions on the its ability to mandate overtime would hamper its ability to provide safe, quality health care (Report to Congress).

In contrast, the highest rates of mandatory overtime found in the literature were those in a study reported by Worthington (2001a). In Worthington's study of 4,826 nurses, representing a broad cross-section of experienced nurses, over 70% of the nurses surveyed cited acute and chronic effects of stress and overwork as one of their top three health and safety concerns. Yet these nurses reported being pushed to work even more, with 67% of them reporting that they work some type of mandatory or unplanned overtime every month—and 10% reporting having to do so as often as eight or more times a month.

Discussion Point

The units most likely to have the greatest problem with mandatory overtime are the operating room and the postanesthesia care units; however, medical–surgical units also report high use of mandatory overtime (Coughlin, 2001). Why do you think it is most prevalent on these units?

Similarly, a study of North Carolina hospitals in 2000 found that 43% of the rural hospitals and 38% of the urban hospitals that had difficulty finding medical–surgical nurses were using mandatory overtime to staff their facilities (Lovern, 2001). In addition, a survey in 2001 of RNs by the Service Employees International Union found that nurses in acute-care hospitals work an average of eight and a half weeks of overtime per year, although the study did not indicate whether the overtime was voluntary (Lovern).

A study by the New Jersey State Nurses Association (NJSNA) found that nearly a third of the respondents had been required to work overtime during the previous year. And yet another study by the Louisiana State Nurses Association (LSNA) found that of the 524 registered nurses surveyed, 38% worked more than 40 hours per week. Twenty-five percent indicated that they were regularly required to work overtime by their employer (LSNA Investigates Mandatory Overtime, 2003).

Similarly, a report from the state Department of Health in Wyoming showed that in 2003, 15.2% of registered nurses in hospitals, 21% in federal and military facilities, and 43% in state health facilities reported being mandated to work overtime within the previous 2 weeks (Allabaugh, 2004).

CHAPTER 11   Mandatory Overtime in Nursing: How Much? How Often?

211

BOX 11.1

Research Study Fuels the Controversy

A Lot of Overtime

This 2001 study examined the number of mandatory overtime hours for nurses and nurse assistants working in veterans hospitals.

> Report to Congress. Report on Mandatory Overtime for Nurses and Nursing Assistants in Department of Veterans Affairs Facilities. (September 2002). Retrieved June 22, 2004 from *http://www.appc1.va.gov/ncvan/docs/Overtime_Report.htm*

Study Findings

During 2001, a total of 55,629 full- and part-time licensed nurses and nursing assistants worked 2.4 million hours of voluntary and involuntary overtime at a cost of $26.6 million, or, on average, about 43 hours of overtime work per employee. Full-time RNs, the largest category of employees involved, worked on average 37.7 hours of overtime during 2001. These figures represent an annual average of less than 1 hour per week, per employee.

Not included in the hours of overtime worked are the approximately 0.8 million hours of voluntary compensatory time off, which is paid time off from the regular work schedule in lieu of overtime premium pay. If voluntary compensatory time off (which reduces the number of hours an employee works in a week) is offset against the total amount of overtime worked, all licensed nurses and nursing assistants worked on average 28.8 hours of overtime, and full-time RNs worked on average 18.3 hours of overtime during 2001.

The Veterans Administration does not maintain an automated database that distinguishes between mandatory and discretionary overtime. To complete the report, it was necessary to gather information from the field. Unfortunately, this resulted in some local inconsistency in distinguishing between mandatory and other overtime. Responses to an *ad hoc* survey of Veterans Health Administration health care facilities indicated that, for the most part, between 0% and 3.5% of overtime was mandatory in nature. One facility reported that mandatory overtime was as high as 20% of all overtime hours; however, that resulted from some positions being left unfilled because of a pending reorganization that would eliminate the vacant positions. The data was both objective and subjective in nature. Responses from Veterans Health Affairs facilities ranged from "mandatory overtime had not been used for several years", to "all overtime met the definition of mandatory overtime."

Data collected in the 2001 All Employee surveys indicate nursing employees identify workplace issues other than mandatory overtime and floating as more important to their job satisfaction (e.g., pay, work and family balance, respect and fairness, quality of care, recognition, shift work, supervisor training, safe work climate, social support, ergonomics, patient/nonpatient violence, and role conflict). Only 7.1% of nurses identified mandatory overtime as their first or second priority for management intervention. However, nursing employees were more likely than other employees to list mandatory overtime and floating as their first or second priority from a list of 19 work-related issues.

*CONSIDER: Nurses report a dramatic increase in the use of mandatory overtime to solve staffing problems, and fear potential consequences for safety and quality of care for their patients (ANA, 2001b).

In a 2000 report, the ANA's House of Delegates asserted that in some areas of the country, hospitals speak of "mandation" as a legitimate way to staff their facilities (Vernarec, 2000). Indeed, the practice of mandatory overtime in nursing has become so widespread and of such concern, that nurses are refusing to work or are seeking legislative intervention to ban the practice. For example, in 2001, nurses at the Brockton Hospital in Massachusetts went on strike, specifying the use of mandatory overtime as a central issue (Lovern, 2001). A Brockton hospital spokesperson said, however, that mandatory overtime accounted for only one-fourth of 1% of all nursing hours for the first half of that fiscal year, and that most of the mandatory overtime was used as a last resort, when nurses called in sick (Lovern).

Discussion Point

Is mandatory overtime simply the "cover" nurses are using to protest current working conditions, or is it the "straw that broke the camel's back"?

Yet, increasingly nurses are reporting that mandatory overtime has become standard operating procedure instead of a last resort to short staffing. Indeed, in some hospitals, mandatory overtime is routinely used in an effort to keep fewer people on the payroll as well as to alleviate immediate shortage needs.

The NJSNA makes a distinction between acute and chronic use of mandatory overtime in their draft definition of "chronic short staffing." NJSNA defines chronic short staffing as a situation in which a facility is unable to meet hospital unit–specific minimum staffing levels through the use of regularly scheduled staff and per diem staff. Therefore, it requires the use of temporary staff and/or voluntary and/or mandatory overtime for greater than 10% of required hours as defined by the hospital unit–specific minimum staffing levels in the previous 30 days or a total of 90 days in the previous year (Torre, 2002). "Regularly scheduled staff" does not include staff working voluntary overtime. It should be noted, however, that administrative representatives of both acute and long-term care institutions in New Jersey disagree with the NJSNA definition and state they would prefer a looser definition (Torre).

*CONSIDER: "Federal regulations have used transportation law to place limits on the amount of time that can be worked in aviation and trucking. Certainly, nursing has as much of an impact on public health and safety as these professions" (ANA, 2004). It seems appropriate that Congress needs to go beyond the FLSA and at least examine the need to create safety parameters around mandatory overtime in nursing.

▶ CONSEQUENCES OF ENFORCING MANDATORY OVERTIME

To date, research on the effects of overtime has been largely limited to studies of those working scheduled 12-hour shifts (Kany, 2001). Yet, according to a study by the National Institute for Occupational Safety and Health Division of Biomedical and Behavioral Science, when staff plan to work additional shifts on a volunteer basis, they are more likely to get plenty of rest immediately before working the extended shift. Overtime mandated by an employer, however, occurs with little or no prior notice, resulting in high levels of fatigue and increased errors (United Steelworkers of America, n.d.). In addition, nurses routinely report working far more than 12 hours when overtime is involved, and also report working erratic schedules that result in disrupted sleep patterns and fatigue (Kany).

A recent study by Rogers, Wei-Ting, Scott, Aiken, and Dinges (2004) found that the risk of making an error greatly increased when nurses had to work shifts that were longer than 12 hours, when they worked significant overtime, or when they worked more than 40 hours per week. Nurses who worked shifts of 12.5 hours or longer were three times more likely to make errors than those who worked an 8.5-hour day.

In addition, logbooks completed by the 393 hospital staff nurses in the study (Rogers et al.) revealed that participants usually worked longer than scheduled and that approximately 40% of the 5,317 work shifts they logged exceeded 12 hours. Fourteen percent of respondents worked at least 16 consecutive hours at least once during the 4-week period studied, suggesting that double shifts or longer are not confined to rare emergencies. The longest shift worked was nearly 24 hours (Rogers et al.). Working overtime increased the odds of making at least one error, regardless of how long the shift was originally scheduled (Rogers et al., 2004).

These findings reinforced those of the (2004) Board on Health Care Services (HCS) & Institute of Medicine (IOM) Report, *Keeping Patients Safe: Transforming the Work Environment of Nurses*, which said that nurses' long working hours pose a serious threat to patient safety.

Mandatory overtime induces fatigue and sleep disruption; the effect on the quality of patient care, however, warrants further study. Mee (2001) suggests that mandatory overtime threatens RNs' licenses because working in an exhausted state may represent a risk to public health and patient safety. The ANA (2004) reports that sleep loss influences several aspects of performance, leading to slowed reaction time, delayed responses, failure to respond when appropriate, false responses, slowed thinking, diminished memory, and other effects. Worthington (2001b) concurs, stating that fatigue contributes to poor judgment and errors and can affect a nurse's personal safety. One source goes so far as to suggest that mandatory overtime is linked to a host of patient problems and that it is perhaps the single worst practice to emerge from the era of downsizing and managed care (Worst Practices, n.d.).

Discussion Point

How many hours can the typical nurse work before she or he might be considered unsafe? How much individual leeway is feasible in making this determination?

In contrast, a study by the VA National Center for Patient Safety information systems, examining the relationship between nursing staff overtime and adverse events or close calls ("near misses"), showed that less than 1% of nursing staff overtime was involved in an adverse event or close call. In no case was nursing staff overtime identified as the primary cause of an adverse event (Report to Congress, 2002).

What is clearer in the literature is that there is a positive relationship between the use of mandatory overtime and nurse dissatisfaction and turnover. Indeed, working conditions are often cited as the primary cause for nurses leaving the profession or reducing work hours. In fact, a recent study by the Ohio Nurses Association reported that approximately 60% of the nurses it surveyed have considered leaving nursing because of mandatory overtime (Widowfield, 2004).

Similarly, the USWA (n.d.) reports that recent studies show that one in five nurses are considering leaving nursing; when polled on their reasons for leaving, mandatory overtime was always listed in the top 10 reasons. Mandatory overtime also discourages nurses from accepting employment in the first place. Perhaps that is why mandatory overtime is almost universally banned by magnet hospitals.

*CONSIDER: "Health care workers, especially nurses, are leaving their profession because of workplace stresses, long work hours and depreciation of their essential role in the delivery of quality, direct patient care" (2004 Mandatory Overtime Bill, 2004, para 3).

Finally, although mandatory overtime may be thought of as a cost-saving measure, it often generates very large costs, even if sometimes unaccounted for, in the form of increased turnover, lower productivity, longer patient stays, and higher rates of treatment errors that in turn necessitate more extended and costly solutions (Worst Practices, n.d.).

For these reasons, Mee (2001) argues that mandatory overtime must be eliminated or the nursing shortage will worsen and the quality of patient care will further erode. Calarco (2001) agrees, stating that the human toll of mandatory overtime is clear and that forcing staff to work long hours increases their fatigue, erodes morale, and in the end, has the potential to undermine the safety of both staff and patients. It also disrupts the lives of these nurses' families, and the stress generated by this disruption often reverberates back onto the nurse and exacerbates the feelings of guilt, anger, helplessness, and "burn-out" already experienced. "Certainly, the use of forced overtime flies in the face of the current generation's need to balance work life with home and their desire to choose jobs or careers with ever-increasing flexibility and control" (Calarco, p.34).

*CONSIDER: In an age of severe nursing shortages, creating an environment that is attractive to nursing is not a luxury. It's a necessity (Hensinger, Minerath, Parry, & Robertson, 2004).

Calarco goes on to suggest that although mandatory overtime is neither efficient nor effective in the long term, it has an even more devastating short-term impact in terms of staff perceptions of a lack of control and its subsequent impact on mood, motivation, and productivity. Vernarec (2000) concurs, stating that nurses who are forced to work overtime do so under the stress of competing duties—to their job, their family, their own health, and their patients' safety. Clearly, mandatory overtime should be a last resort and not standard operating procedure caused by an institution not having enough staff.

Yet Nevidjon (2001) states that there are situations in which all other strategies have been exhausted and there are patients who need care. In these situations, Nevidjon argues that what is of utmost importance is how the organization designs, communicates, and implements such a process.

Regardless of how an employer chooses to deal with an inadequate number of staff, Marquis and Huston (2006) argue that certain minimum criteria must be met. These criteria are shown in Box 11.2. When possible, however, employers should do whatever they can to adhere to the ANA's Principles for Nurse Staffing. In addition, they should follow the advice of the National Institute for Occupational Safety and Health as outlined in their booklet, *Plain Language About Shiftwork* (Worthington, 2001b).

CHAPTER 11 Mandatory Overtime in Nursing: How Much? How Often?

215

BOX 11.2

Minimum Criteria for Staffing Decisions

- Decisions made must meet state and federal labor laws and organizational policies.
- Staff must not be demoralized or excessively fatigued by frequent or extended overtime requests.
- Long-term as well as short-term solutions must be sought.
- Patient care must not be jeopardized.

Source: Marquis, B., & Huston, C. (2006). *Leadership roles and management functions* (5th ed.). Philadelphia: Lippincott Williams & Wilkins.

▶ PATIENT ABANDONMENT

Many staff members who have worked mandatory overtime report feeling as if they have been held hostage by their employer under threat of "patient abandonment" charges. Indeed, nurses are the only health care professionals who can lose their license if found guilty of patient abandonment (ANA, 2004). Therefore, many nurses believe they have no actual choice when confronted by a request for overtime, despite the fact that they are already working shifts in excess of 12 hours.

*CONSIDER: In some facilities, nurses are being threatened with dismissal or with the charge of patient abandonment if they refuse to accept overtime.

It is imperative that nurses know and understand the provisions of the Nurse Practice Act in their state as well as the position statements or advisory opinions that have been issued by their state board on mandatory overtime and patient abandonment (Vernarec, 2000). For example, the Michigan Board of Nursing (Michigan Nurses Association [MNA], 2001) unanimously passed a resolution that removes the threat of patient abandonment when nurses refuse to work mandatory overtime because they do not believe they are able to provide safe care. The board resolution emphasizes that nurses are educated to make critical decisions based on their analytical skills and are the best judges of their ability to provide safe care (MNA).

Discussion Point

What position statement or advisory opinion has your state board of nursing issued regarding mandatory overtime and patient abandonment? Do you feel it is adequate to protect both nurses and patients from unsafe working conditions?

Similarly, the Board of Registration in Nursing (BORN) in Massachusetts has issued a position statement that says "in general, it would not consider that patient abandonment has occurred when a nurse is asked to work beyond the nurse's established work schedule and informs the employer that she or he is unable to do so" (Massachusetts Nursing Association, 2004, para 12).

BOX 11.3   Four Elements That Must Be Present for Patient Abandonment to Occur

Specifically, the nurse must have:

1. Accepted responsibility for patient care,
2. Voluntarily withdrawn the care,
3. Failed to give reasonable notice that the care was being withdrawn so that continuing care arrangements could be made, and
4. Failed to report essential patient information to an appropriate person.

Source: Massachusetts Nurses Association, (2004). News. The latest developments in the Massachusetts nursing environment. Retrieved April 25, 2005, from *http://www.mass-nurses.org/News/2001/001003/bornmtg2.htm.*

Rachael Tierney, chairperson for the BORN in Massachusetts, was even more explicit in her discussion of the board's position when she presented testimony on the new regulations before the Special Commission on Nursing. Tierney stated that four critical elements must be present for patient abandonment to occur. These four elements are shown in Box 11.3. Tierney went on to state that given that all four elements must be present before disciplinary action would be taken, "the Board finds it difficult to foresee adequate grounds to support a complaint of patient abandonment in connection with any nurse declining to work an additional shift" (Massachusetts Nursing Association, 2004, para 13).

The California Board of Registered Nursing (BRN) issued a similar advisory in November 2001, stating, "A fatigued and/or sleep deprived RN may have a diminished ability to provide safe, effective patient care. Refusal to work additional hours or shifts would not be considered patient abandonment by the BRN" (Hawaii Government Employees Association [HGEA], 1996–2003).

Similarly, the Oregon State Board of Nursing (OSBN), in its disciplinary sanctions for patient abandonment, does not consider refusal to work an additional shift (double shift) or a refusal to float to an unfamiliar unit to be patient abandonment. Instead, the Oregon SBN believes that these are employer–employee issues (HGEA, 1996–2003). Other state regulatory bodies that have determined that refusal to work overtime is not considered patient abandonment include Arkansas, North Dakota, Ohio, Pennsylvania, and Rhode Island (HGEA).

In contrast, the Hawaii Board of Nursing has yet to issue an advisory or decision on the refusal by a nurse to work overtime because of fatigue or illness. It should be noted that under the Hawaii Administrative Rules 16-89-60 (6) (G), leaving a nursing assignment or abandoning a patient without properly notifying appropriate personnel is considered unprofessional conduct (HGEA, 1996–2003).

Generally speaking, most state boards of nursing suggest that refusal to work mandatory overtime is not patient abandonment; in a situation where a nurse has accepted a patient or assignment, the nurse must simply notify the supervisor that he or she is leaving and report off to another nurse. Usually, however, nurses have less likelihood of losing their license if an assignment (mandatory overtime) is never accepted in the first place than if the assignment is accepted and then the nurse changes his or her mind. This is because accepting the assignment suggests that a nurse–patient relationship has been established. Sample language from the California BRN (2001) regarding the link between nurse–patient relationships and patient abandonment is shown in Box 11.4.

Mee (2001) argues that even *threats* of patient abandonment are "the ultimate insult," and questions whether a supervisor would truly notify the board if an RN refused to work additional hours. Mee says likely not, and that instead the facility itself could come under fire for routinely using mandatory overtime to meet staffing needs. In addition,

BOX 11.4

The Link Between Nurse-Patient Relationships and Patient Abandonment

"A nurse-patient relationship begins when responsibility for nursing care of a patient is accepted by the nurse. Failure to notify the employing agency that the nurse will not appear to work an assigned shift is not considered patient abandonment by the BRN, nor is refusal to accept an assignment considered patient abandonment. Once the nurse has accepted responsibility for nursing care of a patient, severing of the nurse-patient relationship without reasonable notice may lead to discipline of a nurse's license."

Source: California Board of Registered Nursing. (2001). *Abandonment of patients*. Retrieved April 25, 2005, from *http://www.rn.ca.gov/policies/pdf/npr-b-01.pdf*.

in June 2000, the ANA House of Delegates voted 541 to 11 for a measure opposing mandatory overtime under any circumstances and declared that refusing overtime did not constitute patient abandonment (Kany, 2001; Vernarec, 2000).

*CONSIDER: Although boards of nursing can rule that patient abandonment is not cause for loss of licensure, they have no jurisdiction over employment and contract issues. Refusing to work mandatory overtime therefore may result in termination of a nurse's employment. "Ironically, while this preserves the institution's power, it only adds to the original problem, a shortage of nurses to provide care" (DeWolf Bosek, 2001, p. 102).

▶ PROFESSIONAL DUTY AND CONSCIENCE

DeWolf Bosek (2001) suggests that mandatory overtime and patient abandonment must not be examined just as a legal issue, but as part of a bigger concept—that of professional duty. A professional duty is the direct result of others having welfare rights, such as the right to safe care. Because people have a right to such care, nurses have an associated duty to ensure that the nurse–patient ratio is adequate to see that care is safe. If nurses accept that patient safety is a primary ethical duty, then they must place the well-being of their clients ahead of every other consideration, both the professional's own interests and all other obligations and concerns the professional might have (DeWolf Bosek, 2001).

DeWolf Bosek goes on to say that nurses also have a right to question whether the nurse's professional duty has limits and to ask how much risk a professional nurse is expected to assume in fulfilling a professional duty. For example, the practice of mandatory overtime is grounded in the commitment to prevent harm to patients by guaranteeing adequate nurse–patient ratios, yet the overfatigued nurse may pose even greater risk of harm to patients by agreeing to work.

Discussion Point

Who bears the risk or the consequences of risk when an overworked nurse makes errors that contribute to patient harm?

Charles (2002) concurs that the decision to comply with mandatory overtime has ethical ramifications because it involves an appeal to *conscience*. A conflict of conscience is created when a person faces two conflicting moral demands, neither of which can be met without at least partially violating the other. In the case of mandatory overtime, there is both a conflict of obligation and a conflict of interest. Nurses perceive they have an obligation to do whatever is necessary to help patients, but may find this to be in conflict with personal needs, issues, or wants.

Charles (2002) suggests that appeals to conscience may be addressed by reflecting on the moral imperatives, such as those promulgated in the ANA's *Code of Ethics* (2001a). Yet, this is still problematic. The *Code of Ethics* states that nurses should care for all people without discrimination and maintain and foster nursing competence and professional development. Yet the code also says that the nurse is to maintain conditions of employment that are conducive to high-quality nursing care.

Sister Carol Taylor (1998, p. 71) wrote "In the not so distant past, one could safely assume when speaking to practicing nurses that each nurse in the audience shared as a valued starting assumption that nursing was a moral practice. I no longer find this to be true." Taylor goes on to say that what many nurses challenge today is the assumption that professional nursing demands a service orientation that entails altruism.

Salladay (2002) suggests that one option nurses should consider if they do not want to work mandatory overtime is to file for *conscientious objection*. The purpose of conscientious objection is to protect the rights of employees who refuse to participate in procedures that conflict with their ethical or religious beliefs. Originally, these types of policies were developed to address the hospital's responsibility to respect the moral convictions of nurses and other staff who refused to assist with certain patient-care procedures, such as abortion, blood transfusion, or withdrawing or withholding life support. Today, these policies can take on a new role as nurses address the conflict of conscience that mandatory overtime presents (Saladay).

▶ UNIONS AND MANDATORY OVERTIME

Because collective bargaining agreements can require greater protections beyond those outlined in the FSA, the position of most collective bargaining agents is that the practice of mandatory overtime should be eliminated entirely. Yet, there are differences between union contracts.

For example, the HGEA Unit 09 contract simply states that *no* mandatory overtime is allowed (HGEA, 1996–2003). This differs from other nurse contracts in Hawaii. Unit 09 employees have the right under Article 20, Personal Rights and Representation, to refuse overtime for good cause, and HGEA continues to advocate that fatigue or illness constitute good cause to refuse overtime (HGEA). Dependent care issues, such as caring for an infant, a young child, or an elderly parent, can also be considered good cause because excessive overtime on a regular basis creates a tremendous burden on nurses who are primary care providers for family members (HGEA).

Model language by the Federation of Nurses and Health Professionals, American Federation of Teachers states that "notwithstanding any provisions of the general laws to the contrary, no health care facility shall require any employee to accept work in excess of eight (8) hours per day or in excess of forty (40) hours per week, the acceptance of such work in excess of forty (40) hours per week or eight (8) hours per day shall be strictly voluntary, and the refusal of any employee to accept such overtime work shall not be a grounds for discrimination, dismissal or discharge or any other penalty upon the employee" (AFL-CIO, 2002, para 5).

Yet, the Health Professionals and Allied Employees, AFT, Local 5091, contract states that hospitals "have the right to require overtime provided it is of reasonable duration, commensurate with employee health, safety and endurance and the direction is issued under reasonable circumstances" (AFL-CIO, 2002, para 5). The contract goes on to state:

> *Employees can be required to work emergency overtime only in cases of unforeseen emergent circumstances and only when the following alternatives have been employed without success and are documented. Such documentation shall be available to the union.*
> *1. Volunteers sought from all available staff, including per diem.*
> *2. Outside agency personnel are utilized.*
> *In the event that no one is available, the supervisor may require employees on a rotating basis, in order of reverse seniority, to work emergency overtime and only for the time necessary to meet the emergency. If the employee works more than one-half of an extra consecutive shift, the time worked for the entire extra shift shall be paid at time and one-half of pay (AFL-CIO, 2002, para 5).*

Because union contract language regarding mandatory overtime varies as much as state board of nursing position statements on patient abandonment, nurses should be aware of the contract provisions set by their place of employment.

▶ ALTERNATIVES TO MANDATORY OVERTIME

There are many successful alternatives to mandatory overtime that share commonalities—the provision of incentives that induce employees to willingly work extra hours and giving employees some degree of control over when they work.

One alternative intended to reduce staffing shortages is *shift bidding*. In shift bidding, a health care organization "sets the opening price for a shift, and then nurses come along and bid down the price" (LeMaire, 2004). If the organization receives more offers to work than are needed, it notifies the nurse with the highest bid via e-mail message or pager of the current bid to give them an option to resubmit a lower bid (LeMaire). Typically, nurses are notified 24 hours in advance as to whether their bids are accepted.

Generally speaking, administrators choose the nurse who bids the lowest, yet exceptions to this rule include denying bids from nurses who are working too much overtime or those who do not have an adequate break between shifts worked (Trossman, 2004a). Yet the "lowest bids" do not come cheap. At St. Peter's Health Care Services in Albany, New York, the average bid is $37 an hour, approximately 30% higher than the base rate paid to RNs, but less than the average $49 an hour agency nurses get (Chang, 2003a). Approximately two-thirds of the bidding comes from St. Peter's employees seeking more work. Part-time nurses are the main bidders, while salaried nurses who bid are paid overtime. When nonhospital nurses bid, they must first pass an orientation process and are added to the payroll as bidders (Chang).

Shift bidding has been implemented successfully at many hospitals across the United States. Since 2001, St. Peter's has filled more than 127,000 hours and saved more than $1.7 million through online bidding, and the overall nurse vacancy rate has dropped from 11% to 5% (Chang, 2003b). Similarly, since implementing shift bidding in May 2003, Mercy Hospital in Pittsburgh has virtually eliminated its use of agency nurses and mandatory overtime to meet staffing needs (Trossman, 2004a).

In addition, Spartanburg Regional Healthcare System in South Carolina created a bidding site in 2002, after learning about St. Peter's success (Chang, 2003b). The system's three hospitals currently allow RNs and LPNs to bid; similar opportunities to bid are expected to be offered in the future. Spartanburg Regional Medical Center, the system's largest hospital with 588 beds, saw its nurse vacancy rate plummet from 20% to 7% after it went online. The hospital also decreased the number of outside nurses by more than 90%, saving between $10,000 and $20,000 a week, and planned to phase out using agency nurses altogether by the end of 2003 (Chang, 2003b).

Cheryl Peterson, a senior policy fellow in the ANA Nursing Practice Department, cautions, however, that although shift bidding "can be a creative tool to allow nurses to have some control over their schedules, hospital management should not use it as a primary means to solve staffing problems, many of which are complex and deep-rooted" (Trossman, 2004a, p. 1). The bottom line is that many facilities don't have enough permanent staff, and shift bidding relies on nurses to pick up extra shifts and likely work more than they should. In addition, ANA is concerned that some facilities might permit nurses to bid for shifts on units where they are not adequately trained to work.

New York State Nurses Association Executive Director Lois Fehr summarizes these concerns best in the following comment:

> *How can we sanction a practice within health care that says the nurse who'll take care of patients for the lowest bid wins? It shouldn't be about a race to the bottom. How can that be in the best interest of RNs? (Trossman, 2004a, p. 8)*

221

Discussion Point

Do you believe shift bidding is in the best interest of RNs? Does the need for flexibility and choice in scheduling outweigh the idea that the "cheapest" RN is the one who will work?

Lambrinos, LaPosta, and Cohen (2004) describe another alternative successfully used at an academic medical center that increased nursing hours while decreasing costs. Implemented in February 2002, this *Pay Enhancement Program* included a monetary incentive program and a new premium pay structure. The incentive program was based on committed hours, as well as the actual number of hours worked each pay period by full time and 0.9 status nurses. Nurses who worked 80 or more hours in a 2-week period received bonuses of $150–$200 per pay period.

Premium pay for last-minute call-ins was redesigned so that full-time nurses were eligible for a premium rate of 2.0, while nurses at 0.9 status could receive premium at a rate of 1.75. Nurses working between 0.5 and 0.8 status were limited to premium pay of 1.5 times their normal rate of pay. Both the incentive program and premium pay options were reported to have encouraged nurses to work more, meaning that mandatory overtime would be decreased.

Other alternatives to mandatory overtime include internal and external per diem staffing agencies, traveler nurses, and management of patient volume (Nevidjon, 2001).

> **CONSIDER:** "Every nurse and nursing administrator must become involved in creating proactive beneficent staffing policies not only at the unit or institutional level but also through state and national organizations and governmental venues" (DeWolf Bosek, 2001, p. 102).

▶ CONCLUSIONS

The mandatory overtime dilemma, like so many in nursing, comes down to a conflict between costs, availability of resources, and safety (Larson, 2002, para 5) states:

> *Mandatory overtime is a lightning rod issue for both nurses and hospital administrators. Worried that there won't be enough nurses on the floor to care for all the patients, administrators feel they must compel nurses to stay late and work an extra shift. On the flip side, nurses contend that they get so tired from working extra that they may make potentially dangerous mistakes.*

Despite this, most nurses and administrators can agree on two goals: 1) that staffing should be at least minimally adequate to assure that all patients receive safe care, and 2) that nursing staff should not be placed at personal or legal risk to provide that care.

The problem is that the onus is on management to ensure there is appropriate staffing, and most health care institutions state there simply aren't enough resources to meet the first goal without jeopardizing the second.

Clearly, more alternatives such as shift bidding and pay enhancement programs need to be explored. Neither health care administrators nor nurses should have to choose between meeting the needs of patients and meeting the needs of nurses. Calarco (2001) suggests that long-term solutions are needed to ensure that patient care needs are safely met without depleting staff reserves or usurping their ability to control their own lives. Both management and staff want safe patient care, but nurses want to be "partners in solving this dilemma, not pawns" (Calarco, p. 35).

The bottom line is that workers should have the right to refuse overtime without fear of repercussion, especially when staffing shortages and mandated overtime are the norm and not the exception. Sadly, given the severity and duration of the current nursing shortage, the use of mandatory overtime as a means of meeting minimum staffing needs is an issue that will plague the nursing profession for some time to come.

FOR ADDITIONAL DISCUSSION

1. How does the presence of a collective bargaining agreement affect a hospital's ability to require mandatory overtime? How much power do unions currently have in negotiating this aspect of working conditions?
2. Would passage of a national ban on mandatory overtime "tie the hands" of hospitals to assure that staffing is at least minimally adequate during periods of acute nursing shortages?
3. Does the use of mandatory overtime really save hospitals money in terms of recruitment and benefits?
4. How do the rates of mandatory overtime in nursing compare with other professions?
5. Why is nursing the only profession at risk for loss of licensure if found guilty of patient abandonment?

6. Are charges of patient abandonment legally and morally appropriate if a nurse works his or her required shift, but refuses to stay and work longer?

7. Given the severity and scope of the current nursing shortage, what is the likelihood that mandatory staffing will continue to be used for both emergency and routine staffing needs?

REFERENCES

2004 Mandatory Overtime Bill (S.B. 251). Nurses overtime bill passes. (2004). Retrieved April 25, 2005, from http://www.wvnurses.org/PDFs/Mandatory_Overtime_Bill.pdf

AFL-CIO Safety and Health Department. (2002). Restrictions on mandatory overtime: Examples of contract language. Retrieved April 25, 2005, from http://www.aflcio.org/yourjobeconomy/safety/issues/otexamples.cfm.

Allabaugh, D. (2004). State panel to air issues of mandatory OT for nurses. Medi-Smart. The Citizens Voice. Retrieved April 25, 2005, from http://www.medi-smart.com/topnews5.htm.

American Association of Critical Care Nurses [AACN] Public Policy. (2002). Public policy update—mandatory overtime. Retrieved April 25, 2005, from https://www.aacn.org/aacn/pubpolcy.nsf/72fe271374e4c5338825688e00776c20/4d7899d5029a1f9f88256b6700069ed2#Mandatory%20Overtime.

American Nurses Association. (2001a). Code of ethics for nurses with interpretive statements. Washington, DC: American Nurses Publishing. Retrieved April 25, 2005, from http://www.nursingworld.org/ethics/code/protected_nwcoe303.htm.

American Nurses Association. (2001b). Position statements. Opposition to mandatory overtime. Retrieved April 25, 2005, from http://www.nursingworld.org/readroom/position/workplac/revmot2.htm.

American Nurses Association. (2004). *Government affairs. 107th Congress. Registered nurses and mandatory overtime*. Retrieved April 25, 2005, from http://www.nursingworld.org/gova/federal/legis/107.ovrtme.htm.

American Nurses Association. (July 8, 2004). Press release: ANA calls for action on legislation to limit mandatory overtime. Retrieved April 25, 2005, from http://www.nursingworld.org/pressrel/2004/pr0708.htm.

Battle brews over bill to ban mandatory overtime. (April 16, 2001). Retrieved April 25, 2005, from http://www.nurseweek.com/onlinecareerfair/mandot.asp.

Board on Health Care Services (HCS) & Institute of Medicine (IOM). (2004). *Keeping patient safe: Transforming the work environment of nurses*. National Academies Press. Retrieved April 25, 2005, from http://www.nap.edu/books/0309090679/html/.

Calarco, M. M. (2001). Point/counterpoint. Given the nursing shortage, is mandatory overtime a necessary evil? *Nursing Leadership Forum, 6*(2), 33–36.

California Board of Registered Nursing. (2001). Abandonment of patients. Retrieved April 25, 2005, from http://www.rn.ca.gov/policies/pdf/npr-b-01.pdf.

Chang, A. (2003a). Nurses use web to choose shifts and pay. *Information Week*. Retrieved April 25, 2005, from http://www.informationweek.com/story/showArticle.jhtml?articleID=16600293.

Chang, A. (2003b). The right shift. *The Washington Times*. Retrieved June 25, 2004 from http://www.washtimes.com/business/20031208-094434-5138r.htm.

Charles, J. (2002). Ethical considerations. Mandatory overtime: Conflicts of conscience? *JONA's Healthcare Law, Ethics, and Regulation, 4*(1), 10–12.

Coughlin, C. (2001). Professional responsibility versus mandatory overtime. *Journal of Nursing Administration, 31*(6), 290–291.

DeWolf Bosek, M. S. (2001). Spotlight on . . . Mandatory overtime: Professional duty, harms, and justice. *JONA's Healthcare Law, Ethics, and Regulation, 3*(4), 99–102.

Dixon, M. E. (2004). Connecticut limits mandatory overtime. *Advance for Nurses*. Retrieved April 25, 2005, from http://nursing.advanceweb.com/commom/EditorialSearch/AViewer.aspx?cc=35604.

Efforts to continue to preserve overtime pay. (September/October 2004). *The American Nurse*. p. 1,3.

Fandray, D. (2000). Eight days a week. *Workforce, 79*(9), 34–40. Retrieved April 25, 2005, from http://articles.findarticles.com/p/articles/mi_m0FXS/is_9_79/ai_6565077.

Golden, L. & Jorgensen, H. (January 2002). *Time after time. Mandatory overtime in the U.S. economy*. Economic Policy Institute. Retrieved May 28, 2004 from http://www.epinet.org/briefingpapers/bp120.pdf.

Hawaii Government Employees Association. *Unit 9: Stop the use of "mandatory overtime."* Retrieved April 25, 2005, from http://aloha.hgea.org/webnews.asp?id=588.

Hensinger, B., Minerath, S., Parry, J., & Robertson, K. (2004). Asset protection: Maintaining and retaining your workforce. *Journal of Nursing Administration, 34*(6), 268–272.

Kany, K. (2001). Issues update. Mandatory overtime. New developments in the campaign. *American Journal of Nursing, 101*(5), 67–71. Retrieved April 25, 2005, from http://www.needlestick.org/AJN/2001/may/Issues.htm.

Lambrinos, J., LaPosta, M. J., & Cohen, A. (2004). Increasing nursing hours without increasing nurses. *Journal of Nursing Administration, 34*(4), 195–199.

Larson, J. (2002). State nursing organizations press for legislation. Retrieved April 25, 2005, from http://www.nursezone.com/Job/MedicalNewsAlerts.asp?articleID=8584.

LeMaire, B. (2004). Ken Dion, on health care staffing solutions. *Nurseweek, 17*(5), 6.

LSNA investigates mandatory overtime. (2003). *Pelican News, 59*(4), 4.

Lovern, E. (2001). The overtime debate goes center stage. *Modern Healthcare, 31*(36), 7–9.

Marquis, B. & Huston, C. (2006). *Leadership roles and management functions* (5th ed.). Philadelphia: Lippincott Williams & Wilkins.

Massachusetts Nursing Association. (2004). News. The latest developments in the Massachusetts nursing environment. Retrieved April 25, 2005, from http://www.massnurses.org/News/2001/001003/bornmtg2.htm.

Mee, C. L. (2001). Dear colleague. Mandatory madness. *Nursing 2001, 31*(9), 6.

Michigan Nurses Association. (2001). Mandatory overtime resolution clarified. Retrieved April 25, 2005, from http://www.minurses.org/news/Opress/pr041601.shtml.

Nevidjon, B. (2001). Point/counterpoint. Due to the nursing shortage, mandatory overtime is a necessary evil. *Nursing Leadership Forum, 6*(2), 32, 37–38.

Nurses progress further than ever before on mandatory overtime. (2003). *West Virginia Nurse, 7*(2), 1, 4.

Phillips, K. (2004). *Overtime rules receive praise, scrutiny.* Nursezone.com. Retrieved May 20, 2004 from http://www.nursezone.com/job/MedicalNewsAlerts.asp?articleID=12344.

Report to Congress. *Report on mandatory overtime for nurses and nursing assistants in Department of Veterans Affairs facilities.* (2002). Retrieved April 25, 2005, from http://www.appc1.va.gov/ncvan/docs/Overtime_Report.htm.

Rogers, A., Wei-Ting, H., Scott, L. D., Aiken, L. H. & Dinges, D. F. (2004). The working hours of hospital staff nurses and patient safety. *Health Affairs, 23*(4), 202–212.

Salladay, S. (2002). Ethical problems. Mandatory overtime: New role for conscientious objectors. *Nursing, 32*(12), 65–66.

Taylor, C. R. (1998). Reflections on "nursing considered as moral practice." *Kennedy Institute Ethics Journal, 8*(1), 71–82.

Torre, C. T. (2002). Mandatory overtime, *New Jersey Nurse, 32*(8), 2.

Trossman, S. (2004a). Move over ebay? A potential trend involving bidding for shifts online. *The American Nurse, 36*(3) 1, 8, 12.

Trossman, S. (2004b). New overtime regulations may harm RNs. *The American Nurse,* 1, 3, 18.

United Steelworkers of America. (n.d.). Facts on mandatory overtime. Retrieved April 25, 2005, from http://www.uswa.org/uswa/program/content/515.php.

Vernarec, E. (2000). Just say "no" to mandatory overtime? *RN, 63*(12), 69–72, 72, 74, 76.

Widowfield, J. (2004). Safer nurses; Safer care: Ban on mandatory overtime proposed. *Ohio Nurses Review, 79*(2), 1, 10.

Worst practices. Mandatory overtime. (n.d.). Retrieved April 25, 2005, from http://www.afscme.org/una/sns10.htm.

Worthington, K. (2001a). American Nurses Association/NursingWorld.org on-line health and safety survey. Retrieved April 25, 2005, from http://www.nursingworld.org/surveys/keyfind.pdf.

Worthington, K. (2001b). The health risks of mandatory overtime: The hidden costs of this all-too-common practice. *American Journal of Nursing, 101*(5), 96.

BIBLIOGRAPHY

ANA commends IOM report outlining critical role of nursing work environment in patient safety: Study reinforces call to eliminate mandatory overtime; improve staffing levels, work environment. (2004). *Alabama Nurse, 30*(4), 25.

Center for Policy Alternatives. (2004). Safe staffing for hospital care. *2004 Policy Toolkit.* [Electronic version], 284-292. Retrieved April 25, 2005, from http://www.stateaction.org/issues/issue.cfm/issue/SafeStaffing.xml.

Clarke, S. P. (2003). Balancing staffing and safety. *Nursing Management, 34*(6), 44–48.

McManis & Monsalve Associates. (2004). *Healthy work environments: Striving for excellence* (Vol. II). Washington, DC: American Organization of Nurse Executives & McManis & Monsalve Associates. Retrieved April 25, 2005, from http://www.hospitalconnect.com/aone/docs/hwe_excellence_full.pdf.

Kany, K. (2001). Mandatory overtime. *American Journal of Nursing, 101*(5), 67–71.

Kaufman, S. (2000). Desperate strategies for last-minute staffing. *Nursing Management, 31*(1), 35.

Klitch, B. A. (2000). Staffing strategies for survey success. *Nursing Homes: Long-Term Care Management, 49*(3), 12–17.

Michigan Nurses Association. (June 2004). *The business case for reducing patient-to-nursing staff ratios and eliminating mandatory overtime for nurses.* Retrieved April 25, 2005, from http://www.minurses.org/spc/MNA%20Report%200607.pdf.

Nelson, R. R. & Fitzpatrick, J. J. (2004). State labor legislation enacted in 2003. *Monthly Labor Review, 127*(1), 3–29.

Price of professional status. (2003). *Advance Online Editions for Nurses, 5*(15), 7.

Under pressure. (2003). *Nursing, 33*(10), 12.

White, K. (2003). Effective staffing as a guardian of care. *Nursing Management, 34*(7), 20–24.

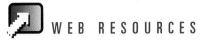

WEB RESOURCES

Academy of Medical Surgical Nurses (AMSN) Official Position Statement On: Mandatory Overtime

http://www.medsurgnurse.org/position/ot.htm

American Nurses Association Position Statement: Opposition to Mandatory Overtime (Oct. 17, 2001)

http://www.nursingworld.org/readroom/position/workplac/revmot2.htm

Colorado Nurses Association Position Statement on Mandatory Overtime (March 2003)

http://www.nurses-co.org/Article_feature.asp?story=272

Emergency Nurses Association (ENA) Position Statement: Staffing and Productivity in the Emergency Care Setting (2003).

http://www.ena.org/about/position/staffingproductivity.asp

Kansas State Board of Nursing Position Statement: Mandatory Overtime (May 16, 2002)

http://www.ksbn.org/positionstatements/Mandatory%20overtime%20position%20statement.doc

Massachusetts Organization of Nurse Executives Position Statement: Mandatory Overtime

http://www.massone.org/main/Position%20Statements/Mandatory%20Overtime.htm

Mississippi Board of Nursing Position Statement: Patient Abandonment

http://www.msbn.state.ms.us/p14.htm

Position of the Pennsylvania State Nurses Association on Mandatory Overtime (March 30, 2001)

http://www.psna.org/c_PosStat_OT.htm

Safe Nursing and Patient Care Act (H.R. 745/S. 373) (proposes limitations on mandatory overtime in hospitals)

http://www.seiu.org/health/nurses/mandatory_overtime/mot_details.cfm

Solving the Nursing Shortage. Worst Practices: Mandatory Overtime

http://www.afscme.org/una/sns10.htm

U.S. Department of Labor: Fair Labor Standards Act (FLSA)

http://www.dol.gov/esa/whd/flsa/

Violence in Nursing: The Expectations and the Reality

Charmaine Hockley

12

N urses, wherever employed, in whatever capacity or area of expertise, may experience various forms of violence at work. A recent international study reported that although workplace violence has the potential to affect all sectors and all categories of workers, the health sector is at major risk (Di Martino, 2002).

Violence in the workplace, particularly in the health care sector, is not a new phenomenon, but only in the past decade or so have researchers and practitioners been reporting on the seriousness and magnitude of this issue. According to various researchers, violence in the workplace is becoming a human rights issue, a public health challenge, and a potential impact on primary health care at a national and international level, and in industrial and developing nations (Cooper, 2002; Di Martino, 2002; Hockley, 2002b).

Although health care facilities generally contain many health care professionals, including physicians, pharmacists, physiotherapists, and social workers—all of whom have the potential to be targeted at work—studies show that nurses are most at risk for experiencing workplace violence (Di Martino, 2002). Ironically, nurses face the possibility of being targeted by the very same people they seek to assist. However, it is important to note that not all violence comes from patients and their families. At times the violence is caused by their health care colleagues (Di Martino; Hockley, 2003c).

There is a scarcity of specific research into violence in nursing compared to the reporting of workplace violence, particularly in the health care arena. Thus, it is difficult to estimate the extent and severity of workplace violence in the health care sector because "comprehensive and unequivocal evidence does not exist" (Mayhew & Chappell, 2001a, p. 3). Comparative data are generally drawn from other countries reporting on violence in nursing.

Therefore, it has been necessary at times in this chapter to draw nursing data from research directed at violence within the health care arena. With this in mind, the terms *violence in nursing, workplace violence*, and *workplace violence in the healthcare sector* have been used to source nursing data. In addition, although many of the major studies on workplace violence are not specific to violence in nursing, it is clear from the literature that if it is occurring in the health care arena, it is highly probable that nurses must be included in the statistics.

CONSIDER: Violence in nursing is an important professional issue for all nurses.

Although the following data are U.S.-based, these figures are likely comparable to those of other countries experiencing workplace violence. The National Institute for Occupational Safety and Health (2002a) reported that each year from 1993 to 1997, "an average of 1.7 million people were victims of violent crimes while working on duty in the United States" (p. 1). Another report by the U.S. Department of Labor, Bureau of Labor, showed that in the year 2000 in the United States, 677 work-related homicides occurred; this was the third leading cause of occupational fatality for women (Gerberich et al., 2004). These statistics are particularly relevant considering that the nursing population is more than 90% female. Furthermore, in the United States, 85% of all nonfatal assaults occur in the retail and service industries. Within the service sector, health care workers face 16 times the risk of violence from patients/clients that other service workers face

227

(Cooper, 2002, p. v). Moreover, the "violence often takes place during times of high activity and interaction with patients, such as meal times, during visiting hours and patient transportation. Assaults may occur when services are denied, when a patient is involuntary admitted, or when a health care worker attempts to set limits on eating, drinking, or tobacco or alcohol use" (NIOSH, 2002b, p. 4).

▶ PERSPECTIVES ON THE ISSUE

A Global Perspective on Violence in Nursing

Until the mid-1990s, research on violence in nursing was mainly centered in North America (Diaz & McMillin 1991) and the United Kingdom (McMillan, 1995). Since the mid-1990s, other countries, such as Australia, New Zealand, and South Africa, have shown a growing interest in researching the topic of violence in health care (Geyer, 2003; Lyneham, 2000; McKenna, Poole, Smith, Coverdale, & Gale, 2003). The first major international study was commissioned by the International Labour Organization (ILO), International Council of Nurses (ICN), World Health Organization (WHO), and Public Services International (2002) to investigate the prevalence and nature of violence in the health care workplace. Table 12.1 shows a selected perspective of the results (Di Martino, 2002).

U.S. data on general and health care workplace violence are collected and reported by the Bureau of Justice Statistics. The data are collected from an annual survey that is not dependent on police reports, which Gershon (2002) asserts "is important since many workplace violence incidents may go unreported both to the employer and the police" (p. 25).

Although many developed nations have reporting systems similar to that of the United States, there are no international databases on either workplace violence or, more specifically, health care workplace violence (Gershon, 2002, p. 25). This lack of international databases adds to the difficulty in making precise comparisons between countries because of differences in the completeness of data and attitudes in reporting workplace

TABLE 12.1 Global Perspective of Violence in Nursing

Nation	Researchers' Comments
Brazil	Nurses constituted the group with the largest proportion of victims (62%).
Bulgaria	Half of the nurses interviewed had experienced verbal abuse and bullying in the previous 12 months.
Portugal	Seventy-four percent of nurses in health centers and 54% in hospitals had been exposed to at least one type of violence in the previous year.
South Africa	Fifty-eight percent of nurses had been victims of verbal abuse during the same period.
Australia	Up to 67% of the nurses interviewed reported that they had been subjected to verbal abuse, 13% to threats, 9% to assaults, 6% to bullying, and 5% to some other form of violence.

Source: Di Martino, 2002.

violence. Studies show that workplace violence is very complex because it is "multifaceted, poorly enumerated, without monocausal explanations, and not amenable to simple preventative solutions" (Mayhew & Chappell, 2001b, p. 1). Nevertheless, although international and national evidence is "patchy," a common thread appears to be developing—that violence in nursing occurs along a wide continuum from nonphysical (e.g., emotional and psychological) to physical harm (including homicide).

A comparison of the international literature regarding violence in nursing is also difficult because of the differences in research methods, definitions, and research perspectives. For example, international, national, or local approaches to researching this topic must take into account the differing standards and expectations for acceptable and unacceptable workplace behavior in the range of societies and workplace cultures around the world. Different countries, each with their own cultures, have different rules about acceptable behaviors at work.

Given the diverse views regarding what constitutes violence in nursing, researchers find it difficult to identify common operational terms for their studies. Researchers studying workplace violence in the health care sector reported that "sometimes it is simply a matter of finding the terms most appropriate to the specific situation, such as in the case of Portugal where workplace violence in the health care sector was typified as *verbal, moral, against property, discrimination (including racial harassment and physical and sexual),* . . ." (Di Martino, 2002, p. 12).

Table 12.2 reports on other countries' interpretation of workplace violence in health care. Researchers in the International Labour Office (ILO) et al. (2002) study reported that although the different interpretations of workplace violence were culturally significant, a general understanding of the concept could be reached. Nevertheless, as Di Martino (2002) points out, "within this general shared understanding, cultural and linguistic differences are certainly in operation that need to be taken into full account and properly addressed" (p. 13).

TABLE 12.2   Global Interpretation of Workplace Violence

Nation	Interpretation
Thailand	Thai researchers had to broaden their definition of workplace violence to include violent incidents that occur to employees living onsite. In Thailand, many health care workers live on campus, and any violence that occurred outside working hours was still considered workplace violence if it occurred on campus.
Brazil	In Brazil, the contracts and established agreements that were not fulfilled between employer and employee were considered workplace violence.
South Africa	Many of the male participants in a South African study questioned the inclusion of sexual harassment as workplace violence, even though the researcher claimed that this country "has the highest incidence of rape in the world."
Lebanon	The researcher from Lebanon stated that in her country the definition of sexual harassment is restricted to an actual physical act, which had the potential to hide the magnitude of the phenomenon.

Source: Di Martino, 2002.

An interesting point to raise here is that two Australian researchers reported that "while there may sometimes be a fine dividing line between bullying behaviors and sexual harassment, sexual violence at work is not normally included within definitions of occupational violence" (Mayhew & Chappell 2001b, p. 2).

Regardless of how violence is defined or measured, it is important for nurses to continue to reiterate the gravity and scope of the problem and the extent of the damage, emphasizing that this is not only a local issue, but also a national and international one. Until there are global nurse population-based studies that investigate violence in nursing, there will always be difficulty in estimating the magnitude of the problem.

Violence in Nursing

Leather (2002) states that once it was acknowledged by various researchers that nurses were particularly at risk of workplace violence, the research focus changed from researching other health professionals such as psychiatrists, social workers, and psychologists to researching nurses' experiences. Indeed, violence in nursing has attracted media attention. Although the incidents reported are primarily attacks on nurses from external sources and to a lesser degree client-initiated attacks, the incidents that gain the most media and community attention are nurse-initiated violence and when a nurse is killed on duty.

One extreme case of violence in nursing was reported as follows:

> *In the wake of the tragic murder of a nurse by a patient who was being admitted to a psychiatric hospital in Port St. Lucie, FL, the American Nurses Association (ANA) is calling for federal standards mandating a safer work environment for the nation's health care workers. "No nurse should have to fear for her life while providing care to her patients," ANA President Mary Foley, MS, RN, said referring to the murder of registered nurse Alda Ellington by a psychiatric patient last week (Price, 2001).*

However, when discussing various forms of violence in nursing, the reality is that physical attacks do not occur as often as nonphysical attacks. Researchers show that ongoing verbal abuse and similar nonphysical behaviors cause the most concern to nurses, but such behaviors do not get the same attention as severe physical abuse from other sources.

The type of violence reported has changed in recent years from patients and doctors being the main perpetrators of violence to colleagues within formalized working relationships causing violence. For example, a recent survey commissioned by the American Association of Occupational Health Nurses reported that employee-on-employee violence was "the most common source of threats or assaults on the workplace violence continuum" (McDuffee, 2003, p. 2). This survey was not specific to nurses, but the results were similar to many other studies involving nurses.

Although there may be some difficulty in constructing a consistent definition of workplace violence generally, and violence in nursing specifically, there is some common ground in what constitutes this phenomenon. Most definitions focus on either the antisocial workplace behaviors or the outcomes of the incidents of violence, particularly the personal, professional, social, financial, mental, and spiritual harm done to an individual. How the concept of harm is interpreted varies from country to country and from one legal system to another. For example, in Australia the law recognizes three types of harm: physical, economic, and psychological (Wallace, 2001).

231

Discussion Point

What are the essential features of violence in nursing?

DEFINING WORKPLACE VIOLENCE

The term *workplace violence* is gradually being recognized as the most appropriate term to collectively describe the various antisocial behaviors and incidents that lead a person to believe they have been harmed by the experience. However, one of the continuing difficulties in considering why the concept of violence is not attributed to many workplace incidents may be due to people's reluctance to expand their understanding of the meaning of violence.

> ***CONSIDER:** Violence has penetrated every sector of society including the workplace, and yet there continues to be difficulty in defining incidents as violent when they occur in the nursing workplace.

In common usage, *violence* is still considered to mean harm done to a person through physical force or the threat to use physical force. Terms used to describe violence often have some element of physical interpretation such as *wild, brutal, savage, fierce, ferocious,* or *frenzied* (*Oxford Dictionary and Thesaurus,* 1997, p. 1755). Early researchers in violence reinforced these interpretations in their studies, which focused on the physical aspects of violence by patients (Lanza, 1983).

Hockley (1999; 2003c) reported in her study that, during the early to mid-1990s, nurses rarely used the term *violence*, instead using metaphors and euphemisms or generally ignoring the terms usually associated with violence, such as *victim, perpetrator, bullying*, and *mobbing* when discussing violent behavior among their female colleagues. She stated that the reluctance to use unequivocal language when discussing workplace violence contributed to the issue remaining poorly recognized and poorly addressed, and increased the negative impact of workplace violence on the health and well being of the individual. Moreover, the vocabulary that was used to describe violence among female nurses often carried with it different connotations from that common in general society (Hockley, 2000).

However, by the late 1990s, and particularly recently, the language used to define this phenomenon changed notably, for example when violence in the workplace generally, and in nursing specifically, is discussed, the nonphysical aspects (sometimes known as *psychological violence*) are now being included. Terms describing antisocial workplace behaviors such as *verbal abuse, violence, bullying, mobbing, harassment*, and *stalking*, to name a few, are now often used interchangeably. Although bullying continues to be the preferred term by many researchers, contemporary literature on this phenomenon is beginning to use the term *workplace violence*. However, the choice of terms appears to be specific to the country, with the United Kingdom (UK) and Australia preferring the term *bullying* in their legislation, and northern Europe preferring the term

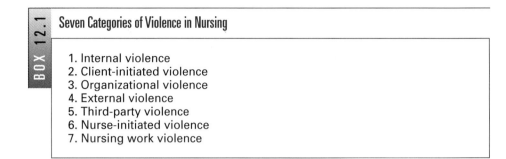

BOX 12.1

Seven Categories of Violence in Nursing

1. Internal violence
2. Client-initiated violence
3. Organizational violence
4. External violence
5. Third-party violence
6. Nurse-initiated violence
7. Nursing work violence

mobbing. North American nurses often refer to this bullying behavior as *horizontal violence*.

Nevertheless, defining this phenomenon often depends on the researcher's or practitioner's perspective. For example, the late Andrea Adams, a well-known UK antibullying activist, defined her own workplace bullying experiences in the following quote:

> *Bullying at work is like a malignant cancer. It creeps up on you long before you or anyone else are able to appreciate what it is that is making you feel the ill effects (Adams, 1992, p. 9).*

The WHO identified nonphysical abuse that has the potential to lead to severe psychological and career consequences in their definition of workplace violence that follows: "the intentional use of power, threatened or actual, against another person or against a group, in work-related circumstances, that either results in or has a high degree of likelihood of resulting in injury, death, psychological harm, mal-development or deprivation" (WHO, cited in Cooper & Swanson, 2002, p. v).

▶ TYPOLOGY OF WORKPLACE VIOLENCE

Typologies have been developed (Bowie, 2002; Mayhew & Chappell, 2001b) to delineate the various categories of workplace violence. Box 12.1 lists seven basic categories specific to nursing that have been modified and/or added to these authors' typologies.

It may not be possible to develop a statement that covers all the categories in the typology in Box 12.1; however, the definition that follows is a start:

> *Violence in nursing is the outcome of any act that causes harm to a nurse. Along a continuum, these acts can range from nonphysical, such as abuse of power, to physical, including homicide. Violence is not so much the act itself; it is the outcome of a harmful experience. Harmful experiences may include professional, social, economic, or personal harm, such as loss of career, ostracism, loss of wages, or third party victims' experience of third party violence (Adapted from Hockley, 2002b).*

*CONSIDER: Clarification is necessary as to what type of behaviors or incidents are being referred to when discussing *violence in nursing*.

What do nurses mean when discussing violence in nursing, as compared to the rest of the population?

Internal Violence

Internal violence occurs in formalized working relationships; for example, those between employers and employees (nurse manager–registered nurse) or colleagues (nurse–nurse) (adapted from Mayhew & Chappell, 2001a). In this form of violence, the perpetrators are employees within the same organization.

Box 12.2 lists some of the nonphysical antisocial workplace behaviors that can lead to causing another person harm. These various behaviors can, over a prolonged time, cause a person to develop low self-esteem, to feel worthless, or to feel frustrated. When an individual does decide to report these incidents, they are often difficult to prove unless there are witnesses, and even then, there is no guarantee of support from colleagues. Moreover, even when there is evidence, such as e-mail messages, it is often dismissed as the sender "being too busy," by protestations of misreading, "I didn't mean it as it has been interpreted," by trivializing particular incidents, "I was only joking," or by accusations of personal deficiencies in the recipient, "Can't you take a joke?" (Hockley, 2003c).

Client-Initiated Violence

This type of violence is committed by individuals who have, or had, some form of service relationship with the organization (Mayhew, 2002). Within nursing, client-initiated violence originates mainly from patients/clients and their families and is directed toward nursing staff. The reporting of this violence shows that often a nurse is the victim of an attack simply because of being in the wrong place at that time. In other words, these attacks are not personal; but the perpetrators are acting out their aggression, possibly

---

BOX 12.2 **Antisocial Workplace Behaviors**

- Sending abusive email messages and posters
- Being verbally abusive
- Engaging in favoritism
- Setting a worker up for failure
- Withholding necessary information
- Denying workers promotional opportunities
- Supervisors acting disinterested or interacting in ways perceived to be discouraging, criticizing, excluding, alienating, intimidating, sabotaging, stalking, threatening, or humiliating
- Bullying
- Playing "humorous" pranks (sometimes perceived as initiation or rites of passage)

Source: Hockley, 2003a.

because of stress, substance abuse, illness, or feeling vulnerable. Moreover, these attacks against nurses are generally one-time incidents, except in the case of patients who are unstable (e.g., substance abuse), have a disability (e.g., brain injury), or have a long-term mental health problem (e.g., dementia).

How these aggressive behaviors are perceived often depends on the context. For instance, consider spitting, which may be perceived as an antisocial behavior; if a person is seen spitting in the parking lot, another person may be offended but is not harmed by it. Yet, if a person spits at a staff member in anger, the staff member may be harmed by this behavior. How a person responds to various intimidating and threatening antisocial workplace behaviors, and whether they are personally or professionally harmed, will vary from person to person. For some nurses, despite the fact that some of these incidents can be traumatic, even aberrant in nature, the perception is that this is a "part of the job" (Bain, 2000).

> *CONSIDER: The impact that these antisocial workplace behaviors have on a person depends on that person. Not everyone is personally or professionally harmed by these behaviors or incidents.

Organizational Violence

This type of violence refers to the harm that may occur to nursing staff when an organization is experiencing economic pressures resulting in restructuring, redundancy, redeployment, or resignations (adapted from Bowie, 2002). Generally, organizational violence is not a single incident but a series of incidents, and is symptomatic of organizational crisis.

One of the characteristics of this form of violence is that it impacts the whole organization, not only the perpetrator and victim. When organizational violence occurs, the organization's reputation is often tarnished with low staff morale, increased absenteeism, reduced efficiency, and spiraling recruiting and legislative costs. There is also the possibility of retaliatory violence by staff via strikes, picket lines, deliberate damage such as arson, computer hacking, and in the worst cases, random killings.

On occasion, health care facilities that experience this type of violence may be "named" on the Internet, sometimes through various nursing chat groups, or by a "whistleblower." A health care facility that receives bad publicity will find it difficult to attract qualified staff and may, in fact, attract the "wrong" type of staff to meet nursing staffing needs. This increases the potential for staff members to take future legal action against the employer for negligent hiring.

External Violence

External violence is perpetrated by outsiders entering the workplace with criminal intent, such as armed robbery for drugs or gang reprisals in emergency departments. This form of violence includes incidents that occur while a nurse is going to or returning from work. In these incidents, the assailant may not have any personal or workplace relationship. This form of violence is often random and can include rape, robbery, homicide, or attempted homicide.

Third-Party Violence

Until recently, legislation and research into violence in nursing mainly recognized two parties: perpetrator and victim. However, it is now recognized that there is a third party: the witnesses to these behaviors and incidents who may be affected.

A definition of third-party violence is that it:

▶ *is the outcome of workplace violence and can include those who directly or indirectly witness the event(s) such as those with a professional relationship (e.g., colleagues), personal relationship (e.g., family members) and indirect relationship (e.g., case managers) (Hockley, 2002b, p. 71).*

When a nurse bullies another nurse in the workplace, others may witness this behavior. Nurses, as witnesses, can support the bully's actions, ignore these actions, or become third-party victims of the behavior. However, other third parties—those with a personal or indirect relationship; are also drawn into these incidents.

Research shows that third-party witnesses experience similar emotions and feelings of being harmed in some way to those of the primary target. Some nurses, for example, may be reluctant to be seen speaking with a nurse who is being targeted because of the fear of becoming the next target; that is, fearing guilt by association (Hockley, 2002b). Nearly all of the reports on third-party violence showed that this form of workplace violence systematically undermined the individual; therefore, the perpetrator was inflicting damage not only on the primary target, but also on secondary targets—the third person.

Additionally, there is the potential for another manifestation of third-party violence in nursing: the family member who cares about the person who is the primary target. Research shows that living with a person who has been bullied at work can contribute to poor health and changes in financial status and socialization of that individual (Hockley, 2002a; 2003a). One nurse in Hockley's study describes her experiences and how they exacerbated her precarious mental state. She explained her own situation while caring for her partner—the primary target—who was also a nurse.

▶ *I had recently been assaulted. I was unfit for work, suffering post-traumatic stress disorder severely, with depression, episodes of dissociation, intrusive thoughts about the trauma, hyper vigilant, and anxiety.*

My witnessing my partner in this state, and with myself in an emotional mess with my illness was a very crippling experience. . . . In the ensuing weeks, with both of us depressed (and on one occasion both feeling suicidal simultaneously), we found it was best for both of us to live separately in the same house, because our depressed states seemed to worsen each other's mood (Hockley, 2002a, p. 158).

*CONSIDER: Violence in nursing is not a single incident but a symptom of nursing in crisis.

Occupational health and safety (OHS) legislation varies from state to state and country to country. Nevertheless, the general consensus within OHS legislation is that the employer has a duty of care to its employees.

Nurse-Initiated Violence

This form of violence occurs when nurses are violent toward those in their professional care. Although there have been studies into the various forms of violence toward nurses, there has been little research into the causes and effects of nurse-initiated violence toward patients. Violence by nurses against people in their care goes against the professional code of ethics, and it is important to identify the issues that cause nurses to act in this way (Hockley, in press).

More than 6 years ago, Hockley's (1999) research into violence among female nurses in their formalized working relationships demonstrated that nurses are violent toward patients as well as colleagues. Her study showed that the patients were at a higher risk in some health care settings than in others. For example, patients in aged care and mental health settings were more at risk than those in the acute care sector, with one respondent reporting that she observed psychiatric nurses abusing their patients more than when she worked in the general nursing sector. One nurse's report of nurse-initiated violence follows:

> *Patients being abused? I have seen that. . . . There was a bruise on his face. He was a diabetic—lost his big toe nail because the nurse had been standing on his feet (Hockley, 2003c, p. 66).*

*CONSIDER: Further work needs to be done to develop an instrument that can accurately predict which nurses are at risk of causing harm to those in their care.

Nursing Work Violence

This type of violence focuses on the nurse's experience in times of extreme emergencies, such as biochemical assaults, terrorist attacks, attacks on civil society, or violence related to armed conflict or other major disasters. This form of violence may occur once (e.g., a terrorist attack; schoolyard or work massacres) or at special events (e.g., the final games of the football [soccer] season). Many issues are emerging, in part, because of the changing trends in the different types of violence that are occurring in society. To date, there is a scarcity of nursing research on the impact on nurses managing large numbers of trauma cases caused by exceptional violent acts.

Acts of terrorism are not new. Nevertheless, it is relevant to expand briefly on this issue because of the impact it has on nurses and contemporary nursing. Terrorist acts in the 1970s and 1980s mainly targeted specific groups of people, such as the Israeli Olympic team at the 1972 Munich Olympic Games, or high-profile people such as the Italian Prime Minister, Aldo Moro. However, in the 1990s and the early 21st century, the direction of attacks changed, with terrorists launching their attacks on civilians. In these attacks, hundreds and sometimes thousands of civilians are targeted at work, and nurses, along with other health professionals, are being called upon to take care of these traumatized people and their families.

Little is known about the impact this type of violence is having on nurses. What can be assumed from studies of workers traumatized by events—for example, servicemen in Vietnam and Iraq; firefighters and police officers in New York following September 11, 2001; rescue workers after the Bali bombing on October 11, 2002, and the train bombing in Madrid in 2004—is the potential for serious health and mental health issues to arise, such as posttraumatic stress disorder (PTSD).

The ICN recognizes "the need for information resources to assist in coping with the aftermath of these attacks and the climate of fear and uncertainty they have created" (ICN, 2002b, p. 1). However, until further research is undertaken, the strategies used are from other contexts. That is not to say they are not appropriate, but many of the participants are from male-oriented occupations, such as police officers, firefighters, paramedics, and the armed services. With nursing being a predominantly female occupation, the health and mental health issues may be different from the male-oriented occupations.

Although the true extent of violence in nursing is considered to be greater than the statistics indicate, studies show that violence against female nurses is greater than that against male nurses. Studies into violence against males in other contexts tend to focus on rites of initiation of apprentices, college fraternity rites of passage (hazing), and armed service "bastardization" practices. However, the question of whether workplace violence against male nurses is an outcome of the same forces identified in studies into workplace violence in female nurses is open to further research. Because the statistics show that males are often the major perpetrator of violence in society and in the workplace (except possibly for *internal* violence in nursing), the very fear that some male nurses may experience violence could also create more violent incidents in the workplace, generating a cycle of violence.

Clearly, nursing work associated with violent situations can be very stressful (McVicar, 2003) and may lead to job dissatisfaction (Happell, Martin, & Pinkahana, 2003; Moyle, Skinner, Rowe, & Gork, 2003). In these studies the main focus was stress, however defined, and how it related to a nurse's specific area of practice. What is missing from this scholarly writing is the voices of nurses working in highly volatile areas of practice and the traumatizing effects it had on them.

The consequences of working in volatile areas have been acknowledged in studies on other groups, such as paramedics, firefighters, and police officers. The lack of acknowledgment of nurses working in extremely violent situations was noticeable in the coverage by the international media following the events of September 11 in New York City, as almost all attention was focused on other services—firefighters and police officers. In contrast, nurses' work was highly publicized in the Australian media following the Bali bombings in 2002. Nevertheless, with or without media attention, the impact of these events on nurses has not been fully studied in the short or long term.

▶ THE IMPACT OF WORKPLACE VIOLENCE ON NURSES AND NURSING

The impact of violence on nurses often depends on the type they have experienced and over what period of time. Research shows that nurses, including student nurses, may suffer a wide range of physical, mental, and psychological problems (Randle, 2003; Taylor & Martin, 2002). Although it is recognized that some nurses may not be harmed by their work practices, for others these practices may have a profound, negative effect on their health and well being. For example, nurses who are bullied over a long time may experience greater health and mental problems than nurses coping with an isolated incident.

Various researchers have reported nurses contemplating or committing suicide because of destructive ongoing bullying behavior by senior nursing staff. Even though not all nurses experience or witness extreme incidents, the literature shows that non-physical violence can make them feel as powerless, alone, and frightened as physical violence.

The literature shows that many of the health problems developed by those who have been targeted at work, such as anxiety, depression, PTSD, stress-related skin conditions, suicidal thoughts, and suicide, can also be experienced by others close to them, including colleagues and families (Hockley, 2002b). The decision about whom to consult for these health problems is determined by many factors, which, in turn, can exacerbate the level of anxiety (Hockley 2002a).

Unfortunately for some nurses, words seldom convey their intense feelings because they have been severely traumatized by the damaging workplace behaviors. Hockley (2002b) reported that some respondents in her study discussed the shame they felt. Therefore, they did not tell colleagues or their families at all, or they withheld reporting the behaviors until they had been under attack for a prolonged time.

*CONSIDER: Increasingly, behavioral problems in society are being reflected in the workplace, including violence in nursing.

▶ STRATEGIES TO ADDRESS THE PROBLEM

At an international level, the World Health Assembly (WHA) declared in 1996 that violence, including violence in the workplace, was a global public health problem, and proposed that strategies be developed to address this problem (WHA, 1997). Some national governments have recognized that all forms of violence are unacceptable, regardless of a worker's gender, age, sexuality, identity, cultural or religious beliefs, and where they live or work. Some federal governments may need a mandate to address this issue because they do not have appropriate legislative power over the state governments. Thus, individual and community lobbying may be needed to specifically include workplace violence on the agenda.

Professional nursing associations acknowledge that violence in nursing occurs, and have provided guidelines on how to address the problem (e.g., Royal College of Nursing [RCN], 2002). The workplace organizations that acknowledge workplace violence have developed policies and procedures to address this important issue; it is vital that these policies are implemented in the spirit that they were written. At the individual level, the development of survival strategies is paramount for personal protection and the maintenance of personal integrity. There are also some nurses who advocate tougher laws on workplace violence as a safety strategy (Connolly, 2001).

International Intervention

In 2002, joint ILO guidelines for addressing workplace violence in the health sector were published. A variety of strategies to address five key areas were proposed. Box 12.3 lists these five key areas of recommended action. For example, the ILO group emphasized the need for governments, employers, workers, professional bodies, and the wider community to participate. To achieve this broad mandate they suggested that an integrated, participative, cultural and gender sensitive, nondiscriminatory, and systematic approach be considered (ILO et al., 2002, pp. 7–8). A further strategy was to identify the violence that is occurring, the organizations at risk, and the potential perpetrators and victims, followed by assessment of risk factors, intervention, and evaluation of outcomes.

BOX 12.3 **Key Areas for Addressing Violence in Nursing**

- Prevention of workplace violence
- Dealing with workplace violence
- Management and mitigation of the impact of workplace violence
- Care and support of workers affected by workplace violence
- Sustainability of initiatives undertaken

Source: International Labour Office, International Council of Nurses, World Health Organization, & Public Services International, 2002.

*CONSIDER: Violence in nursing undermines the right to work in a safe environment in a manner compatible with human dignity.

Organizational Intervention

Violence in nursing may not be completely eliminated, but by measuring the risks between the various causative factors and violence and identifying those that can be modified, there is the potential for these behaviors and incidents to be prevented, or at least minimized. The success of these strategies often depends on the philosophy of those implementing the plans as well as their leadership qualities.

Some people and groups propose a public health approach to prevent violence in nursing and support strategies grounded within the framework of human rights. A public health approach serves to support the government's requirements that employers have a duty of care towards their employees. Because violence in nursing can undermine an individual physically and psychologically, the consequences have the potential to bear heavily on the individual, the organization, the health care sector, and the health care system.

Discussion Point

Is violence in nursing a "part of the job"?

Individual Intervention

The literature on how to survive violence in nursing shows that there is no "one wrong way" or no "one right way" to respond to these experiences (Arnetz & Arnetz, 2000; Ulrich, 2001). Compared to the national and international approach, an individual's strategy may range from ignoring the issue to becoming "institutionalized" to survive. An individual, for example, may choose not to report the incidents or he or she may choose to be compensated for his or her experiences and require medical support.

The literature shows that targeted nurses consulted with a variety of health professionals—general practitioners, psychologists, psychiatrists, endocrinologists, neurologists, dentists, lawyers, counselors, mediators, and therapists—to survive. Hockley (2003c) revealed that although some nurses were looking for answers to resolve these issues, others were looking for retribution; that is, "someone will pay for what I have gone through." However, that was rare.

The literature reports that one of the best strategies for an individual seeking to deal with violence is counseling; however, it is apparent nurses were reluctant to consult with other health professionals, particularly if they lived in a small community. When they did, they preferred to meet with psychologists rather than psychiatrists to help them address their workplace issues. A possible reason for this approach is that conditions associated with violence in nursing are more closely aligned to psychology than psychiatry (Hockley, 2003a). In addition, it could be that psychologists, such as Heinz Leymann (1998), were the pioneers in researching workplace violence and therefore became *de facto* custodian or pioneer parameters setters.

The strategy nurses use depends mainly on the type of violence and whether their employing organization will support them. For example, the more physical the violence, the more support the workplace appears to give the staff, in keeping with OHS legislation. The literature shows, however, that in many instances, the victims of *internal violence* do not appear to receive the same support as victims of *external violence*. *Ad hoc* information from nurses asserts that the violence that occurs within the workplace; that is, all the other categories of violence except external violence, is often ignored, supported, or condoned. There are reports that even extreme nurse-initiated violence is covered up by providing good references for the accused nurse so that he or she can be transferred out of the employing facility or discharged with confidentiality.

Commitment at all levels is required to address this problem, and yet some nurses remain reluctant to report this destructive behavior, so only the tip of the iceberg is revealed. Box 12.4 outlines possible reasons why a targeted nurse may be hesitant to report these incidents.

Some studies show that the frequency of the exposure to aggression in the workplace has a cumulative effect on the targeted persons (Rippon, 2000), whereas other studies show that some individuals who have experienced child abuse, domestic violence, and violence in nursing recognize the signs and prepare themselves (Hockley, 2003c). What can be deduced from the different studies and various interventions proposed is that addressing violence in nursing is not straightforward. Violence in nursing is a complex

240

BOX 12.4 **Reasons for Reluctance to Report Violence in Nursing**

- Denial, as a way of coping
- Confidentiality and/or breaches of privacy legislation
- Stigma attached to troublemakers
- Too much documentation to submit
- Poor or ineffective reporting systems
- Peer pressure not to report, to avoid administration retaliation
- Lack of support by management, colleagues, other staff, union, or professional association
- Fear of official repercussions—loss of privileges, promotion, or leave
- Poor health
- Personal apathy
- Low self-esteem
- Belief of not receiving "fair" treatment
- Lack of trust in the processes; and/or
- Believing the perpetrator is right

Sources: Hockley, 2004; Rippon, 2000.

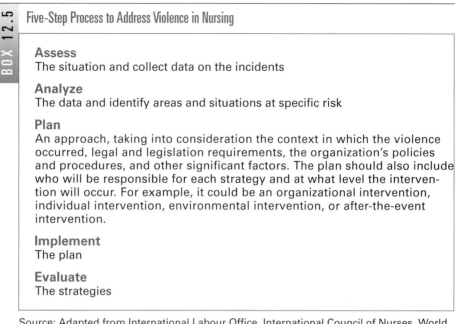

BOX 12.5

Five-Step Process to Address Violence in Nursing

Assess
The situation and collect data on the incidents

Analyze
The data and identify areas and situations at specific risk

Plan
An approach, taking into consideration the context in which the violence occurred, legal and legislation requirements, the organization's policies and procedures, and other significant factors. The plan should also include who will be responsible for each strategy and at what level the intervention will occur. For example, it could be an organizational intervention, individual intervention, environmental intervention, or after-the-event intervention.

Implement
The plan

Evaluate
The strategies

Source: Adapted from International Labour Office, International Council of Nurses, World Health Organization, & Public Services International, 2002.

issue and may need complex solutions. To address the problem, a process, similar to the nursing process, may help to ensure that all steps are included in achieving a successful outcome. These steps are outlined in Box 12.5.

*CONSIDER: Nurses who bully are seen as powerful, and at times brave, because they appear to be at the cutting edge by flouting the system.

▶ NURSING CODE OF ETHICS

The ICN recognizes violence in nursing in its assertion that "[R]egrettably, a small number of nurses have also been known to be perpetrators of violence, patient or colleague abuse in violation of nursing's code of conduct" (ICN, 2002a, p. 1). The nurses' code of conduct may vary from country to country, from professional associations to registering bodies and from generalist to specialist groups. Nevertheless, a common thread runs through these codes. They have been developed as an ethical and moral guide for nurses. The guide is flexible, but within the law, to protect the public from unacceptable practice, and can be used for determining if unprofessional conduct has occurred (American Nurses Association, 2001).

The ICN Code of Ethics for Nurses (2000) has four main elements that outline ethical conduct for nurses. Box 12.6 outlines the third section of the fourth element, which has an approach focusing on the development of policies by three key stakeholders to minimize abuse by health care personnel.

A Three-Prong Approach to Addressing Nonprofessional Conduct

Practitioners' and Managers' Roles

Develop mechanisms to safeguard the individual, family, or community when their care is endangered by health care personnel.

Educators' and Researchers' Roles

Instill in learners the need to safeguard the individual, family, or community when care is endangered by health care personnel.

National Nurses Association's Role

Provide guidelines, position statements, and a discussion forum related to safeguarding people when their care is endangered by health care providers.

Source: International Council of Nurses, 2000.

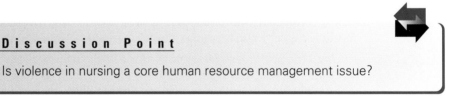

D i s c u s s i o n   P o i n t

Does nursing have a culture of "never complain and never explain"?

▶ WHAT SHOULD BE DONE?

A famous Danish philosopher wrote, "Life can only be understood backwards; but it must be lived forwards" (Kierkegaard, cited in Storm, 2004). To demonstrate that violence in nursing is not only a contemporary issue but also an enduring one, it has been necessary to review past research on the topic, what is currently occurring, and where this research is leading so that key directions can be planned.

D i s c u s s i o n   P o i n t

Is violence in nursing a core human resource management issue?

One of the major issues facing employers and employees is the traditional view of the workplace as "a quite benign environment where, despite certain levels of robust confrontation and dialogue, people usually manage to resolve their dilemmas in a peaceful and constructive way" (Chappell & Di Martino, 1998, p. 142). Although this view continues, unwanted and unwarranted forms of violence in nursing still occur.

The various forms of violence nurses experience continues to be a growing concern and urgently needs to be addressed by individuals, organizations, and governments. Although studies suggest some answers to addressing violence by showing its scope, causes, and how it may be prevented, researchers state that violence in nursing often goes unreported. Violence in nursing is not only a contemporary issue, but also an enduring one as researchers and practitioners identify the damage and the cost to the individual, organization, community, and government.

▶ CONCLUSIONS

Although all types of violence can occur in one workplace, not all nurses may witness or experience the seven categories discussed in this chapter. However, there is the potential for nurses to do so. At some time in their career, most nurses may experience or witness at least one of these categories.

In the 21st century, the focus of research into violence in nursing is expanding. Although all categories need further research, three areas in particular need urgent attention because evidence-based information is so scarce: third-party violence, nurse-initiated violence, and nursing work violence.

Third-party violence is an important issue because witnesses to this behavior suffer consequences (Box 12.7). Third parties are acknowledged in other contexts—third-party vehicle insurance for example—but are not recognized in OHS legislation except for those employed by the organization where the violence is occurring. Therefore, those affected who are not employees of the offending organization (which employs the bully) are not covered by legislation.

Nurse-initiated violence has the potential for extensive harm to the nursing profession as the community loses trust in what it considers one of the most trustworthy professions. Nursing work violence is a category that needs study because of the way nurses become involved in the aftermath of large-scale attacks on society. Trauma that was previously confined to the battlefield is becoming more common on "soft" targets.

There remains a need for further study, particularly through evidence-based literature searches, on the causes of violence in nursing. At a macro level, further studies are required into possible factors contributing to this behavior, such as the history of nursing, biological factors, mental illness, media influences, substance abuse, or personality issues. At an individual level there could be biological, psychological, or social factors needing further study.

It is important to acknowledge the legacy of early researchers on violence in nursing and the achievements of nurse leaders in addressing this problem. Nevertheless, there is much to be achieved. Some nurses still believe that violence has to be physical and that workplace bullying is similar to school bullying. Therefore, it is vital that all nurses acknowledge that bullying is inappropriate behavior; that it is a problem and that the problem begins in nursing.

Finally, the profession needs to recognize that addressing violence in nursing is a shared responsibility, requiring a diverse, integrated, and systemic approach including organizational, community, government, professional, and union intervention. Research, education, and training are essential elements in ensuring that the negative behaviors and their impact are greatly reduced and the outcomes of these strategies reflect the values and guiding principles of nurses' ethical and moral codes of professional practice.

BOX 12.7

Research Study Fuels the Controversy

Costs of Third-Party Violence

This study challenged the traditional views about the victim of workplace violence and employer–employee relationships. Since the introduction of occupational health, safety, and welfare legislation in Australia in the mid-1980s, an organization's duty of care has been between two parties: the employer and the employee. However, it is proposed that in circumstances of violence in the workplace there is a third party, the witnesses to these behaviors, in particular the families who indirectly witness the impact that workplace violence has on the targeted person.

> Hockley C. (2003). The impact of workplace violence on third party victims: A mental health perspective. *The Australian e-Journal for the Advancement of Mental Health, 2*(2)1–11.

Study Findings

Early results from this ongoing study showed that workplace violence has huge human costs not only on the primary targets, but also on those close to them, such as colleagues and family members. The results show that, depending upon the relationship with the primary target, the impact of workplace violence on third parties varies between groups, although there may be some overlap. For example, family members as third-party victims were more likely to suffer financial and health problems than colleagues of the primary target. Colleagues, on the other hand, were more likely to experience professional issues. Both groups of participants experienced social isolation.

One of the reasons why colleagues' financial and health status may be less affected was because they continue to work in paid employment and, if necessary, receive counseling assistance from the workplace through employee assistance programs. In contrast, family members may initially experience financial difficulties through time lost from employment caring for the bullied person who faces unemployment, or could be in ill health and unable to function either physically or emotionally. At times, family members may also require medical treatment for the parallel stress they are experiencing. In some circumstances, family members have contemplated suicide. One of the major recommendations from the study is for employers to have a holistic approach to mental health promotion in the workplace because any disruption that damages an individual's ability to interact with workmates, colleagues, and managers can have a profound effect on their family relationships as well as their work status.

FOR ADDITIONAL DISCUSSION

1. What is your interpretation of violence in nursing?
2. What are the advantages and disadvantages of having general definitions to cover all categories of violence in nursing?
3. Does a person have to experience professional or personal harm for it to be considered violence in nursing?
4. Why do some nurses indicate that they are surprised and "more hurt" when the perpetrators are their colleagues rather than other health professionals or patients?
5. How could a nurse overcome fears of reporting these incidents?

6. What could an organization do to encourage staff to report all incidents of violence, even if they are not harmed by the experience or consider it as "a part of the job?"

7. Why do some nurses initiate violence on the very people they are committed to care for?

8. Is it paradoxical that those whose responsibility it is to provide care and promote an environment where the human rights, values, customs, and spiritual beliefs of those in their care are respected should act in this manner?

9. How does your professional association define unprofessional conduct?

10. Are bullying, horizontal violence, stalking behaviors, and mobbing violent behaviors? If not, why not?

REFERENCES

Adams, A. (1992). *Bullying at work*. London, UK: Virago.

American Nurses Association. (2001). Code of ethics for nurses with interpretive statements. Silver Spring, MD: American Nurses Publishing.

Arnetz, J. & Arnetz, B. (2000). Implementation and evaluation of a practical intervention program for dealing with violence towards health care workers. *Journal of Advanced Nursing, 31*(3), 668–680.

Bain, E. (2000). Task force concludes: Workplace violence is not "part of the job." Retrieved January 2, 2004 from http://www.massnurses.org/News/2000/000003/workvio.htm.

Bowie, V. (2002). Defining violence at work: A new typology. In Gill, M., Fisher, B., & Bowie, V. (Eds.), *Violence at work: causes patterns and prevention*. Devon, UK: Willan.

Chappell, D. & Di Martino, V. (1998). *Violence at work* (2nd ed.). Geneva, Switzerland: International Labour Office.

Connolly, A. (2001). Nurses want tougher laws on workplace violence. Boston Business Journal. Retrieved April 26, 2005, from http://boston.bizjournals.com/boston/stories/2001/03/05/story5.html.

Cooper, C. L. (2002). Introduction. In Cooper, C. L. & Swanson, N. (Eds.). *Workplace violence in the health sector. State of the art. (p. 1)* Geneva, Switzerland: International Labour Organization, International Council of Nurses, World Health Organization, and Public Services International.

Cooper, C. L. & Swanson, N. (2002). Workplace violence in the health sector. State of the art. Geneva, Switzerland: International Labour Organization, International Council of Nurses, World Health Organization, and Public Services International.

Diaz, A. & McMillin, J. (1991). A definition and description of nurse abuse. *Western Journal of Nursing Research, 13*(1), 97–109.

Di Martino, V. (2002). *Workplace violence in the health sector. Country case studies. Brazil, Bulgaria, Lebanon, Portugal, South Africa, Thailand and an additional Australian study. Synthesis report*. Geneva, Switzerland: International Labour Organization, International Council of Nurses, World Health Organization, and Public Services International.

Gerberich, S. G., Church, T. R., McGovern, P. M., Hansen, H., Nachreiner, N. M., Geisser, M., Ryan, A. D., Mongin, S. J., & Watt, G. D. (et al.) (2004). An epidemiological study of the magnitude and consequences of work-related violence: The Minnesota nurses' study. *Occupational and Environmental Medicine, 61*(6), 495–503.

Gershon, R. R. M. (2002). Information collection and reporting of violence at work in the health sector. In Cooper, C. L. & Swanson, N. (Eds.), Workplace violence in the health sector. State of the art. Geneva, Switzerland: International Labour Organization, International Council of Nurses, World Health Organization, and Public Services International, 19–25.

Geyer, N. (2003). Violence in the workplace: Management's role. Nursing Update, 27(9), 20–23.

Happell, B., Martin, T., & Pinkahana, J. (March 2003). Burnout and job satisfaction: A comparative study of psychiatric nurses from forensic and a mainstream mental health service. *International Journal of Mental Health Nursing, 12*(1), 39–47.

Hockley, C. (1999). Violence among nurses: An ethnomethodological perspective of nurses' experiences. Unpublished doctoral dissertation. Faculty of Nursing, University of South Australia.

Hockley, C. (2000). The language used when reporting interfemale violence among nurses in the workplace. The Collegian. *Journal of the Royal College of Australia, 7*(4), 24–29.

Hockley, C. (2002a). The impact of workplace violence on third party victims: A mental health perspective. In L. Morrow, I. Verins, & E. Willis (Eds.), Mental health and work: Issues and perspectives (pp. 149–165). South Australia: Auseinet and Flinders University.

Hockley, C. (2002b). *The silent third party victims of workplace bullying: Family members*. Paper presented at the Adelaide International Workplace Bullying Conference—Skills for survival, solutions and strategies. Adelaide, South Australia.

Hockley, C. (2003a). The impact of workplace violence on third party victims: A mental health perspective. *The Australian e-Journal for the Advancement of Mental Health, 2*(2)Retrieved April 26, 2005, from http://auseinet.flinders.edu.au/journal/vol2iss2/index.php.

245

Hockley, C. (2003b). Positive outcomes by looking backwards before moving forward. Paper presented at the Work Trauma Foundation/Denosa Gauteng International Conference on the Management of Psychosocial Problems in the Workplace. Gauteng, South Africa.

Hockley, C. (2003c). *Silent hell, workplace violence and bullying*. Norwood, South Australia: Peacock.

Hockley, C. (2004). If you did not write it then it did not happen. Paper presented at the AUSMED Publications Conference. Adelaide, South Australia.

Hockley, C. (in press). Staff violence against those in their care. In B. Fisher, V. Bowie, & C. Cooper (Eds.), *Countering the many faces of workplace violence*. Devon, UK: Willan.

International Council of Nurses. (2000). The ICN code of ethics for nurses. Geneva, Switzerland: ICN. Retrieved April 26, 2005, from http://www.icn.ch/icncode.pdf

International Council of Nurses. (2002a). Position statement. Abuse or violence against nursing personnel. Geneva, Switzerland: ICN. Retrieved April 26, 2005, from http://www.icn.ch/psviolence00.htm

International Council of Nurses. (2002b). Resources for coping with terrorism. Geneva, Switzerland: ICN. Retrieved April 26, 2005, from http://.icn.ch/terrorism.htm.

International Labour Office, International Council of Nurses, World Health Organization, & Public Services International. (2002). Framework guidelines for addressing workplace violence in the health sector. Joint program on workplace violence in the health sector. Geneva, Switzerland.

Lanza, M. (1983). The reactions of nursing staff to physical assault by a patient. *Hospital and Community Psychiatry, 34*(1), 44–47.

Leather, P. (2002). Workplace violence: Scope, definition and global context. In C. L. Cooper & N. Swanson (Eds.), *Workplace violence in the health sector. State of the art.* (pp. 3–18) Geneva, Switzerland: International Labour Organization, International Council of Nurses, World Health Organization, and Public Services International.

Leymann, H. (1998). Some historical notes: Research and the term mobbing. The Mobbing Encyclopaedia. Retrieved April 26, 2005, from http://www.leymann.se/English/frame.html.

Lyneham, J. (2000). Violence in New South Wales emergency departments. *Australian Journal of Advanced Nursing, 18*(2), 8–17.

Mayhew, C. (2002). *Preventing violence within organizations: A practical handbook*. Canberra, Australia: Australian Institute of Criminology.

Mayhew, C. & Chappell, D. (2001a). "Internal" violence (or bullying) and the health workforce. Taskforce on the prevention and management of violence in the health workplace. Working paper series 141. School of Industrial Relations and Organization Behavior and Industrial Relations Research Center. December. University of New South Wales, Sydney.

Mayhew, C. & Chappell, D. (2001b). 'Occupational violence: types, reporting patterns and variations between health sectors,' Working paper series no. 139, School of Industrial Relations and Organizational Behavior and the Industrial Relations Research Center. Paper written for the Task Force on the Prevention and Management of Violence in the Health Workplace. University of New South Wales, Sydney.

McDuffee, J. (2003). Critical warning signs of workplace violence not what employees expect: AAOHN and FBI deliver workplace violence prevention tips and tools to prepare workforce. Retrieved April 26, 2005, from http://www.workplaceviolence911.com/docs/20040115-04.htm.

McKenna, B. G., Poole, S. J., Smith, N. A., Coverdale, J. H., & Gale, C. K. (2003). A survey of threats and violent behavior by patients against registered nurses in their first year of practice. *International Journal of Mental Health Nursing, 12*(1), 56–63.

McMillan, I. (1995). Losing control. Bullying in the workplace. *Nursing Times, 19*(5), 40, 42–43.

McVicar, A. (2003). Workplace stress in nursing: A literature review. *Journal of Advanced Nursing, 44*(6), 633–642.

Moyle, W., Skinner, J., Rowe, G., & Gork, C. (2003). Views of job satisfaction and dissatisfaction in Australian long term care. *Journal of Clinical Nursing, 12*(2), 168–176.

National Institute for Occupational Safety and Health. (2002a). Occupational violence. Retrieved April 26, 2005, from http://www.cdc.gov/niosh/injury/traumaviolence.html.

National Institute for Occupational Safety and Health. (2002b). Violence. Occupational hazards in hospitals. Retrieved April 26, 2005, from http://www.cdc.gov/niosh/2002-101.html.

Oxford Dictionary & Thesaurus. (1997). Oxford, UK: Oxford University Press.

Price, C. (2001). American Nurses Association demands stricter violence protections for health care workers. Murder of Florida psychiatric nurse prompts profession's call to action. Retrieved April 26, 2005, from www.nursingworld.org/rnrealnews.

Randle, J. (2003). Experiences before and throughout the nursing career. Bullying in the nursing profession. *Journal of Advanced Nursing, 43*(4), 395–401.

Rippon, T. J. (2000). Aggression and violence in health care professions. *Journal of Advanced Nursing, 31*(2), 452–460.

Royal College of Nursing. (2002). Dealing with bullying and harassment at work: A guide for RCN members. London, UK: RCN. Retrieved April 26, 2005, from http://www.ren.org.uk/news/congress2002/congressitems/bullying.php

Storm, D. (2004). D. Anthony Storm's commentary on Kierkegaard. Retrieved April 26, 2005, from http://www.sorenkierkegaard.org/

Taylor, M. & Martin, D. (2002). Students in clinical areas: Debate continues . . . Students must be treated better in clinical areas. *British Journal of Nursing, 11*(19), 1234.

Ulrich, B. (2001). Risky business. As workplace violence rises, nurses and facilities must put safety first. Nurse Week. Retrieved April 26, 2005, from http://www.nurseweek.com/ednote/01/080601a.html

Wallace, M. (2001). Health care and the law. (3rd ed.) Pyrmont, New South Wales: Law Book.
World Health Assembly. (1997). World Health Assembly endorses plan of action to deal with violence as a public health issue. April 26, 2005, from http://www.who.int/entity/occupational_health/en/oeh49wha.pdf.

BIBLIOGRAPHY

Ashanasy, N. M., Hatel, C. E. J., & Zerbe, W. J. (Eds.). (2000). *Emotions in the workplace: Research, theory and practice*. Westport, CT: Quorum.

Barling, J., Rogers, A., & Kelloway, E. (2001). Behind closed doors: In-home workers' experience of sexual harassment and workplace violence. *Journal of Occupational Health Psychology*. 6(3), 255–269.

Barnadi, L. M. (2001). Management by bullying: The legal consequences. *Canadian Manager, 26*(3), 13–15.

Curbow, B. (2002). Origins of violence at work. In C. L. Cooper & N. Swanson (Eds.). *Workplace violence in the health sector. State of the art*, pp. 35–48. Geneva, Switzerland: International Labour Organization, International Council of Nurses, World Health Organization, and Public Services International.

Hockley, C. (1998). *Wildside of nursing: Horizontal violence*. Paper presented at Australian Nurses Federation (ANF) South Australian Branch Delegates Conference, Adelaide, South Australia.

Hockley, C. (1999). *Road to survival: An ethnomethodological perspective of nurses' experiences*. Paper presented at Sigma Theta Tau International Convention, San Diego, California.

Hockley, C. (2000). *Women stalking women at work: A preliminary study on nurses' experiences*. Paper presented at the Australian Institute of Criminology. Stalking: Criminal Justice Responses. Sydney, Australia.

Hockley, C. (2002a). *Bullying in the workplace*. Paper presented at the Aggression and Violence in the Workplace, You Can Make a Difference Conference, North Adelaide, South Australia.

Hockley, C. (2002b). *Staff hostility and aggression in the workplace*. Paper presented at the Night Duty Nursing Conference, North Adelaide, South Australia.

Hockley, C. (2003a) *Vertical solution for horizontal violence: What to do when staff are destructive and negative and try to undermine your authority*. Paper presented at the "IN CHARGE" Nurse Managers' Conference, Adelaide, South Australia.

Hockley, C. (2003b). *Workplace violence: A collaborative approach to a global issue*. Paper presented at the International Council of Nurses Conference, Building Excellence Through Evidence. Geneva, Switzerland.

Hockley, C. (2004a). *Aggressive incidents reports*. Paper presented at the Nursing Documentation and Risk Conference, Adelaide, South Australia.

Hockley, C. (2004b) *Vertical solutions for horizontal violence*. Paper presented at the Human Resource Management Conference, Adelaide, South Australia.

Lee, M. B. (2001). Oppression and horizontal violence: The case of nurses in Pakistan. *Nursing Forum, 36*(1), 15–24.

Madison, J. & Minichiello, V. (2000). Recognizing and labeling sex-based and sexual harassment in the health care workplace. *The Journal of Nursing Scholarship, 32*(4), 405–410.

Madison, J. & Minichiello, V. (2001). Sexual harassment in healthcare: Classification of harassers and rationalizations of sex-based harassment behavior. *The Journal of Nursing Administration, 31*(11), 534–543.

Mayhew, C. & Chappell, D. (2001). *Prevention of Occupational violence in the health workplace*. Working paper Series no. 140. School of Industrial Relations and Organizational Behavior and the Industrial Relations Research Center, paper written for the Task Force on the Prevention and Management of Violence in the Health Workplace, University of New South Wales, Sydney.

Namie, G. & Namie, R. (2003). *The bully at work*. Naperville, IL: Sourcebooks.

Nazarko, L. (2001). Bullying and harassment. *Nursing Management, 8*(1), 14–15.

Nurses Board of South Australia. (2003). *Code of professional conduct*. Adelaide, South Australia.

Queensland Workplace Bullying Taskforce. (2001). Workplace bullying. Issues paper. Queensland, Australia: Queensland Government.

Robertson, J. (2003). Changing a culture of horizontal violence. *Community Management, 5*(2), 18–20.

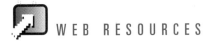

WEB RESOURCES

Australian Institute of Health & Welfare	http://www.aihw.gov.au
Beyond Bullying Association, Australia	http://www.connectqld.org.an
Bully OnLine, UK	http://www.bullyonline.org
International Council of Nurses	http://www.icn.ch
International Labour Organization	http://www.ilo.org
Massachusetts Nurses Association, USA	http://massnurses.org
Royal College of Nursing, Australia	http://www.rcna.org.au
Violence in the Workplace, National Institute for Occupational Safety & Health, USA	http://www.cdc.gov/niosh/violcont.html
World Health Organization	http://www.who.org

Technology in the Health Care Workplace: Benefits, Limitations, and Challenges

13

Carol J. Huston

Technology is everywhere and it is continually transforming health care, particularly nursing care. From improving patient care processes, to enhancing interdisciplinary communication, to improving the work environment and job satisfaction of registered nurses, technology has become an imperative for the health care industry (Bradley, 2003).

With advances in technology come new challenges, opportunities, and problems. Clearly, technology can cut costs, support compliance efforts, optimize data scrutiny, reduce medical errors, streamline workflow, and guarantee information accessibility, whether from remote locations or at the point of care (Simpson, 2001). Yet determining what technology should be developed in an era of limited resources, and how it should be used, is not clear.

Kremsdorf (2003) argues that the central focus of innovative technology should always be on the patient's need for care. Bradley (2003) agrees, suggesting that newly developing technology should be directed at improving the work environment for nurses so that the patient care process can be supported and improved. To do so, Bradley argues that health care must prioritize its technology investment toward solutions that address the key leverage points shown in Box 13.1.

This chapter will address many of these key leverage points, beginning with the use of technology such as robotics, computers, and wireless communication to improve the utilization of human resources. Biometrics, point of care testing, and computerized data access/entry are presented as technology approaches directed at improving documentation and knowledge acquisition. Electronic health records and telehealth are introduced as strategies for overcoming geography of care issues, and provider computer order entry (PCOE) is discussed both as a strategy to improve existing care processes and as a means for decision support. Finally, the Internet's impact on both patients and providers is explored, including the concept of "expert patient" and the resultant need for nurses trained in consumer health informatics.

▶ NEW TECHNOLOGIES IN HEALTH CARE

Most baby boomers remember the TV show *Star Trek*, where the spaceship crew and aliens dematerialized into tiny atoms for transport between locations and where sensors were waved over patients in the sick bay, rendering an immediate diagnosis and treatment.

BOX 13.1

Key Leverage Points in Technology Investment

✓ Improving use of human resources and increasing access to and mobility of technology (e.g., portable handheld devices)
✓ Improving current technology or existing care processes and outcomes (e.g., documentation, medication delivery systems)
✓ Overcoming geography of care issues (e.g., Internet-based care, telehealth)
✓ Improving access to and application of information and knowledge acquisition (e.g., decision support, artificial intelligence)

Source: Bradley, C. (2003). Technology as a catalyst to transforming nursing care. *Nursing Outlook, 51*(3), S14–S15.

Although technology has not yet reached this point, much of the futuristic thinking envisioned on *Star Trek* may well become a reality.

Nelson (2003) provides a glimpse into such a future, suggesting that someday, computer-based diagnostic tools will give unprecedented images of soft and hard tissues in the body, eliminating exploratory surgery and invasive procedures. Biologic markers of disease and genetic markers will facilitate forecasting of disease and disability and patients will wear health watches to detect new signs and symptoms before they develop into emergencies. In addition, health monitoring devices will be installed in showers to complete daily body scans and full body examinations, and microbots and nanodevices will circulate in the body and repair systems early in the disease process.

Nelson goes on to report that room sensors will be developed that will automatically charge for all supplies. In addition, such sensors will charge for human health care resources based on the number of minutes health providers interact with patients. Automated voices will announce the exact time that providers will see patients. All assessments and diagnostics will be automatically recorded in the patient's record and automated recognition systems will reduce errors (Nelson).

Finally, Nelson (2003) suggests that health care teams will cover all specialties, and will be aided by *expert systems* (defined as a computer application that performs a task otherwise performed by a human expert) that both constrain decisions and improve patient outcomes. In addition, synthetic life forms (robots) will have developed to the point that the differences between what these life forms and humans can do will be few.

Robots and Health Care

The use of robots as described by Nelson (2003) may not be as futuristic as it sounds. Indeed, the use of robotics in contemporary health care is no longer science fiction. Domrose (2004) describes contemporary high-tech "smart suites" in operating rooms, where computers announce when everything is ready and activated; room lights dim or brighten on voice command; robots hold cameras in place; and video monitors show clear, clean pictures of the simulated model patient and procedure from three angles. Indeed, robots such as the DaVinci surgical system actually perform surgery, manipulated from a distance by the surgeon (Domrose). Similarly, Richards and McMannus (2002) describe both robotic open heart surgery where a robot's "wrists" mimic the surgeon's motions and a console that offers high-definition, magnified three-dimensional images of the surgical site provided by an endoscope.

Discussion Point

Can nurses be replaced by technology? How important is the "caring" element of nursing?

Nativio (2000) describes similar high-tech robotic environments in Japan, where navigation-equipped robots have been developed to carry and clear food trays, and in Ireland, where robotic technology has been applied to a wheeled, walker-like apparatus (the Smart Zimmer frame) to help frail, visually impaired individuals walk safely without caretaker assistance. Nativio suggests that prototype nurse robots, termed "nursebots" can be used as an adjunct to traditional nursing care by verbally reminding patients who need prompting to eat, take fluids or medications, or go to the bathroom on a scheduled voiding protocol.

Robots (in the form of automated drug dispensing devices and related technology) are currently being used in hundreds of pharmacies in the United States. Their use has decreased the annual cost of maintaining drug inventories by more than 48% (Felder, 2003). If robotics were used to assist in filling the 2.6 billion prescriptions issued in the United States every year, more than $3 billion could be saved (Felder). In addition, the efficiency of drug distribution could be improved by linking the pharmacy information system to these devices.

Finally, Feldman (2003) describes the use of robots for picking up and delivering equipment, specimens, pharmaceuticals, and food within the hospital, arguing that in a typical 550-bed hospital, such delivery services can cost more than $1.2 million annually. In a predictive model using six robots as couriers, Feldman forecast a 30% improvement in delivery time as well as a cost savings of $250,000 per year compared to the use of human couriers.

Biometrics

Simpson (2001, 2002) also describes a health care environment that is rapidly being transformed by new technology as a result of the need to comply with the Health Insurance Portability and Accountability Act of 1996 (HIPAA). HIPAA calls for a tiered approach to data access in which staff members have access to only the information they need to know to perform their jobs, so new technology to assure that access is both targeted and appropriate is being developed.

One such new technology is *biometrics,* the science of identifying people through physical characteristics such as fingerprints, handprints, retinal scans, voice recognition, and facial structure. The implications of biometric technology are enormous. Cline (2004) reports that drivers' licenses in the near future will use machine-readable biometrics, possibly including facial and fingerprint patterns. In addition, numerous government initiatives around the world are in place to augment identity and travel documents, such as passports, with biometric identifiers (Kirwan, 2004). Indeed, as of September 30, 2004, citizens of 27 countries (including Ireland, the United Kingdom, Australia, Japan, Italy, France, and Germany) considered visa-waiver countries by the United States, must be fingerprinted and digitally photographed before they can gain entry to the U.S. (Kirwan).

Fingerprint biometrics is still the most common type of biometrics in health care, primarily because of their ease of use, small size, and affordable price. All of these factors make fingerprint biometrics an attractive option in health care's multiple-workstation environment (Tabar, 2003). Another type of biometrics currently being investigated for use in health care are matrix codes placed on fingernails to label patients (Felder, 2003).

Simpson (2001, 2002) predicts biometrics will become even more commonplace in the near future due to decreasing costs, increasing accuracy, increasing public acceptance, and the need to comply with HIPAA. Indeed, technology analysts have predicted "unprecedented growth for the biometrics market" as a result of increased security concerns (Tabar, 2003; Nine Tech Trends, 2003). This prediction was confirmed in a study conducted by PricewaterhouseCoopers and CIO magazine in 2004 of 8,000 senior information technology (IT) executives in 62 countries (Ware, 2004). Identity management was deemed to be a major factor affecting purchasing decisions and best practice organizations stated they expected to increase spending for identity management and information security in the future.

Other developing technology directed at preserving client confidentiality includes voice recognition data input systems and low-cost, centrally managed computers with no local storage, no local processing, and no local opportunity to gain access to sensitive data (Simpson, 2001).

"Smart cards," devices with a chip, stored memory, and an operating system that record a patient's entire clinical history, are also being developed. Such cards provide access to reading devices in physicians' offices, primary care centers, hospitals, and other medical institutions, eliminating concerns about easily lost, compromised, and exposed paper records (Simpson, 2002).

Point-of-Care Testing

Nelson and Pennington (2001) suggest that *point-of-care testing* (POC) is another recent technologic advance that is improving bedside care and promoting positive patient outcomes. In POC testing, caregivers gather and test specimens near the patient or at the bedside using handheld analyzers, pulse oximeters, and blood glucose monitoring systems. Then, by networking via the Internet and downloading results to a central clinical lab, manual documentation of test results can be eliminated.

POC testing also works for consumer use in the home. Patients can precisely monitor their laboratory values, first by deciding which test to perform and then by obtaining results electronically within seconds or after mailing them to a lab (Nelson & Pennington, 2001).

Yet, POC testing represents only a small portion of clinical laboratories' total testing volume, and evaluation challenges exist for all POC programs in terms of accuracy, ease of use, quality control, and accurate data management. Indeed, delivering diagnostic tests at the bedside may be prone to errors as a result of failure to follow procedures, inappropriate documentation, improper patient identification, and failure to perform required quality control tests (Felder, 2003). Yet, Nelson and Pennington (2001, p. 64) suggest that "healthcare decision makers should devise and implement pilot programs to evaluate them, and keep in mind that this technology's rapid turnaround time results in more timely decision making and patient treatment."

Automated Medication Administration

Automated medication administration is another technology that shows great promise for reducing medication errors and improving quality of care. POC bar coding, the least expensive method of electronic patient labeling, has been developed to help caregivers ensure the right medication, in the right dose, is given to the right patient at the right time, and by the right route (the "five rights"). Bar coding works by requiring the nurse to match his or her nametag, the bar code on the patient's identification band, and the medication to be given. When one of the five "rights" does not match, an alert is issued or the medication will not be dispensed from its storage system.

Unfortunately, according to an American Society of Health-System Pharmacists national survey, only 5% to 6% of hospitals are currently using bar code technology for drug administration (Grissinger & Globus, 2004). In addition, in a survey by the Institute for Safe Medication Practices in 2000, fewer than half of the 1,435 hospitals responding had even discussed the possibility (Grissinger & Globus).

Hospitals are, however, increasingly turning to so called "smart" pumps for intravenous (IV) therapy infusions. These smart pumps have safety software inside an advanced infusion therapy system that prevents IV medication errors through minimum and maximum dose limits, as well as preset limits that cannot be overridden at a clinician's discretion (Kremsdorf, 2003).

Computerized Data Entry

Computerized physician/prescriber order entry (CPOE) is also a rapidly growing technology. Part of this growth has occurred as a result of its designation as one of three key patient safety initiatives by the Leapfrog Group, a conglomeration of non–health care Fortune 500 company leaders committed to modernizing the current health care system (Milstein, Galvin, Delbanco, Salber, & Buck, 2000). In addition, the 1999 Institute of Medicine study, *To Err Is Human,* recommended the use of CPOE to address medical errors.

CPOE is a clinical software application designed specifically for providers to write patient orders electronically rather than on paper (Case, Mowry, & Welebob, 2002). With CPOE, providers produce clearly typed orders, reducing medication errors based on inaccurate transcription. In addition, there are safety nets in place when the nurse logs on to verbally enter orders (Case et al.).

The Agency for Healthcare Research and Quality (2001) estimates that computerized monitoring systems such as CPOE can reduce medication errors and prevent anywhere from 28% to 95% of adverse drug events. A similar study by the Leapfrog Group for Patient Safety (2004) suggested that 55% of prescribing errors in hospitals could be eliminated with CPOE.

CPOE also gives providers vital *clinical decision support* (CDS) via access to information tools that support a health care provider in decisions related to diagnosis, therapy, and care planning of individual patients. For example, physicians might access evidence-based medicine databases electronically for CDS when writing medication orders. If the provider has ordered a test or treatment that is contraindicated for a particular patient or condition, the CDS will inform that provider of the potential danger at the time the order is entered. The real power of CDS, then, is its ability to work in real time, generating feedback based on the information entered into the system (Case et al., 2002).

D i s c u s s i o n   P o i n t

Should health care organizations require providers to use CPOE or should this be left to the discretion of the provider?

A Gartner Group survey in 2001 found that 88% of health care organizations that currently did not have CPOE, planned to implement it within the next 2 to 3 years (Hieb & Handler, 2001). According to the Dorenfest Complete Integrated Healthcare Delivery System Database, nearly 40% of 441 health care delivery systems were considering CPOE in 2002; another 2002 study of 517 hospitals by the Leapfrog Group found that 25% planned to implement CPOE by 2004 (May, 2003).

The reality, however, is that intent has not translated to action, at least not to speedy action. A study by the Leapfrog group in 2004 suggests that only 2% to 3% of U.S. hospitals have fully implemented CPOE systems (Tough Medicine, 2004). Cost is a significant factor as are workflow problems, inadequate training, and the added time required for computer entries (Tough Medicine). There also may be cultural obstacles to

BOX 13.2

Requirements for Full Compliance With Leapfrog's CPOE Standard

1. Hospitals must ensure that physicians enter at least 75% of medication orders via a computer system with prescribing-error prevention software.
2. Hospitals must demonstrate that their inpatient CPOE system can alert physicians to at least 50% of common, serious prescribing errors, using a testing protocol now under development by First Consulting Group and the Institute for Safe Medication Practices.
3. Hospitals must require physicians to electronically document a reason for overriding an interception prior to doing so.

Source: Leapfrog Group for Patient Safety, 2004.

CPOE; for example, a physician may not want to order prescriptions by computer, preferring to write orders by hand (Leapfrog Group for Patient Safety, 2004). In addition, the requirements to fully meet Leapfrog's CPOE standards are stringent (Box 13.2).

Still, institutional and clinician adoption of CPOE is crucial to helping caregivers reduce medical errors and enhance patient safety (Meadows & Chaiken, 2002), and health care institutions must commit the necessary human and fiscal resources to make this technological innovation a reality.

Electronic and Wireless Communication

Computers are increasingly a part of interdisciplinary team communication and care documentation in acute care hospitals. Computerized charting has become commonplace, with more institutions moving toward the use of *tablet personal computers*—flat-panel laptops that use a stylus pen or touch screen technology. In fact, futurists predict that computers in the not too distant future will essentially be invisible, replaced with *smart objects* (everyday objects injected with easy to use software) that give devices limited intelligence (Microsoft Teases, 2002; Nelson, 2003).

For example, in his keynote address at the 2003 International Consumer Electronics Show, Microsoft Corporation Chairman and Chief Software Architect Bill Gates outlined his vision of wristwatches that would allow access to personal messages and appointments, and provide up-to-date news, traffic, weather, and sports information. According to Gates, these smart objects "would extend the power of personal computing in a natural—and fashionable—way" (Bill Gates Showcases, 2003, para 3).

In addition, *personal digital assistants* (PDAs)—mobile, handheld devices such as the Palm series and Handspring Visors—that give users access to text-based information are becoming more common. The latest advancements include institution-wide documentation systems in which everyone uses the same documentation software and the information is transferred to and retrieved from a central server via "hot synching" (putting the PDA into a cradle or connecting it via cable to the central server) (Enger & Segal-Isaacson, 2001). In addition, the PDA can serve as a reference library, especially for drug information, and as a calculator for computing drug dosages.

PDAs, however, are not cheap, typically costing between $200 and $600 each (Enger & Segal-Isaacson, 2001). In addition, PDAs can be lost or stolen, posing concerns about patient confidentiality. Finally, some nurses feel uncomfortable using such technology in front of patients and some just feel uncomfortable with the technology itself (Case et al., 2002). However, the quality and number of PDA applications continues to grow, as does their use.

> ***CONSIDER:** "In the old days, every nurse had a bandage, scissors, a watch and a couple of other things. The PDA is like the bandage and scissors. It's always in your pocket in case you need to access information" (Scully, 2004, p. 20).

The use of *wireless local area networking* (WLAN) is also growing. WLAN uses spread spectrum radio frequency modulation technology, instead of hardwired systems or paper-based records, to document care where it is provided, eliminating errors that happen in translation (Simpson, 2002). WLAN also allows caregivers to access, update, and transmit critical patient and treatment information between buildings where the installation of new wires proves either impractical or impossible (Simpson). By 2004, it was estimated that 50% of all hospital physicians would use wireless, handheld devices for data access and consultation (Felder, 2003).

Phillips (2004) illuminates even more advanced applications of this technology in her discussion of Bluetooth wireless connections to the Logitech® io™ pen, which enables writing to be transferred directly to a computer screen, and then converted to Word text.

Electronic Health Records

Even health records have changed as a result of technology. The Healthcare Information and Management Systems Society (HIMSS) (2003) defines the *electronic health record* (EHR) as a "secure, real-time, point-of-care, patient-centric information resource for clinicians." Importantly, it can audit access, thereby guaranteeing patient health information confidentiality and security. The EHR is available 24 hours a day, 7 days a week, can integrate with the clinician's workflow, and can be accessed at inpatient and ambulatory care sites, as well as remotely (HIMSS).

> ***CONSIDER:** "Integration of information at the point of care frees up nurses from being data enterers to being data analyzers" (Case et al., 2002, p. 19).

In May 2003, the U.S. Department of Health and Human Services asked the Institute of Medicine (IOM) to provide guidance on the key care delivery–related capabilities of an EHR system. According to Birz (2004), the IOM report stated that an EHR system has eight core functions (Box 13.3) and should include:

- Longitudinal collection of electronic health information for and about people, where health information is defined as information pertaining to the health of an individual or health care provided to an individual.

BOX 13.3   Eight Core Functions of an Electronic Health Record

- Health information and data
- Result management
- Order management
- Decision support
- Electronic communication and connectivity
- Patient support
- Administrative processes
- Reporting

Source: Birz, 2004.

- Immediate electronic access to person- and population-level information by only authorized users.
- Provision of knowledge and decision support that enhance the quality, safety, and efficiency of patient care.
- Support of efficient processes for health care delivery. Critical building blocks of an EHR system are the EHRs maintained by providers (e.g., hospitals, nursing homes, ambulatory settings) and by individuals (also called personal health records).

Despite this clarification of core functions and guidelines and the obvious potential benefits of EHRs, a review of the literature revealed limited success stories regarding their use. Perhaps this simply reflects normal resistance to change because a number of behavioral and procedural changes are required to rework such a fundamental aspect of normal operations. In addition, there is a period of implementation that must be accommodated by the staff, and financial support is required from the organization (Korst, Eusebio-Angeja, Chamorro, Aydin, & Gregory, 2003).

Or perhaps the delay in implementation is because the introduction of EHRs is labor intensive and thus potentially expensive. One drawback cited has been that nurses must frequently "double chart" during system implementation, meaning that they must enter the same data elements both electronically and on paper, and this increased documentation can increase staffing requirements and costs. Yet research by Korst et al. (2003) found that the additional time required to "double chart" did not seem excessive when compared to estimates of time required for charting on paper alone.

Other Electronic Data Repositories and Intranets

Just as the electronic medical record can be used to record everything that happens with a patient, the same framework has been applied to record information about nurses. LeMaire (2004) describes an education data repository for nurses that tracks education any time it occurs, from the time a representative comes onto the unit to the more formal classroom.

In addition, electronic data repositories have been created within organizations as a way of cataloging internal reference materials, such as policy and procedure manuals. This increases the likelihood that staff will be able to find such resources when they need them and that they are as up to date as possible. In such a system, references are typically converted to the portable document format and launched electronically via an Intranet. *Intranets* are internal networks (not normally accessible from the Internet), that allow workers and departments to share files, use websites, and collaborate. Using the electronic format is more operationally efficient, results in high staff satisfaction levels, eliminates the need for paper reference materials, and saves money on materials and their manual replacements (Kasoff, 2003).

▶ TELEHEALTH AND TELENURSING

Given declining reimbursement, the current nursing shortage, and an increasing shift in care to outpatient settings, home care agencies are increasingly exploring technology-aided options that allow them to avoid the traditional 1:1 nurse-patient ratio with face-to-face contact. *Telehealth*, also called remote monitoring technology, telemedicine, telenursing, telecare, telehomecare, telemanagement, and telephone care, allows nurses to care for patients over a distance, using a combination of telecommunication and multimedia technologies.

A retrospective chart review by Wooten et al. (1998) suggested that as many as 45% of home care episodes in the United States might be suitable for telehealth of some form. Whitten, Doolittle, Mackert, and Rush (2003) suggest that telehealth is an underutilized method of providing hospice care because only 15% of the dying in this country use telehospice, and many individuals living in rural areas would not have access to hospice expertise if telehospice did not exist.

Even more amazing is the prediction that most health care in the future will essentially be removed from traditional office environments and provided either virtually through videophones and monitoring equipment or at ambulatory centers in places such as shopping centers and kiosks. The focus of primary care then will become "forecast, prevent, and manage" (Nelson, 2003, p. S28).

*CONSIDER: In the near future, health kiosks at local malls may provide access to health care providers and eliminate the need to go to the health care provider's office for medical care (Lewis & Pesut, 2001).

For nurses, telehealth has meant greater ubiquity—nurses can now practice across geographical boundaries and expand their involvement in patient care (Simpson, 2003). For patients, telehealth has meant increased flexibility and often, more personalized care. For health care providers, telehealth has provided opportunities to reduce costs and improve quality of care (Simpson).

Discussion Point

What, if anything, is "lost" when there is no face-to-face meeting between the nurse and the patient? Can technology overcome this loss? What does technology offer that face-to-face visits do not?

How Telehealth Works

In more advanced telehealth, providers interact with patients through computer stations hooked up in the patient's home that typically include a video monitor; a moveable color video camera; a speakerphone and microphone; and one or more medical peripherals for patient self-monitoring, such as blood pressure and pulse meter, stethoscope, pulse oximeter, scale, and glucometer. Patients record their heart rates, blood pressures, blood glucose levels, and other readings periodically and then transmit this data to a provider with a computer station similar to theirs. This gives the provider a real-time picture of the patient's health status.

Lee, Friedman, Cukor, and Ahern (2003, p. 277) suggest that interactive voice response systems, often described as "a telephone connected to a talking computer," interact with patients for data collection and can deliver recorded telephone messages related to medication compliance or behavior modification.

*CONSIDER: Telehealth provides greater opportunities for nurse-patient encounters, particularly for homebound, isolated individuals.

In less sophisticated telehealth programs, assessment, intervention, and evaluation occur by fax, e-mail message, or simply by telephone alone. Indeed, consumer access to telephone nurse lines in the United States increased from 2 million Americans in the early 1990s to approximately 35 million in a 5-year span (Sabin, 1998).

Telehealth and Telenursing Outcomes

Because telehealth and telenursing are relatively new, the identification of performance indicators and appropriate measures of quality is still in the neophyte stage. Larson-Dahn (2001) suggests that the relative newness and autonomous nature of telephone nursing should raise questions about its safety and appropriateness, and that formalization of the processes of telephone nursing practice and evaluation of those processes is needed. To address this concern, the American Academy of Ambulatory Care Nursing (AAACN) (1997) published telephone nursing practice standards to guide program design and implementation, and to further define the scope of practice.

> *CONSIDER: The practice of telephone nursing has not yet been standardized and there are few standardized tools to assess outcomes.

Waldo (2003) suggests that the jury may still be out on what kind of telehealth system—or what mix of telehealth and in-home visits—adds the most value both clinically and financially, but adds that there is little dispute that data and images captured via telehealth equipment improve the quality of the patient's record. Other common indicators thought to represent telephone nursing practice quality are time and cost savings for staff, competencies, documentation, and the use of protocols (Hoare, Lacoste, Haro, & Conyers, 1999; Larson-Dahn, 2001).

Desired patient outcomes for telehealth nursing are a little better defined. They include decreases in travel time, reduced costs, decreased visits to patients' homes, and increases in both the number of patient encounters and the amount of data that can be added to the patient's medical record (Waldo, 2003). In addition, patient satisfaction, increased involvement in health care decision making, and knowledge acquisition must be considered desirable patient outcomes in telehealth.

Despite the lack of clarity about what constitutes quality in telenursing, researchers are examining outcomes. Whitten et al. (2003) report that within weeks of their telehospice program launch, staff reported significant savings in time and travel, particularly for unexpected and unscheduled visits. Staff also reported an increased ability to supplement services and increase care quality as well as an "expansion of the circle of loved ones" (p. 38).

Greenberg and Schultz (2002) reported that patient satisfaction is high with telenursing; patients stated that they value the convenience of telephone access, the personalized and collaborative care, and the information shared. Patients also reported that telenursing created a personal connection with their health care providers, and that this was a vital component of their care. In addition, although patients expressed a preference to speak with their physician, they also expressed that they would change clinics if a telephonic nursing program were not available.

Johnson-Mekota et al. (2001) also reported high levels of satisfaction among patients receiving telehealth care, despite having some trouble hearing and seeing nurses electronically; 55% of patients were "very satisfied" with telecommunications visits versus 40% who were "very satisfied" with on-site visits. Similarly, Dansky, Palmer, Shea, and Bowles (2001) reported that telehomecare patients were enthusiastic about the technology and

BOX 13.4

Research Study Fuels the Controversy

In a study funded by the U.S. Department of Commerce's Telecommunications Information Infrastructure Assistance Program, the Visiting Nurse Association (VNA) of Greater Philadelphia used a combination of 25-minute video visits and home visits to monitor patients with diabetes and educate them about heart disease.

> Bowles, K., & Dansky, K. H. (2002). Teaching self-management of diabetes via telehomecare. *Home Healthcare Nurse, 20*(1). 36–42.

Study Findings

Study group participants received an average of 23.9 combined home and video visits, compared with 17.5 home visits for patients in the control group. The video group improved its self-management of diabetes by a statistically significant factor over the usual care group. The study concluded that short video visits with a one-on-one focus provided focused opportunities for increased patient teaching. In addition, patient independence and empowerment were fostered as a result of self-monitoring.

The researchers concluded that telehomecare is an effective way to improve patient education and self-management outcomes, particularly when visits focus on teaching and monitoring. In addition, the cost-effectiveness of this technology makes it an attractive medium for reaching patients who require close monitoring, reinforced teaching, and reassurance. Telehomecare also provides unique opportunities to support caregivers and connect socially isolated individuals with their care providers.

felt it empowered them. Their research also demonstrated that, although telehomecare imposed additional expenses for care delivery, it contributed substantial savings without compromising quality, and the financial benefit increased exponentially as the duration of the patient care episode increased.

Some studies have compared outcomes of patients receiving both telenursing care and traditional home visits. A study by Bowles and Dansky (2002) concluded that short video visits, in combination with face-to-face visits, resulted in increased patient teaching, patient self-empowerment, and improved opportunities to connect socially isolated individuals with their care providers (Box 13.4).

Finally, Sipe, Marthinsen, Baker, Harris, and Opperman (2003) argue convincingly that telehealth and its associated virtual meetings have a tremendously positive impact on patients, families, nurses, and health care providers and enhance the health care delivery process. This is because patients and families can be offered a variety of information resources that they might not otherwise have access to, including consultation with members of the multidisciplinary health care team and specialists contacted by the local facility, patient education, and reporting.

*CONSIDER: If the benefits of telemedicine are to be fully realized, providers need a standard interface specification to easily merge telehealth data with information from other clinical systems, creating a single, inclusive record that contains all of the patient's data, regardless of how or where it is gathered (Waldo, 2003).

IS TECHNOLOGY WORTH THE COSTS?

The market for mobile computing in health care was $50 million in 2002 and is expected to grow to $1.2 billion by 2006 (Scully, 2004). Domrose (2004) suggests that although this state of the art technology is expensive and requires more education, it also generally saves time, creates less room for error, reduces the amount of pushing and lifting that nurses must do, and gives nurses more time to do nursing. Similarly, in a study of 100 physicians, nurses, and administrators, Spyglass Consulting Group of Menlo Park, California, reported that nurses who use such technology say it helps them work more efficiently and provides a higher quality of care (Scully).

Priselac (2003) goes so far as to say that health care organizations that invest in cutting-edge technology to improve clinical practice environments are becoming employers of choice. "Such high-tech organizations attract and retain nurses by recasting their role as clinicians who use sophisticated information and scientific technology to provide the best care while enhancing their skill set and work life" (p. S12).

Not all critics agree, however. Some argue that technology is not only expensive (both initially and in terms of maintenance and technical support), but also needs constant upgrades, and the education needed to truly be competent in the use of all this technology is never ending. In addition, Scully (2004) states even simple questions, like how technology such as PDAs should be used and where, still need to be answered.

In addition, not all nurses embrace technology. Simpson (2003) states that perhaps this reticence to adopt important technology comes from a belief that caring for patients is the supreme mission, not balancing on the cutting edge of technology. Bradley (2003) argues, however, that some nurses fail to embrace new technology because they have not been adequately involved in priority identification, solution development, and practical application within the care environment.

Abrahamsen (2003) suggests that organizations face a significant learning curve in applying the new communication technologies available to them because there is such great diversity in user educational needs and motivation to adopt these new technologies. Additionally, Abrahamsen asserts that "technology holds great promise for the health care environment while presenting it with countless challenges" (Abrahamsen, p. 50).

One must also remember that not all technology is worth the cost (Domrose, 2004). "In making technology decisions, financial concerns must be weighed against the benefits of technology, such as increased patient safety through medication administration, improved patient care through access to information and standards, and greater efficiency for nurses through automated documentation and easier modes of communication" (Case et al., 2002, p. 22). Still, technology is like a rolling freight train—it's very difficult to stop it and even more dangerous to get in the way.

THE INTERNET AND HEALTH CARE

The Exponential Growth of the Internet

The growth of the Internet as an information source for all types of information, including health, has grown exponentially. Personal computer use increased from less than 5% in 1981 to more than 51% in 2000 and is expected to exceed 80% in 2005 (National Telecommunications and Information Administration, 1999).

Worldwide, 592 million people had Internet access in 2002, with an annual rate of growth of 20% in 2002 (Rhode, 2003). In a national telephone survey between March 12 and May 20, 2003, the Pew Internet & American Life Project (2004) found that more than 53 million American adults have used the Internet to "publish their thoughts, respond to others, post pictures, share files and otherwise contribute to the explosion of content available online." Additionally, one out of every four online U.S. households is connected by some form of high-speed access—an 82% increase in a 7-month period (Sabia, 2001).

Consumers, however, use the Internet in different ways for different purposes. One typology that has been developed for classifying consumer use of the Internet was done by Shay who suggests that health care on the Internet can be classified into three generations. The first generation of Internet health care uses involved passive applications that simply described products, services, and resources that were available from various types of health care vendors (Shay, 2000). They were the online equivalent of magazine advertising. Examples of first-generation websites include *www.webmd.com* and *www.drkoop.com.*

Second-generation health care uses of the Internet have been directed at e-commerce involving electronic data interchanges, such as enrolling for health insurance, paying health insurance claims, and purchasing prescription drugs online. Second-generation online activity is far more interactive than the first generation, yet transactions still only involve the exchange of fairly neutral information and not clinical judgment.

As technology continues to evolve, Shay (2000, para 12) suggests that "the Internet will be used in complex health management programs—the emerging third generation of health care on the Internet." Clinical judgment is required in the third judgment. For example, a third-generation use of the Internet in health care would be telehealth—allowing patients to electronically transmit their personal health data, such as blood pressure or glucometer readings, to an online database that can be accessed and monitored by their doctors or pharmacists. Shay warns, however, that this third generation of Internet use will likely pose the greatest challenges to those who attempt to regulate health care on the Internet. This is because health care providers must rely on technology rather than on what they can directly observe by sight, sound, and touch. In other words, the "human element" and "the laying on of hands" is missing.

The Impact of the Internet on Provider–Patient Relationships

Historically, providers were recognized as the keepers of medical information. This allowed them to be the primary health care decision maker, often relegating patients to a somewhat passive and dependent role. Steffan-Dickerson and Brennan (2002) suggest that the Internet has changed these dynamics because it has expanded the power and control of health information from a privileged few to many people, including patients themselves. Indeed, the Internet, which is growing faster than any other medium in the world, has great potential to improve Americans' health by enhancing communications and improving access to information for care providers, patients, health plan administrators, public health officials, biomedical researchers, and other health professionals.

Not surprisingly, some providers have been cautious about embracing the Internet. Physician user numbers have grown, but many remain skeptical about the role of the Internet in their practices (Shay, 2000).

The "Expert Patient"

The Internet has also changed health care access, education, and information sharing as we know it. According to a Louis Harris and Associates poll, 60 million people searched for health-specific information online in 1998, and 91% reported finding what they were looking for (Hartman, 1999). The end result is that patients today have electronic access to medical information on virtually any topic, any time.

Theoretically, this means that consumers are better informed and are more likely to be active participants in their own decision making. Concerns abound, however, regarding the accuracy and currency of information patients find on the Internet, and many patients do not fully understand the information that is available to them, even when it is accurate. Some providers are concerned that patients will inappropriately self-diagnose, leading them to seek inappropriate treatment or no treatment at all. Other providers simply are not sure they want to share decision-making power with patients.

Expert patient is a term that was coined by the chief medical officer of England and refers to patients who have the confidence, skills, information, and knowledge to play a central role in the management of their health care. Shaw and Baker (2004, p. 723) suggest that many providers are suspicious of expert patients, imagining that such a patient is "the one clutching a sheet of printouts from the internet, demanding a particular treatment that is unproved, manifestly unsuitable, astronomically expensive, or all three. Or possibly, worst of all, a treatment the doctor has never heard of, let alone personally prescribed."

Discussion Point

Empowering patients and involving them in their own health care decision making is a socially encouraged value in health care today. Do you believe that most providers value and appreciate increased numbers of "expert patients"?

Shaw and Baker (2004) argue, however, that health care providers need to act on what they already know—that all patients are experts, however uninformed or misinformed they may be about health issues, and that patients who have the resources to find out about their illness and want to take an active part in managing their care should be welcomed as allies and partners. Providers then will need to transition from being the primary source of information to patients to helping patients sort out the information they have access to (Hartman, 1999). Students in health care programs will need to be taught to not only recognize patient expertise, but also to actively encourage and support it. Finally, patients will need to become experts at retrieving health care information and deciphering it to better empower themselves in health care decision making.

Nursing Informatics

This transition will not be easy for either patients or providers. At least partly as a result of these changing relationship dynamics, new nursing specialties have emerged, including *nursing informatics* (NI). NI was first recognized as a specialty by the American Nurses Association in 1992, and the number of nurses specializing in NI has grown 20% annually since then (Briggs, 2004). The American Nursing Informatics Association (2001–2004) states that NI combines nursing science with computer science as well as information processing theory and technology.

Similarly, the American Nurses Association (ANA) (2001, p. vii) *Scope and Standards of Nursing Informatics* defines NI as a:

> *. . . specialty that integrates nursing science, computer science, and information science to manage and communicate data, information, and knowledge in nursing practice. Nursing informatics facilitates the integration of data, information and knowledge to support patients, nurses and other providers in their decision-making in all roles and settings. This support is accomplished through the use of information structures, information processes, and information technology.*

The *consumer health informatics* (CHI) nurse is charged with understanding the implications and consequences of technologies for nursing practice and for assuring that health care represents a seamless network of data, services, information, and connectivity (Lewis & Pesut, 2001). This requires competencies and skill sets that support nursing knowledge and roles in the consumer health information age. In addition, skills in organization, critical thinking, and problem solving are critical for NI nurses (Briggs, 2004).

The education required to become a CHI nurse has changed over time. Before the ANA's designation of NI as a specialty in 1992, most nurses involved in informatics were self-educated because very few graduate NI programs were available (Klein, n.d.) In 1988, however, the first graduate program in nursing informatics was established at the University of Maryland School of Nursing in Baltimore, and numerous other graduate programs have proliferated since then. In addition, NI certification became available in 1995 through the American Nurses Credentialing Center (ANCC).

CONCLUSIONS

Richards and McMannus (2002) state that new technologies offer great opportunities to provide exceptional patient care, but that technology alone isn't the answer. Regardless of the system that is deployed, health care organizations must consider the uniqueness of each unit as well as the tools currently in place to accomplish workload (Case et al., 2002). Successfully adopting and integrating new technology will require that care providers be involved in the design, selection, and implementation of the new methods and devices (Richards & McMannus).

Technology, despite its multiple benefits, will never replace the human element of care. Simpson (2003) argues this is the case because computers cannot and do not care. "Care involves feelings and human communication that transcend technology. Caring is the job of nurses and this alone will probably be the reason nursing will survive" (Simpson, p. 115).

Yet nurses need to overcome their "technophobia" because clearly, nursing care can be improved with the appropriate use of technology and ironically, it is technology that will likely give nurses more time to do "nursing." Technology holds promise and potential for addressing some of nursing's and health care's greatest challenges (Bradley, 2003, p. S14). Nurses must therefore keep the improvement of patient care first and foremost in their technology development agenda. In addition, nurses must embrace technology, understand it, and bend it to their own purposes, so that nursing can take its rightful place in the provider hierarchy (Simpson, 2003).

1. Is there a place for technology development in health care, even when it does not contribute to the improvement of patient outcomes? In other words, should the technology itself ever be the desired goal?

2. Are nursing schools adequately preparing students with the skill sets and competencies they will need to function successfully in a progressively more technological workplace?

3. How should organizations deal with "technophobic" nurses? Should health care employers let nurses decide what level of expertise they wish to aquire?

4. What safeguards are in place to assure confidentiality of the electronic health record? Do you believe confidentiality is greater with electronic or paper records?

5. What technology do you believe has the greatest potential to reduce the current nursing shortage? Why?

6. What technologies, currently in use, would you predict to be obsolete in 10 years?

7. What barriers exist in health care environments that will impede the development of technology in years to come?

8. What safeguards do consumers have that the health information they find on the Internet is accurate and appropriate?

REFERENCES

Abrahamsen, C. (2003). Patient safety: Take the informatics challenge. *Nursing Management, 34*(4), 48–51.

Agency for Healthcare Research and Quality. (2001). *Research in action, issue 1: Reducing and preventing adverse drug events to decrease hospital costs.* AHRQ Publication Number 01-0020. Rockville, MD: The Agency for Healthcare Research and Quality.

American Academy of Ambulatory Care Nursing. (1997). *Telephone nursing practice administration and practice standards.* Pitman, NJ: Author.

American Nurses Association. (2001). *American Nurses Association scope and standards of nursing informatics practice.* Washington, DC: American Nurses Publishing.

American Nursing Informatics Association. (2001–2004). *Nursing Informatics.* Retrieved April 27, 2005, from http://www.ania.org/nrsg%20info.htm.

Bill Gates showcases new technology for "smart living" in the digital decade. (2003). Retrieved April 27, 2005, from http://www.microsoft.com/presspass/press/2003/jan03/01-08CES2003OverallPR.asp.

Birz, S. (2004). The electronic health record: An information resource for clinicians. Retrieved April 27, 2005, from http://www.nursezone.com/job/DevicesandTechnology.asp?articleID=12433.

Bowles, K. & Dansky, K. H. (2002). Teaching self-management of diabetes via telehomecare. *Home Healthcare Nurse, 20*(1). 36–42.

Bradley, C. (2003). Technology as a catalyst to transforming nursing care. *Nursing Outlook, 51*(3), S14–S15.

Briggs, B. (2004). Information technology fits nurses like a glove. *Health Data Management.* Retrieved April 27, 2005, from http://www.healthdatamanagement.com/html/current/CurrentIssueStory.cfm?PostID=14051.

Case, J., Mowry, M., & Welebob, E. (2002).*The nursing shortage: Can technology help?* First Consulting Group. California Healthcare Foundation. California: Ihealthreports.

Cline, J. (2004). Get ready for the U.S. national ID card. *Computerworld.* Retrieved April 27, 2005, from http://www.computerworld.com/printthis/2004/0,4814,89491,00.html.

Dansky, K. H., Palmer, L., Shea, D. G., & Bowles, K. H. (2001). Cost analysis of telehomecare. *Telemedicine Journal and e-Health, 7*(3), 225–232.

Domrose, C. (March 8, 2004). Working smart. *Nurseweek, 17*(6), 13–15.

Enger, J. C. & Segal-Isaacson, A. E. (2001). The ABCs of PDAs. *Nursing Management, 32*(10), 60–62.

Felder, R. (2003). Medical automation—A technologically enhanced work environment to reduce burden of care on nursing staff and a solution to the healthcare cost crisis. *Nursing Outlook, 51*(3), S5–S10.

Greenberg, M. E. & Schultz, C. (August, 2002). Telephone nursing: Client experiences and perceptions. *Nursing Economics, 20*(4), 181–187.

Grissinger, M. & Globus, N. J. (2004). How technology affects your risk of medication errors. *Nursing, 34*(1), 36–41.

Hartman, G. (1999). The Internet: New frontier or Pandora's box? *Physician Magazine.* Retrieved April 27, 2005, from http://www.family.org/physmag/issues/a0010666.cfm.

Healthcare Information and Management Systems Society (HIMSS). (November 2003). *HIMSS electronic health record definitional model version 1.0.* Retrieved April 27, 2005, from http://www.himss.org/content/files/EHRAttributes.pdf.

Hieb, B. & Handler, T. (2001). *The critical role of orders in the delivery of healthcare.* Stamford, CT: Gartner.

Hoare, K., Lacoste, J., Haro, K., & Conyers, C. (1999). Exploring indicators of telephone nursing quality. *Journal of Nursing Care Quality, 14*(1), 38–46.

Johnson-Mekota, J., Maas, M., Buresh, K., Gardner, S. E., Frantz, R., Specht, J., et al. (2001). A nursing application of telecommunications: Measurement of satisfaction for patients and providers. *Journal of Gerontological Nursing, 27*(1), 28–33.

Kasoff, J. (2003). Nursing references at the point of care. *Journal of Nursing Administration, 33*(1), 10.

Kirwan, M. (2004). Biometrics: Ready for prime time? Retrieved April 27, 2005, from http://www.globetechnology.com/servlet/story/RTGAM.20040412.gtkirwanapr12/BNStory/Technology/.

*Klein, J. A. (n.d.). *Nursing informatics education; Past, present, and future.* Nursing Network. Retrieved April 27, 2005, from http://www.nursingnetwork.com/education.htm.

Korst, L. M., Eusebio-Angeja, A. C., Chamorro, T., Aydin, C. E., & Gregory, K. D. (2003). Nursing documentation time during implementation of an electronic medical record. *Journal of Nursing Administration, 33*(1), 24–30.

Kremsdorf, R. (2003). Using innovation technology to enhance patient care delivery. *Nursing Outlook, 51*(3), S16–S20.

Larson-Dahn, M. L. (2001). Tel-enurse practice: Quality of care and patient outcomes. *Journal of Nursing Administration, 31*(3), 145–152.

Leapfrog Group for Patient Safety. (2004). Fact sheet. Computer physician order entry. Retrieved April 27, 2005, from http://www.leapfroggroup.org/media/file/Leapfrog-Computer_physician_order_Entry_Fact_Sheet.pdf

Lee, H., Friedman, M. E., Cukor, P., & Ahern, D. (2003). Interactive voice response system (IVRS) in healthcare services. *Nursing Outlook, 51*(6), 277–283.

LeMaire, B. (2004). Ken Dion, on health care staffing solutions. *Nurseweek, 17*(5), 6.

Lewis, D. & Pesut, D. J. (2001). Future think: Emergence of consumer health informatics. *Nursing Outlook, 49*(1), 7.

May, S. (February 2003). Computerized physician order entry. Retrieved April 27, 2005, from http://www.healthcare-informatics.com/issues/2003/02_03/cover.htm.

Meadows, G. & Chaiken, B. P. (2002). Computerized physician order entry: A prescription for patient safety. *Nursing Economics, 20*(2), 76–77, 87.

Microsoft teases "smart personal objects" initiative. (2002). Retrieved April 27, 2005, from http://www.windowsfordevices.com/news/NS4829506693.html.

Milstein, A., Galvin, R., Delbanco, S., Salber, P., & Buck, C. (2000). Improving the safety of healthcare: The Leapfrog initiative. *Effective Clinical Practice, 3*(6), 313–316. Retrieved April 27, 2005, from http://www.acponline.org/journals/ecp/novdec00/milstein.pdf.

National Telecommunications and Information Administration. (1999). Falling through the net: Defining the digital divide. Retrieved April 27, 2005, from http://www.ntia.doc.gov/ntiahome/fttn99/contents.html.

Nativio, D. G. (2000). Advanced practice. Robots and nurses. *Nursing Outlook, 48*(4), 154–155.

Nelson, A. (2003). Using simulation to design and integrate technology for safer and more efficient practice environments. *Nursing Outlook, 51*(3), S27–S29.

Nelson, L. R. & Pennington, C. (2001). What's new at the point of care? *Nursing Management, 32*(12), 63–64.

Nine tech trends. (2003). Retrieved April 27, 2005, from http://www.healthcare-informatics.com/issues/2003/02_03/cover.htm.

Reports: Online activities and pursuits. (2004). Retrieved April 27, 2005, from http://www.pewinternet.org/reports/toc.asp?Report=113.

Phillips, K. (2004). Technology options abound for nurses. Retrieved April 27, 2005, from http://www.nursezone.com/job/DevicesandTechnology.asp?articleID=12391.

Priselac, T. M. (2003). Information technology's role in improving practice environments and patient safety. *Nursing Outlook, 51*(3), S11–S13.

Rhode, L. (2003). Worldwide growth in Internet use continued in '02, says UN. Retrieved April 27, 2005, from http://www.computerworld.com/developmenttopics/websitemgmt/story/0,10801,87449,00.html.

Richards, N. M. & McMannus, S. (2002). Match critical care situations with savvy devices. *Nursing Management, 33*(12), 38–39.

Sabia, A. (2001). *What economic slowdown? US consumer demand for Internet access breaks records.* Stamford, CT: Gartner.

Sabin, M. (1998). Telephone triage improves demand management effectiveness. *Journal of Healthcare Financial Management Association, 52*(8), 49–51.

Scully, J. M. (2004). Get smart. Mobile technology streamlines documentation and helps nurses deliver more efficient, higher quality patient care. *NURSEWEEK*, 20, 40.

Shaw, J. & Baker, B. (2004). "Expert patient"—dream or nightmare? *British Medical Journal, 328*(328), 723–724.

Shay, E. F. (March 2000). Evolving uses of health care on the Internet. Retrieved April 27, 2005, from http://www.physiciansnews.com/computers/300.html.

*URL no longer active

Simpson, R. (2001). Techno-marvels just around the corner. *Nursing Management, 32*(12), 50–52.

Simpson, R. (2002). Eyeing IT trends and challenges. *Nursing Management, 33*(12), 46–47.

Simpson, R. (2003). Got technology? How IT can—and can't—make a difference in the nursing shortage. *Policy, Politics & Nursing Practice, 4*(2), 114–119.

Sipe, M., Marthinson, J., Baker, J., Harris, J., & Opperman, J. (2003). Using technology to improve patient care. *Nursing Outlook, 51*(3), S35–S36.

Steffan Dickerson, S. & Brennan, P. F. (2002). The Internet as a catalyst for shifting power in patient-provider relationships. *Nursing Outlook, 50*(5), 195–203.

Tabar, P. (2003). *Biometrics.* Retrieved April 27, 2005, from http://www.healthcare-informatics.com/issues/2003/02_03/cover.htm.

Tough medicine (2004). Retrieved April 27, 2005, from http://www.redcoatpublishing.com/features/f_07_04_hcsup_ToughMedicine.asp.

Waldo, B. (2003). Telehealth and the electronic medical record. *Nursing Economics, 21*(5), 245–246.

Ware, L.C. (2004). The state of information security 2004. Retrieved April 27, 2005, from http://www2.cio.com/research/surveyreport.cfm?id=75.

Whitten, P., Doolittle, G., Mackert, M., & Rush, T. (2003). Telehospice carries end-of-life care over the lines. *Nursing Management, 34*(11), 36–39.

Wooten, R., Loane, M., Mair, F., Allen, A., Doolittle, G., Begley, M., et al. (1998). A joint US–UK study of home telenursing. *Journal of Telemedicine and Telecare, 4*(Suppl. 1), 83–85.

BIBLIOGRAPHY

Bland, M. (2003). PDAs: A nurse's new best friend. Retrieved April 27, 2005, from http://www.nursingspectra.com/StudentsCorner/StudentFeatures/PDAs_stk.htm

Burgiss, S., Dimmick, S., & Robbins, S. (2001). *Cost of care reductions using telehealth: A comparative analysis.* Presented at Telemedicine Association 6th Annual Meeting. Ft. Lauderdale, FL.

Carr, D. M. & Dimitrakakis, J. (2003). Explore all-encompassing electronic health records. *IT Solutions. A premier supplement to the Journal of Nursing Administration,* 24–25.

Coyle, G. & Heinen, M. (2002). Scan your way to a comprehensive electronic medical record. *Nursing Management, 33*(12), 56–59.

Dansky, K. H., Yant, B., Jenkins, D., & Dellasega, C. (2003). Qualitative analysis of telehomecare nursing activities. *Journal of Nursing Administration, 33*(7/8), 372–375.

Dienemann, J. & Van de Castle, B. (2003). The impact of healthcare informatics on the organization. *Journal of Nursing Administration, 33*(11), 557–562.

Glaser, J. (2002). *The strategic application of information technology in health care organizations* (2nd ed.). San Francisco: Jossey-Bass.

Greenberg, M. E. & Cartwright, J. P. (2001). Identifying best practices in telehealth nursing: The telehealth survey. *Nursing Economics, 19*(6), 283–285.

Heinen, M. G., Coyle, G. A., & Hamilton, A. V. (2003). Barcoding makes its mark on daily practice. *IT Solutions. A premier supplement to the Journal of Nursing Administration,* 18–20.

Im, E. O. & Chee, W. (2003). Issues in Internet research. *Nursing Outlook, 51*(1), 6–12.

Kennedy, R. (2003). The nursing shortage and the role of technology. *Nursing Outlook, 51*(3), S33–S34.

Larson-Dahn, M. L. (2000). Tel-eNurse practice. A practice model for role expansion. *Journal of Nursing Administration, 30*(11), 519–523.

Larson-Dahn, M. L. (2002). Tel-eNursing practice. Setting standards for practice across the continuum of care. *Journal of Nursing Administration, 32*(10), 524–530.

Laughlin, J. & Van Null, M. (2003). Boost regulatory compliance with electronic nursing documentation. *Nursing Management, 34*(12), 51–52.

McConnell, E. A. (2000). Where it's at: Point-of-care testing yields results—stat. *Nursing Management, 31*(12), 44–45.

Meadows, G. (2001). The Internet promise: A new look at e-health opportunities. *Nursing Economics, 19*(6), 294–295.

Networking health: Prescriptions for the Internet. (2000). The National Academies Press. Available free online at http://www.nap.edu/books/0309068436/html/.

Newbold, S. K. (2003). New uses for wireless technology. *IT Solutions. A premier supplement to the Journal of Nursing Administration,* 22–23, 32.

Shabot, M. M. (2003). Closing address: Breaking free of the past: Innovation and technology in patient care. *Nursing Outlook, 51*(3), S37–S38.

Simpson, R. (2003). Today's challenges shape tomorrow's technology, part 2. *Nursing Management, 34*(12), 40–44.

Strohecker, S. (2003). Polished automation tools allow patient safety to shine. *Nursing Management, 34*(12), 34–38.

Valanis, B., Moscato, S., Tanner, C., Shapiro, S., Izumi, S., David, M., et al. (2003). Making it work. Organization and processes of telephone nursing advice services. *Journal of Nursing Administration, 33*(4), 216–223.

Valanis, B., Tanner, C., Randles Moscato, S., Shapiro, S., Izumi, S., et al. (February 2003). A model for explaining predictors of outcomes of telephone nurse advice. *Journal of Nursing Administration, 33*(2), 91–95.

Wilven, D. N. Jr. (2001). *Telehomecare: How an agency benefits financially, clinically and with the community.* The Remington Report.

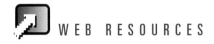 WEB RESOURCES

American Nursing Informatics Association	**http://www.ania.org**
American Telemedicine Association	**http://www.atmeda.org**
Association of Telehealth Service Providers	**http://www.atsp.org**
British Computer Society Nursing Specialist Group	**http://www.bcsnsg.org.uk**
Canadian Society of Telehealth	**http://www.cst-sct.org**
Consumer Health Informatics Research. U.S. Library of Medicine/National Institutes of Health (July 2003)	**http://lhncbc.nlm.nih.gov/cgsb/research/chr/**
Healthcare Information and Management Systems Society (HIMSS)	**http://www.himss.org/ASP/index.asp**
Health Care and Intellectual Property	**http://www.cptech.org/ip/health/**
Health Technology Advisory Committee	**http://www.health.state.mn.us/htac/**
HIPAAdvisory	**http://www.hipaadvisory.com**
HIPAAlert	**http://www.hipaadvisory.com/alert/**
Medical Privacy	**http://www.epic.org/privacy/medical/**
Medical Records Institute	**http://medrecinst.com**
Office for the Advancement of Telehealth	**http://telehealth.hrsa.gov**
TelehealthNet	**http://telehealth.net**
Telemedicine Information Exchange	**http://tie.telemed.org**

Medical Errors: An Ongoing Threat to Quality Health Care

14

Carol J. Huston

Quality health care has emerged as a critically important, yet underachieved goal in this country. One of the most significant threats to achieving quality health care is the scope and prevalence of medical errors. Indeed, former President Bill Clinton stated that "for all of its strengths, our health care system is plagued by avoidable errors" (Quality Interagency Coordination [QuIC] Task Force, n.d., para 6). Dr. John Eisenberg, Director for the Agency for Healthcare Research and Quality (AHRQ), concurred, likening the problem of medical errors to an epidemic, that we are only in the first stage of understanding (Eisenberg, 2000).

Although medical errors have surely occurred since medicine began, the problem in the United States did not receive nationwide attention until several highly publicized cases in the mid-1990s. One such case involved Betsy Lehman, a *Boston Globe* reporter who died following multiple chemotherapy administration errors. The news media jumped on the story because it demonstrated repeated widespread communication and dispensing errors, despite multiple safeguards in place to keep them from happening.

Libby Zion's case occurred about this same time. Zion, 18 years old, died 8 hours after entering a New York emergency department with seemingly minor complaints of fever and earache. Her death from drug interactions brought attention both to the all-too-narrow range between effective and toxic doses of some drugs and the danger of drug-drug interactions, even when all drugs are administered in doses that are considered safe when administered individually. The case also brought attention to the lack of supervision of residents and interns in this country, as well as the excessive work hours forced on them and the errors that occur as a result.

Finally, there was the story of Willie King, a diabetic man from Tampa, Florida, who had the wrong leg amputated. This case, which has become known as the "wrong leg" case, captures our collective dread of wrong site surgery, but it is a medical error that occurs too frequently as a result of the symmetry of the human body.

Discussion   Point

Do you believe the general public considers itself to be at risk for harm when receiving health care? Do you personally know someone who has been harmed by a medical error?

Perhaps it was the clustering of these high profile cases that made Americans stop and look at the problem of medical errors, or maybe it was just time to do so. The end result was that an unprecedented number of seminal research studies delving into medical errors were undertaken in the late 1990s, attempting to discover how many errors were occurring, what was causing them, and what their financial and human costs were.

The results were disconcerting to say the least. Most studies highlighted multiple concerns about quality of care including "high rates of iatrogenic [provider-induced] injury, unnecessary and inappropriate care, and failure to provide interventions proven to be efficacious" (Mechanic, 2002). Many studies found the number of errors in health care to be unacceptably high. And the seminal study of this time, *To Err Is Human*, published by the Institute of Medicine (IOM) in 1999, provided evidence that the public was highly vulnerable to human error in American health care institutions, an arena in which many thought they were safe.

In addition, unlike most health care research, which generally receives little if any national press, medical error research findings in the late 1990s were published and analyzed in almost every media forum in the country. Consumers were barraged with study findings suggesting that the quality of health care in this country was inadequate and that medical errors were a significant problem leading to increased morbidity and mortality.

Discussion Point

Do you believe the quality of health care has declined in the past few decades, or is it simply better monitored and more openly reported on today?

As a result, consumers, providers, and legislators stepped forward to voice their concerns and to demand, at minimum, a safer health care system than they currently had. The government listened and directed providers to re-examine how quality health care was provided, measured, and monitored. In addition, a national agenda was established to reduce medical errors, rebuild the public's trust, and create cultures of safety within all health care organizations (Hemman, 2002).

This chapter examines seminal research on medical errors, medication errors, and adverse events published during the past decade as well as the directives that emerged as a result of their findings. Mechanisms for achieving four goals put forth by the IOM as part of *To Err Is Human* are identified. Finally, strategies for creating a culture of safety management in health care are identified, as are the challenges of changing a system that all too often focuses on individual errors rather than on the need to make system-wide changes.

▶ SEMINAL RESEARCH ON MEDICAL ERRORS

In reviewing the literature on medical errors, medication errors, and adverse events in health care, it is helpful to first define common terms. *Medical errors* are defined by the IOM as the failure to complete a planned action as intended or the use of a wrong plan to achieve an aim (Kohn, Corrigan, & Donaldson, 2000). The National Coordinating Council for Medication Error Reporting and Prevention defines a *medication error* as "any preventable event that may cause or lead to inappropriate medication use or patient harm while the medication is in the control of the health care professional, patient, or consumer. Such events may be related to professional practice, health care products, procedures, and systems, including prescribing; order communication; product labeling, packaging, and nomenclature; compounding; dispensing; distribution; administration; education; monitoring; and use" (Center for Drug Evaluation and Research, 2004). Finally, *adverse events* are defined by the AHRQ as injuries caused by medical management rather than by the underlying disease or condition of the patient.

One of the earliest large-scale studies suggesting that medical errors were a significant problem in health care was published by Brennan, Leape, Laird, Hebert, Localio, Lawthers et al. (1991) in the *New England Journal of Medicine*. This benchmark study involved more than 30,000 hospital patients in New York state. Nearly 5 of every 100 patients suffered an adverse event caused by a medical error of omission or commission. Of these adverse events, approximately one in four involved negligence. The overwhelming majority of iatrogenic occurrences, however, resulted from organization, system, or process failures.

This study, extrapolated to the national population, suggested that 1.3 million people were injured each year in hospitals; of that number, 180,000 would die from those injuries. Providing additional cause for alarm, the report also suggested that most of those injuries were actually preventable.

Leape, Brennan, Laird, Localio, Barnes et al. (1991) also reported that drug complications represented 19% of these adverse events, and that 45% of these adverse events were caused by medical errors. In this study, 30% of the individuals with drug-related injuries died.

In another study, Leape (1994) reported that the average intensive care unit (ICU) patient experienced almost two errors per day. One of five of these errors were potentially serious or fatal. Surprisingly, this translates to a level of proficiency of approximately 99%, which seems reasonable. Yet, if performance levels of 99.9%—substantially better than those found in the ICU by Leape—were applied to the airline and banking industries, it would equate to two dangerous landings per day at O'Hare International Airport, or 32,000 checks deducted hourly from the wrong account (Leape, 1994).

*CONSIDER: The safety record in health care is a far cry from the enviable record of the similarly complex aviation industry. "A person would have to fly nonstop for 438 years before expecting to be involved in a deadly airplane crash, based on recent airline accident statistics. That, the IOM says, places health-care at least a decade behind aviation in safeguarding consumers' lives and health" (Nordenberg, 2000, para 8).

271

Discussion Point

Should the health care industry be willing to accept higher error rates than the banking or airline industries? Why or why not? Is the public willing to do so?

Another seminal study in the late 1990s involving medical errors was completed by Thomas, Stuoidert, Newhouse, Zbar, Howard, Williams et al. (1999), based on a chart review of 14,732 medical records from 28 hospitals in Colorado and Utah. This study found that 265 of 459 (57%) adverse events were preventable. The total cost of adverse events was $661,889,000 with preventable adverse events costing an additional $308,382,000. In addition, the study estimated the national costs of all preventable adverse events to be just under $17 billion (in 1996 dollars). A more recent study by Bates et al. (2002) reaffirms both the high incidence rate of medical errors and the subsequent costs as reported by Thomas. In their study of two prestigious teaching hospitals, Bates and colleagues found that approximately 2 patients of every 100 admitted to the hospital experienced a preventable adverse drug event. In addition, these adverse drug events resulted in average increased hospital costs of $4,700 per admission or approximately $2.8 million annually for a 700-bed teaching hospital.

A high incidence of medication errors was also found in a Commonwealth Fund study in 2002. This study found that 1.5 million American families had experienced a serious drug error, 33% of them during a hospitalization (Commonwealth Fund, 2002).

A study by Rothschild, Bates, and Leape (2000) suggested the outcomes are equally grim in outpatient settings, where 8% to 24% of ambulatory patients receive prescription drugs that are inappropriate or contraindicated. Finally, the Massachusetts State Board of Registration in Pharmacy reported that in a 1-year period, 2.4 million prescriptions were filled improperly in that state alone (News Briefs, 2002).

To Err Is Human

Many of the studies done in the 1990s laid the foundation for what is perhaps the best known and largest study ever done on the quality of health care: *To Err Is Human* (Kohn, Carrigan, & Donaldson, 2000). This study, completed by the IOM, a congressionally chartered independent organization, found that:

- At least 44,000 Americans die each year as a result of medical errors, and the number may be as high as 98,000.
- Even when using the lower estimate, deaths due to medical errors could be considered the eighth leading cause of death in 1999.
- More people die in a given year as a result of medical errors than from motor vehicle accidents, breast cancer, or AIDS (Kohn et al., 2000).

The IOM study also examined the types of errors that were occurring. Many of the adverse events were associated with the use of pharmaceutical agents, and were potentially preventable. Medication errors alone, both in and out of the hospital, were estimated to account for more than 7,000 deaths in 1993, and one of every 854 inpatient hospital deaths was the result of a medication error (Kohn et al., 2000; Phillips, Christenfeld, & Glynn, 1998). Children experienced harmful medication errors three times more often than adults (5.7% of medication orders for pediatric patients), and the rate was higher yet for neonates in the neonatal intensive care unit (Kaushal, Bates, Landrigan, McKenna, Clapp, Federico, & Goldmann, 2001). In addition, ICU patients suffered more life-threatening medication errors than any other patient population (Kaushal et al.) (Box 14.1).

Within a short time of the IOM report's release, some people began to question the numbers, asking whether the problem of medical errors could be as serious as it seemed. Richardson (2001) argued that indeed it was, stating that the conclusions of the IOM report were based on more than 30 studies, including 30,000 medical records from the Harvard Medical Practice Study (Leape et al., 1991) and 15,000 records from Thomas et al.'s (2000) study in Colorado and Utah. In addition, Richardson argued that most studies identify errors from information that is documented in handwritten medical errors and that it is likely that many errors never even get documented in medical records.

The reliability of the IOM figures was also confirmed in a July 2004 study by Lakewood, Colorado–based HealthGrades, Inc. HealthGrades looked at 3 years of

BOX 14.1

Medication Errors Affecting Children

In this study of 1,120 pediatric patients admitted to two urban teaching hospitals in 1999, researchers examined clinical staff reports, medication order sheets, medication administration records, and patient charts to identify medication errors, potential adverse drug events (ADEs), and acutal ADEs.

Kaushal R., Bates D. W., Landrigan C., McKenna K. J., Clapp M. D., Federico F., & Goldmann, D. A. (2001). Medication errors and adverse drug events in pediatric inpatients. *Journal of the American Medical Association. 285*(16), 2114–2120.

Study Findings

The researchers found that errors occurred in 5.7% of medication orders. In addition, the rate of potential ADEs—errors caught before medication was administered to a child—was three times the rate of potential ADEs found in a similar study of hospitalized adults. There were 26 actual ADEs, five (19%) of which were deemed preventable.

Physicians at both hospitals still wrote orders by hand, and copies of their orders were sent to the pharmacy. Physician reviewers judged that computerized physician order entry and decision support (with automatic checks on patient drug allergies, drug dosage, and drug-drug interaction) could have prevented 93% of potential ADEs. Also, ward-based clinical pharmacists participating in ward rounds could have prevented 94% of potential ADEs. A full 79% of potential ADEs occurred at the stage of drug ordering, and 34% involved incorrect dosing.

The researchers emphasized that medication administration is even more problematic in children than in adults for several reasons. Weight-based dosing is needed for virtually all pediatric drugs, and pharmacists often must dilute stock solutions. Young children do not have the communication skills to warn clinicians about potential mistakes in administering medications or about adverse effects that they experience. Finally, children, especially neonates, may have more limited internal reserves than adults with which to buffer errors.

273

Medicare data in all 50 states and Washington, D.C., and found that as many as 195,000 people a year are dying in U.S. hospitals because of easily prevented errors—an estimate that doubles IOM figures (*www.slackdavis.com*, 2004). HealthGrades's study included failure to rescue dying patients and the death of low-risk patients from infections as preventable causes of death, neither of which were included in the IOM report.

"The HealthGrades study also found that about 1.14 million 'patient-safety incidents' occurred among the 37 million hospitalizations. 'Of the total 323,993 deaths among Medicare patients in those years who developed one or more patient-safety incidents, 263,864, or 81 percent, of these deaths were directly attributable to the incidents. . . . One in every four Medicare patients who were hospitalized from 2000 to 2002 and experienced a patient-safety incident died'" (*www.slackdavis.com*, 2004). Perhaps most startling, however, was the conclusion by Dr. Samantha Collier, vice president of medical affairs at HealthGrades, that "if the Centers for Disease Control and Prevention's annual list of leading causes of death included medical errors, it would show up as number six, ahead of diabetes, pneumonia, Alzheimer's disease and renal disease" (*www.slackdavis.com*, 2004).

It is important when reading all of these studies to remember that formal reporting of medical errors has occurred for more than a quarter of a century (Hudon, 2003); however, it was not until the IOM study that significant public attention was drawn to the issue. Indeed, *To Err Is Human* received more publicity than any report ever issued by the National

Academy of Science, and a committee member, Lucian Leape, who authored the report stated that he had "under-estimated the emotional significance of the issue" (Buerhaus, 2001, p. 74). In fact, Jacott (2003) stated that no report from the federal government has created such a flurry of activity since the signing of the Declaration of Independence.

Discussion Point

Why did the IOM report receive so much media attention and spur such action? Was it the message, the timing, or both?

The Response to the Institute of Medicine Report

Within weeks of the report's release, the Senate held its first hearings on the issue, and additional hearings were conducted by committees of both the House and Senate (Richardson, 2001). Local and national as well as private and public sector leaders all took notice, and professional groups such as the American Medical Association (AMA), American Nurses Association (ANA), American Hospital Association (AHA), and American College of Physicians/American Society of Internal Medicine took immediate action (Richardson). Indeed, Bates and Gawande (2000, p. 765), in discussing the impact of the IOM report, stated:

> *The sleeping giant has awoken. Both the public and purchasers are increasingly aware of the safety problems in medicine, and they are applying pressure. As a profession, we are at a crossroads. We have solid epidemiologic data to demonstrate that iatrogenic injury is a major problem. Leaders are now recognizing that the traditional response—that physicians do the best they can—is no longer enough.*

Grol, Baker, and Moss (2002) agreed, asserting that everyone—authorities, policy makers, and professionals—seemed to accept the need for change after the IOM report was released, and new initiatives aiming to cure the ailing system were generated in droves. The significance of the IOM report as a catalyst for change cannot be understated.

That said, however, it is important to note that the problems of medical errors and patient safety were not totally unrecognized before *To Err Is Human* was published. Four months before the IOM report was released, the AMA's National Patient Safety Foundation (NPSF), the AHA, and the Joint Commission for Accreditation of Healthcare Organizations (JCAHO) convened a policy forum about patient safety (Jacott, 2003). Attendees, who included many leaders in the patient safety arena, called for the development of a national policy agenda to improve patient safety.

Perhaps, then, the most significant aspect of the IOM study was that it summarized the high human cost of medical errors in language that was understandable and personal to the public, something not generally done in the health care system (Buerhaus, 2001). In addition, previously, an assumption was made that most patient injuries were the result of negligence, incompetence, or corporate greed. But the IOM report indicated that errors are simply a part of the human condition and that instead of expecting people not to make mistakes and punishing them when they do, efforts need to be redirected at redesigning basic flaws in the way health care is organized and delivered so that it is more difficult to make errors and easier to recover when one is made (Buerhaus).

BOX 14.2

Institute of Medicine Safety Recommendations

- Establish a national focus to create leadership, research, tools, and protocols to enhance the knowledge base about safety.
- Identify and learn from medical errors through both mandatory and voluntary reporting systems.
- Raise standards and expectations for improvements in safety through the actions of oversight organizations, group purchasers, and professional groups.
- Implement safe practices at the delivery level.

Source: Kohn, Corrigan, & Donaldson, 2000.

As a result of these findings, the IOM recommended a national goal of reducing the number of medical errors by 50% over 5 years (Kohn et al., 2000). To that end, it outlined a four-pronged approach to reducing medical mistakes nationwide (Box 14.2). The strategies needed to achieve this national goal and attend to each of the four approaches are numerous, however, and only a few are detailed in this chapter.

WORKING TO ACHIEVE THE INSTITUTE OF MEDICINE GOALS

The first of the IOM's four-pronged approach to reducing medical errors was to "establish a national focus to create leadership, research, tools, and protocols to enhance the knowledge base about safety" (Kohn et al., 2000, p. 6). The second was to "raise standards and expectations for improvements in safety through the actions of oversight organizations, group purchasers, and professional groups" (p. 6). Work to achieve both of these goals began almost immediately after the IOM report was published.

> *The ink on the first copies of the report [To Err Is Human] was still moist when Congress began hearings, President Clinton established the Quality Interagency Coordination Task Force, members of the medical profession debated the numbers, hospitals formed committees, the quality-control folks said, "I told you so," the media went into a feeding frenzy, and attorneys salivated more than usual (Jacott, 2003, p. 15).*

Indeed, a number of national committees and groups were formed as a result of governmental or legislative intervention. These groups "proposed reporting systems, databases, legislative acts, guidelines, recommendations, and other studies to ultimately decrease the number of medical errors in health care facilities across the United States" (Tackett & Birk, 2001, para 1). Some of the committees, groups, and legislative efforts spearheading the task to reduce medical errors are outlined here.

Quality Interagency Coordination Task Force

The Quality Interagency Coordination (QuIC) Task Force was established by President Clinton in 1998 "to ensure that all federal agencies involved in purchasing, providing, studying, or regulating health care services were working in a coordinated manner toward the common goal of improving quality care" (Tackett & Birk, 2001, para 2). In December

1999, the task force began to evaluate the IOM recommendations and develop strategies for identifying threats to patient safety and reducing medical errors.

The final report, *Doing What Counts for Patient Safety: Federal Actions to Reduce Medical Errors and Their Impact*, was delivered to the president in February 2000. The report proposed to take strong action on all of the IOM recommendations to "reduce errors, implement a system of public accountability, develop a robust knowledge base about medical errors, and change the culture in health care organizations to promote the recognition of errors and improvement in patient safety" (QuIC, n.d, para 15).

On September 11, 2000, the QuIC Task Force also sponsored a national summit to help set a research agenda on medical errors and patient safety. During the summit, five panels of experts offered suggestions for what types of research the government and the private sector need to conduct to help reduce and prevent future errors.

The National Forum for Health Care Quality Measurement and Reporting

Consistent with the QuIC's recommendations, the National Forum for Health Care Quality Measurement and Reporting was launched by former Vice President Al Gore in 2000. Known as the National Quality Forum (NQF), it is a broad-based, private, not-for-profit body that establishes standard quality measurement tools to help people better ensure the delivery of quality services (NQF, n.d.b; QuIC, n.d.). "The mission of the NQF is to improve American health care through endorsement of consensus-based national standards for measurement and public reporting of health care performance data that provide meaningful information about whether care is safe, timely, beneficial, patient-centered, equitable, and efficient" (NQF, n.d.a, para 1). Strategic and organizational goals identified by the NQF are shown in Box 14.3.

BOX 14.3   Strategic and Organizational Goals of the National Quality Forum

Strategic Goals

1. National Quality Forum (NQF)–endorsed standards will become the primary standards used to measure the quality of health care in the United States.
2. The NQF will be the principal body that endorses national health care performance measures, quality indicators, and/or quality of care standards.
3. The NQF will increase the demand for high quality health care.
4. The NQF will be recognized as a major driving force for and facilitator of continuous quality improvement of American health care quality.

Organizational Goals

1. Promote collaborative efforts to improve the quality of the nation's health care through performance measurement and public reporting.
2. Develop a national strategy for measuring and reporting health care quality.
3. Standardize health care performance measures so that comparable data is available across the nation (i.e., establish national voluntary consensus standards).
4. Promote consumer understanding and use of health care performance measures and other quality information.
5. Promote and encourage the enhancement of system capacity to evaluate and report on health care quality.

Source: National Quality Forum.

Floyd D. Spence National Defense Authorization Act of 2001

In October 2000, President Clinton signed into effect the Floyd D. Spence National Defense Authorization Act (NDAA) of Fiscal Year 2001, specifically requiring the Department of Defense to establish a centralized process for reporting, compiling, and analyzing errors in health care (within the defense health program) (Tackett & Birk, 2001). It also mandated the creation of a Patient Safety Center at the Armed Forces Institute of Pathology to analyze patient care errors and to develop and execute plans to reduce and control those errors.

Department of Defense Patient Safety Work Group

Established in January 2000, the Department of Defense's Patient Safety Work Group set forth its initial goal: to create a process for tracking and reporting errors for use by all military health care facilities. Its second goal was to incorporate specific legislative mandates set forth in the NDAA (Tackett & Birk, 2001). Both mandatory and voluntary reporting systems were to be used as part of the process, similar to that done in the Veterans Affairs (VA) Patient Safety Reporting Program.

*CONSIDER: Although few organizations would argue the benefits of well-developed and well-implemented quality control programs, quality control in health care organizations has evolved primarily from external impacts and not as a voluntary monitoring effort.

The National Patient Safety Foundation

The National Patient Safety Foundation (NPSF) was also formed in response to the IOM report. The mission of the NPSF is to measurably improve patient safety in the delivery of health care by its efforts "to identify and create a core body of knowledge; identify pathways to apply the knowledge; develop and enhance the culture of receptivity to patient safety; raise public awareness and foster communications about patient safety; and improve the status of the Foundation and its ability to meet its goals" (NPSF, 2004). It is also dedicated to serving as a catalyst for transition from a culture of blame to a culture of safety in health care and the community (Hemman, 2002). Basic beliefs of the NPSF are shown in Box 14.4.

Joint Commission for Accreditation of Healthcare Organizations

New organizations were not the only ones that responded to the recommendations of the IOM. The JCAHO, in existence since 1951, accredits hospitals, long-term care facilities, psychiatric facilities, ambulatory care programs, and home health operations. It has made patient safety a centerpiece of its accreditation activity and has developed and implemented new patient safety standards (Jacott, 2003). Indeed, five of six new standards were designed for hospital leadership to demonstrate JCAHO's commitment to patient safety (Hemman, 2002).

The JCAHO's National Patient Safety Goals, implemented in January 2003, set forth clear, evidence-based recommendations to focus health care organizations on significant documented safety problems. Accredited health care organizations that provide care

BOX 14.4

Basic Beliefs: National Patient Safety Foundation

- Patient safety is central to quality health care as reflected in the Hippocratic Oath: "Above all, do no harm."
- Prevention of injury, through early and appropriate response to evident and potential problems, is the key to patient safety.
- Continued improvement in patient safety is attainable only through establishing a culture of trust, honesty, integrity, and open communication.
- An integrated body of scientific knowledge and the infrastructure to support its development are essential to advance patient safety significantly.
- Patient involvement in continuous learning and constant communication of information between caregivers, organizations, and the general public will improve patient safety.
- The system of health care is fallible and requires fundamental change to sustainably improve patient safety.

Source: National Patient Safety Foundation, 2004.

relevant to the goals are evaluated for compliance with these goals (Joint Commission President Testifies, 2003).

JCAHO also maintains one of the nation's most comprehensive databases of sentinel (serious adverse) events by health care professionals and their underlying causes (Joint Commission President Testifies, 2003). JCAHO has standardized formats and data elements on medical error data, allowing it to 1) combine and track data over time, 2) lessen the burden on health care organizations, and 3) facilitate communication with consumers and purchasers about patient safety (Kohn et al., 2000). Information from the JCAHO database is regularly shared with accredited organizations to help them take appropriate steps to prevent medical errors.

Another JCAHO priority is the development of a *root cause analysis* with a plan of correction for the errors that do occur (Jacott, 2003). In completing root cause analysis, organizations must determine which errors happened, why they occurred, and what should be done to prevent them from happening again, thereby helping to "build a culture of safety and move beyond the culture of blame" (VA National Center for Patient Safety, 2002, para 2).

*CONSIDER: National legislation designed to keep such error analyses confidential is a critical, but thus far unrealized, step. Until such legislation is passed, health care organizations will be reluctant to share root cause analyses, which may be used against them in a law suit (Jacott, 2003).

Centers for Medicare and Medicaid Services

The Centers for Medicare and Medicaid Services (CMS), formerly the Health Care Financing Administration (HCFA), is also playing an active role in setting standards and measuring quality of health care. With the introduction of the Medicare Quality Initiative (MQI) in November 2001, a new era of public reporting on quality began, giving consumers access to health outcomes data (Harris, 2003).

Harris describes the four-pronged approach inherent in the MQI. First, the state survey agencies and CMS conduct regulation and enforcement activities as usual. Second, information is made available to all consumers via a variety of media on the quality of care in target settings. Third, ongoing community-based improvement programs are conducted for the agencies that report outcomes data for the various quality initiatives. Finally, all stakeholders act as collaborators and partners, including quality improvement organizations, state survey organizations, and service providers. Many believe that this initiative may become the new benchmark in terms of measuring health outcomes and making quality reports readily available to the consumer (Harris, 2003).

Patient Safety Task Force

One of the newest government appointed groups to address the IOM goals is the Patient Safety Task Force (PSTF). This task force was established in April 2001 at the direction of Tommy Thompson, former secretary for the Department of Health and Human Services (Roark, 2004). The PSTF is composed of representatives from the AHRQ, the Centers for Disease Control and Prevention (CDC), the Food and Drug Administration (FDA), and the CMS. This group is responsible for coordinating both the integration of data collection on medical errors and adverse events, as well as the research and analysis efforts. In addition, the PSTF is charged with promoting collaboration within the Department of Health and Human Services in an effort to improve health care quality by preventing the adverse events associated with health care delivery (AHRQ, 2003).

The PSTF plans to complete several projects. First, a series of "demonstration projects will help identify the best methods to detect errors and adverse events, encourage accurate reporting, determine the underlying causes of errors, evaluate the impact of errors on patients, and evaluate the most successful strategies to help clinicians and health care agencies prevent errors" (AHRQ, 2003, para 14). AHRQ will also combine data on adverse events from the CDC's National Healthcare Safety Network and the FDA's reports into one coordinated system (AHRQ 2003).

Finally, the demonstration projects will develop national benchmarks and other comparative data to create accurate assessments of certain classes of adverse events. The goal is to collect reliable information regarding patients' risks of errors. This information can then be used to compare progress in error reduction among similar facilities, alerting facilities as to their need to improve their error reduction efforts and the integration of patient safety into their standard of care (AHRQ, 2003).

Mandatory Report Cards

In response to the demand for objective measures of quality including the number and type of medical errors, several health plans, health care providers, employer purchasing groups, consumer information organizations, and state governments have begun to formulate health care quality report cards. In the early 1990s, California mandated the development of report cards for all hospitals licensed in the state; Ohio and Pennsylvania have similar laws that mandate the dissemination to the public of health care institutions' quality performance data (Huston, 1999). Most states have laws requiring providers to report some type of data. AHRQ also is exploring the development of a report card for the nation's health care delivery system.

It is important to remember, however, that currently most report cards do not contain information about the quality of care rendered by specific clinics, group practices, or physicians in a health plan's network (Huston, 1999). In addition, most report cards focus on service utilization data and patient satisfaction ratings and have minimal data regarding medical errors. Critics of health care report cards also point out that health plans may receive conflicting ratings on different report cards. This results from using different performance measures as well as how each report card pools and evaluates individual factors. Report cards may also not be readily accessible or may be difficult for the average consumer to understand.

CREATING A CULTURE OF SAFETY MANAGEMENT

In response to public forces and professional concerns, patient safety has become one of the nation's most pressing challenges and a mandate for every health care organization. Indeed, the final recommendation of the IOM report was to implement safe practices at the delivery level (QUIC, n.d, para 15). The strategies that have been recommended to achieve this goal are overwhelming both in scope and quantity. In addition, there are insufficient outcome studies to determine which strategies in current use are achieving their stated goals.

Testifying before the U.S. Senate Committee on Governmental Affairs, JCAHO President Dennis S. O'Leary, M.D., outlined six crucial strategies for the creation of a true culture of safety within health care institutions (Box 14.5). Other strategies discussed in this chapter include: the Six Sigma approach (a customer-based, management philosophy) to error management; mandatory/voluntary reporting of errors; increasing confidentiality of reporting to reduce fear of legal liability for reporting errors that do occur;

BOX 14.5

JCAHO's Six Strategies for Creating a True Culture of Safety

- Create a blame-free, protected environment that encourages the systematic surfacing and reporting of serious adverse events.
- Reinforce the "systems approach" to preventing medical errors, whereby health care organizations assess the weak points in their systems of care and redesign care processes by putting safeguards into place to keep mistakes from reaching the patient.
- Reform the professional educational system to produce health care professionals who are proficient in executing a "systems approach" to patient safety and are trained in team approaches to patient care.
- Invest in the information infrastructure of health care organizations in order to make critical patient information available on a timely basis and thereby support the safe and appropriate delivery of medical care to patients.
- Establish performance incentives for achieving safety objectives through federal adoption of the Joint Commission's National Patient Safety Goals, and align reimbursement for health care services with the provision of safe, high quality care.
- Enact patient safety legislation that would encourage the voluntary reporting of health care errors and their causes by affording confidentiality protections for such reports.

Source: Joint Commission president testifies before U.S. Senate on critical strategies for reducing medical errors. (August 1, 2003). *Nevada RNformation, 12*(3) 14. Retrieved April, 2005, from EBSCO Host.

Leapfrog recommendations; bar coding and changing organizational cultures from that of "individual blame" to error identification and system modification.

> ***CONSIDER:** Because quality health care is a complex phenomenon, the factors contributing to quality in health care are as varied as the strategies needed to achieve this elusive goal.*

A Six Sigma Approach

One approach that has been taken to create a culture of safety management at the institutional level has been the implementation of a Six Sigma approach. "Sigma" is a statistical measurement that reflects how well a product or process is performing. "Higher sigma values indicate better performance, while lower values indicate a greater number of defects per unit" (Seecof, 2000, para 5). Six Sigma uses an approach called DMAIC, which stands for define, measure, analyze, improve, and control (Jones, 2002).

Historically, industry has been comfortable striving for three-sigma processes (where all the data points fall within three standard deviations). By achieving six sigma, the failure rate is minimized to 3.4 defects (errors) per million opportunities or a 99.9996% success rate (Lanham & Maxson-Cooper, 2003). Organizations aim for this lofty target by carefully applying Six Sigma methodology to every aspect of a particular product or process. This approach allows companies to redirect "time, energy, and resources toward activities that bring real value to customers instead of forestalling and fixing defects in order to perform at a minimally acceptable level" (Seecof, 2000, para 5).

Discussion Point

Is a Six-Sigma failure rate a reasonable goal for all health care organizations? Should some health care organizations be expected to have higher failure (defect) rates than others? What variables might impact an organization's ability to achieve this goal?

For example, Jones states that many hospitals have used the Six Sigma approach to reduce prescription errors. One hospital in Milwaukee used Six Sigma to map a prescription from the time it originated with a doctor's handwritten note, moved on to be filled by the pharmacy, and then was administered by nurses. It turned out that most errors occurred because of difficulty reading the doctors' handwriting. In response, the hospital implemented a computer-based program in which doctors typed each prescription into a computer. This program successfully decreased the error rate (Jones 2002).

Mandatory Reporting of Errors

The third prong of the IOM's four-pronged approach to creating a safer health care system is "to identify and learn from medical errors through both mandatory and voluntary reporting systems" (Kohn et al, 2000, p. 6). To accomplish this, the IOM report recommended "developing a nationwide mandatory reporting system to collect standardized information from state governments about adverse events that result in death or serious harm" (Tackett & Birk, 2001, para 7). For states that choose not to implement the mandatory reporting system, the IOM report suggested that the Department of Health and Human Services serve as the responsible entity. As of 2004, a total of 21 states had implemented some type of mandatory reporting system for medical errors (Robeznieks, 2004).

It is important to note, however, that Dr. Lucian Leape, member of the IOM committee who authored *To Err Is Human*, suggests that medical professional societies and Congress seemed to fixate on the mandatory reporting issue, when in fact, it was only a small part of what was recommended (Buerhaus, 2001). Yet, it is readily apparent that there must be more mandatory reporting of medical errors as well as voluntary efforts if quality goals are to be achieved.

It is also important to note that the IOM report did suggest more options be created for limited voluntary reporting systems in all 50 states, and suggested that these systems build on existing options and focus on selected areas, such as medications, surgery, and pediatrics, or use a sampling technique that allows them to collect the full range of information from a subset of health care providers (QuIC, n.d.). The IOM also recommended that more research be conducted on how best to develop voluntary reporting systems that complement proposed mandatory reporting systems. Thus, potential precursors to errors could be identified, preventing patient harm (QuIC).

Increased mandatory and voluntary reporting must also occur at the institutional level as well as by individual providers. Tackett and Birk (2001) stress that health care professionals need to be aware of the extent of preventable errors and must help design systems that decrease the potential for error. They also need to do a better job of identifying what errors are occurring, categorizing those errors, and examining and reworking the processes that led to the errors (Chaiken, 2001). As a result, the IOM report suggested that mandatory adverse event reporting should initially be required of hospitals and eventually of other institutional and ambulatory care delivery facilities (Kohn et al., 2000). This was the impetus for the subsequent JCAHO action for sentinel event reporting as part of the accreditation process.

It will be more difficult, however, to enforce greater disclosure and reporting at the individual provider level. Ethical and professional guidelines suggest that providers have a responsibility to disclose medical errors (American College of Physicians, 1998; AMA Council on Ethical and Judicial Affairs, 2000; Medical Professionalism, 2002).

In fact, a study by Mazor, Simon, Yood, Martinson, Gunter, Reed, and Gurwitz, suggested that full disclosure after a medical error reduced the likelihood that patients would change physicians, improved patient satisfaction, increased trust in the physician, and resulted in a more positive emotional response. Full disclosure was also apt to reduce the likelihood that patients would seek legal advice under some, but not all, circumstances; the specifics of the case and the severity of the clinical outcome also affect patients' responses (Mazor et al., 2004).

In addition, recent standards link disclosure of adverse events to hospital accreditation (JCAHO, 2004). Yet, the literature suggests that disclosure to patients and families after medical errors often does not occur (Allman, 1998; Blendon, Des Roches, Brodie, Benson, Schneider et al., 2002).

In a multi-method study of 29 small rural hospitals in 9 Western states over 3 years, Cook, Hoas, Guttmannova, and Joyner (2004) found that even when there was overwhelming agreement (97%) among participants that an error had occurred, only 64% stated they would disclose the error to the patient affected.

Discussion Point

Do you believe that error disclosure rates differ between nurses and physicians? If so, which professional group is more likely to disclose errors and why?

Perhaps this failure to disclose the errors that do occur is a major contributor to the disconnect that exists between consumers' perceptions of the quality of their own health care and the actual quality provided. Even consumers who are aware of medical error statistics often report they believe medical errors to be a problem, but believe such errors will not happen to them because they trust and believe in their personal health care provider.

McGlynn and Brook (as cited in Lee & Estes, 2003) suggest reports on medical errors have come closest in recent times to breaking through this cognitive dissonance. Yet they suggest that we need to continue to find ways to use the dialogue that has begun around errors to promote a shared understanding of the quality problem without fundamentally undermining trust in the health care system.

Discussion Point

Do you consider the care you receive from your primary care provider to be high quality? Are your perceptions subjective or do you have objective data to back up your impression? Have you actively searched for such data on your own primary care provider?

Legal Liability and Medical Error Reporting

If quality health care is to be achieved, the medical liability system and our litigious society must be recognized as potential barriers to systematic efforts to uncover and learn from mistakes that are made in health care (Huston, 2003). One recommendation of the IOM panel was to encourage learning about safety from cross-institutional reporting systems for errors. This reporting is inhibited by fears that such data will be discovered in liability lawsuits. Provider liability fears stemming from disclosure are usually identified as a primary reason why adverse events are under-reported (Chaing, 2001). Indeed the American Hospital Association vigorously opposed President Clinton's 2000 proposal requiring mandatory reporting of fatal and other serious medical errors, arguing that it would open up caregivers to "lawyers and lawsuits" (Hospital Association Opposes, 2000).

The provision of stronger confidentiality protections likely would improve the voluntary sharing of data (House Committee on Veterans' Affairs, 2000). In 2002, the *Patient Safety Improvement Act* was introduced to the House of Representatives. This bill provides legal protections for medical error reporting, stating that error information voluntarily submitted to patient safety organizations cannot be subpoenaed or used in legal discovery (Duff, 2002). It also generally requires that the information be treated as confidential;

violators would be sanctioned (Duff, 2002; AAMC Government Affairs and Advocacy, 2002). Even though the House overwhelmingly passed its version of this legislation and after several revisions, the Senate has yet to act as of March, 2005 (AMA, 2005).

Federal legislation has been proposed to protect the voluntary reporting of ordinary injuries and "near misses"—errors that did not cause harm this time but easily could the next time. This would be like what is done in aviation where near misses are confidentially reported and can be analyzed by anyone. This seems a good idea, and for near-miss data, confidentiality would not deny liability claimants any information now available (House Committee on Veterans' Affairs, 2000).

Discussion Point

Given the known incidence of medical errors and adverse events that result in patient injury and the challenges inherent in tracking the errors that are already made, how difficult will it be to track "near misses"? What resources would be needed to accomplish this goal?

Legislation is occurring at the state level as well. Eighteen states currently have liability shields for error reporting (Robeznieks, 2004). New Jersey, one of the most recent states to enact such a law, now requires reporting all "serious, preventable adverse events" to the state and to patients or family/guardians. It also allows for confidential, anonymous reporting of near misses, and shields analysis of the errors and near misses from being used as evidence. Although private medical practices are excluded, the law extends beyond the traditional hospital setting to include outpatient clinics, nursing homes, and diagnostic centers (Robeznieks).

Discussion Point

Have you ever encouraged a family member, friend, or colleague to seek legal redress for medical errors? If so, do you think this was the most appropriate means of redress?

Leapfrog Group

The Leapfrog Group is a conglomeration of non-health care Fortune 500 company leaders who are committed to modernizing the current health care system (Milstein, Galvin, Delbanco, Salber, & Buck, 2000). The group has advised the health care industry that big leaps in patient safety and customer value will be recognized. These companies are making safer medicine a top priority by steering their employees to those hospitals that make the fewest mistakes (Tackett & Birk, 2001).

Based on current research, the Leapfrog Group has identified three evidence-based standards they believe have the greatest potential to reduce medical errors:

▶ Computerized physician (or prescriber) order entry (CPOE)
▶ Evidence-based hospital referral (EHR)
▶ Intensive care unit physician staffing (IPS) (Hudon, 2003).

"An understanding of these medically based standards provides nursing an opportunity to consider the potential and actual concerns that span multiple disciplines in their implementation and motivation for future nursing research related to their effect" (Hudon, p. 234).

CPOE is a promising technology that allows physicians to enter orders into a computer instead of handwriting them. Because CPOE fundamentally changes the ordering process, it can substantially decrease the misuse of health care services (Kuperman & Gibson, 2003). CPOE is discussed further in Chapter 13.

The QuIC (n.d.) states that the Department of Defense and the Department of Veterans Affairs, which serve more than 11 million patients, have begun to implement CPOEs because they have proved effective in reducing medical errors. In the past three years, the VA has created an error reporting system, established four Centers of Inquiry for Patient Safety, and implemented bar code technology to reduce medication errors (QuIC). (See the next section for more information on bar coding.) The VA has also created a computerized medical record, in use in all of its 172 hospitals, which provides complete information about patients at the point of care, thus reducing errors.

EHR involves making sure that patients with high-risk conditions are treated at hospitals whose characteristics are associated with better outcomes. The Leapfrog Group believes this method could help prevent unnecessary deaths (Leapfrog Group, 2004a).

IPS examines the level of training of ICU medical personnel. Evidence suggests that quality of care in hospital ICUs is strongly influenced by whether "intensivists" (those familiar with ICU complications) are providing care and how the staff is organized (Leapfrog Group, 2004b). The Leapfrog Group (2004c) argues that there is a direct correlation between the level of training of ICU personnel and the quality of patient care. "When ICUs are staffed with physicians who have credentials in critical care medicine or when intensive care specialists are available to respond to 95% of pages within five minutes, the risk of patients dying in the ICU has been shown to reduce by more than 10%" (Leapfrog Group, 2004c). Only about 10% of ICUs in the United States meet this standard (Leapfrog Group, 2004b).

Bar Coding Medications

In addition, Leapfrog has endorsed the use of bar coding to reduce point-of-care medication errors. Per the U.S. Food and Drug Administration's new rule, passed in April 2004, all prescription and over-the-counter medications used in hospitals must contain a national drug code number (Dohnalek, Cusaac, Westcott, Langeberg, & Sandler, 2004), which "uniquely identifies the drug, its strength, and its dosage forms" (Roark, 2004, p. 63). The FDA suggests that a bar code system coupled with a CPOE system would greatly enhance the ability of all health care workers to follow the "five rights" of medication administration—that the *right* person receive the *right* drug, in the *right* dose, via the *right* route at the *right* administration time (Roark).

In addition, JCAHO originally proposed in its *2005 National Patient Safety Goals and Requirements*, that accredited organizations would have to implement bar code technology to identify patients and match them to their medications or other treatments by January 2007. This proposal was lauded by some members of the health care community as a bold step for patient care, although many worried that the deadline for implementation was too ambitious (Broder, 2004). Because of such implementation concerns, this proposal was abandoned by JCAHO in July 2004 (JCAHO Abandons Proposal, 2004).

As of 2003, only 1.5% of all U.S. hospitals were fully using bar codes to monitor drug administration and the cost to a hospital to install the technology often exceeds $1 million (Haugh, 2003). In addition, the FDA estimates that it would take about 20 years for all U.S. hospitals to fully adopt bar coding. If approved, however, JCAHO's goals could go a long way toward spurring bar code technology adoption in health care (Broder, 2004). Bar coding is also discussed in Chapter 13.

Changing Organizational Cultures

Perhaps the most significant change that must occur before a nationwide culture of safety management can exist is that organizational cultures must be created that remove blame from the individual and, instead, focus on how the organization itself can be modified to reduce the likelihood of such errors occurring in the future. Indeed, Wolf and Serembus (2004) found that organizational culture is pivotal to systems improvement.

The literature clearly shows that a punitive approach to medical errors is not productive and that errors will not be reported if workers fear the consequences.

Employees and patients need to feel comfortable in reporting hazards that can affect patient safety without fear of personal risk. Using discipline and reprisals for employees who report errors counteracts opportunities for improving systems of patient care (Wolf & Serembus, 2004). In addition, ignoring the problem of medical errors, denying their existence, or blaming the individuals involved in the processes does nothing to eliminate the preventable morbidity, mortality, and waste of resources that poor processes generate each day (Chaiken, 2001).

[***CONSIDER:** "The industries that provide the highest level of safety have made safety management organization-wide, comprehensive, pervasive, and visible" (Goodman, 2004, p. 44).]

Organizations must develop a systems approach to medical errors that examines all causes of failure, including components, subsystems, processes, interactions, and functions. Only then will they be able to move beyond blaming individuals, and instead redesign or develop systems that prevent errors (Tackett & Birk, 2001).

▶ CONCLUSIONS

Medical errors are not the only indicator of quality of care. They are, however, a pervasive problem in the current health care system and one of the greatest threats to quality health care that exists today. Tackett and Birk (2001, para 18) state that the "processes for improving quality over the past two decades have done little to actually prevent the system-related errors that injure and kill patients in the course of their treatment." Jacott (2003) agrees, arguing that despite the countless commissions, task forces, coalitions, and work groups on patient safety that have been assembled at the national, state, and local levels, the response has been ineffective. Clearly, the IOM national goal of reducing the number of medical errors by 50% in 5 years was not met.

Yet movement toward the IOM goals is occurring. It is likely that there has never been another time when the public, providers, and government have worked together so closely to achieve a shared health care goal. Janet Woodcock, M.D., the head of the FDA's Center for Drug Evaluation and Research, suggested that if everyone from drug manufacturers to consumers plays a role in improving the health system, the health care system in the United States should become safer (Nordenberg, 2000, para 31). In addition, the health care industry can learn much from other industries who have solved their safety problems.

Yet, much remains to be done. McGlynn and Brook (as cited in Lee & Estes, 2003) call for a "war on poor quality" that has the same level of public commitment as the war on cancer or the campaign to put a man on the moon. This will require sustained public interest to create the momentum necessary to systematically change the health care system in a way that reduces our vulnerability to medical errors. In addition, although there has been a lot of talk about taking a systems approach to the problem of medical errors, there has not been much discussion regarding exactly how this integration is to be accomplished. The bottom line is that Americans should expect, at a minimum, that they will emerge from their encounters with health care providers better for them, and certainly no worse off (Richardson, 2001).

FOR ADDITIONAL DISCUSSION

1. If cost containment and quality goals conflict, which do you think will take precedence in health care organizations today?
2. Why do so many providers, despite stated dissatisfaction levels, state they feel helpless about reducing medical errors and improving the quality of health care?
3. Why have quality control efforts in health care organizations evolved primarily from external requirements and not as voluntary monitoring efforts?
4. Where does individual responsibility and accountability begin and end in a culture where medical errors are recognized as being a failure of the system itself to protect both patients and providers?
5. How common is it that medical error documentation is used against employees as part of the performance appraisal process? If so, does this discourage reporting?
6. Does the average consumer have access to and an accurate understanding of health care report cards?
7. Given that most individuals can quickly identify medical errors that have happened to themselves, a friend, or a family member, why does the American public seem so reluctant to accept that medical errors constitute a threat to the quality of their health care?
8. Has your fear of legal liability ever influenced your decision to report a medical error?

REFERENCES

AAMC Government Affairs and Advocacy. (2002). House bill creates legal protections for medical errors reporting. Retrieved April 27, 2005, from http://www.aamc.org/advocacy/library/wash-high/2002/061402/_4.htm.

Agency for Healthcare Research and Quality. (2000). *Medical errors: The scope of the problem.* Retrieved April 27, 2005, from http://www.ahcpr.gov/qual/errback.htm.

Agency for Healthcare Research and Quality. (2003). *Fact sheet. Patient safety task force.* Retrieved April 27, 2005, from http://www.ahrq.gov/qual/taskforce/psfactst.htm.

Allman, J. (1998). Bearing the burden or baring the soul: Physician's self-disclosure and boundary management regarding medical mistakes. *Health Communication, 10,* 175–197.

American College of Physicians. (1998). Ethics manual (4th ed.). *Annals of Internal Medicine, 128,* 576–594.

American Medical Association. (2005). *National legislative activities.* Retrieved May 6, 2005, from http://www.ama-assn.org/ama/pub/category/6301.html.

American Medical Association Council on Ethical and Judicial Affairs. (2000). *Code of medical ethics: Current opinions.* Chicago: American Medical Association.

Bates, D. W. & Gawande, A. A. (2000). Error in medicine: What have we learned? *Annals of Internal Medicine, 132*(9), 763–767.

Bates, D. W., Spell, N., Cullen, D. J., Burdick, E., Laird, N., & Petersen, L. A. (2002). The costs of adverse drug events in hospitalized patients. *Journal of the American Medical Association, 277*(4), 307–311.

Blendon, R. J., Des Roches, C. M., Brodie, M., Benson, J. M., Rosen, A. B., Schneider, E., et al. (2002). Views of practicing physicians and the public on medical errors. *New England Journal of Medicine, 347,* 1933–1940.

Brennan T. A., Leape, L. L, Laird, N. M, Hebert, L., Localio, A. R., Lawthers, A.G., et al. (1991). Incidence of adverse events and negligence in hospitalized patients. Results of the Harvard medical practice study 1. *New England Journal of Medicine, 324*(6), 370–376.

Broder, C. (2004). *JCAHO proposal would mandate bar code technology by 2007.* Retrieved July 19, 2004 from http://www.bridgemedical.com/04_22_04.shtml.

Buerhaus, P. I. (2001). Follow-up conversation with Lucian Leape on errors and adverse events in health care. *Nursing Outlook, 49*(2), 73–77.

Center for Drug Evaluation and Research. (2004). Medication errors. Retrieved April 27, 2005, from http://www.fda.gov/cder/drug/MedErrors/default.htm.

Chaiken, B .P. (2001). Patient safety: Is it really a problem? *Nursing Economics,* 19(4), 176–177.

Chaing, M. (2001). Promoting patient safety: Creating a workable reporting system. *Yale Journal on Regulation, 18,* 396–401.

Commonwealth Fund. (2002). *Room for improvement: Patients report on the quality of their health care.* Retrieved April 27, 2005, from http://www.cmwf.org/publications/publications_show.htm?doc_id=221270.

Cook, A. F., Hoas, H., Guttmannova, K., & Joyner, J. C. (2004). An error by any other name. *American Journal of Nursing, 104*(6), 38–39.

Dohnalek, L. J., Cusaac, L., Westcott, J., Langeberg, A., & Sandler, S. G. (2004). The code to safer transfusions. *Nursing Management, 35*(6), 33–36.

Duff, S. (2002). Medical-errors reporting system proposed. *Modern Healthcare's Daily Dose.* Retrieved April 27, 2005, from www.bridgemedical.com/patient_psqia.shtml.

Eisenberg, J. (2000). *Summary: Opening remarks.* National Summit on Medical Errors and Patient Safety Research. Retrieved April 27, 2005, from http://www.quic.gov/summit/sumopening.htm.

Goodman, G. R. (2004). A fragmented patient safety concept: The structure and culture of safety management in healthcare. *Nursing Economics, 22*(1), 44–46.

Grol, R., Baker, R., & Moss, F. (2002). Quality improvement research: Understanding the science of change in healthcare. *Quality & Safety in Health Care, 11,* 110–111.

Harris, M. J. (2003). Medicare quality initiative. *Policy, Politics & Nursing Practice, 4*(4), 263–265.

Haugh, R. (2003). Bar code bandwagon. *Hospital & Health Networks.* Retrieved April 27, 2005, from http://www.aha.org/hhnmag/jsp/articledisplay.jsp?dcrpath=AHA/PubsNewsArticle/data/0305HHN_FEA_BarCode&domain=HHNMAG.

Hemman, E. A. (2002). Creating healthcare cultures of patient safety. *Journal of Nursing Administration, 32*(7/8), 419–427.

Hospital association opposes mandatory reporting of medical errors. (2000). CNN.com.Health. Retrieved April 27, 2005, from http://archives.cnn.com/2000/HEALTH/02/22/medical.errors/.

House Committee on Veterans' Affairs. (2000). *Testimony of Randall R. Bovbjerg, principal research associate, the Urban Institute.* Retrieved July 21, 2004 from http://veterans.house.gov/hearings/schedule106/feb00/2-9-00/RBovberg.htm.

Hudon, P. S. (2003). Leapfrog standards: Implications for nursing practice. *Nursing Economics, 21*(5), 233–236.

Huston, C. (1999). Outcomes measurement in health care: New imperatives for professional nursing practice. *Nursing Case Management Journal, 4*(4), 188–195.

Huston, C. (2003). Quality health care in an era of diminished resources: Challenges and opportunities. *Journal of Nursing Care Quality, 18*(4), 295–301.

Institute of Medicine. (2001). *Crossing the quality chasm: A new health system for the 21st century.* Retrieved April 27, 2005, from http://books.nap.edu/books/0309072808/html/index.html.

Jacott, W. (2003). Guest editorial. Medical errors and patient safety: Despite widespread attention to the issue, mistakes continue to occur. *Postgraduate Medicine, 114*(3), 15–16, 18.

JCAHO abandons proposal to require hospital bar codes. (2004). *NurseWeek* (California edition), p. 6.

Joint Commission on Accreditation of Healthcare Organizations. (2004). *2004 comprehensive accreditation manual for hospitals (CAMH). The official handbook.* Oakbrook Terrace, IL: Author.

Joint Commission president testifies before U.S. Senate on critical strategies for reducing medical errors. (2003). *Nevada RNformation, 12*(3), 14.

Jones, D. (October 30, 2002). *Taking the Six Sigma approach.* Retrieved April 27, 2005, from http://www.usatoday.com/money/companies/management/2002-10-30-sigside_x.htm.

Kaushal, R., Bates, D. W., Landrigan, C., McKenna, K. J., Clapp, M. D., Federico, F., & Goldmann, D. A. (2001). Medication errors and adverse drug events in pediatric inpatients. *Journal of the American Medical Association, 285*(16), 2114–2120.

Kohn, L. T., Corrigan, J. M., & Donaldson, M. S. (eds.). (2000). *To err is human: Building a safer health system.* Executive Summary, pp. 1–6. Retrieved April 27, 2005, from http://print.nap.edu/pdf/0309068371/pdf_image/6.pdf.

Kuperman, G. J. & Gibson, R. F. (2003). Improving patient care. Computer physician order entry: Benefits, costs, and issues. *Annals of Internal Medicine, 139*(1), 31–39.

Lanham, B. & Maxson-Cooper, P. (2003). Patient safety. Is Six Sigma the answer for nursing to reduce medical errors and enhance patient safety? *Nursing Economics, 21*(1), 38–41.

Leape, L. L. (1994). Error in medicine. *Journal of the American Medical Association, 272,* 1851–1857.

Leape, L. L, Brennan, T. A., Laird, N., Lawthers, A. G., Localio, A. R., Barnes, B. A., et al. (1991). The nature of adverse events in hospitalized patients: Results of the Harvard Medical Practice Study II. *New England Journal of Medicine, 324*(6), 377–384.

Leapfrog Group. (2004a). *Fact sheet. Evidence-based hospital referral.* Retrieved April 27, 2005, from http://www.leapfroggroup.org/media/file/Leapfrog-Evidence-Based_Hospital_Referral_Fact_Sheet.PDF.

Leapfrog Group. (2004b). *Fact sheet. ICU physician staffing.* Retrieved April 27, 2005, from http://www.leapfroggroup.org/media/file/Leapfrog-ICU_Physician_Staffing_Fact_Sheet.pdf.

Leapfrog Group. (2004c). *Leapfrog patient safety initiatives.* Retrieved April 27, 2005, from http://www.premierinc.com/frames/index.jsp?pagelocation=/all/advocacy/leapfrog/ips.htm.

Lee, P. R. & Estes, C. L. (2003). *The nation's health* (7th ed.). Boston: Jones and Bartlett.

Mazor, K. M., Simon, S. R., Yood, R. A., Martinson, B. C., Gunter, M. J., Reed, G. W. & Gurwitz, J. H. (2004). Health plan member's views about disclosure of medical errors. *Annals of Internal Medicine, 140,* 409–418.

Mechanic, D. (2002). Improving the quality of healthcare in the United States of America: The need for a multilevel approach. *Journal of Health Services Research & Policy, 7,* Suppl 1, S1:35–S1:39.

Medical professionalism in the new millennium: A physician charter. (2002). *Annals of Internal Medicine, 136,* 243–246.

Milstein, A., Galvin, R., Delbanco, S., Salber, P., & Buck, C. (2000). Improving the safety of health care: The Leapfrog initiative. *Effective Clinical Practice, 3*(6). Retrieved April 27, 2005, from http://www.acponline.org/journals/ecp/novdec00/milstein.pdf.

Morales, J., Hommand, H., & Englert, F. (2000). Survey shows that medical errors and malpractice are among public's top measures of health care quality. Retrieved April 27, 2005, from http://www.ahrq.gov/news/press/pr2000/kffsurvpr.htm.

National Patient Safety Foundation (NPSF). (2004). *About the foundation.* Retrieved April 27, 2005, from http://www.npsf.org/html/about_npsf.html.

National Quality Forum. (n.d.a). National Quality Forum Mission. Retrieved April 27, 2005, from http://www.qualityforum.org/mission/default.htm.

National Quality Forum (n.d.b). Welcome to the National Quality Forum. Retrieved April 27, 2005, from http://www.qualityforum.org.

News briefs. (2002). *Clinical Journal of Oncology Nursing, 6*(3), 124–125.

Nordenberg, T. (2000). Make no mistake. Medical errors can be deadly serious.. *FDA Consumer Magazine.* Retrieved April 27, 2005, from http://www.fda.gov/fdac/features/2000/500_err.html.

Oermann, M. H. & Templin, T. (2000). Important attributes of quality health care: Consumer perspectives. *Journal of Nursing Scholarship, 32*(2), 167–172.

Phillips, D. P, Christenfeld, N., & Glynn, L. M. (1998). Increase in U.S. medication-error deaths between 1983 and 1993. *Lancet, 351*(9103), 643–644.

Quality Interagency Coordination Task Force (QuIC). (n.d.). *Doing what counts for patient safety.* Retrieved April 27, 2005, from http://www.quic.gov/report/mederr2.htm#national.

Richardson, W. C. (2001). *Reconceiving health care to improve quality.* The Tanner Lectures on Human Values. Presented at University of California Santa Barbara.

Roark, D. C. (2004). Bar codes drug administration. *American Journal of Nursing, 104*(1), 63–66.

Robeznieks, A. (May 17, 2004). *New Jersey law expands reporting of medical errors.* Retrieved April 27, 2005, from http://www.ama-assn.org/amednews/2004/05/17/prsb0517.htm.

Rothschild, J. M., Bates, D. W., & Leape, L. L. (2000). Preventable medical injuries in older patients. *Archives of Internal Medicine, 160*(18), 2717–2728.

Seecof, D. (2000). Applying the six sigma approach to patient care. *Healthcare Services, 2*(5). Retrieved April 27, 2005, from http://www.gehealthcare.com/prod_sol/hcare/resources/insights/mins0500.html.

Slack & Davis. News Room–Recent Notes. (July 28, 2004) *Study: Hospital errors cause 195,000 deaths.* Retrieved May 6, 2005 from http://www.slackdavis.com/newsarticle.php/newsid/argval/770/argname/backlink/argval/recentnews.

Tackett, S. & Birk, C. C. (2001). The patient safety mandate: Rebuilding the trust and creating a reporting system. *Legal Medicine 2001.* Retrieved April 27, 2005, from http://www.afip.org/Departments/legalmed/legmed2001/patient.htm.

Thomas, E. J., Studdert, D. M, Newhouse, J. P., Zbar, B. I. W., Howard, K. M., Williams, E. J., et al. (2000). Costs of medical injuries in Colorado and Utah in 1992. *Inquiry, 36,* 255–264.

VA National Center for Patient Safety. (2002). Root cause analysis. Retrieved April 27, 2005, from http://www.patientsafety.gov/tools.html.

Wolf, Z. R. & Serembus, J. F. (2004). Medication errors. Ending the blame-game. *Nursing Management, 35*(8), 41–47.

BIBLIOGRAPHY

Benner, P., Sheets, V., Uris, P., Malloch, K., Schwed, K., & Jamison, D. (2002). Individual, practice, and system causes of errors in nursing. *Journal of Nursing Administration, 32*(10), 509–523.

Black, J. (2003). What can we do to reduce the rate of medical errors? *Plastic Surgical Nursing, 23*(1), 11, 24.

Chang, B. L., Lee, J. L., Pearson, M. L., Kahn, M. L., Elliott, M. N., & Rubenstein, L. L. (2002). Evaluating quality of nursing care. The gap between theory and practice. *Journal of Nursing Administration, 32*(7/8), 405–418.

DeLise, D. C. & Leasure, A. R. (2001). Benchmarking: Measuring the outcomes of evidence-based practice. *Outcomes Management for Nursing Practice, 5*(2), 70–74.

Gabel, R. A., Hayward, R. A., Leape, L. L., Berwick, D. M., & Bates, D. W. (2002). Counting deaths due to medical errors. *Journal of the American Medical Association, 288*(19), 2404–2405.

Gallagher, T. H., Waterman, A. D., Ebers, A. G., Fraser, V. J., & Levinson, W. (2003). Patients' and physicians' attitudes regarding the disclosure of medical errors. *Journal of the American Medical Association, 289*(8), 1001–1007.

Gurwitz, J. H., Field, T. S., Harrold, L. R., Rothschild, J., Debellis, K., Seger, A. C., et al. (2003). Incidence and preventability of adverse drug events among older persons in the ambulatory setting. *Journal of the American Medical Association, 289*(9), 1107–1116.

Hughes, C. M., Honig, P., Phillips, J., Woodcock, J., Anderson, R. E., McDonald, C. J., et al. (2000). How many deaths are due to medical errors? *Journal of the American Medical Association, 284*(17), 2187.

Kuzel, A. J. (2003). Making the case for a qualitative study of medical errors in primary care. *Qualitative Health Research, 13*(6), 743–780.

Landon, B. E., Zaslavsky, A. M., Beaulieu, N. D., Shaul, J. A., & Cleary, P. D. (2001). Health plan characteristics and consumers' assessments of quality. *Health Affairs, 20*(2), 274–286.

Lassetter, J. H. (2003). Medical errors, drug-related problems, and medication errors: A literature review on quality of care and cost issues. *Journal of Nursing Care Quality, 18*(3),175–183.

Layde, P. M., Maas, L. A., Teret, S. P., Brasel, K. J., Kuhn, E. M., Mercy, J. A. et al. (2002). Patient safety efforts should focus on medical injuries. *Journal of the American Medical Association, 287*(15), 1993–1997.

Leape, L. L. (2000). Institute of Medicine medical error figures are not exaggerated. *Journal of the American Medical Association, 284*(1), 95–97.

Leape, L. L. & Berwick, D. M. (2000). Safe health care: Are we up to it? *British Medical Journal, 320*(7237), 725–726.

Marsa, L. (2001a). Demanding overhaul of US health care: A new report by a think tank pushes for standardized guidelines, saying today's patients are at the mercy of a medical industry prone to errors. *Los Angeles Times*, S3.

Marsa, L. (2001b). Health care industry riddled with mistakes, survey shows. *Los Angeles Times*, S3.

McDonald, C. J., Weiner, M., & Hui, S. L. (2000). Deaths due to medical errors are exaggerated in Institute of Medicine report. *Journal of the American Medical Association, 284*(1), 93–95.

Pierluissi, E. (2003). Discussion of medical errors in morbidity and mortality conferences. *Journal of the American Medical Association, 290*(21), 2838–2842.

Servais, C. (2003). Best practices and medical errors. *ACCESS, 17*(6), 13.

Thomas, E. J., McNutt, R., Layde, P. M., Cortes, L. M., Teret, S. P., Brasel, K. J., et al. (2002). How best to improve patient safety? *Journal of the American Medical Association, 288*(6), 697–698.

Thomas, E. J., Sherwood, G. D., & Helmreich, R. L. (2003). Patient safety. Lessons from aviation: Teamwork to improve patient safety. *Nursing Economics, 21*(5), 241–243.

Tieman, J. (2003). Little room for errors: Bill protecting providers that report medical errors passes House, but hopes dim on road to Senate. *Modern Healthcare, 33*(11), 8–9, 16.

Weeks, W. B. & Wallace, A. E. (2003). Broadening the business case for patient safety. *Archives of Internal Medicine, 163*(9), 1112.

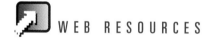

WEB RESOURCES

Agency for Healthcare Research and Quality	http://www.ahcpr.gov
American Nurses Association's National Center for Nursing Quality (NCNQ)—National database of quality nursing indicators	http://www.nursingworld.org/quality/
Council for Affordable Quality Healthcare	http://www.caqh.org
Department of Veterans Affairs	http://www.va.gov
Institute for Healthcare Improvement	http://www.ihi.org/IHI
Institute for Safe Medication Practices	http://www.ismp.org
JCAHO Patient Safety Goals for 2004 and 2005	http://www.jcaho.org/ accredited+organizations/patient+safety/ npsg.htm
Joint Commission on Accreditation of Healthcare Organizations	http://www.jcaho.org
The Leapfrog Group	http://www.leapfroggroup.org
Making Health Care Safer: A Critical Analysis of Patient Safety Practices	http://www.ahcpr.gov/clinic/ptsafety/ summary.htm
National Association for Healthcare Quality (NAHQ)	http://www.nahq.org/

National Committee for Quality Assurance (NCQA)	http://www.ncqa.org
National Guideline Clearinghouse	http://www.guideline.gov
National Patient Safety Foundation	http://www.npsf.org/html/about_npsf.html
National Quality Forum	http://www.qualityforum.org
National Quality Measures Clearinghouse	http://www.qualitymeasures.ahrq.gov
Quality Healthcare Network—Canada	http://www.qualityhealthcarenetwork.ca
U.S. Food and Drug Administration	http://www.fda.gov

Legal and Ethical Issues

4

Whistle-blowing in Nursing

Carol J. Huston

E nron and the artificial manipulation of gas prices . . . Martha Stewart and insider trading . . . WorldCom and accounting fraud . . . Bridgestone and Firestone tires . . . Dow Corning and silicone breast implants . . . Watergate and break-ins. . . . All of these high-profile cases, involving some degree of ethical malfeasance, have led the American public to an increased sense of moral awareness about what is right and what is wrong. In addition, these cases have all come to the attention of the American public as the result of "whistle-blowing."

Whistle-blowing refers to the disclosure of illegal, immoral, or illegitimate practices that are under employer control by either former or current organization members to persons or organizations that may be able to effect action (Near & Miceli, 1995). Kao (2001) states that whistle-blowing is the act of "going public" and exposing a serious wrongdoing, such as negligence or maltreatment that exists in the workplace and Wilmot (2000) defines it simply as the public exposure of organizational wrongdoing.

It is believed that the term "*whistle-blowing*" was first coined during the 1963 publicity surrounding the Otto Otopeka case in the United States (Petersen & Farrell, 1986). Otopeka released confidential documents concerning security risks in the new administration to the chief council of the Senate Subcommittee on Internal Security. As a result, then Secretary of State Dean Rusk fired Otopeka from his State Department job "for conduct unbecoming" (Vinten, 2000).

It is normally accepted that there are two types of whistle-blowing: internal and external. *Internal whistle-blowing* typically involves reporting concerns up the chain of command within an organization in hopes that whatever the problem is, it will be resolved. *External whistle-blowing* involves reporting concerns outside the organization, and in particular, to the media. In many cases, whistle-blowing becomes external only if inadequate action is taken at the organizational level to address the concerns of the whistle-blower. In some cases, however, whistle-blowing becomes external in an effort to embarrass an organization publicly or to seek financial redress.

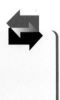

Discussion Point

Is it ever appropriate to whistle-blow externally before attempting to resolve the problem internally?

Terms used for whistle-blowing are conscientious objector, principled organizational dissenter, ethical resister, mole or informer, corruption fighter, concerned employee, rat, company traitor, or licensed spy (Vinten, 2000). These terms indicate the ambiguity of feeling toward whistle-blowers. In fact, Peternelj-Taylor (2003) suggests that the word *whistle-blowing* in itself is unfortunate and that its connotation is so emotionally laden that it has become a powerful deterrent to speaking up.

*__CONSIDER:__ Although the American public wants corruption and unethical behavior to be unveiled, the individual reporting such behavior is often looked upon with distrust and considered to be disloyal.

In an era of managed care, declining reimbursements, and the ongoing pressure to remain fiscally solvent, the risk of fraud, misrepresentation, and ethical malfeasance in health care organizations has never been higher. As a result, the need for whistle-blowing has also likely never been greater.

This chapter will explore the impact of "groupthink" on the likelihood that whistle-blowers will come forward. In addition, select cases of whistle-blowing involving nurses are presented. Personal risks associated with whistle-blowing are described as are the mixed feelings many Americans hold about whistle-blowing. Whistle-blowing is also explored as a failure of organizational ethics, and strategies are identified to create an organizational climate that both discourages the need for whistle-blowing in the first place and supports the whistle-blower when it is necessary for him or her to come forward. Finally, legal protections for whistle-blowing are discussed.

▶ GROUPTHINK AND WHISTLE-BLOWING

Being a whistle-blower takes great courage and self-conviction because it requires the whistle-blower to avoid *groupthink,* an inappropriate conformity to group norms. Going outside of groupthink often carries significant personal and professional risks.

Colvin (2002) recounts how Sherron Watkins, an accountant, first blew the whistle on Enron's complex special-purpose entities. She detailed them in a memo to then-CEO Ken Lay, her boss's boss's boss. She understood that something wrong was going on, something everyone else seemed to think was perfectly okay, and that public revelation would be disastrous.

What Colvin argues was most important in this scandal, was that Watkins had access to the same facts as many other people inside Enron, yet somehow she was able to escape the groupthink that ensnared her colleagues. Soon after writing the memo, she identified herself as its author and met with Mr. Lay. When her memo eventually became public, the wrongness of what happened was apparent even internally (Colvin, 2002).

Colvin details a similar story at WorldCom, where Cynthia Cooper, another internal auditor, saw something that didn't look right and took matters into her own hands. In this case, Cooper began investigating some of the company's capital expenditures and discovered bookkeeping entries that would eventually uncover what is likely the largest accounting fraud in U.S. history (Colvin, 2002).

Faced with disturbing facts, Cooper discussed her findings with the company's controller and with Scott Sullivan, the Chief Financial Officer. Sullivan tried to explain to her why costs that had previously been expensed were suddenly being capitalized. Then he asked her to stop the audit, which was being conducted early, and to put it off until the third quarter. She didn't. Instead, she continued—and immediately went over her boss's head and called the chairman of the board's audit committee. He arranged to meet with her and the company's new auditor, KPMG. Two weeks later, WorldCom announced it would restate earnings by $3.9 billion—the largest restatement ever.

Again Colvin (2002) suggests that the importance of Cooper's refusal to postpone her audit, as Sullivan had asked, is even greater than it may appear. Facts uncovered about the company, combined with the memo Sullivan wrote to the board in a last-ditch attempt to defend himself, show that if Cooper had "been a good soldier," the whole problem might have been concealed forever.

Similarly, in a high-profile whistle-blower case in New Mexico, six nurses at Memorial Medical Center in Las Cruces independently voiced concerns to their nurse managers over a 6-year period, regarding inadequate and inappropriate care being given by an osteopathic physician on staff (Bitoun Blecher, n.d.). In addition, the nurses brought the alleged shortcomings of this particular doctor to the attention of other physicians. The doctor in this case was later accused of negligence and incompetence after one of her patients died from sepsis and another suffered a serious injury.

But for reasons that are still unclear, the hospital failed to act on the nurses' complaints. Instead, the hospital challenged the nurses' actions, citing a provision in state regulations that prohibited the sharing of any patient information, regardless of how it might be used (American Nurses Association [ANA], June 19, 2001).

The hospital also retaliated after the case was filed and the nurses agreed to testify against the doctor. One of the nurses retired and later heard that she had been blackballed by the institution, while a second nurse allegedly was offered a management position in the hospital after being identified as a potential witness for the hospital (ANA, June 19, 2001). The ANA responded by filing an *amicus curiae* ("friend of the court") brief on behalf of the nurses. This brief cited conflict and ambiguity in New Mexico law and urged the court to protect the nurses, who were exercising their ethical responsibility. The ANA argued that the application of the state regulation in question limited the ability of the nurse to report incompetent practice, which is a statutory mandate.

"Sometimes the atmosphere in a hospital is set up so that you cannot work through the system, and that's what happened here—the system failed," said Judith Dunaway, RNC, MSN, HNC, of the New Mexico Nurses Association and a clinical instructor at New Mexico State University in Las Cruces (Bitoun Blecher, n.d.). "If that system refuses to address the complaints, then the process starts breaking down. We're not exactly sure where the breakdown occurred in this case. Supposedly, the complaints never got to the very top. Whether that's true or not, we don't know" (Bitoun Blecher).

*CONSIDER: Mary Foley, ANA President, 2001, stated:"The Memorial Medical Center case is particularly disturbing because it overwhelmingly points to the dangers and ambiguities inherent in a health care system that does not protect health care workers who speak up to safeguard their patients" (ANA, June 19, 2001, para 7).

Perhaps the most frightening aspect of these three cases is that the responses by management at Enron, WorldCom, and the Memorial Medical Center are not unique. In fact, an analysis of business crises between 1990 and 2000 by the Institute for Crisis Management revealed that "management is frequently aware of problem situations, which are ignored until either a crisis-precipitating event occurs or a current or former employee blows the whistle on the activity, often to external audiences such as media or government authorities" (Brujiins & McDonald, 2002, para 3).

Mohr and Horton-Deutsch (2001) suggest that nurses sometimes take comfort in thinking that anyone who evidences a lack of moral responsibility for patients and their care cannot be an introspective professional. The reality, however, is very different. It must be acknowledged that a schism often exists between what one should do, and what one actually does (Peternelj-Taylor, 2003). Similarly, Fiesta argued that "the courage to speak out is something we honor more often in theory than in fact" (Fiesta, 1990, p. 16). This is particularly disconcerting, and those who bear witness are required to overcome groupthink despite their moral distress.

▶ EXAMPLES OF WHISTLE-BLOWING IN NURSING

With the current nursing shortage, complaints about unsafe staffing and the use of unlicensed assistive personnel to perform nursing tasks outside their scope of practice are common. Worse yet, some nurses claim that they have been told to participate in illegal or unethical activities—things such as fraudulently altering medical records, falsifying Medicare or Medicaid claims, and even covering up unfair employment practices (Sloan & Ventura, 1999). In fact, fraud constituted 58% of internal whistle-blowing cases in the United States in 1998 (Figg, 2000).

A review of the literature reveals multiple case studies of whistle-blowing by nurses. Fletcher, Sorrell, and Silva (1998) tell the story of Barry Adams, a registered nurse in a New England hospital, who blew the whistle on short staffing leading to adverse patient events in his work setting in 1996. For 3 months, Adams and other nurses followed the organization's established procedures for reporting concerns to administrators, with the only response being criticism for collecting such documentation. Adams was eventually fired for his actions, although he successfully sued the hospital for wrongful termination.

Blunt (2001) tells the story of nurse Jill Stanek, a labor and delivery nurse for 6 years at Advocate Christ Medical Center in Oak Lawn, Illinois. Stanek disclosed in 1999 that newborns who were alive after abortions in her hospital were left to die without medical care. Stanek's lawyer says the hospital accused Stanek of making "false, defamatory, and misleading statements" when she testified before Congress and again when she was interviewed on Jerry Falwell's *Listen America* program.

Under a 1981 Illinois Supreme Court decision, whistle-blowers who "reasonably believe a crime is occurring" are supposed to be protected under the law from retaliatory discharge. In addition, under Illinois law, it is a crime to deny medical care to babies who are born showing signs of life (Blunt, 2001). Yet these laws may not have been enough to protect Stanek, because she was subsequently fired in 2001, 2 years after her allegations. The hospital did not specify the reason for her termination.

A whistle-blowing case with the saddest possible ending was that of Mary Hochman, a respected and experienced convalescent home nurse. Hochman committed suicide rather than continue to face the fury directed at her by her supervisors after she reported cases of patient neglect and abuse in the Santa Barbara nursing home where she worked to state regulators (Legislation Helps Nurses, 2001). "Hochman had reported that a nurse's aide hit an 81-year-old patient who suffered from dementia. Her employer allegedly told her to cover up the information, and when she refused to participate in the cover-up, Hochman's supervisors targeted her for retaliation" (Legislation Helps Nurses, para 3).

Whistle-blowing cases involving nurses are not limited to the United States. Armstrong (2002, para 2) tells the story of Kevin Moylan, a senior psychiatric nurse at a Tasmanian (Australia) clinic, who in 1995 became aware of what he described as a "dangerous and dysfunctional" environment for both patients and staff. Moylan alleged illegal and unethical abuse of patients and reported that staff were inadequately trained and provided incompetent service. He also suggested that there were serious problems with workplace health and safety: employment of a temporary psychiatrist who was not registered, police reluctance to provide support to protect staff from dangerous patients, and sexual harassment of patients. Moylan stated that he could not remain silent as patients were diagnosed, prescribed medication, and given electroconvulsive therapy by someone he considered a "fraud" (Armstrong).

When Moylan reported his fears to hospital management, instead of being praised and rewarded for his advocacy role, he says he was isolated and intimidated into silence (Armstrong, 2002). Moylan then wrote to the then Tasmanian Minister for Health, outlining his concerns. Unfortunately, a copy of the letter was delivered to the Tasmanian Shadow Minister for Health, who in raising the matter in the Tasmanian Parliament, named Moylan as the whistle-blower, thus removing his anonymity and privacy.

From that moment on, Moylan says his life changed "forever" and he was threatened, isolated, intimidated, and abused. As a result, Moylan states that he has suffered from disabling post-traumatic stress disorder and he has been unable to work since 1996. After 25 years with an unblemished record as a nurse, Moylan has "nothing left but his car and his dog" (Armstrong, 2002, para 9). The clinic was subsequently closed, and while Moylan received some compensation for his injury, he feels the loss of his health, his reputation, and his livelihood are yet to be addressed (Armstrong, 2002).

The same type of story comes from yet another country, South Wales, United Kingdom. BBC News (2001) reported that in spring 1998, Bernice Pinnington, a South Wales nurse, blew the whistle over a special needs school's alleged "do not resuscitate" policy. Pinnington claims she stumbled across instructions telling staff not to resuscitate a seriously ill 5-year-old child being cared for at the school. She alerted the grandparents of the child about the order and was terminated as a result. Although she won the right to appeal her dismissal, in April 2003, an employment tribunal upheld the dismissal, agreeing with the Swansea Local Education Authority and the school governors that Pinnington lost her job because she was absent through ill health (BBC News, 2003).

Patient advocacy is a central role in nursing. So too is professional advocacy, through which nurses are committed to improving the practice of nursing and maintaining the integrity of the health care profession (Kao, 2001). Both advocacy roles suggest that the nurse is accountable for assuring that at least minimum standards are met. All of these cases depict nurses who believed they were acting honorably in the role of patient advocate. Yet all suffered negative consequences including job loss. Unfortunately, this is more common than not.

▶ WHEN WHISTLE-BLOWING IS APPROPRIATE

Whistle-blowing should never be considered the first solution to ethically troubling behavior. Indeed, it should be considered only after all other avenues of addressing problems have been tried (I See and Am Silent, 1999). Fletcher, Sorrell, & Silva (1998) suggest, in fact, that there are six conditions that should be met before blowing the whistle. These are shown in Box 15.1. Klein suggests, however, that despite any personal risks, nurses have an obligation to be whistle-blowers if any of five possible situations occur (Klein, 2001). These are shown in Box 15.2.

BOX 15.1   Conditions to Meet Before Blowing the Whistle

1. The whistle-blower sees a grave injustice or wrongdoing occurring in his or her organization that has not been resolved despite using all appropriate channels within the organization.
2. The whistle-blower morally justifies his or her course of action by appeals to ethical theories, principles, or other components of ethics, as well as relevant facts.
3. The whistle-blower thoroughly investigates the situation and is confident that the facts are as she or he understands them.
4. The whistle-blower understands that her or his primary loyalty is to client(s) unless other compelling moral reasons override this loyalty.
5. The whistle-blower ascertains that blowing the whistle most likely will cause more good than harm to client(s); that is, clients will not be retaliated against because of the whistle-blowing.
6. The whistle-blower understands the seriousness of his or her actions and is ready to assume responsibility for them.

Source: Fletcher, Sorrell, & Silva, 1998.

*CONSIDER: "In America, there is some evidence that the events of September 11, 2001, have made people more public spirited and more inclined to blow the whistle. The Government Accountability Project, a Washington-based group, received 27 approaches from potential whistle-blowers in the 3 months before September 11th, and 66 in the 3 months after" (Peep and Weep, 2002, para 7).

In addition, for some minority nurses, cultural issues can further complicate the question of whether to report a problem or remain silent. For example, "nurses who with certain cultural backgrounds—for example, some Asians, Filipinos, and Africans—may be more reluctant to blow the whistle because they've been raised to respect a clear chain of command and hierarchy" (Bitoun Blecher, n.d., para 12). The same goes for nurses whose first language is not English. "They fear problems related to communication—whether they accurately communicate the magnitude of the problem and whether

BOX 15.2   Whistle-blowing as an Obligation

Whistle-blowing is an obligation when:

- Serious and considerable harm to the public is involved.
- One reports the harm and expresses moral concern to one's immediate superior.
- One exhausts all channels capable of correcting the situation within the corporation.
- One has "documented evidence" that would convince a reasonable impartial observer.
- One has good reason to think that going public will result in necessary changes.

Source: Klein (2001).

not speaking English as a first language would be used against them if they continue to challenge authority," says Winifred Carson, JD, nurse practice counsel for the ANA (Bitoun Blecher).

The ANA Code of Ethics for Nurses with Interpretive Statements may provide guidance for nurses who are considering becoming a whistle-blower (I See and Am Silent, 1999). The Code of Ethics Provision 3 states that the nurse "promotes, advocates for, and strives to protect the health, safety, and rights of the patient" (ANA Code of Ethics with Interpretive Statements, 2001, para 25). In addition, Section 3.5 states that "as an advocate for the patient, the nurse must be alert to and take appropriate action regarding any instances of incompetent, unethical, illegal, or impaired practice by a member of the health care team or the health care system, or any action on the part of others that places the rights or best interest of the patient in jeopardy" (ANA Code of Ethics with Interpretive Statements, para 32). Ethical codes of conduct from Canada, the United Kingdom, and Australia mandate similar action (Ahern & McDonald, 2002). Such ethical codes bind nurses to the role of patient advocacy, and compel them to take action when the rights or safety of patients are jeopardized. The bottom line is that although whistle-blowing can result in negative consequences for both the employing institution and the whistle-blower, nurses are charged with the responsibility to "act in a manner consistent with their professional responsibilities and standards for practice" (Canadian Nurses Association, 1997, p. 19).

> *CONSIDER: As individuals and as a profession, nurses have a responsibility to uncover, openly discuss, and condemn malfeasance when it occurs, yet there has been a collective silence (Mohr & Horton-Deutsch, 2001).

▶ THE PERSONAL RISKS OF WHISTLE-BLOWING

"Advocating for improved patient care and exposing unethical and incompetent health care providers is not without risk" (Erlen, 1999, p. 70). Indeed, it is filled with risks. Sadly, most whistle-blowers set out believing that their actions will be welcomed only to discover that the problems raised go much deeper than they imagined and the personal consequences can be overwhelming. In fact, Wilmot (2000) goes so far as to suggest that employers frequently treat whistle-blowing as if it were an antisocial or criminal action to justify using negative consequences.

The personal risks of whistle-blowing can take many forms, including negative reactions from coworkers, losing one's job, and, in the extreme, legal retaliation. Kao (2001) adds that whistle-blowers may also experience personal and/or professional isolation and ridicule, especially from their peers and the media. In fact, Vinten (1994) likened whistle-blowers to bees, arguing that a whistle-blowing employee has only one sting, and using it may lead to career death.

Armstrong (2002) states that studies in the United States show that 90% of whistle-blowers lost their jobs or were demoted as a result of their actions, 27% faced lawsuits, 26% had psychiatric or medical referral, 17% lost their homes, and 8% went bankrupt. In another survey of 87 American whistle-blowers from both public service and private industry, all but one experienced retaliation, with those employed longer, experiencing greater retaliation (Soeken & Soeken, 1987). Another survey of 200 whistle-blowers who contacted the National Whistleblower Center (NWC) in 2002 demonstrated that 49.5% alleged they were terminated after they blew the whistle (NWC, 2002).

Bitoun Blecher (n.d.) reports similar findings in a recent Australian survey of 95 nurses. Seventy nurses who reported misconduct suffered severe repercussions. Those who remained silent experienced few professional consequences. "Fourteen percent of the whistle-blowers reported being treated as traitors, 16% received professional reprisals in the form of threats, 14% were rejected by peers, 11% were reprimanded, 9% were referred to a psychiatrist, and 7% were pressured to resign" (Bitoun Blecher, para 6).

Hunt (1995) suggests that even if one does not lose one's position, the experiences of broken promises to do something about an unethical practice, isolation and humiliation, formation of "anti-you" groups, organizational stonewalling, questioning of one's mental health, unusually close observation of what one does and says, vindictive tactics to make one's work more difficult and insignificant, talk about so-called generous severance packages, assassination of one's character, and disciplinary hearings before one has had a chance to address one's concerns are extremely troubling.

*CONSIDER: Dr. Jean Lennane, a Sydney psychiatrist and the national president of Whistleblowers Australia, likens whistle-blowers to the canaries once used in coal mines to detect toxic or explosive gases. More sensitive to toxic gases than humans, the canary would perish, indicating the miners' need to evacuate the mine and management's need to address the problem (Armstrong, 2002).

In many cases, the unnecessary addition of psychological strain, mixed in with an already complex and stressful society, contributes to adverse health problems for whistle-blowers. Research documents that sleeplessness, anxiety, and depression are among the common symptoms associated with the stresses of whistle-blowing (Erlen, 1999).

Kao (2001) suggests that whistle-blowers should never assume that doing the right thing will keep them from getting fired. Instead, potential whistle-blowers should determine their legal duty for reporting and carefully research the specifics of their protection under the law. In addition, they should try to report anonymously when possible. Moreover, they must be prepared to defend their claims.

In addition, prospective whistle-blowers should always at least try to solve problems internally before going public. When that is impossible and there is a clear indication of serious harm, they must document their actions and go public. They should also seek the support and counsel from colleagues regarding the whistle-blowing intent and process before taking any steps (I See and Am Silent, 1999). Other strategies that whistle-blowers might use to reduce their personal risks are shown in Box 15.3.

Bitoun Blecher (n.d, para 1) suggests that "reporting incidents of wrongdoing in the workplace is always a risky business—but for minority nurses who blow the whistle, the stakes are even higher." Winifred "Windy" Carson, JD, nurse practice counsel for the ANA concurs, stating that minority nurses are more apt to be retaliated against, especially if they are working in nonminority settings (Bitoun Blecher, n.d., para 7).

It is clear, then, that whistle-blowers often face both social and work-related retaliation, and that at times this retaliation can be severe and life altering. Yet it must be noted that at least some self-satisfaction and pride must come with the recognition that unethical behavior has been exposed and that at least the potential for correction is possible because of the whistle-blower's actions. Box 15.4 lists some of the pros and cons of whistle-blowing.

BOX 15.3

Guidelines for Blowing the Whistle

- Know your legal rights because laws protecting whistle-blowers vary from state to state.
- First, make sure there really is a problem. Check resources such as the medical library, the Internet, and institutional policy manuals to be sure.
- Seek validation from colleagues that there is a problem, but don't get swayed by groupthink into not doing anything.
- Do follow the chain of command in reporting your concerns.
- Confront those accused of the wrongdoing as a group whenever possible.
- Present just the evidence; leave the interpretation of facts to others.
- Use internal mechanisms within your organization.
- If internal mechanisms don't work, use external mechanisms.
- Document carefully the problem you have seen and the steps you have taken to see that it is addressed.

Sources: Bitoun Blecher (n.d.); Klein (2001).

◗ ETHICAL DIMENSIONS OF WHISTLE-BLOWING

Hook (2001, para 4) suggests that "although the average patient's immediate response to whistle-blowing would probably be a resounding "hurrah!" for nurses, whistle-blowing can create considerable moral distress for nurses as they weigh the consequences of their actions against the duties of their profession." Clearly, nurses have professional commitments not only to the well being of clients, but also to their employer and to other health care professionals. All too often, these commitments to *principle* and *duty* conflict, and

BOX 15.4

Pros and Cons of Whistle-blowing

Pros

- Promotes change
- Improves quality of care
- Affirms self-content and moral/ethical principles
- Satisfies ethical duty
- Boosts credibility
- Offers opportunity to eradicate wrongdoings
- Reinforces trust in legal system
- Gains support from others

Cons

- Poses personal and professional risks
- Puts whistle-blower in line for scapegoating and personal/professional isolation
- Casts doubt on motives
- Presents chance for possible loss of employment
- Drains emotional/physical/psychological resources
- May promote sleeplessness

Source: Kao, 2001.

the loyalties of the nurse are divided (I See and Am Silent, 1999). This conflict is demonstrated in the following two quotes:

> As citizens, nurses are bound by the moral and legal norms shared by other participants in society and as individuals, they have a right to choose to live by their own values as long as those values do not compromise the care of their clients. By accepting employment, nurses assume certain obligations to their employer and to their colleagues. Violation of these obligations is viewed as being disloyal (I See and Am Silent, 1999, Para 17).
>
> Recent labor arbitration notes the importance of loyalty, making nurses' duties quite ambiguous: . . . arbitrators have held that public servants and indeed all employees violate their duty of loyalty if they engage in public criticism that is detrimental to their employer's legitimate business interests (Brown & Beatty, 1994, p. 7).

This divided loyalty was also apparent in research conducted by Ahern and McDonald (2002), which compared belief systems of whistle-blowers with those of non-whistle-blowers. Participants who reported misconduct (whistle-blowers) supported the belief that nurses were primarily responsible to the patient and should protect a patient from incompetent or unethical people. Participants who did not report misconduct (non-whistle-blowers) supported the belief that nurses are obligated to follow a physician's order at all times and that nurses are equally responsible to the patient, the physician, and the employer. This research study is discussed further in Box 15.5.

Wilmot (2000) suggests that the ethics of this divided loyalty can be viewed in relation to its moral purpose, whether that is to achieve a good outcome (a consequentialist view) or fulfill a duty (a deontological view). If we see whistle-blowing as aimed at changing a situation for the better, we are operating implicitly within a consequentialist moral framework. If we see our whistle-blowing action as the fulfillment of a duty to keep promises, tell the truth, and protect patients, then we are more likely to be operating within a deontological framework.

Unfortunately, the *consequentialist* perspective is unable, on its own, to resolve problems arising from the balance of good and harm resulting from the act of whistle-blowing (where considerable harm might be caused) or of responsibility for that harm. A deontological approach provides an analysis of these problems but raises its own problem of conflicting duties for nurses (Wilmot, 2000).

*CONSIDER: Dwyer (1994) concluded that "doubts about the effectiveness of speaking up should not occasion a retreat into silence but a search for the most effective way of voicing one's concern" (p. 17).

Wilmot suggests, however, that a strong argument can be made for the precedence of the nurse's duty to the patient over his or her duty to the employer. Although nurses have made either implicit or explicit promises to both their patients and their employer, the promise to a person (the patient) must take precedence over the promise to the organization. It can even be argued that duty to the employer may in fact justify whistle-blowing by nurses in some circumstances. Wilmot also questions the morality of being duty-bound to an organization that is no longer carrying out its intended goals and objectives of providing safe patient care.

Wilmot (2000) and Frais (2001) do suggest, however, that the utilitarian viewpoint must at least be considered when whistle-blowing is involved, because there may be

BOX 15.5

Research Study Fuels the Controversy

Whistle-blowers' Role as Patient Advocate

This descriptive study used a survey research design to examine the beliefs of nurses in Western Australia who reported misconduct (whistle-blowers) and the beliefs of nurses who did not (nonwhistle-blowers). For purposes of this study, a whistle-blower was defined as "a nurse who identifies an incompetent, unethical, or illegal situation in the workplace and reports it to someone who may have the power to stop the wrong." A nonwhistle-blower was defined as "a nurse who identifies an incompetent, unethical, or illegal situation in the workplace, but does not openly report it."

The research instrument listed statements from current ethical codes, statements from traditional views on nursing and statements of beliefs related to the participant's whistle-blowing experience. Respondents were asked to rate each item on a five-point Likert format that ranged from strongly agree to strongly disagree. Data were analyzed using Pearson's correlation matrix and one-way ANOVA. To further explore the data, a factor analysis was run with varimax rotation.

Ahern, K., & McDonald, S. (May 2002). The beliefs of nurses who were involved in a whistle-blowing event. *Journal of Advanced Nursing, 38*(3), 303–309.

Study Findings

Results indicated that whistle-blowers supported the beliefs inherent in patient advocacy, whereas nonwhistle-blowers retained a belief in the traditional role of nursing. Participants who reported misconduct (whistle-blowers) supported the belief that nurses were primarily responsible to the patient and should protect a patient from incompetent or unethical people. Participants who did not report misconduct (nonwhistle-blowers) supported the belief that nurses are obligated to follow a physician's order at all times and that nurses are equally responsible to the patient, the physician, and the employer.

situations where the harm caused by whistle-blowing is greater than the harm caused by the employer's actions. For example, organizational disruption affecting staffing and patient services might result in greater harm than the original abuses or shortcomings of care. In this case, by a utilitarian argument, whistle-blowing would not be justified.

Discussion Point

Can you think of a situation you have been involved in, in which utilitarianism would support not blowing the whistle on unethical behavior?

WHISTLE-BLOWING AS A FAILURE OF ORGANIZATIONAL ETHICS

Fletcher et al. (1998) present a convincing argument that whistle-blowing is indicative of an ethical failure at the organizational level and that neither the codes of professional nursing associations nor the standards of the Joint Commission on the Accreditation of Healthcare Organizations (JCAHO) provide, in their current forms, mechanisms to overcome the need for whistle-blowing. Fletcher and colleagues state that whistle-blowing would not occur in an ethical organization because internal procedures would be in place to respond to staff concerns.

Klein (2001) concurs, arguing that if an organization needs whistle-blowing, its employees may be morally desensitized. If so, the whistle-blower will need to develop potential allies by providing them with information or by encouraging discussion of problems.

*CONSIDER: The motive of most whistle-blowers is advocacy, not troublemaking.

In addition, steps must be taken to support nurses who act as patient advocates (Ahern & McDonald, 2002). For example, nursing departments within hospitals could provide their nurses with an ethics committee, chaired by a nurse with experience in bioethical issues (not one who has a vested interest in promoting administrative or hierarchical constraints). Nurse managers could reward nurses who uphold the values inherent in patient advocacy, and finally, nursing boards could offer guidance and commendation to nurses who blow the whistle on misconduct (Ahern & McDonald).

The reality is that if an employee is willing to go to the trouble and risk the repercussions of blowing the whistle, those concerns should be taken seriously and investigated. In fact, a University of Massachusetts study investigating validity of employee whistle-blowing complaints concluded that 76% of the employee complaints were true (Figg, 2000).

▶ LEGAL PROTECTION FOR WHISTLE-BLOWERS

At present, there is no universal legal protection for whistle-blowers; the whistle-blower protection that does exist in the U.S. varies from state to state. As of December 2002, only 13 states (Box 15.6) had passed some type of whistle-blower legislation, although a number of other states have since at least introduced such legislation (ANA, 2002). The problem is that although some of these state laws prohibit retaliation, the standards for proving retaliation vary.

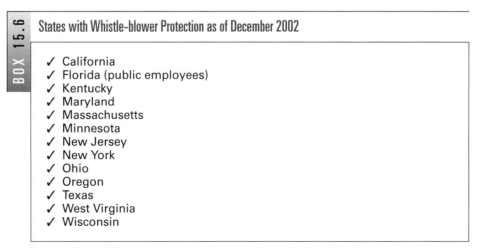

BOX 15.6	States with Whistle-blower Protection as of December 2002

✓ California
✓ Florida (public employees)
✓ Kentucky
✓ Maryland
✓ Massachusetts
✓ Minnesota
✓ New Jersey
✓ New York
✓ Ohio
✓ Oregon
✓ Texas
✓ West Virginia
✓ Wisconsin

Source: ANA (2002).

For example, in Massachusetts, "if an employee reports legitimate violations of policy or patient care standards, state law requires the employer to correct the violations and prohibits them from taking retaliatory action against the whistle-blower, including discharge, suspension, demotion, or denial of promotion. If these actions occur, the employee can report the employer to the attorney general's office, which may act on the public's behalf to protect the employee" (Bitoun Blecher, n.d., para 53).

Because state laws vary so much regarding whistle-blower protection, Polston (1999) suggests that state nursing associations must be actively engaged in advocating for whistle-blower protection at the state level. For example, the NWC (2002) lists patient abuse as one area with little to no whistle-blower protection. Therefore, it continues to support the passage of a comprehensive national Whistleblower Protection Act modeled on the federal protections currently provided to victims of discrimination based on race, gender, and age. In the meantime, the NWC will continue to support piecemeal legislation designed to address specific gaps in employee protections.

Joseph and Herzfeld (2003a) suggest, however, that employees in most states increase their likelihood of whistle-blower protection under general statutes or common law, if they meet criteria similar to those established at the federal level: 1) they must be acting in good faith that the employer or its employees are breaking the law in some way, 2) they must either complain about that violation to the employer or an outside agency, 3), they must refuse to be a party to the violation, and 4) they should be willing to assist in any official investigations of the violation.

Discussion Point

What whistle-blowing protections, if any, exist in the state where you live? Is any legislation pending?

The False Claims Act

Some whistle-blower legislation has been enacted at the federal level, however, to encourage people to report wrongdoings. One such piece of legislation is the *False Claims Act* (FCA), which encourages whistle-blowers to come forward regarding fraud committed against the federal government and to file a lawsuit seeking lost monies in the government's name (Sloan & Ventura, 1999). The individual would file a *qui tam* or whistle-blower lawsuit and provide knowledge that a person defrauded the government.

For example, a whistle-blower may have knowledge of a colleague inappropriately billing Medicare or Medicaid. The FCA provides protection for government whistle-blowers, thereby prohibiting employers from punishing employees who report the fraud or assist in the investigation of the fraud. If the whistle-blower is dismissed or discriminated against in any way as a result of the lawsuit, the whistle-blower can file a claim against that employer for unlawful retaliation (Sloan & Ventura, 1999). To have a case brought to trial under federal law, the whistle-blower must first exhaust his or her internal chain of command, and then file a complaint with the Department of Health and Human Services (DHHS). If DHHS decides that the complaint is valid, the government proceeds with litigation against the employer, and the whistle-blower receives a percentage of the damages awarded.

One of the most well-known cases involving the FCA involved four health care professionals who opened a home infusion company, known as Ven-A-Care, in the Florida Keys (Taylor, 2001). The company provided care to terminally ill patients who had acquired immunodeficiency syndrome (AIDS). When a large national chain, National Medical Care (NMC), moved in, they approached Ven-A-Care about becoming a partner. Ven-A-Care refused because they believed NMC was using fraudulent schemes as part of their business practices. As a result, NMC countered by offering allegedly illegal incentives to local physicians to refer their patients to its Key West clinic, and Ven-A-Care was forced out of business as a result (Taylor).

One of Ven-A-Care's owners contacted government regulators in 1991 about NMC's business practices, but no action was taken. In June 1994, Ven-A-Care filed a civil whistle-blower suit against NMC in Miami. The case was later transferred to the U.S. attorney's office in Boston. The end result was that NMC was partly dismantled, sold, and absorbed by German dialysis giant Fresenius. Fresenius paid the U.S. Justice Department $486 million in civil and criminal fines to settle Ven-A-Care's civil whistle-blower lawsuit. At least three top NMC executives pleaded guilty to criminal kickback and conspiracy charges and received prison sentences and fines, and three NMC divisions pleaded guilty to criminal fraud and kickback charges and were excluded from Medicare and Medicaid programs. None of the Key West doctors ever faced charges for their role in the NMC scheme there. Under the federal FCA, Ven-A-Care and its partners were entitled to a $40 million recovery (Taylor, 2001).

A different whistle-blower suit was brought by the four Ven-A-Care partners in 1995, in Miami federal court, against more than 20 pharmaceutical companies (Taylor, 2001). This suit alleged that drug manufacturers manipulated the benchmark price Medicare uses to reimburse doctors for administering a relatively small number of drugs. That standard, known as the *average wholesale price*, is set and reported by the drug manufacturers and bears little resemblance to the average selling price of a drug.

The suit alleged drug companies set an artificially high average wholesale price to encourage doctors who administer medications to patients with cancer, hemophilia, or AIDS to prescribe their drugs. Then physicians were encouraged to bill government health programs at 95% of average wholesale price, guaranteeing a huge built-in profit. Through that practice, called "marketing the spread," physicians stood to gain hundreds of dollars in profits per dose just for administering a drug, while the drug companies gained a captive market share and fat profits (Taylor, 2001).

Again, the end result was a $14 million settlement in January with New Haven, Connecticut-based drug giant Bayer Corporation. The suit rocked the pharmaceutical industry and further stirred public outrage in Congress and among consumer groups about high prescription-drug prices and illegal marketing practices. It is the first of an expected 20 settlements, and it took more than 5 years from the time the suit was filed until the first drug company settled (Taylor, 2001).

Because the FCA has been so effective in detecting fraud at the federal level, state versions of the FCA have also passed (National Whistleblower Center, n.d.). Under these state laws, whistle-blowers can file lawsuits seeking lost monies in the state or local government's name and share in the proceeds.

Other Federal Legislation Directed at Whistle-blowing

Another piece of legislation, the *Whistleblower Protection Act of 1989*, only protects federal employees who disclose government fraud, abuse, and waste, even though the name of the act suggests it covers everyone who speaks out in the public's interest (Sloan & Ventura, 1999). The *National Labor Relations Act* may also protect employees in the private sector from retaliation when employees act as a group to modify working conditions or ask for better wages.

The best protection for nongovernmental employees in the United States at this time, is likely the *Sarbanes-Oxley Act of 2002*. This act, signed into law by President George W. Bush, dramatically redesigned federal regulation of public company corporate governance and reporting obligations and provided some protection for whistle-blowers who report fraud in publicly traded companies to the proper authorities. It is important to note, however, that claims made under the Sarbanes-Oxley Act have only a 90-day statute of limitations (Joseph & Herzfeld, 2003b).

WHISTLE-BLOWING AS AN INTERNATIONAL ISSUE

Perhaps, however, the most far-reaching whistle-blower law in the world, is the United Kingdom's Public Interest Disclosure Act, which passed in July 1998 and was fully implemented by 2001 (Sloan & Ventura, 1999). Under this act, whistle-blower disclosures to employers, regulatory bodies and the media, are protected from retaliation.

Indeed, the *Public Interest Disclosure Act* "provides individuals in the workplace with full protection from victimization when they raise genuine concerns about malpractice" (Yamey, 2000, para 6). This is because whistle-blowers are viewed as witnesses acting in the public interest and not as people who are merely pursuing a personal grievance (Peep & Weep, 2002). In addition, workers do not have to have proof of a wrongdoing; they simply must have a good faith belief, based on reasonable grounds, that a wrongdoing has occurred (Bradbury, 2003).

Bradbury reports that employment tribunal statistics reveal that approximately 1,200 cases have been filed under the act as of 2003. Many of these were settled before the public hearing stage, so the full usefulness of the act is yet to be determined. Yet, a poll of those individuals who filed cases supports the act as effective in protecting workers who raise concerns (Bradbury, 2003).

CONCLUSIONS

Mohr and Horton-Deutsch (2001) suggest that as individuals and as a profession, nurses have a responsibility to uncover, openly discuss, and condemn malfeasance when it occurs, yet admit that there has been a collective silence about these developments. The reality is that whistle-blowing offers no guarantee that the situation will change or the problem will improve, and the literature is replete with horror stories regarding negative consequences endured by whistle-blowers. The whistle-blower cannot even trust that other health care professionals, with similar belief systems about advocacy, will value their efforts, because the public's feelings about whistle-blowers are so mixed. In addition, state laws vary and protections for the nongovernment employee whistle-blower are often limited.

For all these reasons, it takes tremendous courage to come forward as a whistle-blower. It also takes a tremendous sense of what is right and what is wrong as well as a commitment to follow a problem through until an acceptable level of resolution is reached. Whistle-blowers then are heroes, and should be treated as such; their courage is nothing short of exceptional. How unfortunate that we frequently don't treat them that way.

In the final analysis, Stevens stated: "As a community of professionals, we need to support, rather than ostracize, those who have the courage to call attention to unethical practices. This support takes professionals who are willing to risk their own well-being for the well-being of those who are in our care" (Stevens, 2000, p. 178).

FOR ADDITIONAL DISCUSSION

1. Why do Americans have a "love-hate" relationship with whistle-blowers? Is this dichotomy prevalent in other cultures as well?
2. Which is greater for you personally—your duty to your patients, your duty to your employer, or your duty to yourself?
3. Do you believe that most whistle-blowing must be external before appropriate action is taken?
4. Should whistle-blowers receive compensation under the False Claims Act?
5. Would you personally be willing to bear the risks of becoming a whistle-blower?
6. Do you believe there is more, less, or the same amount of whistle-blowing in health care as in other types of industries?
7. Can you identify a whistle-blowing situation where it might be appropriate to go outside the chain of command in reporting concerns about organizational practice?

REFERENCES

Ahern, K. & McDonald, S. (2002). The beliefs of nurses who were involved in a whistleblowing event. *Journal of Advanced Nursing, 38*(3), 303–309.

American Nurses Association. (2001). *Code of ethics for nurses with interpretive statements*. Washington, DC: ANA Publications. Retrieved April 30, 2005, from http://www.nursingworld.org/ethics/code/protected_nwcoe303.htm.

American Nurses Association. (2001). *ANA files amicus brief in support of six nurse whistleblowers*. Retrieved April 30, 2005, from http://www.nursingworld.org/pressrel/2001/pr0619.htm.

American Nurses Association. (2002). *2002 legislation. Whistleblower protection*. Retrieved April 30, 2005, from http://www.nursingworld.org/gova/state/2002/whistle.htm.

Armstrong, F. (2002). Blowing the whistle: The costs of speaking out. *Australian Nursing Journal, 9*(7), 18–21.

BBC News. (2001). *Whistleblower nurse appeals for job back*. Retrieved April 30, 2005, from http://news.bbc.co.uk/1/hi/wales/1256521.stm.

BBC News. (2003). *School nurse sacking upheld*. Retrieved April 30, 2005, from http://news.bbc.co.uk/1/hi/wales/south_west/2983145.stm.

Bitoun Blecher, M. (n.d.). *What color is your whistle*? Minoritynurse.com. Retrieved April 30, 2005, from http://www.minoritynurse.com/features/nurse_emp/05-03-02c.html.

Blunt, S. H. (2001). Whistleblower fired. *Christianity Today, 45*(13), 11.

Bradbury, J. (2003). Whistle while you work. *Nursing Management (UK), 10* (4) 13–15. Retrieved April 30, 2005, from Academic Search Elite.

Brown, D. J. M. & Beatty, D. M. (1994). *Canadian labour arbitration*. Aurora, ON: Canada Law Book.

Brujiins, C. & McDonald, L. (2002). *Encouraging whistle blowing as a crisis prevention strategy*. IFSAM 2002 Conference. Retrieved April 30, 2005, from http://www.ifsam.org/2002/general-management/Brujins_mcdonald%20%28rev%29PUB.htm.

Canadian Nurses Association. (1997). *The code of ethics for registered nurses*. Ottawa: Canadian Nurses Association.

Colvin, G. (2002). Wonder women of whistleblowing. *Fortune, 146*(3). Retrieved April 30, 2005, from Academic Search Elite.

Dwyer, J. (1994). Primum non tacere: An ethics of speaking up. *Hastings Center Report, 24*(1), 13–18.

Erlen, J. (1999). What does it mean to blow the whistle? *Orthopaedic Nursing, 18*(6), 67–70.

Fiesta, J. (1990). Whistleblowers: Heroes or stool pigeons? Part 1. *Nursing Management, 21*(6), 16–17.

Figg, J. (2000). Whistle blowing. *The Internal Auditor, 57*(2), 30–37.

Fletcher, J. J., Sorrell, J. M., & Silva, M. C. (1998). Whistleblowing as a failure of organizational ethics. *Online Journal of Issues in Nursing*. Retrieved April 30, 2005, from http://www.nursingworld.org/ojin/topic8/topic8_3.htm.

Frais, A. (2001). Whistleblowing heroes—boon or burden? *Bulletin of Medical Ethics, 170*, 13–19.

Hook, K. (Fall 2001). Toward an ethical defense of whistleblowing. *The American Nurses Association. Ethics and Human Rights Issues Update, 1*(2). Retrieved April 30, 2005, from http://www.ana.org/ethics/update/vol1no2a.htm.

Hunt, G. (1995). Conclusion: A new accountability? In G. Hunt (Ed.), *Whistleblowing in the health service: Accountability, law and professional practice* (pp. 155–158). London: Edward Arnold.

I see and am silent. I see and speak out: The ethical dilemma of whistleblowing. (1999). *Canadian Nurse, 95*(10), 5–8. Retrieved April 30, 2005, from http://www.cna-nurses.ca/cna/documents/pdf/publications/Ethics_Prac_See_Silent_November_1999_e.pdf

Joseph & Herzfeld, LLP. (2003a). *Whistleblower.* Retrieved April 30, 2005, from http://www.jhllp.com/CM/Articles/Articles28.php.

Joseph & Herzfeld, LLP. (2003b). *Whistleblower claims.* Retrieved April 30, 2005, from http://www.jhllp.com/CM/Custom/Custom6.asp.

Kao, L. (May-June 2001). Student's corner. Nurses and whistleblowing: Is it worth it? *Maryland Nurse, 2*(3), 7–8.

*Klein, J. A. (2001). The ethical dilemma of whistleblowing. Retrieved April 30, 2005, from http://www.nursingnetwork.com/whistle.htm.

Legislation helps nurses "blow the whistle" on patient neglect and abuse. (2001). Retrieved April 30, 2005, from http://www.nursezone.com/Stories/SpotlightOnNurses.asp?articleID=5892.

Mohr, W. K. & Horton-Deutsch, S. (2001). Malfeasance and regaining nursing's moral voice and integrity. *Nursing Ethics, 8*(1),19–35. Retrieved from Academic Search Elite.

National Whistle-blower Center. (n.d.). Preventing fraud on the taxpayers. Retrieved April 30, 2005, from http://www.whistleblowers.org/html/fca.html.

National Whistleblower Center. (2002). Labor Day report 2002. The national status of whistleblower protection on Labor Day 2002. Retrieved April 30, 2005, from http://www.whistleblowers.org/labordayreport.pdf.

Near, J. P. & Miceli, M. P. (1995). Effective whistle-blowing. *Academy of Management Review, 20*(3), 679–708.

Peep and weep. (2002). *Economist, 362,* 55–57.

Peternelj-Taylor, C. (2003). Whistleblowing and boundary violations: Exposing a colleague in the forensic milieu. *Nursing Ethics, 10*(5), 526–537.

Petersen, J. C. & Farrell, D. (1986). *Whistle blowing: Ethical and legal issues in expressing dissent.* Dubuque, IA: Kendall-Hunt.

Polston, M. D. (1999). Whistleblowing: Does the law protect you? *American Journal of Nursing, 99,* 26–31.

Sloan, A. J. & Ventura, M. J. (1999). Whistleblowing: There are risks. *RN, 62*(7), 65–68.

Soeken, K. & Soeken, D. (1987). *A survey of whistleblowers: Their stressors and coping strategies.* Laurel, MD: Association of Mental Health Specialties.

Stevens, P. (2000). The ethics of being ethical. *The Family Journal: Counseling and Therapy for Couples and Families, 8*(2), 177–178.

Taylor, M. (2001). Four found whistleblowing the best revenge. *Modern Healthcare, 31*(24), 32–33.

Vinten, G. (1994). Whistle while you work in the health-related professions? *Journal of the Royal Society for the Promotion of Health, 114*(5), 256–262.

Vinten, G. (2000). Whistle blowing towards disaster prevention and management. *Disaster Prevention and Management, 9* (1), 18–28.

Wilmot, S. (2000). Nurses and whistleblowing: The ethical issues. *Journal of Advanced Nursing, 32*(5), 1051–1057.

Yamey, G. (2000). Editorials. Protecting whistleblowers. *British Medical Journal, 320,* 70–71. Retrieved April 30, 2005, from http://bmj.bmjjournals.com/cgi/content/full/320/7227/70.

BIBLIOGRAPHY

Adeyinka, E. O. (2004). The code of silence. *American Journal of Nursing, 104*(5), 85–86.

Alderman, C. (2001). A question of conduct. *Nursing Standard, 15*(43), 14–15.

Whistleblowing: Caught between a rock and a hard place (2001). *Nursing Times, 97*(49), 24–25.

Crouch, D. (2001). Taking a stand. *Nursing Times, 97*(45), 22–23.

Despain, D., Gropman, J., & Woodcock, S. (2003). Whistleblowing: When it works—and why. *School Library Journal, 49*(6), 177–184.

Fost, N. (2001). Ethical issues in whistleblowing. *Journal of American Medical Association, 286*(9), 1079.

Haddad, A. (2004). Ethics in action: Warning a patient. *RN, 67*(3), 21–22, 24, 74–75.

Howe, E. G. (2000). How should ethics consultants respond when care providers have made or may have made a mistake? Beware of ethical flypaper. In S. B. Rubin & L. Zoloth (Eds.), *Margin of error: The ethics of mistakes in the practice of medicine.* Hagerstown, MD: University Publishing Group.

Hunt, G. (2003). Comment on whistleblowing and boundary violations. *Nursing Ethics: An International Journal for Health Care Professionals, 10*(5), 539–540.

Mason, D. J. (2004). When silence kills: The Cullen case may erode the public's trust in nurses. *American Journal of Nursing, 104*(2), 11.

McDonald, S. J. & Ahern, K. (2000). The professional consequences of whistleblowing by nurses. *Journal of Professional Nursing, 16*(6), 313–321.

McDonald, S. J. & Ahern, K. (2002). Physical and emotional effects of whistleblowing. *Psychosocial Nursing and Mental Health Services, 40*(1), 14–27.

Miller, K. (2003). The road taken. *Revolution: The Journal for RNs and Patient Advocacy, 4*(5), 18–23.

Mulholland, H. (2001). Whistleblowing: Whistle down the wind. *Nursing Times, 97*(31), 12–13.

Whistleblowing: Nurse who "went through hell" tells of her shame (2001). *Nursing Times, 97*(22), 11.

Payne, D. (2000). Whistleblowing: My message: If in doubt, speak out. *Nursing Times, 96,* (25), 9.

Rhodes, R. & Strain, J. J. (2004). Whistleblowing in academic medicine. *Journal of Medical Ethics, 30*(1), 35–40.

Richardson, B. (2003). Why you should implement a whistleblowing policy. *Nursing & Residential Care, 5*(5), 244–246.

Rohland, P. (2002). Code language: What student nurses are taught about whistleblowing. *Revolution: The.*
Journal for RNs and Patient Advocacy, 3(6), 26–29.
Ryan, C. (2000). Whistleblowing: Seen but not heard. *Nursing Times, 96*(47), 11.
Scottish nurses afraid to speak out. (2004). *Nursing Standard, 18*(26), 9.
Sloan, A. J. (2002). Whistleblowing: Proceed with caution. *RN, 65*(1), 67–68, 70, 80–81.
Trusts must make whistleblowing easier for staff. (2003). *Nursing Standard, 17*(47), 8.
Whyburn, B. (2004). Protected disclosure. *Lamp, 1*, 22–23.

*URL no longer active.

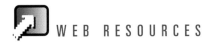

WEB RESOURCES

Blecher, M. B. What color is your whistle? Minoritynurse.com

http://www.minoritynurse.com/features/nurse_emp/05-03-02c.html

Brownsey, D. (March 2001). Nurses and their right to whistle blow. AORN

http://www.aorn.org/JOURNAL/2001/marhpi.htm

Fletcher, J. J., Sorrell, J. M., & Silva, M. C. (December 31, 1998). Whistleblowing as a failure of organizational ethics. *Online Journal of Issues in Nursing*

http://www.nursingworld.org/ojin/topic8/topic8_3.htm

Hook, K. (Fall 2001). Toward an ethical defense of whistle blowing. *The American Nurses Association Ethics and Human Rights Update, 1*(2)

http://www.ana.org/ethics/update/vol1no2a.htm#whistle

National Whistleblower Center

http://www.whistleblowers.org

Protection for Private Sector Employee Whistleblowers

http://www.whistleblowers.org/private.htm

Quyen-Nguyen, B. (July 2001). Workplace rights. Blowing the whistle. *American Journal of Nursing, 101*(7)

http://www.ana.org/AJN/2001/jul/Wrights.htm

Whistleblowers Australia

www.whistleblowers.org.au

The Chemically Impaired Nurse: Discipline or Treatment?

16

Jennifer Lillibridge

"So I don't think there's due consideration given to the grief, and I suppose there's trauma involved in the job. You know, shocking things that you see. It's like you are a nurse, you cope, full stop, that's what you do. It's true we do cope but I think the price you pay is in ways like this. . . . there's always the risk of getting caught and the more desperate you get the more risk there is . . . I sort of knew in the end if I didn't do something soon that I would get caught and then there would really be a lot of trouble" (Lillibridge, Cox, & Cross, 2002, p. 223–224).

The problem of impaired nursing practice is one that has plagued nursing for decades; however, it remains both poorly researched and poorly understood. One explanation for this lack of research may be that nurses find it difficult to talk openly about a situation in which "one of their own" may be engaging in behavior that puts themselves and their patients at risk. The American Nurses Association (ANA) defines an impaired nurse as "one who has impaired functioning which results from alcohol or drug misuse and which interferes with professional judgment and the delivery of safe, high quality care" (ANA, 1984, p. 18).

A discussion about impaired nursing practice often raises more questions than it answers. Two key issues surround impaired nursing practice. The first is concern for the health of the impaired nurse. With denial common, the problem can go without detection or treatment for years. The second is concern for patient safety. When nurses divert drugs for personal use and make poor judgments, the risk for harm to patients is high (Ellis & Hartley, 2004). In addition, questions are also raised about what constitutes impaired practice and how to proceed when impaired practice is suspected. Can confidentiality be maintained to avoid loss of the nurse's license? What are the legal ramifications of reporting an impaired colleague? What happens to the nurse who is able to complete rehabilitation and return to work? Probably the most significant question to be answered is, how can the problem be prevented in the first place? All of these questions highlight the complexity of the problem and the lack of consistent solutions.

▶ PREVALENCE OF THE PROBLEM

Early documentation of chemical dependency in nursing can be found in nursing literature in the 1960s (Garb, 1965; Poplar, 1969). Until the 1980s, impaired nurses were discussed in the literature mainly through testimonial or anecdotal articles. In 1981, when Bissell and Jones published a study about alcoholic nurses, they found there was "little or no reliable data as to the incidence of alcoholism and other drug dependencies within the nursing profession" (1981, p. 96). Their explanation involved speculation that nurses feared both legal and workplace consequences if they admitted their dependency and sought help. The stigma attached to being a nurse with a substance abuse problem 25 years ago encouraged nurses to deny their problem and conceal it from others. Although more options exist today, nurses continue to be influenced by the stigma associated with chemical dependency and the fear of losing their license and their job.

Estimates on the prevalence of substance misuse in the nursing profession are varied; efforts to quantify the prevalence are fraught with problems. It has been suggested that the difficulty in part may be due to the sensitive nature of the information and that "guilt and shame reduce self-disclosure" (Smardon, 1998, para 15). In 1984, the ANA estimated that 6% to 8% of nurses had a problem with alcohol or drugs (ANA, 1984). Trinkoff, Eaton, and Anthony (1991) found that nurses reported substance abuse behaviors less often than or in the same amount as their non-nurse counterparts. This finding was later supported by Blazer and Mansfield (1995) and Trinkoff and Storr (1994). The most recent prevalence study found was published by Trinkoff, Zhou, and Storr (1999) using capture–recapture methods and yielding an estimate that 6.4% of nurses reported a history of substance use problems. Although there is inconsistency in the reporting of substance use problems in the nursing profession, there has been no solid evidence to refute the 1984 ANA estimate of 6% to 8%, which is similar to what one would expect from the general population.

We might ask then, why so much concern? Nurses aren't engaging in these harmful behaviors any more frequently, for example, than lawyers, teachers, or the person next door. Does this increased concern occur because nurses are trusted with providing intimate and often life-saving care to the public? Even one impaired nurse may be the one who takes care of your child or your mother. In recent years nurses have been ranked first and second in Gallup polls for the most trusted and ethical professionals, and other polls have found 84% to 95% of Americans trust, admire, and respect nurses (Domrose, 2002). Is our concern that these nurses have violated that trust, that we actually care about their recovery, or that we are ashamed or embarrassed by our impaired colleagues? Whatever the reason, it is important to explore the nature of substance use problems so that we can find solutions and bring our recovered, impaired colleagues back into the profession.

*CONSIDER: If 6% to 8% of nurses have a substance use problem, every nurse likely will work with chemically impaired colleagues at some time during his/her nursing career.

▶ OVERVIEW OF THE LITERATURE

Literature on the topic of chemical impairment in nursing falls into several subtopics or themes:

- ▶ Prevalence and risk factors of substance misuse among nurses (empirically based research is scarce)
- ▶ Characteristics and experiences of nurses with a substance use problem
- ▶ Nurses' attitudes toward impaired colleagues
- ▶ Different treatment options: discipline versus rehabilitation/diversion
- ▶ Recovery and entry into practice: what are the options? How, when, and with what, if any, license or other restrictions?

One of the problems in reviewing current literature is that there is limited recent published information about substance misuse among nurses. Since 2000, scant research studies have been published; instead, articles focus on discussion that recognizes that there is a problem or on testimonials. With limited recent empirically based research available, there is little to help the profession move closer toward management and resolution of the problem, if indeed resolution is even possible.

Risk Factors for Substance Abuse

Risk factors leading to substance abuse have been identified and explored from various perspectives. Some commonly held beliefs are that health care professionals are at greater risk due to job strain/stress, easy access to mood-altering and narcotic drugs (Ellis & Hartley, 2004; Storr, Trinkoff, & Anthony, 1999; Trinkoff, Zhou, & Storr, 1999; Trinkoff, Zhou, Storr, & Soeken, 2000), and work schedule difficulties that often lead to high levels of fatigue (Trinkoff & Storr, 1994, 1998b), which make nurses vulnerable to self-medication. Some nursing specialties (emergency, oncology, mental health, and administration) have also been noted as being at increased risk of substance misuse, especially alcohol and illicit drugs such as marijuana and cocaine (Storr, Trinkoff, & Hughes, 2000).

West (2002) compared substance-impaired and nonimpaired nurses in order to study early risk indicators of substance abuse among nurses. Findings included that nurses who abuse substances may share common characteristics, but differences are manifested in "development, progression, and severity" (p. 192). West suggested that these differences help to explain each nurse's distinctive pathway to addiction. These findings suggest that treatment options focus on the whole person, not just substance abusing behaviors, as well as how the person interacts with the environment.

The very nature of the work of nurses seems to be challenged when risk factors are considered. Nurses have constant access to narcotics, and fatigue seems to come with the job, no matter what shift is worked. It is difficult to avoid job strain in the current health care environment, which is in the middle of the worst nursing shortage ever reported. Despite the difficulties inherent in the practice setting today, many nurses do work hard to get experience and increase knowledge so they can become specialists, only to find this, too, can put them at higher risk of turning to drugs or alcohol when coping is difficult. These issues highlight the complexity of the problem for the profession, requiring that all nurses become more aware of how to prevent it from occurring.

Discussion Point

Due to long work hours, overtime (often mandatory), and job strain, is the nursing shortage contributing to the prevalence of nurses who misuse substances?

Characteristics and Experiences of Nurses Who Misuse Substances

Many studies outlining or discussing characteristics of nurses who misuse substances are dated and suffer from methodological weaknesses. Smardon (1998) summarized the literature on substance abuse among nurses from 1981 to 1997. She cites several characteristics frequently described in research studies. One common finding was that nurses who abuse substances are often diagnosed with mental health problems rather than substance abuse problems. Valentine (cited in Smardon, 1998) found that nurses with substance abuse problems often are also diagnosed with depression, anxiety, work stress, and family problems. Women are often treated, and sometimes overtreated, with prescription medications for sleep disturbance problems, anxiety, and depression. Anecdotal evidence suggests that nurses' problems with substances often start from legitimate treatment, such as pain medication for a back injury or sedatives for sleep (Danis, n.d.).

Trinkoff and colleagues have also conducted multiple studies about nurses and substance abuse from a variety of perspectives and over an extended time (Storr et al., 1999; Trinkoff et al., 1991, 2000; Trinkoff & Storr, 1994; Trinkoff & Storr, 1998a, 1998b;

BOX 16.1

Research Study Fuels the Controversy

Nurses in Recovery

This Australian study explored substance misuse from the perspectives of nurses who had identified themselves to researchers as having a history of substance abuse. At the time of the study all but one of the 11 participants was in recovery.

> Lillibridge, J., Cox, M., & Cross, W. (2002). Uncovering the secret: Giving voice to the experiences of nurses who misuse substances. *Journal of Advanced Nursing, 39*(3), 219–229.

Study Findings

Five themes were reported. Nurses defended their substance use as being necessary to deal with work stress. Job complexity, lack of resources, and the often traumatic nature of nursing contributed to nurses' justification for using substances. Nurses reported easy access enabled them to take drugs from the workplace. All nurses identified a fear of being discovered and the stigma that would be linked to them if they were found out. This negatively affected their desire to seek help. These nurses identified a personal meaning about using substances, such as needing substances to feel good about themselves or to deal with the high expectations they felt were placed upon them by the profession, by society, and by themselves. Nurses felt let down by peers in that they believed other nurses ignored their inappropriate behavior and took no action to help them. They saw this as a lack of nurses caring for their own members in the same way they care for others. All nurses identified a turning point that put them on the trajectory toward recovery. Nurses identified that treatment programs often did not address their unique needs as nurses, and they questioned whether confidentiality would be maintained.

This study highlights the complexity of this issue from the perspectives of nurses who have experienced substance abuse first hand and then recovered from it.

Trinkoff, Storr, & Wall, 1999; Trinkoff, Zhou, & Storr, 1999). However, these studies fail to address the characteristics of nurses who misuse substances or present findings about how these nurses perceive themselves. Only one recent qualitative study was found that approached substance misuse from the perspectives of the nurses who had the problem (Box 16.1) (Lillibridge et al., 2002).

Research that explores the perspectives of nurses who abuse substances will add to the body of knowledge because more information will be obtained about both how nurses who abuse substances view personal risk factors and which environmental issues make it easy or more difficult to obtain substances from the workplace. If the profession is serious about helping nurses avoid substances, as well as helping them once they become impaired so that they can recover and return to work, then it is imperative that we listen to what these nurses have to say.

Discussion Point

Why hasn't more qualitative research been conducted that explores the experiences and perspectives of nurses who misuse substances?

Nurses' Attitudes About Impaired Colleagues

Often, the attitudes of nurses who misuse substances are obtained anecdotally rather than from research reports. Two recent articles highlight the uniquely personal aspect of the experience. Both are anecdotal, with one being a testimonial of an impaired nurse and her colleague. The anguish felt by both is evident. One article tells the story of the discovery of a friend and colleague misusing medications, of missing narcotics, and of confrontation and denial that finally led to the nurse being fired (DeVries, 2004). The second story is told by a nurse who writes of rejecting a nurse in recovery on her return to work, only to find herself in that impaired nurse's position years later. She states "I wished I knew why we, as nurses, couldn't make a team effort to support one another in the face of substance abuse" (Taylor, 2003, p. 10). Unfortunately this attitude is echoed all too often. Lillibridge et al. (2002) found similar attitudes regarding impaired practice in that nurses with substance use problems were often ignored or rejected by colleagues despite obvious impairment. Firing following discovery was frequently the response to the substance misuse problem.

> *CONSIDER: Nurses are praised and looked up to by clients, society, and other nurses. Yet, a nurse with a substance abuse problem does not seem to receive that same caring attitude from his or her peers.

A common experience both for the impaired nurse and for colleagues is denial of the problem. Smith and Hughes (1996) and Smith, Taylor, and Hughes (1998) suggest that coworkers are often confused by the impaired nurse's actions and often respond initially with enabling behaviors, such as "making excuses, covering up, or attempting to help solve the chemically dependent's problems" (pp. 106–107). However, without intervention or treatment, enabling behaviors may help to escalate the problem, leaving coworkers feeling powerless and discouraged.

319

Discussion Point

You suspect a coworker/friend is diverting drugs for personal use. You find yourself covering up for her because you know she is depressed, exhausted, and having family problems. Your supervisor makes a casual comment with similar suspicions. Your first instinct is to make excuses for your friend; what would you do?

Discipline Versus Treatment

It is the responsibility of every nurse to be aware of reporting requirements when a nurse is suspected of chemical dependency or of diverting drugs for personal use. No uniform agreement exists among the states as to what those reporting requirements are. Information regarding reporting requirements can be found from each state board of nursing, which often can be easily accessed via their website. Before a nurse can be reported

Signs and Behavioral Changes Suggesting Chemical Impairment

Common Signs of Impairment

- Worker appears to be a "workaholic," arriving early, staying late, offering to work extra shifts, and offering to cover for breaks.
- Often works in areas that have a high volume of commonly abused drugs; examples include oncology department, the emergency department, and the operating room.
- Volunteers to care for patients with diminished awareness.
- High reports from patients that pain medication is ineffective; narcotic count errors are common.
- Peers complain about the quality and quantity of the nurse's work.

Behavioral Changes

- Increased irritability with patients and colleagues, often followed by extreme calm.
- Social isolation; eats alone and avoids unit social functions.
- Extreme and rapid mood swings.
- Unusually strong interest in narcotics or the narcotic cabinet.
- Sudden dramatic change in personal grooming or any other personal habits.
- Extreme defensiveness regarding medication errors.

Source: Compiled from Marquis, B. L., & Huston, C. J. (2006). *Leadership roles and management functions in nursing: Theory & application* (5th ed.). Philadelphia: Lippincott Williams & Wilkins; and Ponech, S. (2000). Telltale signs: Clues to employee substance abuse. *Nursing Management, 31*(5), 32–38. Retrieved May 1, 2005, from *http://www.nursing management.com.*

or referred to a treatment program, there must be recognition that the nurse needs help. Recognizing the impaired nurse may not be easy. Some common signs or behavior changes of a chemically impaired nurse are shown in Box 16.2.

The disciplinary approach was the norm in most states through the 1980s. Following the ANA resolution in 1982 to support treatment of chemically dependent nurses, many states began to look at treatment and rehabilitation options instead of discipline. Back in 1992, only 13 state boards of nursing offered treatment as an alternative to disciplinary action (Sloan & Vernarec, 2001). As of 2002, more than 37 states offered treatment and nondisciplinary programs (Blair, 2002).

Ideally, completion of a rehabilitation program prevents revocation of the nurse's license (Blair, 2002). According to Blair, controversy still exists as to whether to treat or punish nurses who have a chemical dependency. One argument on the treatment side is that nondisciplinary options will encourage a higher rate of reporting and self-reporting of chemically dependent nurses.

Arguments on the punishment side may originate as a result of general moralistic views about all substance abuse. Church (2000) suggested that people who view substance abuse from a moralistic perspective will hold that individual accountable for both the problem and the solution. This attitude does not support the impaired nurse getting treatment because addiction is viewed as "willful misconduct as opposed to a disease" (para 5). Similarly, Beckstead (2002) studied the attitudinal antecedents of nurses' decisions to report an impaired colleague. Beckstead reported "the moralistic attitude toward substance use was found related to punitive attitude toward impaired nurses" (p. 548).

*CONSIDER: Some addiction specialists view drug dependence as a chronic medical illness and argue that it should be treated in the same way as diabetes or asthma.

State Diversion Programs

Although most states now offer treatment options, the types of programs vary. Some programs are completely voluntary, which means there is no threat of being reported to disciplinary authorities. Many programs, however, represent a more coercive process; that is, discipline is not implemented as long as the impaired nurse participates in the treatment program. This often requires a 2- to 5-year commitment with rigorous standards (Blair, 2002). The first treatment program offered was the Intervention Project for Nurses (IPN) in Florida in 1983. The IPN currently has a comprehensive website, offering information about the history of IPN, including frequently asked questions and available services (*http://www.ipnfl.org/faq.html*).

California offers a diversion program; information about the program can be retrieved from the California Board of Registered Nursing (California BRN) website (*http://www.rn.ca.gov/div/whatisdiv.htm*). Established in 1985, its goal is to "protect the public by early identification of impaired registered nurses and by providing these nurses access to appropriate intervention programs and treatment services" (CBRN, 2001, para 2). Impaired nurses can be self-referred or can be referred by family, coworkers, or the board. All licensed registered nurses residing in California are eligible to enter the program, but they must agree to enter the program voluntarily. Since 1985, over 800 nurses have successfully completed the diversion program in California. Requirements for completion include "a change in lifestyle that supports continuing recovery and have a minimum of 24 consecutive months of clean, random, body-fluid tests" (para 14). Confidentiality of participants is protected by law, and nurses who successfully complete the program have their records regarding chemical impairment destroyed.

A different approach is seen in the Texas Peer Assistance Program for Nurses. This program offers services to nurses suffering from chemical dependency as well as anxiety and other mental health disorders. It requires abstinence, maintains confidentiality, is strictly voluntary, and is independent of the state licensing board (Texas Nurses Association (TNA), 2004). Information from the TNA website includes how and when to make referrals, how the program works, and important links to services and organizations (*http://www.texasnurses.org/tpapn/index.htm*).

Although it initially offered a voluntary peer assistance program, Michigan has moved away from this approach and now encourages health professionals with chemical dependency problems to be admitted into the health professional recovery program (HPRP). To use this service, nurses must be willing to "acknowledge their impairment, agree to participate in a recovery plan that meets the criteria developed by the HPRP, and voluntarily withdraw from or limit the scope of their practice as determined necessary under the criteria established by the committee" (Fletcher, 2004, p. 92). The benefit of this program, as with the Texas approach, is that treatment reports are confidential and independent of the state licensing board.

*CONSIDER: Although most states lean toward treatment rather than discipline for chemical dependency, many nurses think impaired nurses should be punished and not allowed to return to work.

Haack and Yocom (2002) recently investigated two different approaches to treating nurses with substance use disorders. One group had traditional disciplinary action taken against their license whereas the other group received treatment. They found that the "alternative sample (treatment) had more nurses with active licenses, fewer with criminal convictions, and more nurses employed in nursing" (p. 89). There were no differences between the treatment and discipline groups in terms of relapse. The authors concluded that treatment offers a more humane process and overall is more rehabilitative.

> ***CONSIDER:** Disciplinary policies are based on deterrence and punishment. This prevents nurses from employment, health insurance, and the financial means to help them recover (Haack & Yocom, 2002).

The National Council of State Boards of Nursing (NCSBN) is currently undertaking a study of chemically impaired nurses that will "discover the elements of traditional disciplinary action and alternative-to-discipline programs that are most effective in protecting the public and in returning rehabilitated nurses to safe practice" (NCSBN, 2004, para 1). It is clear the trend is moving in the direction of peer assistance and treatment options and away from the disciplinary process for the impaired nurse. This potentially increases chances of recovery, which in turn increases the chances of the impaired nurse returning to nursing and becoming a functioning member of the profession again.

The Recovered Nurse: Returning to Work

When a nurse has completed a treatment or rehabilitation program and is ready to return to work he or she encounters a number of issues. These issues include whether the nurse's practice is limited or restricted in some way, how long the nursing board has a right to invade the nurse's privacy to ensure recovery is ongoing, where organizational responsibility ends, who bears the cost if the nurse does not return to work at full capacity, and ensuring that confidentiality is maintained (Box 16.3).

Although many anecdotal or discussion articles were found on the topic of what constitutes a disciplinary or treatment approach to impaired practice, few recent articles could be found that addressed the concerns of re-entry of the impaired nurse to the practice setting. There are, however, some general considerations that should be taken into account when a recovered nurse returns to work.

To protect patient safety, practice restrictions may be in place for a varying time, depending on whether the program is treatment-based or disciplinary. Nurse-managers are key to a successful integration of the recovered nurse back into practice. Problems

---

BOX 16.3

Issues to Consider When the Recovered Nurse Returns to Work

- Should nurses returning to work following rehabilitation have their practice limited or restricted in some way?
- How long does the board of nursing have a right to "invade the privacy" of a recovered nurse?
- Where does the organizational responsibility end?
- Who bears the cost if the recovered nurse is not able to return to work not at full capacity?
- Can confidentiality be maintained?

with nursing staff can be avoided if open and honest communication takes place and if nurses are identified who will be willing to exchange specific work tasks that are part of restricted practice for the recovering nurse (Windle & Wintergill, 1994). This approach also diminishes the cost associated with a nurse who has practice restrictions in place. Windle & Wintergill authors suggest that establishing a trusting relationship between the nurse-manager and the returning nurse is critical to a successful re-entry. Recovering nurses need to be reassured that their records are confidential and that they are kept separate from general personnel records. It is also deemed important that staff nurses realize the commitment of the recovering nurse to re-establish his or her career and continue in the profession.

Most board of registered nursing websites offer little information about the re-entry process. Instead, they focus primarily on what should be done if you suspect an impaired colleague, how to report it, the treatment or disciplinary action once impairment is identified, and the specific aspects of each program. A question that is left unanswered is how long the board follows a recovered nurse in terms of random drug testing. Some hospitals or health care agencies already do random drug testing, so the question of invasion of privacy has in some instances already been dealt with.

Smith and Hughes (1996) suggested a "return to work" contract is useful because it puts in writing the expectations of the nurse. This would be a voluntary agreement between the returning nurse and the nurse-manager. Another suggestion is for the nurse to attend a support group for chemically dependent nurses.

Discussion Point

You just came from a staff meeting where the nurse-manager informed everyone that a recovered nurse would begin working on the unit in a few weeks. Some nurses had the attitude that the nurse not be allowed back to work because he or she could not be trusted. How would you respond to your colleagues?

323

▶ HOW CAN WE STOP LOSING NURSES TO SUBSTANCE ABUSE?

Preventative health care is finally receiving much needed attention in the media and in practice. Insurance companies are increasingly paying for prevention and screening procedures, yet in many areas of health care we still lag behind what would be ideal for preventative practices. The issue of preventing substance abuse is no exception to this situation. How can nurses individually and as a profession help prevent the cycle of nurse addiction from starting?

Some of the risk factors for substance abuse that have been identified are difficult to modify. Nurses will always have easy access to narcotics, will do shift work, and will suffer from fatigue. The ongoing stress that has worked its way into clinical settings due to the nursing shortage seems a long way from dissipating. What, then, can we do to diminish the effects of these factors so that nurses do not turn to substances as an inappropriate coping mechanism?

Perhaps one avenue is to more fully explore the experiences of nurses who do not turn to substances. Although much has been written about self-care to prevent burnout (Marquis & Huston, 2006), no evidence could be found that linked burnout to harmful coping strategies, such as substance abuse. Do nurses who use self-care strategies to prevent burnout also use those same strategies to avoid harmful substance use? Perhaps this information about how nurses cope with difficulties of the workplace when they do not turn to drugs or alcohol will contribute to prevention. Most research focuses on the nurse who abuses drugs, when we could learn a lot about positive coping behaviors from nurses who manage stress without abusing drugs.

Where does the education about substance abuse begin? Student nurses need not only to be made aware of the risks of substance abuse, but also be self-aware about their attitudes and beliefs regarding those who do abuse substances, whether those people are patients or colleagues. Nursing school is an incredibly stressful time for students. Studies reported by Spier, Matthews, Jack, Lever, McHaffie, and Tate (2000) have suggested that nursing students demonstrate an increased use of depressants and narcotics and that many use alcohol on a daily or weekly basis. They also report that recovering nurses often identify that their abuse of drugs began as nursing students. Not only could appropriate education in nursing school help prevent substance abuse from beginning, but it may also allow students to explore their feelings and beliefs about impaired practice. This increased self-awareness may help students have empathy toward impaired nurses and encourage them to take the appropriate steps to assist a nurse in getting help.

Nursing is going through a very tumultuous time. The nursing shortage is never far from the minds of most nurses as they struggle on a daily basis with low staffing levels and a stressed work setting. How this stress is channeled can lead a nurse to have positive or negative coping strategies. What are hospitals doing to acknowledge and diffuse this stress? Are nurses too stressed to seek counsel from each other when they have a particularly bad day? Are nurses debriefing with each other or at home, so they can let go of the often traumatic nature of work and move forward? Nurses and nurse-managers need to answer these questions for their particular work settings to know if they are doing enough for themselves, their colleagues, and their staff.

▶ CONCLUSIONS

Losing one nurse to substance misuse is one nurse too many. We are a profession known for its caring nature toward others, yet often we fail to care for ourselves. The harmful coping strategies that lead to substance abuse can begin even before nursing school. Educating our students may help us to increase awareness about this ever-present problem. If new graduates bring current information to their nursing practice and are self-aware about their attitudes, beliefs, and coping strategies, then perhaps they come armed with more positive strategies to help them when times get tough. Do we teach our students, new graduates, and seasoned nurses to ask for help when they need it, or do we expect them to "do it all"?

Nurses who suspect an impaired colleague need to take action and not engage in enabling behaviors, which have been shown to both be ineffective and further isolate the impaired nurse from colleagues (Lillibridge et al., 2002). If all nurses are aware of the problem of chemical dependency and take the initiative to confront or intervene when they suspect a colleague of impaired practice, we are one step closer to decreasing the incidence of substance abuse in the nursing profession.

Finally, responsibility rests not just with individual nurses, but also with employers to create a positive work environment, to know employees so that confrontation can occur early, to increase awareness about substance abuse so that nurses are not afraid to ask for help, and finally to provide a process that helps nurses to return to work following recovery.

FOR ADDITIONAL DISCUSSION

1. Explore your own attitudes and beliefs about impaired nursing practice. How would you treat a colleague suspected of diverting drugs for personal use?
2. What kind of peer support exists in your work setting? How do staff "debrief" from stressful situations?
3. What do you think is the best approach to deal with impaired practice—treatment or discipline? Did morals play a part in your decision?
4. Should recovered nurses who return to work have a limited practice? If so, for how long, and with what types of limitations?
5. What practices are in place in your work setting that could deter a nurse from diverting drugs for personal use?
6. Have you known a colleague who was caught stealing drugs from work? If so, how was it handled? Did the nurse seek treatment and return to work? Could it have been managed better?
7. You are a nurse-manager for an intensive care unit and have been asked to talk to student nurses about impaired practice. What key points would you make?

REFERENCES

American Nurses Association. (1984). *Addiction and psychological dysfunctions in nursing.* Kansas City: Author.

Beckstead, J. W. (2002). Modeling attitudinal antecedents of nurses' decisions to report impaired colleagues. *Western Journal of Nursing Research, 24*(5), 537–551.

Bissell, L. C. & Jones, R. W. (1981). The alcoholic nurse. *Nursing Outlook, 29*(2), 96–101.

Blair, P. D. (2002). Report impaired practice-stat. *Nursing Management, 33*(1), 24–25, 51.

Blazer, L. K. & Mansfield, P. K. (1995). A comparison of substance use rates among female nurses, clerical workers, and blue-collar workers. *Journal of Advanced Nursing, 21*(2), 305–313.

California Board of Registered Nursing. (2001). *What is the BRN's diversion program?* Retrieved May 1, 2005, from http://www.rn.ca.gov/div/div.htm and http://rn.ca.gov/div/whatisdiv.htm.

Church, O. M. (2000). Substance abuse and addictions: Choosing change in the land of steady habits. *Connecticut Nursing News, 73*(2). Retrieved May 1, 2005, from EBSCO Host database.

Danis, S. J. (n.d.). The impaired nurse. *Nursing Spectrum: Education CE, Self-Study Modules.* Retrieved May 1, 2005, from http://nsweb.nursingspectrum.com/ce/ce153.htm.

DeVries, C. (2004). Deception: Disappearing drugs and a fellow nurse in denial. *American Journal of Nursing, 104*(2), 39.

Domrose, C. (2002). Mending our image. Retrieved May 1, 2005 from http://www.nurseweek.com/news/features/02-06/image_print.html.

Elliott Spier, B., Matthews, J. T., Jack, L., Lever, J., McHaffie, E. J., & Tate, J. (2000). Impaired student performance in the clinical setting: A constructive approach. *Nurse Educator, 25*(1), 38–42.

Ellis, J. R. & Hartley, C. L. (2004). *Nursing in today's world: Trends, issues & management.* (7th ed.) Philadelphia: Lippincott Williams & Wilkins.

Fletcher, C. E. (2004). Experience with peer assistance for impaired nurses in Michigan. *Journal of Nursing Scholarship, 36*(1), 92–93.

Garb, S. (1965). Narcotic addiction in nurses and doctors. *Nursing Outlook, 13*(11), 30–34.

Haack, M. R. & Yocom, C. J. (2002). State policies and nurses with substance use disorders. *Journal of Nursing Scholarship, 34*(1), 89–94.

Lillibridge, J., Cox, M., & Cross, W. (2002). Uncovering the secret: Giving voice to the experiences of nurses who misuse substances. *Journal of Advanced Nursing, 39*(3), 219–229.

Marquis, B. L. & Huston, C. J. (2006). *Leadership roles and management functions in nursing: Theory & application* (5th ed.). Philadelphia: Lippincott Williams & Wilkins.

National Council of State Boards of Nursing. (2004). *Regulatory oversight of chemically dependent nurses study*. Retrieved May 9, 2004 from http://www.ncsbn.org/regulation/researchregulation_ D02365F5ED7549D7B8F70D49BFA890E6.htm.

Ponech, S. (2000). Telltale signs: Clues to employee substance abuse. *Nursing Management, 31*(5), 32–37. Retrieved May 1, 2005 from http://www.nursingmanagement.com.

Poplar, J. F. (1969). Characteristics of nurse addicts. *American Journal of Nursing, 69*(1), 117–119.

Sloan, A. & Vernarec, E. (2001). Impaired nurses: Reclaiming careers. *RN, 64*(2), 58–63.

Smardon, M. (1998). An integrative review of substance abuse among nurses from 1981–1997. *The Online Journal of Knowledge Synthesis for Nursing,* Vol. 5, Document 1. Retrieved May 1, 2005 from http://www.stti.iupui.edu/library/ojksn/articles/050001.pdf.

Smith, L. L. & Hughes, T. L. (1996). Re-entry: When a chemically dependent colleague returns to work. *American Journal of Nursing, 96*(2), 32–37.

Smith, L. L., Taylor, B. B., & Hughes, T. L. (1998). Effective peer responses to impaired nursing practice. *Nursing Clinics of North America, 33*(1), 105–118.

Spier, B. E., Matthews, J. T., Jack, L., Lever, J., McHaffie, E. J., & Tate, J. (2000). Impaired student performance in the clinical setting. *Nurse Educator, 25*(1), 38–42.

Storr, C. L., Trinkoff, A. M., & Anthony, J. C. (1999). Job strain and non-medical drug use. *Drug and Alcohol Dependence, 55,* 45–51.

Storr, C. L., Trinkoff, A. M., & Hughes, P. (2000). Similarities of substance use between medical and nursing specialties. *Substance Use & Misuse, 35*(10), 1443–1469.

Sullivan, E., Bissell, L., & Williams, E. (1988). *Chemical dependency in nursing: The deadly diversion.* Menlo Park: Addison-Wesley.

Taylor, A. (2003). Support for nurses with addictions often lacking among colleagues. *The American Nurse, 35*(5), 10–11.

Texas Nurses Association. (2004). *Texas peer assistance program for nurses*. Retrieved May 1, 2005 from http://www.tpapn.org.

Trinkoff, A. M., Eaton, W. W., & Anthony, J. C. (1991). The prevalence of substance abuse among registered nurses. *Nursing Research, 40*(3), 172–175.

Trinkoff, A. M. & Storr, C. L. (1994). Relationship of specialty and access to substance use among registered nurses: An exploratory analysis. *Drug and Alcohol Dependence, 36,* 215–219.

Trinkoff, A. M. & Storr, C. L. (1998a). Substance use among nurses: Differences between specialties. *American Journal of Public Health, 88*(4), 581–585.

Trinkoff, A. M. & Storr, C. L. (1998b). Work schedule characteristics and substance use in nurses. *American Journal of Industrial Medicine, 34,* 266–271.

Trinkoff, A. M., Storr, C. L., & Wall, M. P. (1999). Prescription-type drug misuse and workplace access among nurses. *Journal of Addictive Diseases, 18*(1), 9–17.

Trinkoff, A. M., Zhou, Q., & Storr, C. L. (1999). Estimation of the prevalence of substance use problems among nurses using capture-recapture methods. *Journal of Drug Issues, 29*(1), 187–199.

Trinkoff, A. M., Zhou, Q., Storr, C. L., & Soeken, K. L. (2000). Workplace access, negative proscriptions, job strain, and substance use in registered nurses. *Nursing Research, 49*(2), 83–90.

West, M. M. (2002). Early risk indicators of substance abuse among nurses. *Journal of Nursing Scholarship, 34*(2), 187–193.

Windle, P. E. & Wintergill, C. L. (1994). The chemically impaired nurse's reentry to practice: The nurse manager's role. *AORN Journal, 59*(6), 1266–1273.

BIBLIOGRAPHY

American Association of Colleges of Nursing. (1998). Policy and guidelines for prevention and management of substance abuse in the nursing education community. Retrieved May 1, 2005 from http://www.aacn.nche.edu/ Publications/positions/subabuse.htm.

Burns, C. M. (1998). A retroductive theoretical model of the pathway to chemical dependency in nurses. *Archives of Psychiatric Nursing, 12*(1), 59–65.

Healy, C. M. & McKay, M. F. (2000). Nursing stress: The effects of coping strategies and job satisfaction in a sample of Australian nurses. *Journal of Advanced Nursing, 31*(3), 681–688.

Hrobak, M. L. (2002). Narcotic use and diversion in nursing. Retrieved May 1, 2005 from http://juns.nursing.arizona.edu/articles/Fall%202002/hrobak.htm.

McCall, S. V. (2001). Chemically dependent health professionals. *Western Journal of Medicine, 174*(1), 50–54.

McLellan, A. T., Lewis, D. C., O'Brien, C. P., & Kleber, H. D. (2000). Drug dependence, a chronic medical illness: Implications for treatment, insurance, and outcomes evaluation. *Journal of the American Medical Association, 284*(13), 1689–1695.

Michael, R. & Jenkins, H. J. (2001). Work-related trauma: The experiences of perioperative nurses. *Collegian, 8*(1), 19–25.

Morrison, C. (2000). Fear of addiction. *American Journal of Nursing, 100*(70), 81.

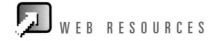

WEB RESOURCES

Addiction Recovery Resources for the Professional   http://www.lapage.com/arr/
California Board of Registered Nurses   http://www.rn.ca.gov/div/div.htm
    Diversion Program
Case Study: The Chemically Impaired Nurse   http://learn.sdstate.edu/vossj/
                                                    Casestudies2002/hatzenbuhler.htm
Intervention Project for Nurses: Florida   http://www.ipnfl.org/faq.html
Kentucky Peer Assistance Program for Nurses, Inc.   http://www.kpapn.org/information.html
National Association of State Alcohol   http://www.nasadad.org
    and Drug Abuse Directors
National Council of State Boards of Nursing   http://www.ncsbn.org
National Institute on Drug Abuse   http://www.nida.nih.gov
Nurses in Recovery   http://brucienne.com/nir/
Nurses Program: Professionals   http://www.clevelandclinic.org/health/
    Helping Professionals   health-info/docs/2000/2008.asp?index=8673
                                                    &src=news
Nursing and Health Care Directories on: http://www.nursefriendly.com/nursing/jobs/
    The Nurse Friendly, Chemical Dependence,   impaired.nurses.chemical.dependence.
    Substance Abuse, Impaired Nurses   substance.abuse.htm
Nursing Spectrum: Education CE Module—   http://nsweb.nursingspectrum.com/ce/
    The Impaired Nurse   ce153.htm
Peer Assistance: American Association   http://www.aana.com/peer/read.asp
    of Nurse Anesthetists

Collective Bargaining and the Professional Nurse

Carol J. Huston

17

* This chapter reproduced in part, with permission, from Marquis, B., & Huston, C. (2006). *Leadership Roles and Management Functions in Nursing* (5th ed). Chapter 22. Understanding Collective Bargaining, Unionization, and Employment Laws. Philadelphia: Lippincott Williams & Wilkins.

T here is likely no greater dichotomy than stereotypical images of nurses dressed in white uniforms and caps, acting as handmaidens to physicians, and angry nurses in picket lines, waving strike placards at passersby. Although both of these images are stereotypical, they are at the heart of the debate about whether nursing, long recognized as a caring and altruistic profession, should be a part of collective bargaining efforts to improve working conditions.

Collective bargaining may be defined as "activities occurring between organized labor and management that concern employee relations. Such activities include negotiation of formal labor agreements and day-to-day interactions between unions and management" (Marquis & Huston, 2006, p. 554). A *labor union* (hereafter referred to as *union*) can be defined as "an organization of employees formed to bargain with the employer" (Hyperdictionary, n.d.).

Many nurses have strong feelings about unions and collective bargaining activities. Often these feelings have to do with their exposure to unions while growing up. Many nurses from working-class families were raised in a cultural milieu that promoted unionization. Other nurses know little about unions and know only what they have seen portrayed in the media. Some nurses, however, have been actively involved in collective bargaining in their place of employment and emerged from the experience with either positive or negative impressions, or a combination thereof.

Despite this tension, collective bargaining and unions are very much a part of many nurses' lived experiences. Although union membership in the private sector is declining, participation in nursing unions is increasing (As Shortages, 2002). Unions once represented approximately one-third of all workers; by 2002, the figure was closer to 13% (Gallagher, 2002). Indeed, Steltzer (2001, p. 35) used the term *exponential* to describe the increased unionization in nursing that occurred in the first 18 months of the 21st century in the Pittsburgh area. Still, fewer than 20% of registered nurses (RNs) belong to collective bargaining units today (Fitzpatrick, 2001).

The issues driving nurses to pursue unionization are "very real and significant" (Fitzpatrick, 2001, p. 41). "Increased nursing workloads and responsibilities and a perception that hospitals aren't responding to nurses' frustration often result in nurses seeing unionization as their only option to gain greater and unified control over their work environments" (Steltzer, 2001, p. 35). Similarly, Bilchik argues that "nurses are now finding a voice through unions..." and, "as a result, are raising the ante in their relationships with health care institutions" (Bilchik, 2000, p. 40).

This chapter will explore the historical development of unions in America, particularly in nursing. The motivations behind nurses' decisions to join or not join unions are explored as are the specific unions that represent the majority of nurses. Union organizing strategies are presented as well as specific steps for starting a union. Emphasis is given to the importance of management creating a work environment that eliminates or reduces the need for unionization in the first place. The chapter concludes with a discussion of the definition of "supervisor" in nursing, types of labor union–management relationships, and whether striking can be viewed as an ethically appropriate action for professional nurses.

HISTORICAL PERSPECTIVE OF UNIONIZATION IN AMERICA

Unions have been present in the United States since the 1790s. "Skilled craftsmen formed early unions to protect themselves from wage cuts during the highly competitive era of industrialization" (Marquis & Huston, 2006, p. 554). "The first American strikes in the late 1700s and early 1800s were by shoemakers, printers, and carpenters led by their trade societies and were generally effective because of the limited labor pool skilled in those trades. The strikers simply refused to work until their pay demands were met. The strikes were generally short, peaceful, and successful" (Labor Unions and Nursing, n.d., para 1).

This changed in the early 1800s with strike activity increasing during economic prosperity and declining during less prosperous economic times. In addition, women began to participate in strikes as early as the 1820s (Labor Unions and Nursing, n.d.). In the mid- to late 1800s, the labor movement began to more closely resemble what we see today. Unions started negotiating with employers, addressing not only wages, but also work rules, hours, and grievances, thus arbitrating contracts between employees and employers (Labor Unions and Nursing, n.d.).

Interestingly, the most important labor organization of the 1800s, the Knights of Labor, discouraged strikes. Craft unions affiliated with the American Federation of Labor (AFL) in the early 1900s also questioned the usefulness of strikes, turning to private mediation groups to help settle disputes (Labor Unions and Nursing, n.d.).

By the 1930s, and after 4 years of the Great Depression, repressive management was the norm and tensions were high between workers and their employers. There were no legal protections for workers, no overtime compensation, no child labor laws, and no health or safety regulations (Forman & Davis, 2002b). Workers attempted to form unions to improve working conditions, but business owners responded by blacklisting organizers and using force to prevent strikes (Franklin D. Roosevelt Presidential Library, n.d.).

President Roosevelt attempted to intervene by establishing the National Industrial Recovery Act but was forced to make an even bolder stand with labor, when the Supreme Cout ruled that act unconstitutional. Instead, Roosevelt enacted the National Labor Relations Act (NLRA), also known as the Wagner Act, in 1935. This act, which was named after New York Senator Robert Wagner, gave workers the right to form unions and bargain collectively with their employers (Box 17.1). It also provided for the creation of the National Labor Relations Board (NLRB) "to oversee union certification, arrange meetings with unions and employers, and investigate violations of the law" (Franklin D. Roosevelt Presidential Library, n.d, para 1).

With this rapid shift in power from management to labor, labor–management relations were turbulent throughout the 1930s and 1940s. "History books are filled with battles, strikes, mass-picketing scenes, and brutal treatment by both management and employees" (Marquis & Huston, 2006, p. 564). The balance of power, however, fell to labor unions.

[***CONSIDER:** The United States has the most violent and bloodiest labor history of any industrialized country (Foner & Garraty, 1991).]

Because of this, it was necessary to pass additional federal legislation to restore a balance of power to management. Passed in 1947, the Taft–Hartley Labor Act, also known as the

BOX 17.1

Unfair Management Practices Identified in the Wagner Act (1935)

1. To interfere with, restrain, or coerce employees in a manner that interferes with their rights as outlined under the act. Examples of these activities are spying on union gatherings, threatening employees with job loss, or threatening to close down a company if the union organizes.
2. To interfere with the formation of any labor organization or to give financial assistance to a labor organization.
3. To discriminate with regard to hiring, tenure, and so on, to discourage union membership.
4. To discharge or discriminate against an employee who filed charges or testified before the NLRB.
5. To refuse to bargain in good faith.

Labor–Management Relations Act, retained the provisions under the Wagner Act that guaranteed employees the right to collective bargaining, but added the provision that employees had the right to refrain from taking part in unions ("closed shops" were illegal) (Box 17.2). In addition, the act permitted the union shop only after a vote of a majority of the employees. It also forbade jurisdictional strikes ("a concerted refusal to work undertaken by a union to assert its members' right to particular job assignments and to protest the assignment of disputed work to members of another union or to unorganized workers" [Wikipedia, n.d.]), secondary boycotts, and forbade unions from contributing to political campaigns.

Discussion Point

The Taft–Hartley Labor Act also required union leaders to affirm they were not supporters of the Communist party. Why was this requirement a part of the act, and how did it mesh with the culture of the time?

BOX 17.2

Unfair Labor Union Practices Identified in the Taft–Hartley Amendment (1947)

1. Requiring a self-employed person or an employer to join a union.
2. Forcing an employer to cease doing business with another person. This placed a ban on secondary boycotts, which were then prevalent in unions.
3. Forcing an employer to bargain with one union when another union has already been certified as the bargaining agent.
4. Forcing the employer to assign certain work to members of one union rather than another.
5. Charging excessive or discriminatory initiation fees.
6. Causing or attempting to cause an employer to pay for unnecessary services.

Eventually, federal legislation such as the Fair Labor Standards Act (1938), the Occupational Safety and Health Act (1970), and the Equal Employment Opportunity Act (1972) were passed, providing federal protection for workers. These acts were important in the history of unions because unions no longer had to be the primary source of security for workers, which reduced "some of their [unions] usefulness" (Forman & Davis, 2002b, p. 376). As a result, there has been little growth of unions in the private and blue-collar sectors since membership peaked in the 1950s. Indeed, an all-time low for union membership was reported in 2003, with unions representing only 12.9% of wage and salary workers and only 8.2% of the private-sector workforce (nonagricultural and nongovernmental) (U.S. Department of Labor, 2004).

To counteract these dwindling numbers, several major unions merged and new affiliations have been formed. In addition, new organizing tactics have been developed and organizers have developed more sophisticated skills (Forman & Grimes, 2004). Nowhere is this turnaround more apparent than in the health care industry, where labor won 61% of the elections in health care in 2002, as compared to 51% in other industries (Bureau of National Affairs, 2003).

▶ HISTORICAL PERSPECTIVE OF UNIONIZATION IN NURSING

Collective bargaining was slow in coming to the health care industry for a number of reasons. "Until labor laws were amended, unionization of health care workers was illegal. In addition, nursing's long history as a service commodity further delayed labor organization in health care settings" (Marquis & Huston, 2006, p. 555).

Discussion Point

Is it appropriate for nurses to organize into collective bargaining units, something historically reserved for blue-collar workers?

Initial collective bargaining in nursing took place in government of public organizations as a result of Kennedy Executive Order 10988. This 1962 order lifted restrictions that prevented public employees from organizing. As a result, city, county, and district hospitals and health care agencies joined collective bargaining in the 1960s.

"In 1974, Congress amended the Wagner Act, extending national labor laws to private nonprofit hospitals, nursing homes, health clinics, health maintenance organizations, and other health care institutions. These amendments opened the doors to much union activity for professions and the public employee sector" (Marquis & Huston, 2006, p. 556). Indeed, a review of union membership figures shows that since 1960, most collective bargaining activity in the United States has occurred in the public and professional sectors of industry, most notably among faculty at institutions of higher education, teachers at primary and secondary levels, and physicians.

TABLE 17.1	Labor Legislation		
	Year	**Legislation**	**Effect**
	1935	National Labor Relations Act/Wagner Act	Gave unions many rights in organizing; resulted in rapid union growth
	1947	Taft–Hartley Amendment	Returned some power to management; resulted in a more equal balance of power between unions and management
	1962	Kennedy Executive Order 10988	Amended the 1935 Wagner Act to allow public employees to join unions
	1974	Amendments to Wagner Act	Allowed nonprofit organizations to join unions
	1989	National Labor Relations Board ruling	Allowed nurses to form their own separate bargaining units

Discussion Point

Why is white-collar union membership growing when the private and blue collar sectors are not? Have societal norms altered perceptions regarding the appropriateness of unionization in white-collar industry?

"From 1962 through 1989, there were slow but steady increases in the numbers of nurses represented by collective bargaining agents. In 1989, the NLRB ruled that nurses could form their own separate bargaining units, and union activity increased. However, the American Hospital Association immediately sued the American Nurses Association (ANA), and the ruling was halted until 1991, when the Supreme Court upheld the 1989 decision by the NLRB" (Marquis & Huston, 2006, p. 557). A summary of the legislation impacting the development of unionization in nursing is shown in Table 17.1.

▶ UNIONS REPRESENTING NURSES

New and increasingly aggressive unions are courting health care employees, and at least 18 different unions already represent nursing personnel (Forman & Merrick, 2002). The Service Employees International Union (SEIU) is the largest union in the health care industry, representing more than 870,000 health care workers, including 110,000 nurses and 40,000 doctors (SEIU, 2003). SEIU is also the largest union of nursing home workers in the United States, representing more than 145,000 employees.

Some of the other unions that represent nurses include the ANA; the National Union of Hospital and Health Care Employees of Retail, Wholesale and Department Store Union; American Federation of Labor–Congress of Industrial Organizations (AFL–CIO); the United Steelworkers of America; the American Federation of

Government Employees; the International Brotherhood of Teamsters; the American Federation of State, County, and Municipal Employees, which operates mostly in the public sector; and the United Auto Workers.

Discussion Point

Is it appropriate for RNs to be represented by nonnursing unions? Why would nurses seek out nonnursing unions for representation?

Union representation varies by state. The states with the most union organizing for all industries, including health care, are New York, California, Pennsylvania, Michigan, and Illinois. The right-to-work states, typically low in union activity, include Arizona, New Mexico, Oklahoma, and Florida (Murray, 2001).

▶ MOTIVATION TO JOIN UNIONS

"Knowing that human behavior is goal-directed, it is important to examine what personal goals union membership fulfills" (Marquis & Huston, 2006, p. 558). Some individuals suggest that health care institutions differ from other types of industrial organizations, yet most nurses work in large and impersonal organizations and the individual nurse often feels powerless and vulnerable.

*CONSIDER: People are motivated to join or reject unions as a result of many needs and values.

Of the many motives for joining a union (Box 17.3), one is economics. In some organizations, pay is neither fair nor competitive (Forman & Merrick, 2002). Most economists agree that joining a union typically is an effective means of raising one's pay. Indeed, people who are members of unions earn approximately 20% more than nonmembers. Figures from the Bureau of Labor Statistics show that wages and salaries for private industry union workers averaged $16.21 per hour in the late 1990s, compared with $13.54 for nonunion workers (Gallagher, 2002).

BOX 17.3 Reasons Nurses Join Unions

1. Wage advantages
2. To increase the power of the individual
3. To increase their input into organizational decision making
4. To eliminate discrimination and favoritism
5. Because they are required to do so as part of employment (closed shop)
6. Social need to be accepted
7. Because they believe it will improve patient outcomes and quality of care

Another reason to join a union is to increase one's individual power. "Employees know that singly, they are more vulnerable than if they are part of a group. Because a large group of employees is generally less dispensable than an individual nurse, nurses generally increase their bargaining power and reduce their vulnerability by joining a union. This is a particularly strong motivating force for nurses when jobs are scarce and they feel vulnerable" (Marquis & Huston, 2006, p. 558).

Union activity also tends to change in response to workforce excesses and shortages. For decades, employment demand for nurses has increased and decreased periodically. High demand for nurses is tied directly to a healthy national economy and, historically, this has been correlated with increased union activity (Marquis & Huston, 2006). Similarly, when nursing vacancy rates are low, union membership and activity tends to decline.

> *CONSIDER: "Unions don't create the climate in which organizing activity thrives; they simply take advantage of it. The roots of union activity lie in the fertile soil of poor relationships between employees and their leaders" (Forman & Davis, 2002a, p. 444).

Murray (1999) reports that from 1995 to 1998, when hospitals were rapidly downsizing and restructuring, petitions by nurses to unionize increased yearly by 39%, 111%, and over 77%, respectively. This is an unprecedented amount of union activity.

> *CONSIDER: The rapid downsizing and restructuring of the 1990s left many nurses feeling that management did not listen to them or care about their needs. This discontentment provides a fertile ground for union organizers because unions thrive in a climate that perceives the organizational philosophy to be insensitive to the worker.

When there are nursing shortages, nurses feel less vulnerable, and other reasons to join unions become motivating factors. One reason nurses in this situation join unions is to "communicate their aims, feelings, complaints, and ideas to others. The desire to have input into organizational decision making is often a reason people join unions. A feeling of powerlessness or the perception that administration does not care about employees is a major driving force for unionization" (Marquis & Huston, 2006, p. 559).

A survey by the Federation of Nurses and Health Professions found that one in five nurses plans to leave the profession within 5 years because of unsatisfactory working conditions (New Survey, 2001). The main reason given by nurses for leaving was severe understaffing with high patient loads and patient acuity. Many of the nurses stated the job was too stressful and physically demanding in addition to issues involving mandatory overtime, irregular hours, low morale, and worsening work conditions (New Survey, 2001). Indeed, while many people think of salary and benefits as being paramount in union negotiations, they are likely two of the less important issues in most labor and management negotiations today.

Nurses also join unions to eliminate discrimination and favoritism: "This might be an especially strong motivator in groups that have experienced discrimination, such as women and minorities" (Marquis & Huston, 2006, p. 559).

Social factors may also act as motivators for nurses to unionize. Another motivation for joining a union stems from a social need to be accepted and sometimes this results from family or peer pressure to join a union.

Discussion Point

If you are a student, do you belong to the state student nurses association? If you are an RN, have you joined your state nurses association? Why or why not?

Another reason nurses join unions is because they must as a condition of employment. Although common among blue-collar workers, the *closed shop*, or requirement that all employees belong to a union, has never prevailed in the health care industry. Most health care unions have *open shops*, allowing nurses to choose if they want to join the union.

Finally, some nurses join unions because they believe that patient outcomes are better in unionized organizations due to better staffing and supervised management practices. Research by Seago and Ash (2002) does suggest a positive relationship between patient outcomes and RN unions that goes beyond wages and number of hours. Factors identified by Seago and Ash as potentially leading to this relationship in RN unions are stability in staff, autonomy, collaboration with MDs, and participation in decisions regarding practice (Box 17.4).

BOX 17.4

Research Study Fuels the Controversy

Bargaining and Mortality

This study examined the relationship between a bargaining unit for registered nurses and the mortality rate for acute myocardial infarction in acute care hospitals in California. The authors also looked into how registered nurse wages, hospital bed size, volume of patients, and other organizational factors may influence and confound this relationship.

Seago, J. A., & Ash, M. (2002). Registered nurse unions and patient outcomes. *Journal of Nursing Administration, 32*(3), 143–151.

Study Findings

Thirty-five percent of hospitals in California have RN unions. Hospitals in California with RN unions had 5.7% lower mortality rates for acute myocardial infarction (AMI) after accounting for patient age, gender, type of AMI, chronic diseases, and several organizational characteristics, including number of beds, AMI-related discharges, cardiac services, staff hours, and wages.

Findings from the study do not rule out the potential nonrandom selection bias regarding the presence of unions; therefore, the authors could not determine causation and argued that the bias could go in either direction.

Although they did not establish a causal relationship, the authors conclude that there is a positive relationship between patient outcomes and RN unions. They also suggest that further research is needed to explore what factors beyond wages and number of hours in union hospitals are predictive of better outcomes.

REASONS NOT TO JOIN UNIONS

Just as there are many reasons to join unions, there also are many reasons nurses reject unions, including societal and cultural factors (Box 17.5). "Many people distrust unions because they believe they promote the welfare state and oppose the American system of free enterprise. Other individuals reject unions because they feel a need to demonstrate that they can get ahead on their own merits; they want to demonstrate individualism and independent excellence" (Marquis & Huston, 2006, p. 560).

Still other nurses reject unions because they believe that unions promote mediocrity and employment of substandard nurses (Forman & Davis, 2002b). They are afraid that under the protection of a union, nurses will become satisfied with providing care that is just "good enough" and that nurses will abandon attempts for improvement because of the difficulty within union organizations in rewarding exceptional individuals.

Other professional employees are reluctant to join unions because of beliefs and values they hold regarding class and education. "They argue that unions were appropriate for the blue collar worker but not for the university professor, physician, or engineer. Nurses rejecting unions on this basis usually are driven by a need to demonstrate their individualism and social status" (Marquis & Huston, 2006, p. 560).

Other employees reject unions because they identify with management and adopt management's viewpoint toward unions. Other nurses reject unions because they fear employer reprisal such as job loss, for their union activity. Finally, some employees reject unions because they fear losing income associated with a strike or walkout. Strikes and walkouts are a reality of unionization; however, they are regulated by law (striking is discussed later in this chapter).

"Once managers understand the needs and driving forces behind nurses' decisions to join or reject unions, they can begin to address them" (Marquis & Huston, 2006, p. 560). Organizations with unfair management policies are more likely to become unionized. Fitzpatrick (2001) maintains that the key issues driving current union activity are layoffs and the quality of the nurses' work lives. It is certainly, then, within managerial power to eliminate some of the needs staff feel for joining unions. Marquis and Huston (2006) suggest that management can encourage feelings of power by allowing subordinates to have input into decisions that will affect their work.

Management also can listen to ideas, complaints, and feelings and take steps to ensure that favoritism and discrimination are not part of organizational life. Additionally, management can strengthen the drives and needs that make nurses reject unions. By building a team effort, sharing ideas and future plans from upper management with the staff, and encouraging individualism in employees, the workers can be encouraged to identify with management (Marquis & Huston, 2006, p. 561).

BOX 17.5

Reasons Nurses Do Not Want to Join Unions

1. A belief that unions promote the welfare state and oppose the American system of free enterprise
2. A need to demonstrate individualism
3. A belief that unionization allows for mediocrity and substandard practice
4. A belief that professionals should not unionize
5. An identification with management's viewpoint
6. Fear of employer reprisal
7. Fear of lost income associated with a strike or walkout

Forman and Merrick argue that it is much easier to prevent unionization than it is to get rid of it once it exists. This is because the NLRB forbids organizations to encourage or support any activity designed to remove a union unless a group of employees officially takes action to remove it. Only then can the employer legally speak with staff about their options and only under specific NLRB guidelines (Forman & Merrick, 2002).

Steltzer (2001) says that when nurses begin showing signs of job dissatisfaction, when they feel frustrated, stressed, or powerless, they are sending a wake-up call to management. "Management must be alert to employment practices that are unfair or insensitive to employee needs and must intervene appropriately before such issues lead to unionization. However, organizations offering liberal benefit packages and fair management practices may still experience union activity if certain social and cultural factors are present. If union activity does occur, managers must be aware of specific employee and management rights so the NLRA is not violated by either managers or employees" (Marquis & Huston, 2006, p. 561).

▶ ELIGIBILITY FOR UNION MEMBERSHIP

The NLRA defines a *supervisor* as:

> ▶ *Any individual having authority, in the interest of the employer, to hire, transfer, suspend, lay off, recall, promote, discharge, assign, reward, or discipline other employees, or responsibility to direct them, or to adjust their grievances, or effectively to recommend such action, if in connection with the foregoing the exercise of such authority is not of a merely routine or clerical nature, but requires the use of independent judgment (Wachtler, 1994, para 2).*

Historically, supervisors and managers have been exempt from NLRA protection and cannot be included in a bargaining unit. Before 1974, however, some states governed collective bargaining within the state, and in some instances, supervisors and managers were included in a bargaining unit. When the law was extended to health care in 1974, the NLRB chose not to disturb those established units (Forman & Davis, 2002b).

In addition, the definition of supervisor in nursing came into question with several administrative and court rulings in the early 1990s. These rulings came about as a result of a case involving four licensed practical nurses (LPNs/LVNs), employed at Heartland Nursing Home in Urbana, Ohio. During late 1988 and early 1989 these LPNs complained to management about what they thought were disparate enforcement of the absentee policy; short staffing; low wages for nurses aides; an unreasonable switching of prescription business from one pharmacy to another, which increased the nurses' paperwork; and management's failure to communicate with employees (Health Care Corporation, 1992). Despite assurances from the vice president for operations that they would not be harassed for bringing their concerns to headquarters' attention, three of the LPNs were terminated as a result of their actions.

In response to what they perceived to be illegal termination, the LPNs filed for protection under the NLRA. The NLRB ruled that because the LPNs had responsibility to ensure adequate staffing, to make daily work assignments, to monitor the aides' work to ensure proper performance, to counsel and discipline aides, to resolve aides' problems and grievances, to evaluate aides' performances, and to report to management, that they should be classified as "supervisors," thereby making them ineligible for protection under the NLRA.

On appeal, the administrative law judge (ALJ) disagreed, concluding that the nurses were not supervisors and that the nurses' supervisory work did not equate to responsibly directing the aides *in the interest of the employer*, noting that the nurses' focus is on the well-being of the residents, rather than on the employer (Wachtler, 1994).

In another turnabout, the United States Court of Appeals for the Sixth Circuit then reversed the decision of the ALJ, arguing that the NLRB's test for determining the supervisory status of nurses was inconsistent with the statute (Wachtler, 1994) and that the interest of the patient and the interest of the employer were not mutually exclusive. The court said that, in fact, the interests of the patient are the employer's business, and argued that the welfare of the patient was no less the object and concern of the employer than it was of the nurses. The court also argued that the statutory dichotomy the NLRB first created was no more justified in the health care field than it would be in any other business where supervisory duties are a necessary incident to the production of goods or the provision of services (NLRB, 1994).

The court further stated that it was up to Congress to carve out an exception for the health care field, including nurses, should Congress not wish for such nurses to be considered supervisors. The court reminded the NLRB that it is the courts, and not the board, who bears the final responsibility for interpreting the law. After concluding that the board's test was inconsistent with the statute, the court found that the four licensed practical nurses involved in this case were indeed supervisors and ineligible for protection under the NLRA (NLRB, 1994).

Wachtler (1994, para 8 & 9) states:

> *It is entirely possible that many RNs working in hospitals and nursing homes can be considered "supervisors," and are therefore unprotected by the NLRA. Both RNs and LPNs who are now represented for purposes of collective bargaining, and who possess the requisite statutory authority, may be removable from their existing bargaining units. . . .*
>
> *Obviously, this situation creates difficult and complicated problems. Health care facilities whose nurses are organized and currently members of existing bargaining units must carefully consider all of the ramifications. It may make health care institutions less vulnerable to work stoppages by nursing personnel because of a potentially larger group of supervisory employees available to perform patient care duties. It will also make it harder for unions to organize health care professionals, since many may be supervisors.*

339

Discussion Point

Would the NLRB's definition of *supervisor* affect nurses' eligibility for union membership at the facility in which you work?

In response to a request from the NLRB, the ANA and its newly created labor arm, United American Nurses (UAN), collaborated on an *amicus* (friend of the court) brief filed with the NLRB on September 22, 2003, regarding its current review of the statutory definition of "supervisor." The request was for briefs discussing how and whether employees use independent judgment and assign and direct work that would classify them as supervisors, and therefore exclude them from bargaining units (ANA, 2004).

▶ UNION ORGANIZING STRATEGIES

Murray (2001) suggests that unions have used 10 primary organizing strategies to promote union membership since the early 1990s (Box 17.6). The first of these strategies

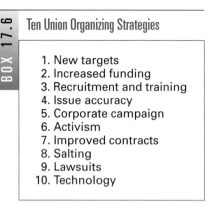

Source: Murray (2001).

is to "identify new targets," including physicians and home care workers. Physicians are increasingly represented in collective bargaining as a result of a 1999 decision by the American Medical Association (AMA) to support the collective bargaining process.

A second strategy has been increased funding. Large unions such as the AFL-CIO have set aside millions of dollars for unions that need financial help in running campaigns and increasing organizing funds. A third strategy is recruiting and training new full-time organizers. For example, the AFL-CIO offers the Organizing Institute, Union Summer, and Seminary Summer programs to promote union organizing (Murray, 2001).

Issue identification is a fourth strategy. Issues identified by unions as critical to nurses include the amount of change in the health care system, health care shortages, reengineering, and managed care. All of these issues have made working nurses question the meaning of loyalty and to ponder whether they have suffered the lion's share on "take-aways" (e.g., lost benefits, weekend plan scheduling changes, staffing shortages, and salary freezes).

The fifth strategy identified by Murray (2001) is corporate campaigns. Unions are refining corporate campaigns with allegations of discrimination, boycotts, rallies, media stories, visits to board members' homes, and 1-day strikes. Thirteen percent of chief financial officers say that their companies experienced a walkout or a strike during 2000, and 25% say they were threatened with one (On Labor Issues, 2000).

A sixth strategy contributing to labor union wins is activism. Central labor councils, local labor unions, and state labor federations are reaching out to community groups, faith-based organizations, and elected officials in an effort to create unrest and to change the environment in which workers organize.

The seventh strategy is focusing contract negotiations on what is deemed most important by workers. The current issues deemed more important by nurses often focus on nonmonetary issues (see "Consider" below). Unions have increasingly recognized this and shifted their contract negotiations accordingly.

*CONSIDER: Although historically, unions focus heavily on wage negotiations, the current issues deemed more important by nurses are often nonmonetary issues, such as guidelines for staffing, float provisions, shared decision making, and scheduling.

"Salting the bargaining unit" is the eighth strategy identified by Murray (2001) as currently being used by unions to increase membership. *Salting* means that an outsider comes in to organize the union. The United States Supreme Court ruled in 1995 that employees cannot discriminate against paid union organizers who seek jobs to organize nonunion workers. Thus, many unions have "salted" potential union sites with individuals who have union organization as their primary motive.

The ninth strategy is filing lawsuits. Labor unions maintain the goal of breaking employer resolve and demonstrate their ability to protect employees by initiating legal action on behalf of employees against targeted employers (Murray, 2001).

The final strategy is technology. The Internet has made finding information about how to organize a union very accessible to interested workers. E-mail has also proved to be an inexpensive and efficient means of mass communication regarding issues critical to the union.

▶ SEEKING UNION REPRESENTATION

The first step in seeking union representation is determining that adequate levels of desire for unionization exist. The NLRB requires that at least 30% of employees sign an interest card before an election for unionization can be held, but most collective bargaining agents will require 60% to 70% of the employees to sign interest cards before they would begin an organizing campaign. Union representatives are generally careful to keep a campaign secret until they are ready to file a petition for election. They do this so they can build momentum without interference from the employer (Forman & Davis, 2002a).

After enough interest cards have been signed, the organization must hold an election. At that time, all employees of the same classification, such as RNs, vote on whether they desired unionization. A choice in every such election is *no representation*, which means that the voters do not want a union. During the election, 50% plus one of the petitioned unit must vote before the union can be recognized.

Unions can also be decertified by a process similar to that of certification. *Decertification* may occur when at least 30% of the eligible employees in the bargaining unit initiate a petition asking to no longer be represented by the union. Employers, by law, are not allowed to instigate or promote decertification, but may provide employees with information regarding their rights to do so, under the NLRA (Forman and Kraus, 2003).

There are important differences, however, between organizing in a health care facility and in other types of organizations. "Generally, the solicitation and distribution of union literature are banned entirely in immediate patient care areas. Managers should never, however, independently attempt to deal with union-organizing activity. They should always seek assistance and guidance from higher-level management and the personnel department" (Marquis & Huston, 2006, p. 564).

Labor and management rights and responsibilities during the organizing and establishment phases of unionization are complex and they have only been touched upon briefly here. Perhaps the most important thing to remember is that power has balanced between labor and management for many years and Congress has attempted to balance this power through legislation. "At times, the balance of power has shifted to management or labor, but Congress wisely eventually enacts laws that restore the balance. The manager must ensure that the rights of management and employees are protected" (Marquis & Huston, 2006, p. 564).

▶ LABOR–MANAGEMENT RELATIONS

In the past 30 years, the relationship between most employers and unions could be characterized as accommodating, if not collaborative. Although contemporary health care organizations have come to accept the reality that unions are here to stay, industry in the United States is still less comfortable with unions than their counterparts in many other countries. "Likewise, unions have come to accept the fact that there are times when organizations are not healthy enough to survive aggressive union demands" (Marquis & Huston, 2006, p. 564).

> *CONSIDER: It is possible to create a climate in which labor and management can work together to accomplish mutual goals.

The bottom line is that employees have a right to participate in union organizing under the NLRA and managers must not interfere with this right. "Prohibited managerial activities include threatening employees, interrogating employees, promising employees rewards for cessation of union activity, and spying on employees. However, if management picks up early clues of union activity, the organization may be able to take steps that will discourage unionization of its employees" (Marquis & Huston, 2006, p. 563).

Once management must deal with a bargaining agent, it can choose to either accept or oppose the union. In opposing the union, some organizations employ active *union-busting techniques*. Other times, the organization is more subtle and simply tries to discredit the union and win employee trust. "Acceptance also may run along a continuum. The company may accept the union with reluctance and suspicion. Although they know the union has legitimate rights, managers often believe they must continually guard against the union encroaching further into traditional management territory" (Marquis & Huston, 2006, p. 564).

> *CONSIDER: "The union isn't the enemy; it's a new reality for nurse leaders" (Porter-O'Grady, 2001, p. 31).

Another type of union acceptance is known as *accommodation*. "Increasingly common, accommodation is characterized by management's full acceptance of the union, with both union and management showing mutual respect. When these conditions exist, labor and management can establish mutual goals, especially in the areas of safety, cost reduction, efficiency, eliminating waste, and improving working conditions" (Marquis & Huston, 2006, p. 564). Porter-O'Grady (2001) believes that this type of relationship has begun to be evidenced between unionized professional nurses and health care organizations, and refers to this more cooperative interaction as a new model of collective-bargaining relationship. Such cooperation represents the most mature and advanced type of labor–management relations.

Discussion Point

When unions are present in the workplace, what should be the relationship between them and management? What is accomplished by having a competitive or hostile relationship?

"The attitudes and the philosophies of the leaders in management and the union determine what type of relationship develops between the two parties in any given organization" (Marquis & Huston, 2006, p. 565). Managers must be rational, flexible, attentive to workplace and staff issues, and try not to overwhelm others with power when they deal with unions. Steltzer (2001) argues that leaders in the health care industry and unions representing nurses should partner with one another to strengthen trust between labor and management.

AMERICAN NURSES ASSOCIATION AND COLLECTIVE BARGAINING

One issue nurse managers face that is typically not encountered in other disciplines is that their professional organization, the ANA, is recognized by the NLRB as a collective bargaining agent at most state levels. Indeed, the ANA represents a significant percentage of union membership at health care organization bargaining tables.

> ***CONSIDER:** The ANA acts as both a *professional association* for RNs and a *collective bargaining agent*. This dual purpose poses a conflict in loyalty to some nurses.

"The use of state associations as bargaining agents has been a divisive issue among American nurses. Some nurse-managers believe they have been disenfranchised by their professional organization. Other managers recognize the conflicts inherent in attempting to sit on both sides of the bargaining table" (Marquis & Huston, 2006, p. 558). Some nurses, do not feel this is a problem, yet, there does appear to be some conflict in loyalty and there are no easy solutions to the dilemma created by the dual role held by the ANA.

Discussion Point

Should the ANA, the recognized professional association for nurses in the United States, also be a collective bargaining agent?

Some nurses think that because of this dual role, the ANA cannot be as action-oriented in collective bargaining as it should be. For this reason, some state unions have broken away from the ANA. They are forming a new national union, the *American Association of Registered Nurses* (AARN) (Forman & Davis, 2002b). The intent of the AARN is to broaden the influence of the "aggressive and action-oriented" California Nurses Association (CNA), which has already broken off from the ANA (Tieman, 2002). The AARN has hired a lobbyist to represent its interests in Washington and has stated its intention to serve as a union for members.

NURSES AND STRIKES

The NLRA (National Labor Relations Act, n.d., para 6) states in part, "Employees shall have the right to engage in other concerted activities for the purpose of collective bargaining or other mutual aid or protection." "Other concerted activities" refers to "working to rule," "blue flu" epidemics, work slowdowns, filing a barrage of grievances, participating in informational or recognition picketing, contacting government agencies such as the Department of Health or Occupational Safety and Health Administration, and striking (Forman & Powell, 2003).

Unions must, however, give employers and the Federal Mediation and Conciliation Service 10 days' notice of their intent to strike (Forman & Powell, 2003). This law is "specifically designed to give the facility time to stop admitting patients, transfer existing patients to other facilities, and reduce medical procedures that require nurse-intensive labor." Problems occur when management continues to admit new patients or maintains normal operations. These actions strain the system and are usually followed by a call for strikebreakers (Bronder, 2001).

Discussion Point

Can striking, walkouts, "blue flu epidemics," and picket lines be considered ethical actions if nurses believe they are the only way they can improve working conditions or assure safe patient care?

Ketter (1997) suggests that the controversy over whether nurses should strike is as long-standing as the debate between those who favor collective bargaining for nurses and those who believe it is not professional. Ketter states that those who oppose the idea of nurses striking often state striking nurses are abandoning their patients, and that it is not ethical, even with the required advance notice given to management.

The ANA supports the rights of nurses to strike as a last resort, and after careful consideration of every factor. Cheryl Johnson, chair of the UAN, concurs, arguing that "the decision to strike is very serious and has far-reaching and long-lasting consequences. Nurses exercise this right infrequently and only as a last resort" (Bronder, 2001, para 3).

This support of striking has divided the membership of the ANA and the nursing profession, although strikes have been used sparingly and effectively by nurses in this country (Ketter, 1997, p. 323). Ironically, both proponents and opponents of strikes in nursing argue that they aim for the same goal: safe patient care. Indeed, the ANA has held consistently for 50 years that nurses not only have a right to strike, but also a "professional responsibility and ethical duty to maintain employment conditions conducive to a high quality of nursing care"—and that sometimes, striking is necessary to achieve those conditions (Ketter, 1997, p. 324). It is important to remember, however, that nurses do have a choice not to participate in strikes or to cross picket lines when strikes occur. Bronder suggests, however, that a decision to do so, "defies logic." Strikebreakers, commonly known as "scabs," enable employers to pursue intimidation and punitive action, designed to break the wills of their nurses, instead of continuing negotiations and resolving problems (Bronder, 2001). The UAN argues that successful strikes can lead to better working conditions and a safer care delivery environment. "By refusing to cross a picket line, you refuse to sabotage nurses who are fighting for patients' and nurses' rights, and you maintain the respect of your nurse colleagues whose fight is your fight" (Cheryl Johnson as quoted by Bronder, 2001).

▶ CONCLUSIONS

The question of whether nurses should participate in collective bargaining has been around since legislation made such organization possible. Advocates on both sides of the issues present earnest, well-reasoned arguments to support their positions. Clearly, nurses working in unionized organizations appear to have some economic advantage, and their individual vulnerability to arbitrary action on the part of their employer is reduced.

Yet, nursing's longstanding struggle to be recognized as a profession underscores some nurses' concerns that the profession's involvement in collective bargaining associations, historically reserved for blue-collar industries, undermines this goal. In addition, union organizing campaigns frequently divide staff, and some nurses think that union activities may draw attention away from patients and patient-related activities (Forman & Merrick, 2002). Union advocates would argue that improving pay, benefits, and working conditions ultimately leads to improved patient care.

There are also issues related to who can belong to a union, what the definition of "supervisor" is in nursing, and whether strikes and walkouts are ethically justified for nursing professionals. In addition, the dual role of the ANA as both the national organization for nurses and a collective bargaining agent poses ethical dilemmas for many nurses. Even unionized nurses cannot agree on the intensity and direction their unions should take, resulting in state unions breaking off from the ANA. Finally, the relationships health care organizations have developed with their collective bargaining agents vary from direct opposition to collaboration. The impact that relationship has upon working conditions and quality of patient care cannot be understated.

Unionization, then, is fraught with challenges. Yet, unionization in nursing is not going to go away. "With job pressures putting more stress on registered nurses, an increasing number are turning to unions to help them find a voice in the workplace" (Forman & Davis, 2002, p. 376) and the "new age" of union-organizing methods are very effective (Forman & Grimes, 2004). "By applying the best practices, committing to good patient care, valuing staff participation at all levels of decision making, and being sensitive to critical issues, leaders and employees can thrive together and deliver great health care. When all is said and done, what other purpose is there?" (Porter-O'Grady, 2001, p. 32).

▶ FOR ADDITIONAL DISCUSSION

1. Does the presence of unions increase the likelihood that management will be more fair and more consistent with employers?
2. How do you feel about the formation of the AARN? Would having this "more aggressive and action-oriented" (Forman & Davis, 2002) nursing union allow the ANA to focus more on professional issues and less on collective bargaining issues?
3. Can the need for unionization be eliminated simply by management being more attentive to worker needs and being willing to provide employees reasonable working conditions and a voice in government?
4. Would you be willing to cross a picket line to work during an authorized strike?
5. Are there other ways in which nurses can increase their "group power" other than by unions? If so, are they as effective?
6. Some state unions are choosing to break off from the ANA. Does this further fragment nursing's collective power in the political arena by diminishing group size, or does it increase the broad-based support of nursing issues?

7. Do you believe the current nursing shortage will accelerate the rate of unionization in nursing?
8. How does a nursing shortage impact a union's power in negotiating wages, benefits, and working conditions?

REFERENCES

American Nurses Association. (2004). Amicus brief. ANA and UAN file brief with NLRB regarding definition of "supervisor." Retrieved May 3, 2005 from http://www.nursingworld.org/readroom/nlrbrief.htm.

As shortages rise, nursing unions swell in California. (June 8, 2002). *The Sacramento Bee.* Abstract retrieved February 9, 2003 from EbscoHost database.

Bilchik, G. S. (2000). Norma Rae, RN. *Health & Hospital Network, 74*(11), 40–44.

Bronder, E. (2001). A decision that defies logic. *American Journal of Nursing, 101*(4), 57–58. Retrieved May 3, 2005, from http://www.needlestick.org/AJN/2001/apr/Issues.htm.

Bureau of National Affairs. (May 2003). *NLRB representation and decertification election statistics. Year end 2002 report: 2000 elections by industry.* Washington DC: BNA Plus.

Cherry, B. & Jacob, S. (2002). *Contemporary nursing: Issues, trends & management* (2nd ed.). St. Louis: Mosby.

Fitzpatrick, M. (2001). Collective bargaining: A vulnerability assessment. *Nursing Management, 32*(2), 40–42.

Foner, E. & Garraty, J. (1991). *The reader's companion to American history.* Boston: Houghton Mifflin. (Eds.) Electronic version licensed by Inso Corporation.

Forman, H. & Davis, G. A. (2002a). The anatomy of a union campaign. *Journal of Nursing Administration, 32*(9), 444–447.

Forman, H. & Davis, G. (2002b). The rising tide of healthcare labor unions in nursing. *Journal of Nursing Administration, 32*(7/8), 376–378.

Forman, H. & Grimes, T. C. (2004). The "new age" of union organizing. *Journal of Nursing Administration, 34*(3), 120–124.

Forman, H. & Kraus, H. R. (2003). Decertification: Management's role when employees rethink unionization. *Journal of Nursing Administration, 33*(6), 313–316.

Forman, H. & Merrick, F. S. (2002). Vulnerability audits: Good insurance in troubled times. *Journal of Nursing Administration, 32*(10), 495–497.

Forman, H. & Powell, T. A. (2003). Managing during an employee walkout. *Journal of Nursing Administration, 33*(9), 430–433.

Franklin D. Roosevelt Presidential Library and Museum. (n.d.). *Our documents: National Labor Relations Act.* Retrieved May 3, 2005, from http://www.fdrlibrary.marist.edu/odnlra.html.

Gallagher, J. (December 27, 2002). Negotiate for more money: Wages often not main union issue. *Detroit Free Press.* Retrieved May 3, 2005, from http://www.freep.com/money/business/union27_20021227.htm.

Health Care Corporation. (January 21, 1992). *Decisions of the National Labor Relations Board.* (306 NLRB No. 11). Retrieved May 3, 2005 from http://www.nlrb.gov/nlrb/shared_files/decisions/306/306-11.txt.

Hyperdictionary. (n.d.). *Labor union.* Retrieved May 3, 2005, from http://www.hyperdictionary.com/dictionary/labor+union.

Ketter, J. (1997). Nurses and strikes: A perspective from the United States. *Nursing Ethics, 4*(4), 323–329.

Labor unions and nursing. (n.d.). Retrieved July 31, 2004, from http://www.freeessays.cc/db/11/bmu374.shtml.

Marquis, B. & Huston, C. (2006). *Leadership Roles and Management Functions in Nursing* (5th ed.). Philadelphia: Lippincott Williams & Wilkins.

Murray, M. K. (1999). Is healthcare reengineering resulting in union organizing of registered nurses? *Journal of Nursing Administration, 29*(10), 4–7.

Murray, M. K. (2001). The new economy and new union organizing strategies: Union wins in healthcare. *Journal of Nursing Administration, 31*(7/8), 339–343.

National Labor Relations Act (n.d.). Retrieved May 3, 2005 from http://home.earthlink.net/~local1613/nlra.html.

New survey says nursing shortage will get worse. (April 19, 2001). Retrieved from http://archives.cnn.com/2001/HEALTH/04/19/nursing.shortage/.

NLRB v. Health Care & Retirement Corp. 114 S. Ct. 1778. (May 23, 1994). Retrieved May 3, 2005, from http://www.sppsr.ucla.edu/ps/pdf/W00/PSM232/PDF/Health.PDF.

On labor issues: Labor gets louder. (2000). *Institutional Investor, 34*(6), 36.

Porter-O'Grady, T. (2001). Collective bargaining: The union as partner. Part 3. *Nursing Management, 32*(6), 30–32.

Seago, J. A. & Ash, M. (2002). Registered nurse unions and patient outcomes. *Journal of Nursing Administration, 32*(3), 143–151.

Service Employees International Union. (2003). *SEIU: America's largest and fastest growing union.* Retrieved May 3, 2005, from http://www.seiu.org/who/closer_look/.

Steltzer, T. M. (2001). Collective bargaining: A wake-up call. Part 2. *Nursing Management, 32*(4), 35–37, 48.

Tieman, J. (2002). New nursing group divides ANA. *Modern Healthcare, 32*(6), 13.

United States Department of Labor, Bureau of Labor Statistics. (January 21, 2004). *Union members summary.* Retrieved May 3, 2005, from http://bls.gov/news.release/union2.nr0.htm.

Wachtler, D. R. (1994). U.S. Supreme Court rules that nurses can be considered supervisors. *FindLaw for Legal Professionals.* May 3, 2005 from http://library.lp.findlaw.com/articles/file/00325/004677/title/Subject/topic/Employment%20Law_Collective%20Bargaining/filename/employmentlaw_2_2791.

Wikipedia: The Free Encyclopedia. (n.d.) *Jurisdictional strike definition.* Retrieved May 3, 2005, from http://en.wikipedia.org/wiki/Jurisdictional_strike.

BIBLIOGRAPHY

Cartmail, G. (2003). Your rights at work: Capturing ideas and enthusiasm. *Journal of Community Practice, 76*(6), 227.

Demoro, R. A. (2003). It's like representation without representation. *California Nurse, 99*(4), 4–5, 8.

Fitzpatrick, M. (February 2001). Collective bargaining: A vulnerability assessment—Part 1. *Nursing Management, 32*(2), 40–42.

Forman, H. & Grimes, T. C. (2002). Living with a union contract. *Journal of Nursing Administration, 32*(12), 611–614.

Forman, H. J. & Powell, T. A. (2003). Management rights. *Journal of Nursing Administration, 33*(1), 7–9.

Johnson, C. L. (2000). Come together. *American Journal of Nursing, 100*(9), 81–82.

Kasoff, J. (2003). Grievance tracking: Targeting an improvement process. *Journal of Nursing Administration, 33*(7/8), 376.

Murray, M.K. (2001). The new economy and new union organizing strategies: Union wins in healthcare. *Journal of Nursing Administration, 31*(7/8), 339–343.

Labor relations: Charge nurses in nursing home are supervisors, not part of the bargaining unit. (2003). *Legal Eye Newsletter for the Nursing Profession, 11*(7), 8.

Martin, S. (2003). Solidarity: Union nurses swarm Capitol Hill. *American Journal of Nursing, 103*(8), 65, 67, 69.

Mason, D. J. (2000). The state of the unions. *American Journal of Nursing, 100*(9), 7.

Meier, E. (2000). Is unionization the answer for nurses and nursing? *Nursing Economics, 18*(1), 36–37.

Our new contract: How we got there and the lesson learned in the process. (2003). *California Nurse, 99*(6), 6, 15.

Parish, C. (2003). Unions win right to query pay review body's advice. *Nursing Standard, 17*(43), 4.

Reynolds, M. (n.d.). *The impact of nursing unions on job satisfaction and patient outcomes.* Indiana-Purdue University at Fort Wayne. Retrieved May 3, 2005, from http://users.ipfw.edu/wellerw/APApaper.pdf.

You can help win better workers compensation: Your union has been lobbying for injured workers to receive the income they would normally take home when they receive workers' compensation. (Autumn 2003). *Enrolled Nurse*, 17.

Zolot, J. S. & Sofer, D. (2001). To supervise or unionize? That is the question. *American Journal of Nursing, 101*(8), 21.

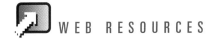 WEB RESOURCES

American Federation of State, County, and Municipal Employees—AFL–CIO	**http://www.afscme.org**
American Federation of Teachers	**http://www.aft.org/healthcare/index.htm**
American Nurses Association/United American Nurses	**http://nursingworld.org/uan/**
Australian Nursing Federation	**http://www.anf.org.au**
California Nurses Association	**http://www.calnurse.org/**
Canadian Federation of Nurses Unions	**http://www.nursesunions.ca/en/index.shtml**
Health and Community Services Union—Australia	**http://www.hacsu.asn.au/about**
National Education Association	**http://www.nea.org/esphome/**
New York Professional Nurses Union (NYPNU)	**http://www.nypnu.org/**
Nova Scotia Nurses Union	**http://www.xpdnc.com/links/locans.html**
Ontario Nurses Association	**http://www.ona.org/index.html**
Service Employees International Union (SEIU)	**http://www.seiu.org/health/nurses/**
Teamsters International Union	**http://www.teamster.org**
United Auto Workers	**http://www.uaw.org**
United Food and Commercial Workers (UFCW)—AFL/CIO	**http://www.ufcw.org**
United Nurses and Allied Professionals (UNAP)	**http://www.unap.org**
United Nurses of Alberta	**http://www.una.ab.ca**

Assuring Provider Competence Through Licensure, Continuing Education, and Certification

18

Carol J. Huston

W hittaker, Smolenski, and Carson (2000, para 1) ask: "What is the best way to determine if a nurse is competent?" They suggest that this question is increasingly being asked by employers, regulators, certifying agencies, insurance companies, and professional associations. Raudonis and Anderson (2002) answer that question in their assertion that the nursing profession has three means of being accountable for the clinical competence of its practitioners. The first of these is state regulation through statutes of the Nurse Practice Act, which includes licensure. The second is the scope and standards of clinical nursing practice developed by professional nursing organizations such as the American Nurses Association (ANA) and specialty nursing organizations; and the third is professional certification.

Additionally, Pearson, Fitzgerald, Walsh, and Borbasi (2002, p. 361) suggest that recency of practice may provide one other means of recognizing competency; however, they also note that "this in itself does not recognize variations in competency levels across nurses who have not practiced for some time, and makes the assumption that nurses who are in current practice, or who have not practiced for some period, are indeed competent." Pearson et al. then argue that other indicators of competency must be required for nurses seeking relicensure.

Unfortunately, in many states, a practitioner is determined to be competent when initially licensed and thereafter unless proven otherwise. "Yet many believe this is not enough and are exploring other approaches to assure continuing competence in today's environment where technology and practice are continually changing, new health care systems are evolving and consumers are pressing for providers who are competent" (Whittaker et al., para 1). Cook (1999) concurs, arguing that graduation from a nursing program and passing a licensure examination does not assure practitioners' competency throughout their careers. Instead, "nurses must maintain competency in practice by updating their knowledge to assure quality care" (Cook, para 1).

In 1995, the Task Force on Healthcare Workforce Regulations of the Pew Health Professions Commission recommended changing how health care professions, including nursing, were regulated and suggested that continued competence should be assured as a regulatory board function (North Carolina Board of Nursing, n.d.). The Citizens Advocacy Center, a public policy organization located in Washington, DC, concurred, as did the 1999 Institute of Medicine (IOM) in its report *To Err Is Human*, which included a recommendation for professional licensing bodies to assume the responsibility for determining licensees' competence and knowledge (IOM's Medical Error Report, 2000).

There is little disagreement, then, that the knowledge health care professionals need must be current and appropriate to their area of practice and that their care should be competent at the minimum. The challenge lies, however, in determining how best to assure that competency and in determining who should be responsible for its oversight.

This chapter explores definitions of competence with particular attention given to that of continuing competence. Licensure, continuing education, and professional certification are examined as potential strategies for assuring provider competence. The chapter also discusses the limitations of each of these strategies for assessing both initial and continuing competence as well as the difficulties inherent in standardizing continuing competence requirements in a health care system composed of varied stakeholders. Finally, capping the chapter is an exploration of a contemporary strategy that allows health care professionals to carry out a self-assessment of their practice, and to develop a personal plan for maintaining competence.

▶ DEFINING COMPETENCE

Competence in nursing can be defined in many ways. In a 1996 position paper, the National Council of State Boards of Nursing (NCSBN), defined competence as "the application of knowledge and the interpersonal, decision-making, and psychomotor skills expected for the nurse's practice role, within the context of public health, welfare and safety" (NCSBN, 1996–2001, para 3). The position statement delineated three standards for competence: 1) application of knowledge and skills at the level required for a particular situation; 2) demonstration of responsibility and accountability for practice and decisions; and 3) restriction and/or accommodation of practice if essential functions of the nursing role cannot be performed safely because of mental or physical disabilities. These standards are further delineated in Box 18.1.

In 1999, the ANA also convened an expert panel that defined three types of competency in nursing: *continuing competence*, *professional nursing competence*, and *continuing professional nursing competence* (Box 18.2). Special attention was given, however,

---

BOX 18.1 Standards for Competence*

Standard 1

Apply knowledge and skills at the level required for a particular situation.

- Determines actions needed to achieve desired outcomes
- Performs nursing activities in a safe/effective manner
- Demonstrates current knowledge necessary to provide safe client care
- Delegates in accordance with established guidelines
- Collaborates with appropriate professionals to attain client health care outcomes

Standard 2

Demonstrate responsibility and accountability for practice and decisions.

- Exhibits ethical behavior
- Assures client welfare prevails
- Establishes and maintain therapeutic boundaries
- Limits practice to current knowledge, skills and abilities
- Clarifies expectations of the role
- Intervenes when unsafe nursing practice occurs
- Practices within the legal authority granted by the jurisdiction
- Implements professional development activities based on assessed needs

Standard 3

Restrict and/or accommodate practice if cannot safely perform essential functions of the nursing role due to mental or physical disabilities.

- Identifies abilities necessary to perform the essential functions of the nursing practice role
- Implements accommodations when needed
- Safely performs essential functions of the nursing practice role
- Limits practice when accommodations are not sufficient to enable safe performance of essential functions of the nursing practice role

*NCSBN 1996 Position Statement.

Similarly, the Canadian Nurses Association and Canadian Association of Schools of Nursing (2004, para 1) define continuing competence as "the ongoing ability of a nurse to integrate and apply the knowledge, skills, judgment and personal attributes required to practice safely and ethically in a designated role and setting." Maintaining this ongoing ability involves a continual process of linking the code of ethics, standards of practice, and lifelong learning (National Framework for Continuing Competence, 2000).

Finally, the Office of the Professions, New York State Education Department (2000, para 3) stated that in its simplest form, "continuing professional competence means that a licensee: 1) is at least as qualified to practice as at the time of licensure, and 2) has kept current with changes and developments in the profession since the time of licensure."

Glazer (1999) expresses frustration at the lack of consensus regarding the definition of continued competence and suggests that this has occurred because each entity defines continued competence in terms of its own stakeholder's perspectives. In many instances, for example, nurses develop high levels of competence in specific areas of nursing practice as a result of work experience and specialization at the expense of staying current in other areas of practice. Yet employers, who espouse support of continuing competence, often ask registered nurses (RNs) to provide care in areas of practice outside their area of expertise because the current nursing shortage encourages them to do so.

In addition, professional nursing organizations fear implementing continuing competence mandates because of "the very real and imagined fear of losing members" (Glazer, 1999, para 5). For example, the American Nurses Credentialing Center (ANCC) continues to offer certification examinations for registered nurses without baccalaureate degrees, despite the recognition that such certification suggests advanced rather than basic practice and a level of competence in practice beyond the entry level measured by licensure (Glazer). What is more, ANA advocates that states defer competence monitoring to the professional association, without governmental involvement in the process, partly because of concern about misconduct charges if state regulators are involved and partly because memberships and revenues are likely to increase if the association monitors competence. Clearly then, stakeholders and politics continue to influence how continuing competence is defined, used, and promulgated.

The issue is also complicated by the fact that there are no national standards for defining, measuring, or requiring continuing competence in nursing. In addition, "while the primary reason for developing continuing competence programs is public protection, there is a major underlying principle of lifelong learning and professional growth and development" that cannot be ignored (Campbell & MacKay, 2001, p. 22).

Glazer (1999, para 4) suggests that "nursing needs a policy statement about continued competence that specialty nursing organizations, state nurses associations, state boards of nursing and professional nursing organizations can agree upon." The reality, however, is that given the multiplicity and variations of the definition of continuing competence; and the number of stakeholders affected by its promulgation; identifying and mandating strategies that assure the continuing competence of health care providers will be very difficult.

---

*CONSIDER: "Competency within a profession such as nursing is vastly complex and difficult to operationalize into pragmatic methods of regulation" (Pearson et al., 2002, p. 361).

BOX 18.2   **Definitions of Competence***

- *Continuing competence* is ongoing professional nursing competence according to level of expertise, responsibility, and domains of practice.
- *Professional nursing competence* is behavior based on beliefs, attitudes, and knowledge matched to and in the context of a set of expected outcomes as defined by nursing scope of practice, policy, Code for Nurses, standards, guidelines, and benchmarks that assure safe performance of professional activities.
- *Continuing professional nursing competence* is ongoing professional nursing competence according to level of expertise, responsibility, and domains of practice as evidenced by behavior based on beliefs, attitudes, and knowledge matched to and in the context of a set of expected outcomes as defined by nursing scope of practice, policy, Code of Ethics, standards, guidelines, and benchmarks that assure safe performance of professional activities.

*ANA (2000) Expert Panel.

to continuing competence because so many assumptions exist regarding the rights and responsibilities of consumers, individual nurses, employers to see that such competence is present and promulgated (Box 18.3). Indeed, it is continuing competence that is a primary focus of this chapter, since initial licensure at least suggests that minimum competency levels were met at that time.

Continued competence was also the focus of the North Carolina Board of Registered Nursing (n.d., para 4), which defined continued competence as "the ongoing application of knowledge and the decision-making, psychomotor, and interpersonal skills expected of the licensed nurse within a specific practice setting resulting in nursing care that contributes to the health and welfare of clients served."

351

BOX 18.3   **Assumptions Regarding Continuing Competence***

1. The purpose of ensuring continuing competence is the protection of the public and advancement of the profession through the professional development of nurses.
2. The public has a right to expect competence throughout nurses' careers.
3. Any process of competency assurance must be shaped and guided by the profession of nursing.
4. Assurance of continuing competence is the shared responsibility of the profession, regulatory bodies, organizations/workplaces, and individual nurses.
5. Nurses are individually responsible for maintaining continuing competence.
6. The employer's responsibility is to provide an environment conducive to competent practice.
7. Continuing competence is definable, measurable and can be evaluated.
8. Competence is considered in the context of level of expertise, responsibility, and domains of practice.

*ANA (2000) Expert Panel.

▶ PROFESSIONAL LICENSURE

Licensure is the process by which a state government agency "grants permission to an individual to engage in a given profession upon finding that the applicant has attained the essential degree of competency necessary to perform a unique scope of practice. Licensing requirements define what is necessary for the majority of individuals to be able to practice the profession safely and validate that the applicant has met those requirements" (Medilligence, n.d., para 7). Licensing is used when regulated activities are complex and require specialized knowledge, skill, and independent decision making (Medilligence). Most health care professionals then must be licensed and this license is assumed to provide at least some assurance that the practitioner is competent in their field at the time of initial licensure.

Licensure Processes in Nursing

One of the most important purposes of the NCSBN and its 61 state boards of nursing is to protect the health, safety, and welfare of the public (Whittaker et al., 2000; Wendt, 2003). This is done by having a regulatory role in the accreditation of nursing education programs, through licensure, and by implementing and enforcing the Nurse Practice Act. In addition, the NCSBN has created and disseminated numerous nursing practice and regulation resources "including position papers, model laws, resource folders, and other documents" on nursing practice and education (NCSBN, 1996–2004, para 4). Moreover, the NCSBN maintains a database on nursing disciplinary actions taken across the nation.

It is the licensing examinations for RNs and licensed practical/vocational nurses (LPNs/LVNs), however, that the NCSBN and its state boards of nursing are probably best known for. "Under the guidance of its membership, the NCSBN has developed two licensure examinations to test the entry-level nursing competence of candidates for licensure as registered nurses and as licensed practical/vocational nurses. These examinations, the National Council Licensure Examinations (NCLEX-RN® and NCLEX-PN®), are administered with the contractual assistance of a national test service" (NCSBN, 1996–2004, para 1).

"When a practitioner is initially licensed, they are deemed by the state to have met minimal competency standards" (Whittaker et al., 2000, para 4). A report of the American Association of Colleges of Nursing (AACN) Task Force on Education and Regulation for Professional Nursing Practice (AACN, 2002) argues, however, that the licensure mechanism has little relevance to the different competencies achieved in the various types of education programs for nurses.

Discussion Point

Does having just one NCLEX for multiple levels of educational levels into practice, argue that the associate degree in nursing provides an adequate knowledge base for competence in all areas of professional nursing practice?

Moreover, the AACN argued that the NCLEX is developed using a process that is retrospective (incumbent job analysis), rather than futuristic in its analysis of the nursing skills necessary for high quality practice. This is because the NCSBN conducts RN job analysis studies every 3 years to collect empirical data from newly licensed nurses that describe what they actually do on the job. A panel of nurse experts, active in clinical practice, then reviews and revises a list of activities representing the full scope of current nursing practice and uses these as the basis for NCLEX questions (AACN, 2002).

> ***CONSIDER:** "Although the NCSBN asserts the need to develop an examination based on descriptions of current practice, other health disciplines in the U.S., and nursing bodies in other countries, have used successfully a more sophisticated and future-oriented approach to assessment of competence for practice" (AACN, 2002, para 30).

Despite these potential flaws, licensure by examination continues to be a highly regarded strategy for assuring competence levels of health care professionals. Indeed, some professional organizations and regulatory bodies suggest that RNs should be required to repeat the NCLEX periodically or that nurses should be required to take examinations similar in scope to the NCLEX for license renewal.

Efforts to implement mandatory reexamination as a prerequisite for license renewal in nursing, however, have met with minimal success. This is because there is little agreement about what such an examination should look like, how it would be administered, and how often it should be required. The Office of the Professions (2000) appropriately questions whether certification examinations that are appropriate for determining the minimum competency of a novice practitioner should be the vehicle for assessing the continuing competence of a seasoned professional. Regardless, 11 states have introduced legislation with varying approaches from retesting to requiring a provider to demonstrate competency in the workplace, but resistance is high and there is little hope that periodic reexaminations to assess competence will be a part of nursing's immediate future.

Licensure Processes in Medicine

In contrast, U.S. medical licensure examinations are developed using a competency-based process that requires examinees to be cognizant of practice changes, the evidence required for practice, and the knowledge necessary to be competent into the future. In addition, to achieve full authority to practice independently, physicians are required to pass three licensure examinations (AACN, 2002). These examinations begin in medical school and are completed during the second year of residency. The National Board of Medical Examiners (NBME) also is currently developing a fourth examination, which will be required of all physicians and will test affective and interpersonal skill levels (AACN, 2002) and both the NBME and Federation of State Medical Boards (FSMB) are planning to require clinical skills examinations for physician relicensure.

However, the American Medical Association (AMA) House of Delegates put forth a resolution in April 2004, arguing that "while the AMA supports clinical skills examinations in the medical school setting, it opposes their use in medical licensure, until such examinations can be shown to accurately predict physician clinical incompetence or moral turpitude" (American Medical Association, 2004, lines 15–17).

In addition, although periodic reexamination was recommended in 1967 by the Bureau of Health Manpower (U.S. Department of Health) for licensure of physicians; in 1971, the Bureau shifted the responsibility for ensuring competence to state professional associations (Office of the Professions, 2000). The result is that routine, periodic reexamination of current physician licensees does not occur at this time in many states.

Licensure Processes in Pharmacy and Dentistry

Pharmacists have also been reluctant to embrace the IOM's *To Err Is Human* recommendation that periodic reexamination of key providers is critical to resolving health care quality problems, especially medical errors. Of the pharmacists surveyed, 58% said that testing is not a valid measure for determining continuing competence (Office of the Professions, 2000).

Indeed, while it embraces the IOM report's major thrust, the National Association of Boards of Pharmacy suggests that retesting is problematic and is not guaranteed to fix the problem (IOM's Medical Error Report, 2000). In addition, the American Pharmaceutical Association supports voluntary self-assessment but opposes state pharmacy boards using competency examinations as a requirement for relicensure (IOM's Medical Error Report). The American Dental Association also opposes mandated reexamination for licensure renewal (Office of the Professions, 2000).

Discussion Point

Why are professional health care organizations reluctant to support re-examination as a means of assuring continuing competency? Who are the stakeholders involved? What are some ramifications of adopting such a mandate?

▶ CONTINUING EDUCATION

"The challenge of licensure boards is to assure practitioners are competent throughout their practice career, not just with initial licensure" (Whittaker et al., 2000, para 4). As a result, many professional associations and states have developed requirements to ensure continued competence including mandated continuing education (CE) for license renewal. Indeed, it is the position of the National Association of School Nurses (NASN) (2003) that nurses must actively participate in professional development and/or CE to meet the increasing and ever-changing demands and expectations of the profession and of the education community. The NASN (para 6) suggests that CE "promotes confidence in the nursing and education professions that competence in the practice of professional school nursing is continuous."

Continuing Education in Nursing

Currently, only 23 states require some form of CE for professional nurse license renewal (Continuing Education Requirements by State/Territory, 2001–2002), and requirements in these states vary from a few hours to 30 hours every 2 years (Box 18.4). Some states, Colorado, for example, required CE at one time, but removed that requirement because it felt that CE did not guarantee competence (Whittaker et al., 2000). Colorado nurses argued that if Colorado did not require CE for pharmacists, the state should not require it for nurses (Berry, n.d.). Similarly, Hawaii discontinued CE requirements for many professions, including nursing and physical therapy, because of high costs of these courses to the individual practitioner, considerable costs to the state to administer the legislation, and the inability to demonstrate positive outcomes (Office of the Professions, 2000).

Sample State Continuing Education Requirements for Nurses

California: 30 hours every 2 years (California Board of Registered Nursing, 2004)

Florida: 25 hours every 2 years with 1 hour dedicated to HIV and 1 hour dedicated to domestic violence (Continuing Education Requirements by State/Territory, 2001–2002)

Indiana: none (Indiana Health Professions Bureau, 2004)

Iowa: 36 hours for a 3-year license and 24 hours for less than 3-year licenses (Iowa Board of Nursing, 1998)

Michigan: 25 hours every 2 years (Michigan Nurses Association, n.d.).

Minnesota: 24 hours every 2 years (Minnesota Board of Nursing, n.d.).

Montana: none (Montana Board of Nursing, n.d.)

New York: 4 hours on infection control every 4 years and 2 hours on child abuse one time (Office of the Professions, 2000)

Ohio: 24 hours every 2 years. At least 1 of these hours must be in the area of the law and rules related to nursing practice in Ohio (Ohio Board of Nursing, n.d.)

Texas: 20 hours every 2 years (Texas Board of Nurse Examiners, 2003)

Discussion Point

Is the need for continuing education greater for one type of health care professional than another? When required, should the minimum number of mandated hours be the same for all health care professionals? If not, how many should be required for each health care specialty?

Continuing Education in Medicine

The Composite State Board of Medical Examiners (n.d.) suggests that physicians and physician assistants must complete Board-approved continuing medical education (CME) of not less than 40 hours biennially for relicensure. The Office of the Professions (2000), however, states that only 33 states currently require CME for physician license renewal and the number of required hours varies dramatically. For example, Louisiana, Mississippi, North Carolina, South Carolina, Tennessee, and Virginia require no CME hours; Oklahoma requires 150 hours every 3 years, and California requires 80 hours annually (Office of the Professions).

A review of state relicensure requirements, provided by the FSMB and the AMA, shows that 31 states have laws that direct the format of CME (Kefalides, 2000). Several states mandate that specific topics be covered. For example, Florida requires that all physicians take CME classes in human immunodeficiency virus (HIV) and acquired immunodeficiency syndrome (AIDS) and domestic violence. Kentucky and Rhode Island also mandate HIV education before relicensure (Kefalides). In New York, child abuse must be covered in CME classes, and in Nevada and Texas, physicians renewing their licenses must receive instruction on ethics and professional responsibility. Massachusetts has an unusual law that requires all physicians to read from the Board of Registrations' book of regulations (Kefalides).

Continuing Education in Other Health Care Professions

All but three states (Colorado, Wisconsin, and Hawaii) require CE for pharmacists with the norm being 15 CE hours annually or 30 over 2 years (Berry, n.d.). Most require the CE be from approved sources such as American Counsel on Pharmacy Education. Sometimes carryover is allowed, and sometimes the type is proscribed; for example, in Connecticut and New Hampshire, five hours must be from live presentations (Berry).

Respiratory care professionals must complete 30 hours of approved CE every 2 years for license renewal (Composite State Board of Medical Examiners, n.d.). Thirty-three states require CE for acupuncturists; 30 states require CE for audiologists for license renewal; and 28 states require CE for licensure for occupational therapists (Office of the Professions, 2002).

Discussion Point

Berry (n.d.) offers the following statistics: All 50 states have mandated CE for certified public accountants, optometrists, and real estate brokers; 47 for nursing home administrators; 46 for insurance brokers; 43 for dentists; 40 for psychologists; 39 for social workers and veterinarians; and 37 states for lawyers. Given these statistics, why do less than half of the states in the United States mandate continuing education in nursing for license renewal? What rationale can be given for why these occupations have a greater need for CE than nurses?

Does Continuing Education Assure Competence?

The CE approach to continuing competence continues to be very controversial. Whittaker et al. (2000) question the effectiveness of CE as a result of the broad parameters for CE and the lack of formal research to support a correlation between CE, continuing competence, and improved patient outcomes. The Office of the Professions (2000) concurs, arguing that "seat time in continuing education programs does not guarantee learning," and that no direct relationship between CE and competence has been proved.

In addition, professional organizations, such as the American Psychological Association, have expressed concern about the quality of mandated CE courses and the lack of courses for experts and specialists (Office of the Professions, 2000). Likewise, there is no agreement on the optimal number of annual credits needed to ensure competence. Until consensus can be reached regarding how CE should be provided, and how much is needed; and until research findings show an empirical link between CE and provider competence, CE cannot be touted as a valid and reliable measure of continuing competence.

▶ CERTIFICATION

As defined by the American Board of Nursing Specialties (ABNS) (2000), certification is the formal recognition of the specialized knowledge, skills, and experience demonstrated by the achievement of standards identified by a nursing specialty to promote optimal health outcomes. Certification then, is a type of credential that affords title protection and recognition of accomplishment, but does not include a legal scope of practice (Medilligence, n.d.).

The ANCC suggests, however, that "certification does protect the public by enabling anyone to identify competent people more readily; aids the profession by encouraging and recognizing professional achievement; recognizes specialization, enhances professionalism and, in some cases, serves as a criterion for financial reimbursement" (2003a, para 2).

Professional certification for nonadvanced practice nurses was first offered in the 1970s and has grown significantly since then. Because certification "signifies attainment of specific criteria and knowledge, skills, and abilities in a specific specialty field," a minority of the professional nurse population would be expected to be certified (ANCC, 2003a). However, more than 350,000 nurses in the United States and Canada currently hold professional certification. This has occurred, at least in part, because the ANCC has made certification accessible to all qualified RNs in the 21st century (ANCC, 2002; Raudonis & Anderson, 2002). More than 151,000 nurses have been certified by ANCC since 1991 and approximately 58,000 advanced practice nurses are currently certified by the ANCC (ANCC, 2003a). Certification, however, is voluntary and participation depends upon the perceived value of the credential (Gaberson, Schroeter, Killen, & Valentine, 2003).

Becoming Certified

To achieve professional certification, nurses must meet eligibility criteria that include years and types of work experience as well as minimum educational levels, active nursing licenses, and successful completion of a nationally administered examination. "A certification board, usually appointed by the parent nursing specialty organization, establishes the eligibility criteria, and maintains the content validity of the certifying examination" (Anderson, Raudonis, & Kirschling, 1999, p. 45). Certifications usually last 5 years.

The American Nurses Credentialing Center

One organization that has driven the promulgation of professional certification in the United States has been the ANCC. The ANCC, a subsidiary of the ANA, is the largest nursing credentialing organization in the United States. There are currently over 145,000 ANCC certified nurses, representing more than 50 nursing specialties (ANCC, 2003b).

The ANCC website (2003b) states that the organization produces quality examinations that are "psychometrically sound and legally defensible" and that "the integrity of the exams are a top priority." In addition, ANCC states that, "the ABNS and the National Commission for Certifying Agencies (NCCA), both well recognized throughout the certification and health care credentialing community, accredit most of ANCC's examinations and processes."

The American Board of Nursing Specialties

However, with more than 50 different nursing certification credentials, and with certification programs often having very different standards, it may be difficult to draw valid conclusions about the value of a particular nursing certification (Spencer-Cisek & Sveningson, 1995; Flarey, 2000). Moreover, a given specialty certification may have different value for the stakeholders in one specialty than in another (Gaberson et al., 2003).

For these reasons, the ABNS was created in 1991. The ABNS, a peer review program for specialty nursing certification, seeks to create uniformity in nursing certification, advocate for consumer protection by establishing specialty nursing certification, and increase public awareness of the value of quality certification to health care. Member organizations of ABNS represent more than a half million certified RNs around the world (ABNS, 2000).

As the only accrediting body specifically for nursing certification, ABNS has been granted deemed status by the NCSBN (ABNS, 2004). The Accreditation Council provides a peer-review process for accrediting nursing certification programs that demonstrate compliance with ABNS standards. The 5-year program approval is renewable for both members and nonmember organizations (ABNS).

Certification and the Advanced Practice Nurse

Advanced practice nurses were the first nurses to use professional certification as a means of documenting advanced knowledge in practice. In 1946, the American Association of Nurse Anesthetists began certifying nurse anesthetists. The American College of Nurse Midwives soon followed in an effort to denote minimum competency to practice in this specialty area (Gaberson et al., 2003).

Currently, many states use certification as an indicator of entry-level competence in advanced practice nursing, which includes clinical nurse specialists (CNS) and nurse practitioners (NP). Indeed, NPs and CNSs are the only exception to ANCC's requirement that RNs have experience in a specialty field before they can take a certifying examination (ANCC, 2003a). Instead, a master's degree is required to take the certification examination.

Even the NCSBN, which originally proposed second licensure for NPs, now recognizes the certification examination as the regulatory mechanism for advanced nursing practice. Certification, then, in the case of the advanced practice nurse, is not really voluntary; instead, it is required to ensure public safety and enhance public health (Whittaker et al., 2000). "As a result, certifying bodies are expected to demonstrate that initial certification exams truly reflect entry level and that the recertification process reflects continuing competence" (Whittaker et al., para 12).

Yet, the regulation of advanced practice nurses varies greatly among boards of nursing and while many state boards of nursing require master's degree educational preparation and national certification, others do not. In addition, recertification of the advance practice nurse is through the completion of CE, not reexamination (Allrefer.com, 2003).

Discussion Point

The AACN currently does not allow educational waivers for the CSN or NP certifying examination (all applicants must have at least a master's degree). Nor does AACN accept contact hours or experience in lieu of graduate credit. Do you support AACN's decision to not "grandfather" advanced practice nurses who completed their educations through certifying programs (no master's degree) and who are currently practicing in an advanced role? Why or why not?

Does Professional Certification Ensure Competence?

Whittaker et al. (2000, para 13) suggest that "the underlying assumptions regarding the use of certification to ensure competence and its inherent value have been increasingly questioned since the late 1970s." Whittaker goes on to say that "there is a dearth of empirical data from nursing and other fields which substantiate the predictive power of certification and recertification exams, which has led to the assertion that certification does not have an impact on patient outcomes" (para 13).

However, the ANCC (2000) Nursing Credentialing Research Coalition completed a study that showed that certification enabled nurses to experience fewer adverse events and errors in patient care than before they were certified. Nurses in the study reported "feeling more confident, after being certified, in their ability to detect early signs and symptoms of complications in their patients and to initiate early and prompt interventions for such complications" (para 3). This resulted in higher patient satisfaction ratings and more effective communication and collaboration with other health care providers. In addition, some certified nurses stated they experienced fewer disciplinary events and work-related injuries compared to their colleagues.

In addition, Gaberson et al. (2003), in a study of 2,750 certified perioperative nurses, found that nurses perceived the value of their certification in three areas: *personal value*, *recognition by others*, and *professional practice*. Respondents perceived that "their certification reflected a level of clinical competence and attainment of a practice standard, validated their specialized knowledge, and enhanced their personal credibility" (p. 275).

Another study by Cary (2001) showed that 72% of certified nurse respondents reported one or more benefits of certification, including a decreased number of errors or adverse events. However, the length of time of certification, the total years of nursing experience, and the respondent's educational levels were confounding variables that were not controlled by study design.

Yet, one must ask whether "basic competence" or "specialized competence" is of greater value in nursing (Whittaker et al., 2000), and whether having specialty certification lulls practitioners into believing they have more encompassing expertise than they do. In addition, one must at least question whether continuing competence can be assessed in a single examination, whether renewal periods of 5 years are too long, and whether recertification should be by licensure and not by the completion of CE. Finally, certification is really only helpful in determining a nurse's continued competence if that nurse is functioning in the areas of his or her certified competence.

Discussion Point

Do employers value professional certification? Do nurses themselves? Does the general public? On what criteria do you base your answer?

▶ REFLECTIVE PRACTICE

Reflective practice is defined by the North Carolina Board of Nursing (n.d., para 7) as "a process for assessing one's own practice to identify and seek learning opportunities to promote continued competence. Inherent in the process is the evaluation and incorporation of this learning into one's practice." Taylor (2003) adds to this definition in her assertion that reflective practice is self-regulatory. "Rather than looking to external sources for answers, individual practitioners are enjoined to look within themselves through a process of reflection" (Taylor, p. 245). Such self-assessment is gaining popularity as a way to promote professional practice and assist nurses to maintain competence and improve their practice (Campbell & MacKay, 2001).

Portfolios and Self-Assessment

Portfolios are one way for the individual RN to be both reflective about his or her practice and to assess or demonstrate competence, or both. Indeed, Berry (n.d.) suggests that the learning portfolio or professional portfolio is key to lifelong learning because it allows a professional to record items or challenges of learning that are unique for each individual.

The ANA was a leader in the push for RNs to develop portfolios, arguing that portfolios should include professional credentials, organization or workplace evaluation, continuing education, leadership activities, and a narrative self-reflection of practice over the preceding three years (MNA Leaders Object, 2000). However, the Minnesota Nurses Association (MNA) spoke out against the portfolio movement, arguing that the ANA should direct its efforts at supporting nurses and reforming the widespread flaws in the current health care system, rather than forcing individual RNs to demonstrate their competence (MNA Leaders Object, 2000). In addition, the MNA stated that portfolios would create unnecessary legal and disciplinary risks for nurses since they could be discoverable as evidence in lawsuits against nurses.

The concept of a professional portfolio was also not acceptable to licensed nurses in Kentucky in the late 1990s and had to be deleted from a legislative proposal to create competency validation options for relicensure other than CE (McGuire & Weisenbeck, 2001) (Box 18.5).

Emden, Hutt, and Bruce (2004, para 7), however, report a basic commitment to the concept in Australia and suggest that "signing to one's competence is a serious undertaking that arguably goes to the heart of professionalism and professional practice."

Similarly, nursing and midwifery experience in the United Kingdom endorse the use of portfolios to assess continuing competence, with references in the literature first appearing in the early 1990s (Emden, et al.). Only time will tell if portfolios will gain the same level of acceptance in the United States.

> *CONSIDER: "The individual registered nurse has a professional obligation and the primary responsibility for maintaining and continually acquiring competence"(Shanks, 2002, p. 16).

▶ WHO'S RESPONSIBLE FOR COMPETENCE ASSESSMENT IN NURSING?

Who, then, has the responsibility for competence assessment in nursing? Should it be the individual, the employer, the regulatory board or the certifying agency? Is it a shared responsibility? If so, are these entities willing to work together to create an integrated and systematic approach to promoting continuing competence in nursing?

Certainly, an individual responsibility for maintaining competency is suggested by the ANA Code of Ethics for Nurses in its assertion that nurses are obligated to provide adequate and competent nursing care. State nurse practice acts also hold nurses accountable for being reasonable and prudent in their practice. Both standards require the nurse to have at least some personal responsibility for continually assessing his or her professional competency through reflective practice.

The role of the professional association also lacks clarity. Whittaker et al. (2000, para 28) states that professional associations do "develop standards and guidelines upon which the performance and competency of the professional nurse is based; provide support to the individual nurse to maintain and enhance performance and competence through education and professional development opportunities, certification

BOX 18.5

Research Study Fuels the Controversy

Validation of Competency

The Kentucky Board of Nursing (KBN), recognizing the potential regulatory implications of the changing health care delivery system, began to reexamine competency issues in 1994. After a 20-year history of mandatory continuing education, nursing organizations still had unanswered questions about the efficacy of this competency assurance strategy. Relevant literature, conference proceedings, and numerous reports were studied and debated. As a result, in 1998, the Board proposed changing relicensure requirements from "mandatory continuing education" to "competency validation." This change was put before the legislature in 2000.

McGuire, C. A., & Weisenbeck, S. M. (Winter 2001). Revolution or evolution: Competency validation in Kentucky. *Nursing Administration Quarterly, 25*(2), 31–38.

Study Findings

This 6-year exploration of competency by the Kentucky Board of Nursing and a number of stakeholders resulted in enactment of a change to the Kentucky nursing laws that refocused continued competency from mandatory continuing education to multiple validation options. The concept of a professional portfolio, however, was not acceptable to the licensed population, and in the consensus-building process, the portfolio option was discarded. The new proposed legislative package, however, incorporated the following competency validation options recommended by the task force:

- Continuation of the 30 contact hours of approved CE earned during the licensure period

- Current national certification or recertification in effect during the licensure period that was related to the nurse's practice role (designated CE as applicable also required)
- Fifteen (15) contact hours of approved CE (including any designated CE requirements) earned during the licensure period and at least one of the following during the licensure period:

1. Completion of a nursing research project as a principal investigator, co-investigator, or project director
2. Publication of a nursing-related article in a refereed professional publication
3. professional nursing presentation
4. nursing employment evaluation satisfactory for continued employment
5. A successfully completed employment competency validation

The planning, consensus-building, and full disclosure efforts to identify new competency validation mechanisms for nurse relicensure in Kentucky were successful and the 2000 General Assembly revised the statutes governing nursing as a result. Kentucky law now defines nursing competency as "the application of knowledge and skills in the utilization of critical thinking, effective communication, interventions, and caring behaviors consistent with the nurse's practice role within the context of the public's health, safety and welfare." New competency validation options are now available to nurses applying for license renewal in Kentucky.

---

examinations; and influences changes in nurse practice acts." There is, however, no oversight function of either initial or continuing competence. Indeed, the ANA is the only agent that has created an organizational mandate to look at continuing competence policies and to represent the interests of all RNs (Whittaker et al.).

Employers contribute to the competence of employees by performing periodic performance appraisals and by carrying out the requirements of the accrediting bodies to ensure the ongoing competencies of employees. In addition, "many employers provide educational opportunities for employees as well as self-insure against liability for incompetent practices" (Whittaker et al., 2000, para 30). Yet employers are often among the first to argue that "a nurse is a nurse is a nurse" when it comes to meeting mandatory staffing or licensure requirements.

Regulatory boards, such as the state boards of nursing, regulate initial licensure, monitor compliance with requirements for license renewal, and take action when professional standards are breached. Yet clearly, licensure and relicensure, in and of itself, does not guarantee competence, particularly in a discipline as broad in scope and practice as nursing.

Finally, certifying organizations do help to identify those individuals who have an expertise in a specific area of practice; however, knowledge expertise does not always translate to practice expertise. A lack of professional certification does not necessarily mean that the nurse lacks continuing competence. Recertification does not ensure continued expertise because recertification is usually a product of meeting CE requirements, rather than reexamination.

> *CONSIDER: "No profession appears to have found a definitive answer to the issue of continuing competence — one that is reasonable to administer, reliable and acceptable to the profession" (Pearson et al., 2002, p. 363).

▶ CONCLUSIONS

The challenge in assuring competence in nursing is that nursing practice is dynamic and thus best practice must be continually redefined as a result of new discoveries. Licensure, continuing education, and professional certification can only assure provider competence then if they reflect the latest thinking, research, and clinical practice needs. In addition, each of these three strategies is limited in its effectiveness as a competency assessment strategy.

Clearly, the NCLEX, as it currently exists, assures only minimum entry-level competence for professional nursing practice. Given that NCLEX content derives from a retrospective model and that technological changes and the rate of knowledge acquisition are increasing exponentially in the 21st century, the newly licensed nurse has a great likelihood of being dated even before examinations are scored. In addition, as long as a single NCLEX exists and there are multiple levels of educational entry into practice, the examination will continue to have to meet educational content directed at the lowest educational level of entry.

In addition, health care professionals, professional organizations, and regulatory bodies are reluctant to implement mandatory reexamination for licensure. One must at least question whether this is because of the fear that many providers would be unable to demonstrate the continuing competence necessary for relicensure.

CE has similar limitations for assuring provider competence. Most states do not require nurses to complete CE. Those that do, demonstrate wide variation in how much CE is required, what content can be included, and how that CE can be provided. In addition, there is no guarantee that completing CE courses results in a change in the provider's knowledge level or practice or even that the content provided in the CE course is current and relevant. States that have attempted to mandate approaches to continuing competence other than CE, have often failed in their efforts due to a lack of funding, inadequate models, and the view that the requirements would be burdensome (Whittaker et al., 2000).

Finally, professional certification does ensure that the nurse has some specialized area of knowledge and practice expertise. The reality, however, is that many nurses perform outside of the area of their certification expertise each and every day in their jobs, particularly if their area of specialty certification expertise is narrow. In addition, there are multiple certifying bodies and numerous types of certification. Determining what exactly the value of that certification is in terms of improving patient care has not completely been ascertained.

The answer as to how best to assure provider competency cannot yet be answered. Efforts that address the need to do so are under way but these efforts have not been coordinated or integrated by the professional associations, regulatory bodies, and stakeholders that are affected. In addition, most professional entities involved in ensuring continuing competence are reluctant to mandate interventions for fear of alienating stakeholders. Individual practitioners, too, seem reluctant to embrace reflective practice or to put the thought and effort into creating portfolios that identify continuing competence in concrete and measurable ways. Until the focus rests solely on the need to protect patients and improve the quality of health care, mandated interventions for continuing competence are likely never to occur and provider competence will not be assured.

▸ FOR ADDITIONAL DISCUSSION

1. Who should be responsible for the cost of assuring provider competency? The provider, the employer, the clients that are served, or some other entity?
2. How likely is that states, professional organizations, professional certifying organizations, and employers will be willing to agree upon standardized measures for assessing professional competence?
3. Would most RNs support mandatory development of a portfolio? Are most RNs actively engaged in reflective practice in an effort to assess their ongoing competence?
4. Why should the entry level examination for nursing be broad/general in scope whereas continuing competence is arguably demonstrated by professional certification in specialty areas?
5. Is cost and access a deterrent to professional certification?
6. Do most nurses view continuing education coursework as a reliable and valid tool for increasing provider competency?
7. Should nurses be required to complete mandated continuing education hours in the area of nursing practice they work in?
8. Are there core competencies all licensed nurses must achieve regardless of the setting in which they practice?

REFERENCES

Allrefer.com. (2003). Nurse practitioner profession (NP). Retrieved May 5, 2005, from http://health. allrefer.com/health/nurse-practitioner-profession-np-info.html.

American Association of Colleges of Nursing (2002). Report of the Task Force on Education and Regulation for Professional Nursing Practice I. Retrieved May 5, 2005, from http://www.aacn.nche.edu/Education/edandreg02.htm.

American Association of Colleges of Nursing (2004). Certification and regulation of advanced practice nurses. Retrieved May 5, 2005, from http://www.aacn.nche.edu/Publications/positions/cerreg.htm.

American Board of Nursing Specialties (2000). Homepage. Retrieved May 5, 2005, from http://www.nursingcertification.org/.

American Board of Nursing Specialties (2004). Fact sheet. Retrieved November 10, 2004 from http://www.nursingcertification.org/pdf/ABNS_Fact_Sheet.pdf.

American Medical Association. (2004). Resolution 307- Opposition to clinical skills examinations for physician medical relicensure. Retrieved May 5, 2005, from http://www.ama-assn.org/meetings/public/annual04/307a04.rtf.

American Nurses Association. (2000). *Continuing competence: Nursing's agenda for the 21st century.* Washington, D.C. American Nurses Association.

American Nurses Credentialing Center. (Feb. 11, 2002). Certified nurses report fewer adverse events. Press release available online at http://www.nursingworld.org/pressrel/2000/pr0211a.htm.

American Nurses Credentialing Center (2003a). Frequently asked questions—about ANCC certification. Retrieved May 5, 2005, from http://www.nursingworld.org/ancc/certification/cert/certfaqs.html.

American Nurses Credentialing Center (2003b). ANCC certification — Opening a world of opportunities. Retrieved May 5, 2005, from http://www.nursingworld.org/ancc/cert.html.

Anderson, C. M., Raudonis, B. M., & Kirschling, J. M. (1999). Hospice and palliative nursing role delineation study: Implications for certification. *Journal of Hospice and Palliative Nursing,* 1, 45–55.

Berry, M. (n.d.) Competency and quality assurance. Retrieved May 5, 2005, from http://www.clearhq.org/berry-pres.html.

California Board of Registered Nursing (2004). Continuing education for license renewal. Retrieved May 5, 2005, from http://www.rn.ca.gov/coned/ce-renewal.htm.

Campbell, B. & MacKay, G. (2001). Continuing competence: An Ontario nursing regulatory program that supports nurses and employers. *Nursing Administration Quarterly, 25*(2), 22–30.

Canadian Nurses Association and Canadian Association of Schools of Nursing (2004). Joint position statement. Promoting continuing competence for registered nurses. Retrieved May 5, 2005, from http://www.cna-nurses.ca/_frames/search/searchframe.htm.

Cary, A. H. (2001). Certified registered nurses: Results of the study of the certified workforce. *American Journal of Nursing, 101*(1), 44–52.

Composite State Board of Medical Examiners (n.d.) Continuing education requirements: All professions. Retrieved May 5, 2005, from http://www.state.ga.us/meb/ced_info.html#phys.

Continuing education requirements by state/territory. (2001–2002). ResourceNurse.com. Retrieved May 5, 2005, from http://www.resourcenurse.com/RN/CE/state_cert.

Cook, C. (1999). Initial and continuing competence in education and practice: Overview and summary. *Online Journal of Issues in Nursing.* Available at: http://www.nursingworld.org/ojin/topic10/tpc10ntr.htm.

Emden, C., Hutt, D., & Bruce, M. (December 2003/January 2004). Portfolio learning. *Contemporary Nurse,* 16 (1/2). Retrieved May 5, 2005, from http://www.contemporarynurse.com/16-1p15.htm.

Flarey, D. L. (2000). Is certification the current gold standard? *JONA's Healthcare Law, Ethics, and Regulation, 2*(2), 43–45.

Gaberson, K. B., Schroeter, K., Killen, A. R., & Valentine, W. A. (2003). The perceived value of certification by certified perioperative nurses. *Nursing Outlook, 51*(6), 272–276.

Glazer, G. (1999). The policy and politics of continued competence. NursingWorld | OJIN: Legislative Column: *Online Journal of Issues in Nursing.* Available at: http://www.nursingworld.org/ojin/tpclg/leg_8.htm.

Indiana Health Professions Bureau (2004). Indiana State Board of Nursing. Retrieved November 11, 2004, from http://www.state.in.us/hpb/boards/isbn/couned.html.

IOM's medical error report reopens smoldering debate on relicensure examinations. (Jan. 3, 2000). Drug Topics Archive. Retrieved May 5, 2005, from http://www.jaapa.com/be_core/content/journals/d/data/2000/0103/d3miom01a.html.

Iowa Board of Nursing (1998). Continuing education: The basic requirements. Retrieved November 12, 2004, from http://www.state.ia.us/nursing/basic_requirement.html.

Kefalides, P. T. (2000). The invisible hand of the government in medical education. *Annals of Internal Medicine, 132*(8), 686.

McGuire, C. A. & Weisenbeck, S. M. (2001). Revolution or evolution: Competency validation in Kentucky. *Nursing Administration Quarterly, 25*(2), 31–38.

Medilligence (n.d.). U.S licensure for nurses. Retrieved May 5, 2005, from http://www.medilligence.com/employ/liceexm.htm#licenseup.

Michigan Nurses Association (n.d.). Continuing education. Retrieved May 5, 2005, from http://www.minurses.org/conted/contedreq.shtml.

Minnesota Board of Nursing (n.d.). Continuing education. Retrieved May 5, 2005, from http://www.state.mn.us/cgibin/portal/mn/jsp/content.do?contentid=536898882&contenttype=EDITORIAL&agency=NursingBoard.

MNA leaders object to proposed continuing competence portfolios. (2000). *Minnesota Nursing Accent, 72*(6), 2.

Montana Board of Nursing (n.d.). License summary for RN. Continuing education requirements. Retrieved May 5, 2005, from http://www.discoveringmontana.com/dli/bsd/license/bsd_boards/nur_board/licenses/nur/rn_lic_summary.asp.

National Association of School Nurses. (June 2003). Position statement: Professional development/continuing education. Retrieved May 5, 2005, from http://www.nasn.org/positions/pdce.htm.

National Council Position Paper, 1996. Retrieved May 5, 2005, from http://www.ncsbn.org/resources/ncsbn_competence_two.asp.

National Council State Boards of Nursing. (1996). Assuring competence. Attachment two: Definition of competence and standards for competence.

National Council State Boards of Nursing. (2004). About NCSBN. Purpose. Retrieved May 5, 2005, from http://www.ncsbn.org/about/index.asp.

National framework for continuing competence programs for registered nurses (2000). Canadian Nurses Association. Retrieved May 5, 2005, from http://www.cna-nurses.ca/_frames/search/searchframe.htm.

North Carolina Board of Nursing (n.d.). Continued competence: North Carolina Board of Nursing fact sheet. Retrieved May 5, 2005. from http://www.ncbon.com/ContCompetence.asp.

Office of the Professions, New York State Education Department (2000). Continuing competence. Retrieved May 5, 2005, from http://www.op.nysed.gov/contcomp.htm.

Ohio Board of Nursing (n.d.). Continuing education requirements for Ohio's RNs and LPNs. Retrieved November 11, 2004, from http://www.nursing.ohio.gov/pdfs/ce.pdf.

Pearson, A., Fitzgerald, M., Walsh, K., & Borbasi, S. (2002). Continuing competence and the regulation of nursing practice. *Journal of Nursing Management, 10*(6), 357–364.

Raudonis, B. M. & Anderson, C. M. (2002). A theoretical framework for specialty certification in nursing practice. *Nursing Outlook, 50*(6), 247–252.

Shanks, J. (2002). Continuing Competence Program for registered nurses in Saskatchewan. *SRNA Newsbulletin, 4*(3),16.

Spencer-Cisek, P. & Sveningson, L. (1995). Regulation of advanced nursing practice: Part Two-Certification. *Oncology Nursing Forum, 22*, 39–42.

Taylor, C. (2003) Narrating practice: Reflective accounts and the textual construction of reality. *Journal of Advanced Nursing, 42*(3), 244–251.

Texas Board of Nurse Examiners (2003). Continuing education requirements for registered nurses. Retrieved May 5, 2005, from http://www.bne.state.tx.us/ceu.htm.

Wendt, A. (July/August 2003). Mapping geriatric nursing competencies to the 2001 NCLEX-RN test plan. *Nursing Outlook, 51*(4), 152–157.

Whittaker, S., Smolenski, M., & Carson, W. (June 30, 2000): Assuring continued competence—Policy questions and approaches: How should the profession respond? Online Journal of Issues in Nursing. Available at: http://www.nursingworld.org/ojin/topic10/tpc10_4.htm.

BIBLIOGRAPHY

Australian Nursing Council, Inc. (2000). Position statement. Continuing competence in nursing. *ANC Newsletter, 11*(20).

Beatty, R. M. (2001). Continuing professional education, organizational support, and professional competence: Dilemmas of rural nurses. *Journal of Continuing Education in Nursing, 32*(5), 203–209.

Bib, S. C., Malebranche, M., Crowell, D., Altman, C., Lyon, S., Carlson, A., et al. (2003). Professional development needs of registered nurses practicing at a military community hospital. *Journal of Continuing Education, 34*(1), 39–45.

Cary, A. H. (2000). Data driven policy: The case for certification research. *Policy, Politics, & Nursing Practice, 1*, 165–171.

Craven, R. F. & DuHamel, M. B. (2003). Certificate programs in continuing professional education. *Journal of Continuing Education in Nursing, 34*(1), 14–18.

Frank-Stromborg, M. & Ward, S. (2002). Does certification status of oncology nurses make a difference in patient outcomes? *Oncology Nurse Forum, 29*(4), 665–672.

Harper, J. P. (2000). Nurses' attitudes and practices regarding voluntary continuing education. *Journal for Nurses in Staff Development, 16*(4), 164–167.

Hart, G., Clinton, M., Edwards, H., Evans, K., Lunney, P., & Posner, N., et al. (2000). Accelerated professional development and peer consultation: Two strategies for continuing education for nurses. *Journal of Continuing Education in Nursing, 3*(1), 28–37.

Lazarus, J. B., Permaloff, A., & Dickson, C. J. (2002). Evaluation of Alabama's mandatory continuing education program for reasonableness, access, and value. *Journal of Continuing Education in Nursing, 33*(3), 102–111.

National Council of State Boards of Nursing. (2001). *Test plan for the National Council Licensure Examination for registered nurses.* Chicago, IL: Author

Postler-Slattery, D. & Foley, K. (2003). The fruits of lifelong learning. *Nursing Management, 34*(2), 34–37.

Prater, L. & Neatherlin, J. S. (2001). Texas nurses respond to mandatory continuing education. *Journal of Continuing Education in Nursing, 32*(3), 126–132.

Schoon, C. G. & Smith, I. L. (2000). *The licensure and certification mission: Legal, social, and political foundations.* New York, NY: Professional Education Services.

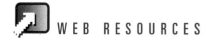 WEB RESOURCES

Alberta Association of Registered Nurses. Continuing Competence Bibliography.
http://www.nurses.ab.ca/practice/contcompBiblio.html

American Board of Nursing Specialties
http://www.nursingcertification.org/

Health Practitioners Competence Assurance Act 2003—Nursing Council of New Zealand
http://www.nursingcouncil.org.nz/hpca.html

National Association of School Nurses (2003). Position Statement. Professional Development/ Continuing Education

National Council State Boards of Nursing

National Council State Boards of Nursing (Provides links to all state boards of nursing)

NCSBN Uniform Core Licensure Requirements. A Supporting Paper. National Council Paper, July 1999

Tennessee Nurses Association. Lenburg, C.B. (2002). Promoting Competence through Critical Self-Reflection and Portfolio Development: The Inside Evaluator and the Outside Context.

http://www.nasn.org/positions/pdce.htm

http://www.ncsbn.org/about/index.asp
http://www.ncsbn.org/regulation/boardsofnursing_boards_of_nursing_board.asp#Iowa
http://www.ncsbn.org/regulation/nursingpractice_nursing_practice_licensing.asp

http://tnaonline.org/portfolio_article.html

Professional
Power

5

The Nursing Profession's Historic Struggle to Increase Its Power Base

19

Carol J. Huston

P ower is an elusive concept. The word "power" is derived from the Latin verb *potere* (to be able); thus, power may be appropriately defined as that which enables an individual or a group to accomplish goals. Power can also be defined as the capacity to act or the strength and potency to accomplish something (Marquis & Huston, 2006). Having power then gives an individual or group the potential to change the attitudes and behaviors of others.

How individuals view power varies greatly. Group and Roberts (2001, para 28) suggest that over time, personal power has come to be associated with political action, which some nurses see as "unprofessional, unworthy, and unwomanly." Indeed, power may be feared, worshipped, or mistrusted, and it is frequently misunderstood (Marquis & Huston, 2006). Women (and thus nurses) have traditionally demonstrated, at best, ambivalence toward the concept of power and until quite recently, have openly eschewed the pursuit of power.

This may have occurred because women historically were socialized to view power differently from men (Marquis & Huston, 2006). As a result, many women believe they do not inherently possess either power (formal or informal) or authority. Instead, that they must rely on others to acquire it (Nikbakht, Emami & Parsa, 2003). Also, rather than feeling capable of achieving and managing power, many women feel that power manages them.

Similarly, the nursing profession has not been the powerful force it could be in dealing with issues that directly affect health care and the profession itself. Indeed nurses are often thought of as an apolitical group. In addition, most nonnurses engage in political action for self-interest purposes, whereas nurses are oriented to the public good (Wilson, 2002). As a result, nursing has often been reactive (rather than proactive) in the policy arena, addressing proposed legislation after its introduction, rather than drafting or sponsoring legislation that reflects nursing's agenda. As a result, external forces (typically male-dominated and medically focused) have, at times, controlled and even subjugated nursing.

All of these factors have contributed to the nursing profession's relatively small power base in the political arena and its historical invisibility as a force in health care decision making. Heineken and Wozniak said that the absence of a power base "has been the singularly most limited force in preventing the [nursing] profession from achieving its overall potential" (1998, p. 591); and Sieloff (2003) suggests there is a continuing lack of empirical research in current literature to assist nurses to systematically improve their power.

This chapter explores six factors that have led to nursing's relative powerlessness as a profession. It also identifies five driving forces that are in place to increase nursing's professional power. The chapter concludes with an action plan to increase nursing's power base so that the profession is recognized as a significant force in health care decision making in the 21st century.

Discussion Point

Why is it that nurses, the largest group of health professionals, with perhaps the greatest firsthand knowledge of the health care problems faced by consumers today, have not been an integral part of health care decision making?

Factors Contributing to Powerlessness in Nursing

1. The oppression of nurses as a group.
2. Nursing's failure to fully align with the feminist movement.
3. Limited collective action by nurses.
4. The socialization of women to view power and politics negatively.
5. The inadequate recognition of nursing as an educated profession with evidence-based practice.
6. The nursing profession's history of being reactive (rather than proactive) in national policy setting.

▶ FACTORS CONTRIBUTING TO POWERLESSNESS IN NURSING

Many factors have contributed to the nursing profession's relative powerlessness in health care policy setting. Six factors are discussed here (Box 19.1).

Oppression of Nurses as a Group

Nursing historically has been controlled by outside forces with greater prestige, power, and status. Generally, these forces were patriarchal and male-dominated such as medicine and hospital administration. Indeed, Ballou (2000) states that the health care environment, particularly hospital bureaucracies and physicians, have had oppressive effects on nursing's voice.

For example, historically, physicians' efforts to exclude women from knowledge emerging from the basic sciences, and their refusal to let nurses use new instrumentation sustained women's subordination in nursing, although many nurses themselves continually and actively sought greater scientific knowledge and techniques and incorporated these into their education. Nevertheless, the relatively powerless position of women in general society allowed physicians to achieve the subordination of nurses and other women health workers (Group & Roberts, 2001; Roberts & Group, 1995).

When a group is oppressed, it tends to have value confusion and low self-esteem. This occurs because the dominant groups identify their norms and values as the "right ones" and use their initial power to enforce them as the status quo. Oppressed groups accept these norms, at least externally, in an effort to gain some power and control.

For example, nursing's oppressors have not always held the same values as nursing (i.e., caring, nurturance, and advocacy). This has led to confusion for some nurses and even at times, contempt for their own profession and what it represents. In fact, Group and Roberts (2001) state that organized nursing and medicine are currently on a collision course, with the American Nurses Association (ANA) often taking positions on nurses' roles, rights, and range of practice in opposition to those espoused by the American Medical Association (AMA).

Discussion Point

Group and Roberts (2001) suggest that nurses cannot afford to "lumber along with an outmoded, gender-derived 'system' that fosters a predominantly male-dominated profession at the expense of the full usage of nurses and the members of other female-dominated professions." Do you agree with Group and Roberts? Is this feminist perspective warranted? Why or why not?

Failure to Align Fully with the Feminist Movement

A second factor contributing to nursing's relative powerlessness in national policy setting is the profession's failure to align fully with the feminist movement. As an occupation comprising primarily of women, nursing has suffered the same effects of gender stereotyping as have all women (Reverby, as cited in Ballou, 2000). Yet, while both nurses and women have improved their status in the past four decades, nursing has not kept pace with the progress women have made in other areas. This has occurred, because, at least in part, nurses have not been fully engaged in the feminist movement.

This occurred for several reasons. One was that many feminists in the 1970s were influenced by a more radical feminism perspective, and as a result, spoke out against women becoming nurses; instead they encouraged women to pursue medicine and other traditionally male occupations (Faludi, 1991). Nurses have also historically "exhibited a concern for gender issues somewhat later than that expressed by women external to nursing" (Group and Roberts, 2001, para 15). In fact, Faludi states that nurses clearly have a fear of public identification with feminism.

Discussion Point

Many nursing leaders in the early 1900s were political activists, actively involved in social issues such as suffrage and public health. At what point did nursing diverge from a sociopolitical agenda and why?

The reality, however, is that nursing continues to be a profession composed of approximately 94% women and this figure has changed very little over time. This is noteworthy given that there have been major gender shifts in virtually all the other traditionally female-dominated professions (such as social work, librarians, K–12 teachers) since the 1970s.

While having female dominance in the profession may have some benefits, it also poses some liabilities. Indeed, some nursing leaders have suggested that nursing will never attain greater status and power until more men join the ranks. Others think that adding men to nursing's ranks is not the answer. Instead, nurses need to accept the responsibility for addressing the problems that have historically plagued the profession and take whatever steps are necessary to proactively build a powerbase that does not depend on gender.

*CONSIDER: Being a female professional in a male-dominated health care system brings the "Ginger Rogers syndrome" to mind. Both Ginger Rogers and her dancing partner, Fred Astaire, were known as wonderful dancers, but Fred Astaire's name always came first and he always received the greater recognition. In reality, Ginger Rogers danced the same steps as Fred Astaire, but she did them backward and in high heels. So, who deserved the greater recognition?

Fortunately, there has been a resurgence of feminism in the past few decades and nurses have become more involved. For example, "feminist issues such as pay equity are now widely espoused by nurses and while an overt feminist analysis is still not common in nursing publications, such efforts could be classified as attempts to achieve greater autonomy and power—both important goals of feminism" (Group & Roberts, 2001, para 15).

Additionally, recognition that assertive, independent nurses cannot exist if they have been socialized to be dependent females is growing. Similarly, it is improbable, if not impossible, for female nurses to implement expanded roles in advanced practice if they are unaware of or unwilling to recognize the social constraints imposed on them because they are women. Indeed, the successes or failures of the nursing profession in its struggle to grow in stature and gain autonomy during its long history cannot be fully understood unless they are integrally linked to the relationship between gender and professional roles as these have changed over time (Group & Roberts, 2001).

Progress is occurring, however. A study by Ledet and Henley (2000) (Box 19.2) suggests that stereotypes of women as passive and dependent are changing and that women may no longer be penalized for using "gender incongruent styles of power" (p. 524) in the workplace.

Nurses need then to continue to examine the progress women have made in other professions and work with them inside and outside of nursing to strengthen power for women everywhere. This holds true for the men in nursing because the relative powerlessness of the profession transfers to them as well, despite gender differences. Both male and female nurses must solve problems, exchange current literature, and network to increase nursing's knowledge base and power, and provide mutual support.

Limited Collective Representation of Nurses

A third factor limiting the development of the nursing profession's power base is the limited collective representation of nurses by groups, such as collective bargaining agents and professional nursing organizations. For example, less than 20% of the nursing workforce is represented by collective bargaining agents (Fitzpatrick, 2001).

BOX 19.2

Research Study Fuels the Controversy

Perceptions of Women's Power as a Function of Position Within an Organization

In this study, introductory psychology students (N = 456) were given vignettes depicting people in a variety of occupations. In addition, they were given an adjective checklist adapted from the Bem Sex Role Inventory (Bem, 1974) and a power style scale by Hinkin & Schriesheim (1989). The students indicated what adjectives they believed represented the character in their vignette as well as that character's ability to use different styles of power

Ledet, L. M., & Henley, T. B. (2000). Perceptions of women's power as a function of position within an organization. *The Journal of Psychology 134* (5), 515–526.

Study Findings

Women in positions of high power were rated as more masculine than those in positions of lower power. In fact, women in high-power positions were perceived to be as masculine as men in such positions. There were no differences in power styles based either on gender or the position level of the vignette character. The authors concluded that "to the extent that perceptions of masculinity stand as a proxy for perceptions of power, this is a positive finding for women in the workplace" (p. 524). The authors also concluded that stereotypes of women as passive and dependent may be changing and that women may no longer be penalized for using "gender incongruent styles of power" (p. 524).

⎡ ***CONSIDER:** Nurses must be represented in mass, in some way, before
they will be able to significantly impact the decisions that directly influence their
own profession. ⎦

In addition, approximately 2,694,540 people living in the United States are educated and
licensed to practice as registered nurses (RNs), and 2,201,813 are employed as RNs
(ANA, 2004a). Yet, only 150,000 RNs are members of the ANA, the recognized professional association for RNs in the United States (ANA, 2004b). This is less than 6% of the
licensed RNs in the United States. This small membership number directly reflects the
money that is available for lobbyists to represent nursing in the political arena. In contrast, the AMA has one of the most powerful lobbying organizations in the United States.

There are many reasons for the small representation of nurses in ANA. The dual
and often conflicting role of the ANA as both a professional organization for nurses and a
collective bargaining agent is certainly one reason (see Chapter 17). Some nurses think
that state nurses associations have been burdened with the task of collective bargaining
under the federation model of the ANA and that other programs have suffered as a result of
funds being used for collective bargaining. Other nurses have expressed concerns about the
cost of membership in ANA or argue that ANA is not responsive enough to the needs of
the nurse at the bedside. Other nurses look upon nursing as a job and not as a career and
have little interest in professional issues outside their immediate work environment.

D i s c u s s i o n   P o i n t

Do you belong to a professional nursing organization? Why or why not? Do
contemporary nursing leaders espouse this as a value? Is it encouraged in
the workplace? In academe?

Whether these issues are valid or not is almost immaterial. The reality is that as
long as ANA has such a limited membership, and thus, limited economic power, its ability to significantly influence policy setting and legislation will be limited. Perhaps even
more importantly, until nurses are willing to work together collectively in some form,
they will be unlikely to increase either their personal or professional power.

⎡ ***CONSIDER:** At times, nurses have lacked pride in their collective groups and
begun to view alignment with other nurses as alignment with other powerless persons, something that does little to advance an individual's professional power. ⎦

This idea is certainly reinforced in Hagbaghery, Salsali and Ahmadi's (2004) study of 44
Iranian nurses, using semi-structured interviews and participant observation methods. In
this study, participants emphasized the importance of unity and its role in professional
power and stated that they considered the unity of nurses and the formation of professional unions and associations as the best strategies for strengthening nursing as a profession. Indeed, all participants in the study pointed out the disunion among nurses and
stated that it was one of the reasons behind their weakness as a professional group.

Although the research of Hagbaghery et al. was conducted in Iran, the implications for American nurses are apparent. Unfortunately, more often than not, nurses in this

country have not acted cohesively, whether it is at the local level fighting for wage increases or at the national level attempting to influence health policy. Even the various professional nursing organizations that nurses belong to have not worked together cooperatively and the reality is that nurses today are widely divided on basic issues such as entry into practice, mandatory staffing ratios, and collective bargaining.

> ✱**CONSIDER:** An analogy for increasing nursing's power base through collective action would be a snowball. Individual snowflakes are fragile but when they stick together, they become a force to be reckoned with.

Socialization of Women to View Power and Politics Negatively

A fourth factor contributing to powerlessness in the nursing profession is the socialization of women to view power and politics negatively. Women in particular, and thus approximately 94% of nurses, often hold negative connotations of power and never learn to use power constructively (Marquis & Huston, 2006). Nurses must recognize that power and politics provide opportunities for change—the chance to make things better for both nurses and clients.

> ✱**CONSIDER:** Changing nurse's view of both power and politics is perhaps the most significant key to proactive rather than reactive participation in policy setting.

Indeed, Ballou (2000) argues that professional nurses practice within a social, economic, cultural and political context. Nursing education, however, has historically focused their attention on the nurse-patient relationship. Ballou argues this is inadequate to meet the needs of society in today's health care environment and that there is a moral and professional obligation to participate in sociopolitical activities. Yet, there is abundant evidence that professional nurses, individually and collectively, are minimally involved at any level.

The phrase "the personal is political" seems appropriate here. Nurses must perceive a need not only to be more knowledgeable about power, negotiation, and politics, but also to be more involved in broad social and political issues. Nurses then must become politically astute. They need to understand what politics means and they need to become experts in using politics to help nursing achieve both its professional goals and the needs of their clients.

Inadequate Recognition of Nursing as an Educated Profession with Evidence-Based Practice

A fifth factor contributing to the nursing profession's relative powerlessness is the inadequate recognition of nursing as a profession driven by research and the pursuit of higher education. While nurses should value highly the caring, intuitive, nurturing part of nursing practice, the nursing profession has been negligent in equally emphasizing their extensive scientific knowledge base and the high level of critical thinking and analysis professional nurses use every day in their clinical practice.

Indeed, the Hagbaghery study found that professional power had a direct and mutual relationship with the application of knowledge and skills in nursing practice. In fact, the study's researchers conceptualized professional power as the nurse's ability to apply professional knowledge and skills and to provide care based on the nurse's diagnosis in response to client needs (Hagbaghery et al., 2004).

Both the art and the science of nursing require highly developed skills and a well-developed knowledge base. The nurse of the 21st century is well educated, with an incredible knowledge base in the sciences as well as the arts. In addition, nurses today must be critical thinkers, because they must continually look for and analyze subtle clues in their client data, make independent nursing diagnoses, and create plans of care. Constant assessment and adjustment to the plan of care is almost always necessary so that nurses must be highly organized and know how to set priorities. In addition, nurses today must have highly refined communication skills, well-developed psychomotor skills, and sophisticated leadership and management skills. This is the image nurses must promote to the public.

Discussion Point

If the public was asked to list five adjectives to describe nursing, what would they be? Would the art or science of nursing be recognized more? Would nurses themselves use different adjectives?

Profession's History of Being Reactive in National Policy Setting

The last factor discussed here as contributing to a relative lack of professional power in nursing is the profession's history of being reactive rather than proactive in national policy setting regarding nursing practice. *Reactive* means waiting until there is a problem and then trying to fix it. *Proactive* is more anticipatory; it means developing appropriate policy before action is taken or a problem occurs.

The level of downsizing and restructuring that occurred in health care in the 1990s was beyond most health care professional's expectations. And the nursing profession, as well as many individual nurses, was far from proactive in shaping its course. In the 1990s, health care became big business. Managed care proliferated and gatekeepers, not providers and consumers, began deciding who needed care and how much care was needed. Hospitals lost their place as the center of the health care universe as client care shifted from inpatient hospital stays to outpatient and ambulatory health care settings. Physicians lost much of their autonomy to practice medicine as they saw fit, as insurers increasingly placed restrictions on not only what physicians patients could see, but also what services the physician was authorized to prescribe.

Patients found themselves with limited choices of providers, longer wait times for care, more rules to follow, and more confusion about what would and would not be a covered expense. And RNs in record numbers, for the first time in history, were downsized, restructured, and often replaced by a cheaper counterpart, in an effort to reduce costs.

Many nurses felt both overwhelmed and helpless with this degree of change. However, these changes did not happen overnight. Many of them were incremental and insidious, and the health care system changes occurred with little concerted effort to stop them.

There is a brief parable that Peter Senge (1990) wrote about in *The Fifth Discipline* that nurses should keep front and foremost when they think about the need to be proactive, even with incremental change. It's called *"The parable of the boiled frog"* and it goes like this:

> *If you place a frog in a pot of boiling water, it will immediately try to scramble out. But if you place the frog in room temperature water, and don't scare him, he'll stay put. Now, if the pot sits on a heat source, and if you gradually turn up the temperature, something very interesting happens. As the temperature rises from 70 to 80 degrees F., the frog will do nothing. In fact, he will show every sign of enjoying himself. As the temperature gradually increases, the frog will become groggier and groggier, until he is unable to crawl out of the pot. Though there is nothing restraining him, the frog will sit there and boil. He will boil to death, oblivious to what is happening to him.*

*CONSIDER: Gradual, but constant change, may be even more dangerous than cataclysmic change because resistance is less organized.

Pierce (2004) argues convincingly that nursing can no longer afford to be reactive in the policy arena. Instead, she states that collectively, the nursing profession must decide what the significant priorities are and then construct a legislative agenda based on these priorities. The priority list can not be an exhaustive laundry list to combat all the profession's issues and woes. It must be strategic and timely to the debates taking place at the national level.

▶ DRIVING FORCES TO INCREASE NURSING'S POWER BASE

So what is the likelihood that the nursing profession will ever be a powerful force in health care decision making and the political arena? The answer is unclear although such a likelihood is increasing because several driving forces are in place to make that happen. Five forces are discussed below (Box 19.3).

Timing Is Right

Timing is everything. Although President Clinton's Health Security Act officially failed in 1993, the political ferment regarding health care reform continues to escalate. Issues of cost and access are paramount. Indeed, Families USA reports that 43.6 million people in the United States were uninsured for 2002 and an astounding 81.8 million people lacked health coverage for all or part of 2002 and 2003 (Byrne, 2004). In addition, the Bureau of the Census announced that the number of uninsured Americans increased by more than

---

BOX 19.3

Five Driving Forces to Increase Nursing's Power Base

1. The timing is right
2. The size of the nursing profession
3. Increasing knowledge base and education for nurses
4. Nursing's unique perspective
5. Consumers and providers want change

1.4 million in 2003 (U.S. Census Bureau, 2004). In addition, as a result of publications like *To Err is Human (1999)*, consumers, health care providers and legislators are more aware than ever of the shortcomings of the current health care system and the clamor for action has never been louder (see Chapter 14).

Woolhandler and Himmelstein (Byrne, 2004, p. 28) echo these concerns in their warning:

> *Our health care system is so sick that even people with good insurance are feeling the fever. . . . Employers have downsized coverage by super-sizing co-payments and deductibles. Insurance is proving to be illusory when it's most needed—payment denials, visit limits, loopholes and policy cancellations leave millions stuck with huge medical bills despite what they thought was good coverage. . . . Seniors can't afford drugs, Medicaid recipients face draconian cuts and everyone's rushed out of the hospital.*

Clearly the public wants a better health care system and nurses want to be able to provide high quality nursing care. Both are powerful elements for change and new nurses are entering the profession at a time when their energy and expertise will be more valued than ever.

Deborah Burger, President of the California Nurses Association, affirmed:

> *I believe that as nurses on the frontline of healthcare delivery who see the crisis up close, we and other health care workers should use this moment to insist that candidates—all of them—at the national, state, and local levels take a forthright stand for meaningful health care reform, universal healthcare with a single standard for all (Byrne, p. 27).*

Size of the Nursing Profession

The second driving force for increasing nursing's professional power base is the size of the profession itself. There are almost 2.7 million RNs in the United States. Numbers are the lifeblood of politics. The nursing profession's size is its greatest asset and its collective voting block is increasingly being recognized as a force to be dealt with.

Discussion Point

Have nurses ever made a concerted effort to vote collectively? What positions have professional organizations such as the ANA taken on recent election issues or candidates for office? Have endorsements by professional nursing organizations influenced how you vote?

One subject in Warner's (2003) phenomenological study of six nurse activists stated, "Individually, we make a difference. Collectively, we make a bigger difference" (p. 140). Another activist stated that when nurses were part of a collective group, they knew their voice was louder and their persuasion was greater.

Yet, the role of the individual in collective action is paradoxical. "Policy change is collective action. But there is no collective action unless individuals do something" (Warner, 2003, p. 141). The collective then does not negate the individual; rather it strengthens the individual.

An Increasing Knowledge Base and Education for Nurses

A third driving force for increasing the power of the profession is nursing's increasing knowledge base. Hagbaghery et al. (2004) affirm that knowledge is power, those having knowledge can influence others, nurses who have professional knowledge and use it in the context of efficient human relations gain credibility and a sense of power. Indeed, in a qualitative content analysis of interviews of 30 nurses, Kuokkanen and Leino-Kilpi (2001) found that expertise (knowing how to do the job) and possessing a wide range of knowledge were associated with the development of professional power.

> *CONSIDER: "Nurses who do not understand the legislative process will not be able to influence the policymaking process. A lack of knowledge about the legislative process further accentuates a sense of oppression and powerlessness" (Deschaine & Schaffer, 2003, p. 267).

Similarly, Warner (2003) found that the most important "currency" nursing activists brought to political interactions was their nursing expertise, which included clinical experiences with policy implications and connections as well as the unique values and skills acquired in nursing socialization. Fawcett (2000) echoes a similar theme in her assertion that nursing knowledge is critical to the overall future success of the profession.

Fortunately, more nurses are being prepared at the master's and doctoral level than ever before. In addition, leadership, management and political theory are increasingly a part of baccalaureate nursing education, although the majority of nurses still do not hold baccalaureate degrees. These are learned skills and collectively, the nursing profession's knowledge of leadership, politics, negotiation, and finance is increasing. This can only increase the nursing profession's influence outside the field.

Nursing's Unique Perspective

A fourth driving force for increasing the nursing profession's power base is the unique philosophical perspective nursing brings to the health care arena. Nursing's perspective is unique as a result of its blending of art and science—a blending of "caring" and "curing," if you will. The caring part of the nursing role is better known and better understood by the public. It's what historically has defined nursing. It is important that nurses not forget or under appreciate the unique values nursing represents because these are the values that make the profession different from all the others. These same values will make nursing irreplaceable in the current health care system.

It truly is a privilege for nurses to care, because it allows them to intimately enter so many lives, helping in very ordinary and yet extraordinary ways. It is important to remember, however, that important work does not always mean that the work is extraordinary. It often is as simple as doing little things like helping elderly patients eat their dinner or teaching a new diabetic patient to test his blood sugar or a new mother how to breast-feed. Sometimes, it's performing highly technological tasks such as inserting an arterial line or monitoring cardiac rhythms. More often, it's holding someone's hand and listening to their pain, grief, hopes, and dreams.

The "science" part of nursing is less understood by the public. Nursing has an extensive scientific knowledge base, and the high level of critical thinking and analysis professional nurses use everyday in their clinical practice is enormous. Nursing practice is increasingly becoming evidence based, meaning that nursing practice reflects what the literature says is "best practice." That is, the practice of nursing is research based and scientifically driven (see Chapter 3). Unfortunately, consumers, legislators, and sometimes even other health care professionals fail to recognize this. Nursing then must do a better job of both explaining and emphasizing both the art and the science of nursing practice.

Consumers and Providers Want Change

Finally, health care restructuring and downsizing is resulting in unrest for health care consumers as well as providers. Limited consumer choice, hospital restructuring, the downsizing of registered nursing, and the Institute of Medicine (IOM) medical errors reports were the sparks needed to mobilize nurses as well as consumers to take action. Nurses began speaking out about how downsizing and restructuring were impacting the care they were providing and the public began demanding accountability. The public does care who is caring for them and how that impacts the quality of their care. The good news, then, is that the flaws of our health care system are no longer secret and nursing has the opportunity to use its expertise and influence to help create a better health care system for the future.

▶ ACTION PLAN FOR THE FUTURE

Based on these driving forces, an action plan can be created to increase the power of the nursing profession in the 21st century. Strategies to achieve this goal are presented in this chapter (Box 19.4).

Place More Nurses in Positions That Influence Public Policy

First, more nurses must be placed in positions that influence public policy. Running for and holding elected office is the ultimate in political activism and involvement. As of October 2003, only 79 nurses held elected office in state legislatures across the country. A mere three nurses were in Congress: Rep Lois Capps (D-CA), Carolyn McCarthy (D-NY), and Eddie Bernice Johnson (D-TX) (Nurses Running for Office, 2003).

Nurses are uniquely qualified to hold public office and more nurses need to seek out this role. One nurse activist stated that during a federal internship, she realized her professional skills, related to leadership, communication, and "the ability to tackle problems and make things happen in a variety of settings," were what equipped her for participation in health policy making (Warner, 2003, p. 138). Another nurse activist reported that the versatility nurses demonstrate as well as the ability to grasp complex issues and keep many things on their plate at one time, are excellent preparation for the legislator role (Warner).

BOX 19.4

Action Plan for Increasing the Power of the Nursing Profession

1. More nurses must be placed in positions that influence public policy.
2. Nurses must stop acting like victims.
3. Nurses must become better informed about all health care policy efforts.
4. Coalition building must occur within and outside of nursing.
5. More research must be done to strengthen evidence-based practice.
6. Nursing leaders must be supported.
7. Attention must be paid to mentoring future nurse leaders and leadership succession.

Because the public respects and trusts nurses, nurses who choose to run for public office are often elected. In Warner's (2003) study of nurse activists, one participant credited her re-election to a partisan committee to the one word descriptor by her name on the ballot: "nurse." The problem then is not that nurses are not elected . . . the problem is that not enough nurses are running for office.

Stop Acting Like Victims

A second part of the action plan is that nurses must stop acting like victims. This is not to say that some nurses have not been victimized. Conti-O'Hare (2002) calls nurses who have been traumatized "wounded healers" and suggests that recognition of such trauma and use of that recognition is essential before nurses can effectively help others.

The reality, however, is that nursing, like any other profession, has its good points and its bad. It is so important, however, that nurses enjoy what they do for a career as it impacts everyone around them. If a nurse is unhappy in nursing, he or she needs to address what is wrong, rather than whine about nursing and act like a victim. There are too many opportunities within nursing that can be explored.

If a nurse is bored, new learning experiences should be sought. Nurses should not stay in jobs that make them unhappy. It only demoralizes everyone around them. They either need to fix what is wrong or leave and find a job that fulfills their expectations.

It is critical that each and every nurse never lose sight of his or her potential to make a difference. Some legislators and nursing employers have argued that "a nurse is a nurse is a nurse." This is wrong. Nurses can be whatever they want to be in nursing and they can achieve that goal at whatever level of quality they choose. The bottom line, however, is that the profession will only be as smart, as motivated, and as directed as its weakest link.

If the nursing profession is to be proactive, it needs to be filled with bright, highly motivated people who want to make a difference in the lives of the clients they work with as well as the health care system itself.

[*CONSIDER: Individuals may be born average, but staying average is a choice.]

Become Better Informed About All Health Care Policy Efforts

The third step of the plan is that nurses must become better informed about all health care policy efforts, but especially those that influence their own profession. This is difficult because no one can do this but nurses. This means grass roots knowledge building and involvement. Nurses need to be better-informed consumers and providers of health care. The skills needed to develop this type of political competence were identified in a phenomenological study conducted by Warner (2003) and included having nursing expertise, networking, persuasive skills, a commitment to collective strength, a "big picture view," and perseverance.

Discussion Point

Review the six skills identified by Warner (2003) that comprise political competence. Can these skills be taught? Do you believe as Warner argued, that political competence is within every nurse's skill set?

Warner (2003, p. 143) stated:

> ▶ | *To continue advancing nursing's collective political development requires more and more practitioners, educators and leaders to hone and express their political competence. Motivation for this growth relates to our commitment to influence the determinants of health, advocate for clients, contribute substantively in the creation of our health care system, and position nursing for its optimal role in delivery care.*

Each nurse, then, needs to decide how directly or indirectly he or she will be involved in politics and policy setting. Fortunately, nurses are in the enviable position of having great credibility with legislators and the public. In Warner's (2003) study, one participant noted that nurses are incredibly good at interpreting policy, talking to their members about it, and making connections. As such, interactions between nurses and elected officials often include clinical stories and data.

For nurses who choose to be directly involved in politics and policy setting, legislators can be lobbied either in person or by writing. There are many good sources on how to do both, including "10 Commandments" developed by NP Central (Influencing Congress, 1998) for meeting face to face with legislators, as shown in Box 19.5. For nurses who choose to write letters, the qualifications for offering input and the position on the issue should be stated clearly and simply (see Chapter 22). The legislator needs to understand why this is an issue that is critical to not only the nursing profession, but to his or her constituents. It is important, then, to create a need for the legislator to listen to what is being said.

Nurses can also give freely of their time and money to support nursing's position in the legislative arena. When giving money to a campaign, nurses should try to give early and to make as large a contribution as possible. It is the early and significant contributions that are remembered most.

Nurses interested in a more indirect contribution to policy development may work to influence and educate the public about nursing and the nursing agenda to reform health care. Either role is helpful—at least the nurse will have made a conscious decision to be involved.

Build Coalitions Inside and Outside of Nursing

The fourth step of the action plan to increase professional power is that the nursing profession must look within itself as well as beyond its own organizations for coalition

BOX 19.5	Influencing Congress: Ten Commandments
	1. Thou shalt know thy members of Congress.
	2. Thou shalt know about thy members of Congress.
	3. Thou shalt not limit visitations to crisis situations.
	4. Thou shalt know the members of Congress' staff people.
	5. Thou shalt have a focused and concise message.
	6. Thou shalt not commit effrontery toward someone else's project.
	7. Thou shalt visit the member of Congress in the District.
	8. Thou shalt get to know who the key members of Congress are.
	9. Thou shalt accept a turn-down or set-back graciously.
	10. Thou shalt not do thy lobbying like a lobbyist.

Source: *Influencing Congress. Ten commandments.* (June 21, 1998). N.P Central. Retrieved from *http://www.npcentral.net/leg/10command.shtml*.

building. One nurse activist in Warner's (2003, p. 138) study stated that networking, defined as establishing and maintaining relationships, is the "backbone of success in policy and politics."

Belonging to professional nursing organizations is one way nurses can network for coalition building. For example, Sigma Theta Tau International (STTI), the honor society of nursing, formed the coalition *Nurses for a Healthier Tomorrow* with leading health care corporations such as the American Red Cross and the Arthritis Foundation. This coalition has awarded numerous grants to members and increased funding that speaks to a host of issues facing nurses today. STTI has also forged coalitions such as the International Academic Nursing Alliance and partnered with Johnson & Johnson to address the nursing shortage.

Other coalitions also exist, such as the Health Professions and Nursing Education Coalition. This informal alliance of more than 50 organizations representing a variety of schools, programs, and individuals dedicated to educating professional health personnel, advocate for adequate and continued support for the health professions and nursing education programs authorized under Titles VII and VIII of the Public Health Service Act (American Association of Colleges of Nursing [AACN], 2002).

Coalitions have been formed within nursing groups as well. The Tri-Council for Nursing is an alliance of four autonomous nursing organizations: American Association of Critical Care Nurses, ANA, American Organization of Nurse Executives, and the National League for Nursing. The Tri-Council focuses on leadership for education, practice and research (AACN, 2002). Similarly, the National Federation for Specialty Nursing Organizations and the Nursing Organizations Liaison Forum, an entity of the ANA, merged in 2001 to become the Nursing Organizations Alliance (The Alliance) (National Gerontological Nurses Association [NGNA], 2003). The mission of the Alliance is "to increase nursing's visibility and impact on health through communication, collaboration and advocacy" (NGNA).

Nurses have not, however, done as well in building political coalitions with other interdisciplinary professionals with similar challenges. Pierce (2004), a nurse and congressional detailee in 2003, states that she saw firsthand other professions that were struggling with professional issues similar to nursing, such as scope of practice, critical provider shortages, use of technology, and serving the poor and underserved. Pierce urged nursing to build coalitions with these other professions and not to restrict problem solving and strategizing "to our professional silo" (p. 115).

Discussion Point

All too frequently, the AMA and the ANA stand in opposition to each other in the legislative arena. Are there current health care issues on which they could partner? Are there current issues on which the ANA and the American Hospital Association could partner?

Nurses have also not done well in building political coalitions with legislators. Most legislators have a great deal of respect for nurses but know little about their qualifications to speak with authority about today's health care system. Nurses need to become experts at political networking, tradeoffs, negotiation, and coalition building. They also need to see the bigger picture of health care. This is not to say that nurses should lose sight of client needs. It is to say that they must do a better job of seeing the bigger picture and of building and strengthening alliances with others before they will be seen as powerful and capable.

Conduct More Research to Strengthen Evidence-Based Practice

Another critical strategy for increasing nursing's power base is to continue to develop and promote evidence-based practice in nursing. Great strides have been made in researching what it is that nurses do that makes a difference in patient outcomes, but more needs to be done. Nursing practice must reflect what research has identified as best practices and a better understanding of the relationship between nursing practice and patient outcomes is still needed.

> ***CONSIDER:** Only relatively recently, has research been able to prove that patients get better because of nurses and not in spite of them.

Fitzpatrick and Smith (2003, p. 113) state: "Nurses and their colleagues must create, invigorate, and sustain environments of practice that promote clinical excellence and quality outcomes for patients. We must build models that reflect the principles of organization supported by the evidence and that are known to positively influence nurse-sensitive outcomes and nurse work life."

Building and sustaining evidence-based practice in nursing will require far greater numbers of master's- and doctorally-prepared nurse researchers as well as entry into practice at an educational level similar to other professions. Social work, physical therapy, and occupational therapy all now have the master's degree as the entry level into practice. Nursing cannot afford to continue debating whether or not a bachelor's degree is necessary as the minimum entry level into professional practice (see Chapter 1).

Support Nursing Leaders

Another part of the action plan to increase the profession's power is that nurses must support their nursing leaders and recognize the challenges they face as visionary change agents. Nurses have often viewed their leaders as rule breakers or deviants. Often, this occurred at a high personal cost to the innovator. Indeed Group and Roberts (2001) state that over the past three centuries, many women who have written powerfully on behalf of women, or activists who have moved politically against discrimination, have taken the brunt of societal condemnation by men and even some women. "In general, women can be activists as long as they agitate in behalf of others—children, sanitation, health, morality, and so on—but not for themselves" (Group and Roberts, para 11).

In addition, nurses often resist change and new ideas from their own leaders, and instead, look to leaders in medicine and other health-related disciplines. Some of this occurs as a result of nurse leaders being discounted, at least in part, due to their female majority, but also in part, to the low value placed on nursing expertise.

It is important to remember that typically, it is not outsiders that divide nursing followers from nursing leaders. Instead, the division of nursing's strength often comes from within. Nursing leaders must be perceived as its best advocates. Differing viewpoints should not only be acknowledged, but also encouraged. There is a proper arena for conflict and argument, but the outward force presented must be one of unity and direction.

Mentor Future Nurse Leaders and Plan for Leadership Succession

Finally, and perhaps most importantly, before nursing can become a powerful profession, nurses must actively plan for leadership succession and care for their young by providing mentoring opportunities. It is the future leaders who face the task of increasing nursing's power base in the 21st century.

Female-dominated professions have a history of exemplifying what is known as the *queen bee syndrome*. The queen bee is a woman, who after great personal struggle becomes successful in her career. Her attitude, however, is that because she had to make it on her own with so little help, that other novices should have to do the same. Thus, there has been inadequate empowering of young nurse leaders by older, more established nurse leaders. In other words, nurses really do "eat their young" sometimes. The mentor system, if used more widely in nursing, would result in an increased number of informed, articulate, and powerful leaders.

Discussion Point

Is the nursing profession proactive in planning its leadership succession or is it a change that occurs by drift?

Remember that it is the young who hold, not only the keys to the present, but also the hope for the future. We are responsible for assuring our leadership succession and are morally bound to do it with the brightest, most highly qualified individuals that we can. Pierce (2004, p. 115) states:

> *Leaders chart the direction, facilitate communication, inspire others, and perhaps, most importantly, provide hope. For the nursing profession to flex its collective political muscle and get involved with the redesign of the nation's health care system, we have to use our leadership to get the professional organizations to think and act collaboratively and to deliver a clear and strategic message to lawmakers. As nurses, as voters, and as constituents, we must be part of the solution.*

▶ CONCLUSIONS

Ballou (2000) states that nurses are the persons closest to and in most frequent contact with the vulnerable public. "As the health provider group with the broadest focus, nursing's perspective fits well with social, cultural, economic, and political impact on human health. Thus nursing is bet positioned to intervene on behalf of and with the public it serves" (Ballou, p. 181).

Yet Hagbaghery et al. (2004) caution that nurses cannot empower clients if they feel powerless. Ballou (2000) agrees, arguing that nursing cannot hope to accomplish sociopolitical change for others until it first empowers itself. Nurses then become empowered to empower others.

Nursing, as a female-dominated profession, will have to work harder and fight longer than male dominated professions to have a strong voice in health care policy. Right now, nursing lobbyists in our nation's capitol are influencing legislation on quality, access to care, patient and health worker safety, health care restructuring, reimbursement for advanced practice nurses, and funding for nursing education. Representatives of professional nursing organizations regularly attend and provide testimony at government agency meetings to be sure that the "nursing perspective" is heard on health policy issues.

More than 45 million people in the United States have no health insurance and another 60 to 100 million have inadequate coverage. Tax dollars paid approximately 85% of the roughly estimated $35 billion in care for the uninsured; yet the uninsured received only about half the medical care as those with health insurance (Jennings, 2004).

In addition, the United States is spending more than $1 trillion on health care annually—more than any other industrialized country, and yet rankings in terms of life span, infant mortality, and teenage pregnancy are much lower than many countries that spend significantly less on health care. The elderly in this country cannot afford prescription coverage and too many people lose their life savings trying to pay for catastrophic medical bills.

Clearly, nurses as health care professionals, need to have greater input into and control over how the health care system evolves in this country. We need a health care system that will guarantee basic, affordable health care coverage for all citizens and where all the members of the multidisciplinary health care team work together to create policy and provide care based on what is best for the patient. We also need a health care system that is accountable for its outcomes—that recognizes that individuality, autonomy, quality, and basic human dignity are essential components of health care services and that the bottom line is not always a number.

The nursing profession must be held accountable for being an integral force in shaping such a health care system. Indeed, nursing has a moral professional obligation, to those within the profession and to the public, to be engaged in social reform and political processes and sociopolitical activism may be necessary for viability of both the public and nursing (Ballou, 2000).

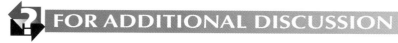

FOR ADDITIONAL DISCUSSION

1. Should the nursing profession target the recruitment of men into nursing in an effort to increase professional power?
2. What partners/external stakeholders should the nursing profession seek out in terms of alliances or coalitions to strengthen our position in the policy arena?
3. What are the priority issues the nursing profession should identify in creating a proactive legislative agenda?
4. Will nursing ever be able to increase its power base if it does not increase its educational entry level to a level similar to that of other health care professionals?
5. Do nursing schools currently provide enough content on politics, policy, and leadership for nurses to develop some degree of political competence? If not, what is missing?
6. Do most nurses internalize the need to be politically competent as a moral and professional obligation?
7. What issues currently being debated in the legislature have the greatest potential impact on nursing and health care?

REFERENCES

American Association of Colleges of Nursing (2002). Health Professions and Nursing Education Coalition (HPNEC). Retrieved May 6, 2005, from http://www.aacn.nche.edu/government/Coalitions.htm.

American Nurses Association (2004a). *Nursing facts. Today's registered nurse–numbers and demographics.* Retrieved May 6, 2005, from http://www.nursingworld.org/about/faq.htm#about.

American Nurses Association (2004b). *Frequently asked questions.* Retrieved May 6, 2005, from http://www.ana.org/readroom/fsdemogr.htm.

Ballou, K. A. (2000). A historical-philosophical analysis of the professional nurse obligation to participate in sociopolitical activities. *Policy, Politics & Nursing Practice, 1*(3), 172–184.

Bem, S. L. (1974). The measurement of psychological androgyny. *Journal of Consulting and Clinical Psychology, 42,* 155–162.

Byrne, M. (2004). Major candidates dodge health care solution. *Revolution–The Journal for RNs and Patient Advocacy, 5*(4), 27–28.

Conti-O'Hare (2002). *The nurse as wounded healer: From trauma to transcendence.* Boston: Jones & Bartlett Publishers.

Deschaine, J. E. & Schaffer, M. A. (2003). Strengthening the role of public health nurse leaders in policy development. *Policy, Politics & Nursing Practice, 4*(4), 266–274.

Faludi, S. (1991). *Backlash: The undeclared war against American women.* New York: Crown.

Fawcett, J. (2000). The state of nursing science. Where is the nursing in the science? *Theoria: Journal of Nursing Theory, 9*(3), 3–10.

Fitzpatrick, M. (2001). Collective bargaining: A vulnerability assessment. *Nursing Management, 32*(2), 40–42.

Fitzpatrick, J. J. & Smith, T. D. (2003). New solutions to new (and old) problems: Challenges facing the nursing workforce. *Policy, Politics & Nursing Practice, 4*(2), 112–113.

Group, T. M. & Roberts, J. I. (2001). *Nursing, physician control, and the medical monopoly.* Bloomington and Indianapolis: Indiana University Press. Retrieved May 6, 2005, from http://iupress.indiana.edu/textnet/0-253-33926-X/0253108616.htm.

Hagbaghery, M.A., Salsali, M., and Ahmadi, F. (2004). A qualitative study of Iranian nurses' understanding and experiences of professional power. *Human Resources for Health, 2*(9). Retrieved May 6, 2005, from BioMed Central at http://www.human-resources-health.com/content/2/1/9.

Heineken, J. & Wozniak, D.A. (1998). Power, perceptions of nurse managerial personnel. *Western Journal of Nursing Research, 10*(5), 591–599.

Hinkin, T. R. & Schriesheim, C. A. (1989). Development and application of new scales to measure the French and Raven (1959) bases of social power. *Journal of Applied Psychology, 74,* 561–567.

Influencing Congress. Ten commandments. (1998). N.P. Central. Retrieved May 6, 2005, from http://www.npcentral.net/leg/10command.shtml.

Jennings, C. P. (2004). "Insuring America's health: Principles and recommendations": IOM report (January 2004). *Policy, Politics, & Nursing Practice, 5*(2). 100–101.

Kuokkanen, L. & Leino-Kilpi, H. (2001). The qualities of an empowered nurse and the factors involved. *Journal of Nursing Management, 9*(5), 273–280.

Ledet, L. M. & Henley, T. B. (2000). Perceptions of women's power as a function of position within an organization. *The Journal of Psychology 134*(5), 515–526.

Marquis, B. & Huston, C. (2006). *Leadership roles and management functions in nursing* (5th ed.). Philadelphia: Lippincott Williams & Wilkins.

National Gerontological Nurses Association [NGNA]. (2003). *Newsletter headlines, 10*(2). Retrieved May 6, 2005, from http://www.ngna.org/html/memberres.htm.

Nikbakht, N. A., Emami, A., & Parsa, Y. Z. (2003). Nursing experience in Iran. *International Journal of Nursing Practice, 9*(2), 78–85.

Nurses running for office. (2003). *Capitol Update, 1*(5). Retrieved May 6, 2005, from http://www.capitolupdate.org/Newsletter/index.asp?nlid=72&nlaid=129.

Pierce, K. M. (2004). Insights and reflections of a Congressional nurse detailee. *Policy, Politics, & Nursing Practice, 5*(2), 113–115.

Roberts, J. I. & Group, T. M. (1995). *Feminism and nursing: An historical perspective on power, status, and political activism in the nursing profession.* Westport, CT: Praeger, Greenwood Publishing Group.

Senge, P. (1990). *The fifth discipline.* New York: Doubleday/Currency.

Sieloff, C. L. (2003). Measuring nursing power within organizations. *Journal of Nursing Scholarship, 35*(2), 183–187.

United States Census Bureau (2004). *Health insurance coverage 2003.* Retrieved May 6, 2005, from http://www.census.gov/hhes/hlthins/hlthin03/hlth03asc.html.

Warner, J. R. (2003). A phenomenological approach to political competence: Stories of nurse activists. *Policy, Politics & Nursing Practice, 4*(2), 135–143.

Wilson, D. M. (2002). Testing a theory of political development by comparing the political action of nurses and nonnurses. *Nursing Outlook, 50*(1), 30–34.

BIBLIOGRAPHY

Black, S. (2002). The joy of nursing. *Nursing Management-UK,* 9(1), 9–12.

Brown, C. L. (2002). A theory of the process of creating power in relationships. *Nursing Administration Quarterly,* 26(2),15–33.

Castledine, G. (2001). Nurse power and regulatory change. *Practical Nursing 12*(8), 309–310.

Hegyvary, S. T. (2003). Foundations of professional power. *Journal of Nursing Scholarship, 35*(2), 104.

Jenkins, S. R. (2000). Introduction to the special issue: Defining gender, relationships, and power. *Sex Roles: A Journal of Research*, 42(7/8), 467–490.

McIntyre, M. & Thomlinson, E. (2003). *Realities of Canadian nursing: Professional, practice, and power issues.* Philadelphia: Lippincott Williams & Wilkins.

Mpumlwana, N. (2000). The monster of professional power. *Teaching in Higher Education, 5*(4), 535–540.

Roberts, S. J. (2000). Development of a positive professional identity: Liberating oneself from the oppressor within. *Advances in Nursing Science, 22*(4), 71–82.

Vance, C. (2000). "Nurse power" transcends boundaries and barriers. *Nursing Spectrum (Washington DC Baltimore), 10*(20), 19.

Venamore, J. (2004). Nurse power. *LAMP, 61*(3), 32–33.

White, C. (2002). More nurse power under GP contract. *Nursing Times, 98*(18), 7.

Zelek, B. & Phillips, S. P. (2003). Gender and power: Nurses and doctors in Canada. *International Journal for Equity in Health, 2*(1).

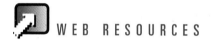 WEB RESOURCES

Academy of Medical Surgical Nurses (AMSN) Official Position Statement on Political Awareness for the Registered Nurse	**http://www.annanurse.org/pos_stat/ politic.htm**
American Nurse. Political Nurse. ANA PAC	**http://www.nursingworld.org/tan/00marapr/ politica.htm**
American Nurses Association	**http://www.nursingworld.org/**
Capitol Update—Nurses Running for Office	**http://www.capitolupdate.org/Newsletter/ index.asp?nlid=72&nlaid=129**
U.S. Congress	**http://www.congress.org/congressorg/ home/**
Fact Sheet on Workforce Issues (RN Voter)	**http://www.nursingworld.org/gova/ votefct3.htm**
Government Affairs—ANA in Action	**http://www.nursingworld.org/gova/**
How to Write to Your Legislator (2004)	**http://nursing.about.com/cs/legalpolitical/ ht/writelegislator.htm**
NP Central. Influencing Congress. Ten Commandments	**http://www.npcentral.net/leg/ 10command.shtml**
Nurse Anesthetists Political Action Committee	**http://www.ndana.org/NAPAC.htm**
Nursingpower	**nursingpower.net**
Nursing's Agenda for the Future	**http://www.nursingworld.org/naf/Plan.pdf**
The Impact of Women in Public Office (2001). Edited by S. J. Carroll	**http://iupress.indiana.edu/~iupress/books/ 0-253-21488-2.shtml**

Professional Identity and Image

Carol J. Huston

20

*I*mage consists of the way a person appears to others and includes appearance, words, behavior, and status (Sullivan, 2004). In other words, image becomes an unknown reality because people only have what they see and think to go on. Sullivan suggests that the public image of the nursing profession is, unfortunately, often one-dimensional and inaccurate.

If asked to describe a nurse, most of the public would use such terms as *nice*, *hardworking*, or *caring*. They would also use the terms *ethical* and *honest*. Indeed, annually, nurses rank very high as a trusted profession in the United States, higher than physicians and other health care workers (Nevidjon & Erickson, 2001). In fact, a 2002 Gallup poll on honesty and ethics places nurses at the top of the list of professions (Jones, 2002). Few people, however, would use the terms *highly educated*, *bright*, *powerful*, *well-educated*, or *independent thinker* to describe a nurse. Even fewer would call the profession *prestigious*. Indeed, Kalisch (2000) states that although physicians routinely rank first in public ratings of prestige, nurses rank 91st as a profession.

Many people would describe a nurse as a caring young woman, dressed in a white uniform dress, cap, and shoes, altruistically devoted to caring for the ill ("angel of mercy"), under the supervision of a physician. Common job functions would be identified as making beds, passing out pills, emptying bedpans, giving shots, and helping doctors. Some people, however, would allude, at least subtly, to a lustier image of sexy young females, dressed in provocative attire, seeking sexual gratification from both patients and physicians. Still others might depict stern, aged "battle axe" females thrusting hypodermic needles into recalcitrant patients, seemingly enjoying the discomfort they have caused and the power that they hold.

What do these portrayals have in common? Almost nothing, and yet everything. All are part of the convoluted, often conflicting stereotypical images of nurses. In addition, all of these images demean the true nature and complexity of nursing, and most are based almost entirely in fiction. Yet these stereotypes are pervasive, and efforts to change them have yielded only slow, but limited progress.

So, it is a strange dichotomy that faces the nursing profession. The public respects nurses and admires them, but does not consider the profession prestigious nor understands what nursing is all about. Many nurses believe nursing's image to be one of the most important issues they face as a profession. Others suggest that professional conversations and energy should shift from a focus on nursing's image to a focus on the spirit and mission of service, because service denotes a higher standard of leadership (Pesut, 1999).

The end result is that little changes. Old stereotypes of nurses as overbearing, brainless, sexually promiscuous, and incompetent women are perpetuated, as are images of nurses as caring, hardworking, altruistic, and selfless. This "image conflict" is an enduring issue for nursing, and the profession's efforts to address the problem have been fragmented and largely unsuccessful.

This chapter explores common historical and contemporary nursing stereotypes. The impact of these inaccurate stereotypes on recruitment into the profession and the collective self-esteem and identity of nurses is examined. In addition, strategies for improving the public image of nursing are presented as well as the challenges inherent in trying to change stereotypes that are ingrained in the profession's history and even in how nurses view themselves.

▶ NURSING STEREOTYPES

Of the many nursing stereotypes, the most common ones are shown in Box 20.1; the nurse as an angel of mercy; the nurse as a love interest (particularly to physicians); the nurse as a sex bombshell or "naughty nurse"; the nurse as a handmaiden to physicians; the nurse as a battle axe; and the male nurse as a gay, effeminate man. All of these stereotypes are profiled in this chapter. In addition, contemporary nursing images, as depicted in movies and on television, are profiled in an effort to better identify what images of nursing are currently before the public, especially the young people who represent the potential future nursing workforce.

Angel of Mercy

One of the oldest and most common nursing stereotypes is that of the nurse as an angel of mercy. When most people think of nurses as angels of mercy, the image of Florence Nightingale bringing comfort to maimed soldiers during the Crimean war comes to mind. Indeed, few individuals outside of nursing would recognize Nightingale as a politically astute, assertive change agent who used her knowledge of epidemiology and statistics to document the effectiveness of nursing interventions. Bargagliotti (2002), however, suggests that the nurse as an angel of mercy stereotype really found its roots in the 1930s as a result of radio programs and movies that depicted nursing almost as a holy vocation.

A more contemporary depiction of a nurse as an angel of mercy occurred in the 1996 movie *The English Patient*. In this film, a man injured in a plane crash was cared for by a nurse named Hana. Hana, at risk to herself, did everything she could to save this man's life. She also demonstrated supreme emotional strength as she watched her patient die, a quality that nurses often learn and gain through practicing their profession (Nursing Stereotypes, n.d.).

Being an angel of mercy is not all bad. Salvage (cited in Bridges, 1990, p. 851) says, "an individual worthy enough to hold the title of angel has a multitude of enviable qualities. The angel is compliant, willing, caring, and dedicated." This isn't far from the truth at all, as many nurses have these qualities.

Unfortunately, however, the angel of mercy image all too often also carries with it the belief that remuneration is not relevant compared with the privilege of doing good, and that any suffering experienced by nurses only adds to their virtue (Cunningham, 1999). This intrapersonal conflict between the values of altruism and pay befitting a professional is still experienced by many nurses today.

Love Interest (Particularly to Physicians)

Another historical stereotype of nurses is that of a love interest, particularly to physicians. Ryan (n.d., para 3) of the Romantic Times Book Club wrote "When doctor and nurse

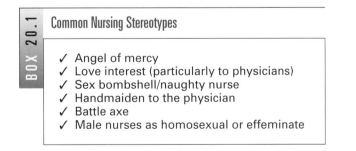

BOX 20.1   Common Nursing Stereotypes

✓ Angel of mercy
✓ Love interest (particularly to physicians)
✓ Sex bombshell/naughty nurse
✓ Handmaiden to the physician
✓ Battle axe
✓ Male nurses as homosexual or effeminate

romances first appeared in the 1930s and 1940s, becoming a nurse was one of the few career opportunities available to women, besides secretarial work and childcare. Nursing was a prestigious profession, requiring a capable and intelligent young woman who had the heart to dedicate her life to caretaking . . . unless, of course, she met a husband."

Once the nurse met her husband (usually a physician), her career would end and she would live happily ever after, devoting the rest of her life to caring for her spouse and children.

With the women's rights movement of the 1970s, women's career opportunities expanded and fewer books were devoted to women as nurses. In addition, readers' interest in medical romances dwindled. Elizabeth Johnson, senior editor at Harlequin/Mills & Boon (and editor of their Doctor & Nurse series of books), acknowledged that "several decades ago, the division was very much between a lordly doctor and a subservient nurse. Now the heroine is quite likely to be a doctor herself, and if not, she is likely to be a 'charge nurse.' That means her knowledge and power often match that of the hero; so the opportunities for tension and rapport are that much greater" (Ryan, para 5).

Romantic relationships between nurses and doctors continue to abound, however, on contemporary television shows such as *Chicago Hope*, *ER*, and *Scrubs*. It could be argued, however, that most of these relationships are not so much love interests, as sexual liaisons.

Romantic relationships between nurses and doctors also continue to be depicted in the movies. In 2000, the movie *Nurse Betty* depicted a waitress from Kansas who witnessed violence perpetrated by hit men. As a result of her trauma, she becomes disoriented and transforms into Nurse Betty—convinced that her favorite soap opera nurse character is real and that she's romantically involved with its lead character, Dr. David Ravell. The point of the movie is that Nurse Betty cannot distinguish medical soap operas from reality, and the implication is that nurses actively seek personal relationships with physicians.

Sex Bombshell/Naughty Nurse

Another common nursing stereotype is that of the nurse as a sex bombshell or "naughty nurse". Indeed, for at least 40 years, nurses have been portrayed as sex objects both on television and in the movies.

One of the most famous portrayals of a lusty nurse during the 1970s was the character Hot Lips Houlihan in the movie *M*A*S*H* (1970) and later in the television series (1972–1983). "The sexual exploits of nurses and physicians and the uncaring Margaret (Hot Lips Houlihan) provided few positive images of nursing" (Bargagliotti, cited in Cherry and Jacob, 2002, p. 32).

At the same time, nurses were increasingly portrayed in motion pictures and on television as "sexual mascots for groups of men, usually physicians" (Bridges, 1990, p. 852). Garbed usually in mini-skirts, sleazy low-cut tops, and high heels, the media-portrayed nurse of the 1960s, 1970s, and 1980s spent most of her time fulfilling someone's sexual fantasies and virtually no time providing care to patients.

More recently in the spring of 2004, a 10-week series entitled *No Angels*, depicting the lives of four young nurses, appeared on television in the United Kingdom. Three nurses who reviewed the show said the characters were "all smoking, all drinking, sexed up independent women, sashaying through the wards en route to another wild night of clubbing or a steamy clinch in the linen cupboard" (Allen, 2004, para 2). In fact, the press release for the show stated that *No Angels* was about the life, death, and lunacy inherent in nursing and the antics that nurses indulge in when they want to let off steam (Allen, 2004).

Nurses are even depicted as sex objects in contemporary television commercials. In 2003, Clairol Herbal Essences shampoo launched a commercial that showed a nurse abandoning her patient to wash her hair in his bathroom and then tossing her hair sensually at the patient as she leaves the room. Many nurses and nursing organizations, including The Center for Nursing Advocacy, condemned the unprofessional stereotype perpetuated in the ad and asked sponsor Procter & Gamble to discontinue it (Procter and Gamble Pulls Offending Ad, 2003).

Procter & Gamble issued an apology to nurses, stating that the company "holds the nursing profession in the highest esteem" (p. 35). The Center for Nursing Advocacy asked the company to counter the "lasting damage" of such an advertisement by running or contributing to a nursing image campaign like the multiyear initiative being sponsored by Johnson & Johnson to attract young people to the nursing profession (Procter and Gamble Pulls Offending Ad, 2003), but this did not occur.

Discussion Point

Do you think that the public truly believes a nurse would abandon patient care duties to wash her hair in a patient's bathroom and then sensually shake her hair at the patient? If not, does the commercial still cause harm?

Handmaiden to the Physician

Perhaps the most pervasive stereotype of nurses is that of handmaiden to physicians. In the handmaiden role, the nurse simply serves as an adoring backdrop to the omnipotent physician, demonstrating little, if any, independent thought or action.

*CONSIDER: Nursing care is frequently conceived of in terms of task performance and not as using independent thought or decision-making skills to fulfill its responsibilities (Schwirian, 1998, p. 38).

Bridges (1990, p. 852) states:

> *Stereotypical nurses in the 1950s and 1960s were weaker, less objective, and less skilled appendages of the medical profession. If ever in any kind of trouble, including personal problems, they would turn to the doctor for help. Since that time, nurses have continued to be shown as weaker beings with the actual nursing care being seen as simple and non-skilled.*

This same view of nurses as a handmaiden to physicians in the 1950s and 1960s was reported by Kalisch & Kalisch, pioneer students of nursing image in the 1970s. Indeed, during the 1970s, nurses generally had no substantial role in television stories, becoming a part of the hospital background in programs that focused on physician characters. When nurses were the focus of a program, the storyline frequently involved the nurse's personal problems, rather than his or her role as a nurse, and attributes such as obedience, permissiveness, conformity, flexibility, and serenity were emphasized (Kalisch & Kalisch, 1982).

Bargagliotti suggests this anti-intellectual view of nursing is influenced, in part, by the marginal percentage of nurses who hold advanced degrees and the public's confusion about the multiple educational entry points for professional nursing. Furthermore, he argues that the way in which nursing students are taught implies that for nurses, knowledge is burdensome (Barnum, 1989; Christman, 1991) "Nursing professors admonish students to learn so that patients will not be harmed or killed, while their medical counterparts teach their students that knowledge enables them to do something and subsequently that knowledge is power" (Bargagliotti, cited in Cherry and Jacob, 2002, p. 39).

Discussion Point

Should beliefs about knowledge building in nursing education be similar to those in medicine? Why have the two professions dealt with this issue so differently?

Battle Axe

Few stereotypes in nursing are as dark or demented as that of the nurse as a battle axe. Bridges (1990, p. 851) states the battle axe stereotype of nurses is that of "an overweight, authoritarian senior nurse who struts around with an air of self-importance, making the junior nurses cry and the patients quake under the sheets." Battle axe stereotypes of nurses have always existed; however, they seemed to hit their peak in the 1970s and 1980s.

*CONSIDER: Cunningham (1999) suggests that in a patriarchal society, men who are ill ridicule nurses as battle axes or sexually provocative people as a way to reverse the power relationship they feel when under the care of nurses.

The movie *One Flew over the Cuckoo's Nest* (1975) provides a perfect example of the battle axe nurse (Nursing Stereotypes, n.d.). Nurse Ratched, a nurse in a mental hospital, fits Bridge's description of a battle axe in almost every way. She craves power and control over all others and forces patients to obey her every whim.

Nurse Diesel, in the movie *High Anxiety* (1978), was another stereotypical battle axe nurse, with the addition of enormous prosthetic breasts. As an overbearing, evil charge nurse, Nurse Diesel continually displayed a dark sneer and a love of domination.

The Male Nurse: Gay or Effeminate

Female nurses are not the only ones who are stereotyped. Male nurse stereotypes are at least as prevalent. Unlike the mixture of positive and negative stereotypical traits for female nurses, the stereotypes for male nurses are virtually all negative, which only adds to the difficulty of recruiting men to the profession (see Chapter 9).

According to research done by Fisher, male nurses are frequently stereotyped as homosexuals, nonachievers, and feminine (Young, 2002). Fisher found that "people believed, regardless of what their sexuality was, that they [male nurses] were homosexual and feminine. Adding to this is a popular stereotype that male nurses are nonachievers for going into nursing, rather than another occupation [sic] such as medicine or physiotherapy" (Young, 2002, para 3).

Male nurse respondents in Fisher's study "also believed they were stereotyped within the profession itself. 'They believed that they were characterized as being lazy, career driven and preferring technical rather than caring tasks,' Fisher said. 'They also stated that they were disproportionately used for manual work—including lots of lifting and also dealing with aggression from patients and relatives'" (Young, para 4).

The most recent effort to depict a male nurse in a major motion picture was in the 2000 movie *Meet the Parents*. Unfortunately, despite the protestations of Greg Focker, the male RN in the movie, that he loves nursing and became a nurse by choice, his future in-laws and other relatives constantly question his sexual orientation and manliness. They also clearly imply that Greg must have become a nurse because his test scores were not high enough for him to qualify for medical school.

The Oregon Center for Nursing has undertaken a campaign to address these negative stereotypes of male nurses and to aggressively recruit men into the profession. The posters they have produced portray a diverse group of male nurses, and ask "Are You Man Enough . . . to Be a Nurse?" (Kleinman, 2004). In addition to the provocative headline, the posters feature pictures of a marathon runner, army veteran, motorcycle rider, Navy Seal, and rugby player—all of whom are nurses.

Contemporary Nursing Stereotypes on Television

Television medical dramas currently provide the greatest number of visual images of nurses at work. Two well-known medical dramas in the past decade have been *Chicago Hope* and *ER*. Both shows have included memorable nursing characters that both reinforce old stereotypes and create new ones.

In its 6-year run from 1994 to 2000, *Chicago Hope* focused on the lives, trials, and tribulations of the medical staff of a Chicago hospital while *ER* (1994–present) focuses on the lives and events of the emergency department staff at County General Hospital in Chicago, a level I trauma center.

As the chief surgical nurse in *Chicago Hope*, Camille Shutt was a drug-addicted, suicidal, man-hungry, chart-carrying charge nurse. She was also married to a doctor but divorced him during the series as she became more and more mentally unstable.

Carol Hathaway was perhaps the most well-known nurse on *ER*. After surviving the September 1994 pilot episode, in which she tried to commit suicide, Hathaway became the charge nurse of the emergency department. She went on to have a sexual relationship with a physician and bore twins out of wedlock. Nurse Hathaway left the show in 1999—supposedly to join her physician love interest in another state.

Interestingly, in a survey of 1,800 children in grades 2 through 10 in 10 cities, conducted by the health care group of JWT Specialized Communications (Sherman, 2000), Carol Hathaway was cited as the strongest image of a nurse. The students, however, felt she was more defined by her romantic involvements than her profession.

Even with the departure of Nurse Hathaway, *ER* continues to provide what are probably the most influential portrayals of nurses on television today. The Center for Nursing Advocacy (Summers, 2003) suggests that *ER* has generally depicted nurses as competent, caring professionals with technical training who contribute to patient outcomes. Yet one of the highest profile nurses remaining on the show is Abby Lockhart, an alcoholic former maternity nurse from a family afflicted with bipolar disorder. She started on the show as a medical student, dropped out of medical school, worked as a nurse, and now recently, has become a doctor. Abby has had sexual relationships with several doctors on the show.

In addition, Samantha Taggart, the newest nurse as of this writing to join the *ER* cast, is a tough, free-spirited, single mother of an 8-year-old child, who has already entered a sexual relationship with one of the physicians. In her introductory scene, Samantha (who has come to the hospital inquiring about employment), grabs a syringe and leaps to sedate an unruly patient through a central vessel in his neck ("*Boo!*" ER's *Abby Lockhart ...*, 2003). This behavior not only earns her a job, but the respect of her soon-to-be coworkers.

HOW NURSES FEEL ABOUT CONTEMPORARY DEPICTIONS

Most nurses are upset about their depiction in contemporary media, but their efforts to respond to and change the situation are fragmented. A more unified voice has been possible since the creation of the Center for Nursing Advocacy in 2001. The Center was created when Sandy Summers and seven other graduate nursing students at the Johns Hopkins University in Baltimore joined forces to address the media's disrespectful portrayal of nursing.

One effort coordinated by the Center for Nursing Advocacy has been to object to how nurses are represented on the television show *ER*. The executive director of the Center for Nursing Advocacy has written that *ER* "portrays nurses as know-nothing hand-maidens who blindly follow without questioning the heroic physicians" (Rester, 2003, para 3). Warner Brothers Television spokesman Phil Gonzalez counters, however, that the show "goes to great lengths to portray medical situations accurately" and that efforts are made to avoid erroneous depictions by having nurses serve as advisors on the set (*Washington Post*, 2003, para 3).

Still, Rester (2003) reports that nurses nationwide have inundated the show's producers with letters asking that they stop portraying nurses in an inaccurate light and suggesting that such portrayals are actively increasing the already critical nursing short-age. An "executive associated with the show [*ER*] who spoke on the condition that his name not be published" responded that *ER* is "'a television show, not a documentary' and asks 'Wasn't there a nursing shortage before *ER*?'" (*Washington Post*, 2003). The Center for Nursing Advocacy responded that *ER* is not the sole cause of the current shortage, but that influential media products like *ER* are one important factor related to the current shortage (*Washington Post*).

HOW INGRAINED ARE NURSING STEREOTYPES?

Increasingly, researchers conclude that inaccurate and negative stereotypes of nurses are not only well ingrained, but also instilled early in life. Indeed, gender stereotyping about career opportunities begins at a very early age. By the age of 3 years, most children already have firmly rooted gender-based ideas about the roles they can and should hold when they grow up.

The reality, then, is that by the end of middle school, many students report having their minds made up about desirable and undesirable careers. Indeed, in a study by Erickson, Holm, and Chelminiak (2004), students reported thinking seriously about career choices as early as 7th grade. Most students stated, however, that they had not considered a career in nursing, because they did not know very much about the field.

An unpublished study by Huston (*Nursing stereotypes engrained by second grade;* Box 20.2) suggests that basic beliefs and stereotypes about professions such as nursing may be ingrained at a far younger age, and that waiting until fifth, sixth, or even seventh grade to address inaccurate or negative images of nursing may be too late. Leonard and Iannone (2000) agree, arguing that recruitment efforts must begin at the

BOX 20.2

Research Study Fuels the Controversy

Second Graders' Image of Nurses

This unpublished study examined stereotypes held by 25 second graders regarding "important" nursing roles and functions. In an effort to introduce students to nonhospital nursing roles, which students stated they already knew, a 30-minute slide show and discussion was held, showing nurses actively engaged in less traditional nursing roles such as cardiac rehabilitation, primary care, flight nursing, education, management, and public health. In addition, nurse practitioners were introduced as primary care providers. Students were shown photos of nurses in all types of garb, except for white uniforms. Efforts were made to assure ethnic and gender diversity in all presentation materials. At the conclusion of the presentation, students were asked to draw a picture of what they thought was the most exciting role that had been presented for nurses.

Huston, C. (unpublished). *Nursing stereotypes ingrained by second grade.*

Study Findings

The caption on the first drawing was "the nurse is doing surgery on a real important disease." In the second, the nurse, with a red cross on her white uniform, was noted to be "rushing" into the hospital. In a third, the nurse, in her white starched cap, was making a hospital bed.

In a fourth drawing, the nurse was giving a hospitalized patient a backrub. In another, a dour nurse, as noted by a capital N on her starched, white cap with red cross on it, enters a hospital nursery. In the sixth, there was a patient in a bed, hooked up to an IV, expressing pain. The smiling nurse is walking away from him.

In the seventh drawing, the nurse was helping the child in the hospital bed and included a caption that the "nurse is in a rush." In another drawing, nurses were scurrying to patients in their hospital beds. Rushing, for nurses, seemed to be a recurrent theme.

In the eighth drawing, the most exciting role for a nurse was noted as transporting a cot from room to room. Similarly, another student noted that the most important thing a nurse did was to transport people to the operating room and yet another student noted that transporting patients in wheelchairs to their car was the most important thing that nurses did.

Several drawings included stern nurses, in white uniforms and caps, with red crosses on their chests, making patients take medicine that tasted bad. Others depicted nurses working in nurseries or teaching mothers how to care for a crying baby. Another depicted a flight nurse taking an injured patient to the hospital and yet another showed a nurse, in a white uniform with a red cross on her chest and wearing a cap, taking blood pressures.

All of the nurses in the drawings were female and white. The overwhelming majority wore white uniforms and caps, and had red crosses on their chests. All but one drawing depicted nurses in hospital settings. Many associated the nurse with pain or an unpleasant experience. Despite the educational intervention, these second graders already held deeply ingrained stereotypes about nursing and nursing roles, which were resistant to change. It suggests that if stereotypes are this difficult to modify in second graders, the challenges in changing the image of nursing with the greater public may be even more difficult.

elementary school level with the understanding that career choice is a process that begins early in life.

This has been clearly borne out in studies of high school students. In the JWT Specialized Communications study (Sherman, 2000), the older students, those in ninth or tenth grade, already had firmly entrenched ideas about nursing. They said they thought of nursing "as being technical as opposed to professional" (para 9). They also reported that they thought nursing was "more like shop, than a college degree" (para 9) and that they were unsure of career advancement opportunities and job security for nurses.

In addition, the students were quick to point out that nursing is a "girls' job" (para 10), and this belief crossed all age and ethnic groups. Indeed, male students had to be asked directly about their thoughts on nursing, because many automatically responded as if the discussion didn't involve them (Sherman, 2000).

The students also said "they had no compelling reason to be a nurse" (Sherman, 2000, para 7). Most knew at least one nurse and some had had an extraordinary experience within the health care system, but the nurses did not stand out in their experience or affect what profession they would choose to enter. Overwhelmingly, the students said they had been "drilled on what was good about becoming a medical doctor as opposed to virtually *no* positive talk about becoming a nurse" (Sherman, para 8). Erickson et al. reported that the young people surveyed in their focus groups, without exception, stated they had clear mental images of a nurse as "a young, sexy woman in a traditional nurse's uniform with a short skirt, white hat, and white shoes" (Erickson et al., 2004, p 83). This unflattering image of nurses created a perception that nurses were unprofessional and that their role in health care was trivial (Erickson et al.). Clearly, an early positive image for students is important if this is the population group the profession hopes will solve the current shortage.

Why the Stereotypes Persist

The domination and pervasiveness of nursing stereotypes is due, at least in part, to what has been called "nursing's invisibility as a profession" (Gordon, 1998, para 57). In 1997, Sigma Theta Tau International (STTI), commissioned *the Woodhull Study on Nursing and the Media*, which was conducted by the University of Rochester School of Nursing. This study analyzed 1 month of health care coverage in the media (2,000 health-related articles published in September 1997) to determine how often and in what context nursing was mentioned. The study found that nurses were mentioned in only 3% of health-related articles found in 16 major news publications, and in only 4% of the seven newspapers surveyed (STTI, Woodhull Study, n.d.). In the four news magazines, nurses were referenced in 5% of the health-related articles. In the five trade publications that focused on the health care industry, nurses were referenced in only 1% of the articles.

When nursing was mentioned, it was mostly just in passing; in many of the stories, nurses and nursing would have been more appropriate for the story's subject matter than the sources used (STTI, Woodhull Study). Recommendations from the study are shown in Box 20.3.

*CONSIDER: "The media will continue to miss major elements of health care news if it continues to disregard the contributions of nurses. By the same token, if nurses merely wait for the media to discover their emerging roles as researchers, educators, problem solvers, and practitioners, they are doing the public—whom they seek to serve—a disservice" (STTI, Woodhull Study, n.d., para 8).

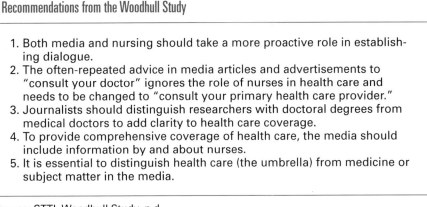

BOX 20.3 Recommendations from the Woodhull Study

1. Both media and nursing should take a more proactive role in establishing dialogue.
2. The often-repeated advice in media articles and advertisements to "consult your doctor" ignores the role of nurses in health care and needs to be changed to "consult your primary health care provider."
3. Journalists should distinguish researchers with doctoral degrees from medical doctors to add clarity to health care coverage.
4. To provide comprehensive coverage of health care, the media should include information by and about nurses.
5. It is essential to distinguish health care (the umbrella) from medicine or subject matter in the media.

Source: STTI, Woodhull Study, n.d.

Beauregard, Deck, Coughlin, Kay, Haynes, Inman, Perry et al. (2003) state that identifying a shared and accurate image of nursing is difficult given the diversity of roles nurses assume today and the lack of a common mode of dress. Indeed, nurses in this country began shedding their white uniforms in the 1960s as part of the anticonformist movement; the end result was that "the clear identity of the RN was blurred" (Mason & Buhler-Willkerson, 2004, p. 11). Patients complain that the nurse is unrecognizable to them or, worse yet, assume that everyone wearing a white uniform in hospitals today is a nurse. Beauregard agrees, arguing that "there is no clear image of nursing that encompasses our diversity" (p. 510).

401

Discussion Point

Is developing a composite nursing image that encompasses the diversity of nursing's responsibilities and its many roles, even possible?

CONSEQUENCES OF INACCURATE OR NEGATIVE IMAGES

Inaccurate or negative public images of nursing have many consequences, particularly because these images influence the attitudes of patients, other health care providers, policy makers, and politicians (Ellis & Hartley, 2004). Perhaps even more critical, given the current, severe nursing shortage, is that negative attitudes about nursing may discourage capable prospective nurses, who will choose another career that offers greater appeal in stature, status, and salary (Ellis & Hartley). The reality is that the *Jobs Rated Almanac for 2001* listed nursing low on career desirability, ranking only 137th of 250 career types (Williams, 2001).

Recruitment Challenges

One significant consequence of the public not understanding both the scope of practice and the skill level required to be a nurse is that it limits the profession's ability to recruit the best and brightest students. Whereas 30 years ago, a significant number of young people would have chosen to be nurse when they grew up, less than 5% of students responded so in a 2004 study (Erickson et al., 2004).

> *It's the public perception that nursing is the assistant to medicine, which is historical but so inaccurate in today's health care system. I think it is one of the major stumbling blocks to having very talented, smart men and women choose nursing today (Kathleen Dracup, in McPeck, 2004, p. 18).*

Like other predominantly female professions, the literature suggests that many clients and their families undervalue nursing and do not understand what it is that nurses do that makes a difference in patient outcomes. Indeed, many nurses will honestly admit they had little factual basis for what nursing would be like when they chose it as a profession. Instead, what drove them to become a nurse were actually images that emphasized the caring, nurturing, and personal rewards associated with the profession.

Self-Concept and Self-Esteem

Another consequence of inaccurate nursing stereotypes is that they may threaten the collective identity and self-esteem of all nurses. Mills and Blaesing (2000) found that nurses who were more likely to be satisfied with their career over time held three values: 1) a sense of professional status, 2) the belief that they made a difference, and 3) pride in their profession. All three of these values are challenged by inaccurate, negative nursing stereotypes.

Indeed, research done by Takase, Kershaw, and Burt (2001) found that nurses perceive the public's image of them as more negative than the way they see themselves. This is because they believe the public's perception of the nursing profession is influenced by negative or inaccurate nursing stereotypes.

Certainly this was the case in a follow-up study done by Takase, Kershaw, and Burt (2002), which showed that public stereotyping of nurses was related to the development of nurses' self-concept, collective self-esteem, and job satisfaction, all of which were associated with their performance. Takase et al. emphasized the importance of encouraging professional socialization and cultivation of positive, personal self-esteem to ward off the negative influences of public stereotypes on nursing practice.

The nurses in Takase's study might have been surprised, however, to see that the public, despite negative or inaccurate stereotypes, still thinks highly of nurses. In a poll of 1,005 Americans aged 21 and older, commissioned by Johnson & Johnson and conducted by Vanderbilt University, 95% of Americans reported that they trust, respect, and admire nurses. Eighty-three percent would encourage a loved one to enter the nursing profession, although only 21% stated they would consider nursing as a career for themselves (Domrose, 2002; Nursing Shortage, 2002). Only one male in 10 stated he would consider a career in nursing.

▶ CHANGING NURSING'S IMAGE IN THE PUBLIC EYE

Changing nursing's image in the public eye will not be easy. Nor will there be a silver bullet. Instead, multiple strategies are needed including active interaction with the media and restriction of the term *nurse* to mean licensed RN. In addition, nurses must increase their efforts to publicly praise and value nursing in addition to emphasizing how nursing uniquely contributes to patients achieving their desired health outcomes. Finally, nurses will need to become even more involved in the political processes that shape their profession.

Accomplishing this will take time and resources, including the time, energy, and funding of coalitions, foundations, and professional nursing organizations. Perhaps most importantly, it will take a concerted effort by individual nurses that will come only by first recognizing that there is a need to take action, and then by doing what is necessary to achieve that goal.

Finding a Voice in the Press

One of the most important strategies needed to change nursing's image is to change the image of nursing in the mind of the image makers. That means proactively seeking positive and accurate media exposure of what nursing really is and what nurses really do. This job cannot be left to professional nursing organizations or to the image makers. Nurses' self-worth needs to be recognized and proclaimed. Margaretta Styles once said, "We shall be vulnerable or invincible depending on our unity, our public visibility, our self-image, our reality orientation, our activism, our product development and salesmanship, and our accountability."

*CONSIDER: "Although some might argue that nurses have better things to do than worry about how the nurse is portrayed in the media, a consistently misrepresented image can negatively affect how the public views nurses" (Ellis & Hartley, 2004, p. 165).

Sigma Theta Tau International (*Benefits of Nurses* n.d.,) suggests that nurses are uniquely qualified to speak with editors, reporters, and producers on topics related to health care because they have a view from the front lines and are able to localize national health care issues. Nurses are also well qualified to simplify medical gibberish, explain the latest health care research, and identify current trends.

Nurses, then, must be taught the basic skills necessary to self-confidently interact with the media. Kalisch says that traditionally, RNs have been uncomfortable with image promotion because it's been considered "unladylike" to speak up about oneself. Yet, Kalisch argues that "the significance of the media in shaping our culture can scarcely be overestimated" and that "the mass media is virtually a 'second God.' It not only answers needs, it creates pseudo needs. It influences the way we feel about the world" (Kalisch, 2000, para 3). Nurses, then, must never pass up the opportunity to work with the media and should always view the media as playing a critical role in changing nursing's image.

*CONSIDER: Nurses are experts in health care. Our invisibility in the media is likely a result of nurses lacking the basic skills and self-confidence to get involved, not that the media doesn't want to talk to nurses.

Nancy Dickenson-Hazard, CEO of STTI, suggests that the Woodhull Study was a catalyst for nursing to learn how to relate to the media and for the media to learn about the contributions of nursing to health care (Manthey, 1999). Dickenson-Hazard argues that nurses must build relationships with the press by initiating contact rather than waiting for a call, and that they must cultivate those relationships on an ongoing basis.

Kalisch (2000), in a presentation to the Sigma Theta Tau chapter at the University of Michigan, sent a similar message in her challenge to members to reshape the image of the nurse through the media. Kalisch says this will require multiple goals and strategies, beginning with:

> *Get rid of modesty! Believe in yourself! Monitor and react to media images. Teach nurses the media skills that will assist them to write news releases; select photos; generate news stories. Hundreds of thousands of stories go untold. Don't wait for someone else to come around to talk to you. Actively influence media images by building strong media relations, including commendation or protest, and letters to the editor. Step up to the challenge to become the concerned health authorities on natural nursing subjects such as prevention and managing chronic illness (as MDs are on medicine). Get on talk shows. Write fiction and books for children. (My Daddy Is a Nurse is one interesting example.) Check the public library shelves for outdated depictions of nurses! If each of us does one thing, together we can make a big difference! Get rid of the stereotypes; do something! (Kalisch, 2000)*

Gordon (2004) suggests that public relation (PR) departments in hospitals also have a responsibility in terms of journalistic coverage of nurses. Journalists generally must call hospital PR departments to find out whom to talk to when covering a particular topic and to get permission for interviews. Yet, according to Gordon, many hospital PR departments conceal the contributions of nurses. In fact, hospital PR departments "are sometimes described as 'nurses' worst enemies,' and when PR staff direct journalists to the 'real' experts on, say, diabetes they are invariably doctors" (Gordon, 2004, para 10).

Gordon (2004) concludes that if the media are to inform the public about nursing, senior nurses must teach their hospital PR staff why nursing is important and what nurses really do—and then direct them to spread the message outside their institutions. Crucially, they must ensure that nurses feel comfortable talking to journalists.

Finally, nurses should recognize that media stereotypes are not limited to nonprofessional sources. A study by Aber and Hawkins (1992) suggested that advertisements in medical and nursing journals often included stereotypical and demeaning nursing images and that nurses were frequently depicted as dependent, passive minor figures on the health care scene. If nurses are not depicted accurately in their own trade publications, how can they expect representation in other types of media to be better?

Reclaiming the Title of "Nurse"

Another strategy needed to improve the image of nursing is to assure that use of the term *nurse* is limited to registered nurses. The International Council of Nurses (ICN) stated in 2004 that the term *nurse* "should be protected by law and applied to and used only by those legally authorised to practice the full scope of nursing" (ICN, 2004, para 1). In addition, all state boards of nursing have passed legislation restricting unlicensed personnel from using the title of "nurse." Unfortunately, however, on a regular basis, nursing aides and attendants either intentionally or unintentionally misrepresent themselves as nurses.

With the increased use of unlicensed assistive personnel and cross-training in the 1990s, a blurring of titles, roles, and responsibilities occurred between RNs, licensed vocational nurses, and unlicensed support staff. Name tags increasingly recognized all staff as "care partners" or "associates," and some hospitals went so far as to prohibit the listing of RN on a name tag. At the same time, a loss of differentiated uniforms further added to the public's confusion about who truly was caring for them.

RNs contribute to the confusion in how they introduce themselves to patients. Typically, nurses introduce themselves using their first name, followed by the statement that they are that patient's nurse for the day. Curtin (1994, p. 10) humorously notes that other professionals would never introduce themselves by saying "Hi, I'm Dick. I'm your doctor" or "Hi, I'm Larry, the lawyer." Nurses then must proactively introduce themselves to their patients, using their full names, and as the "registered nurse" providing their care. Bargagliotti (2002) points out that some nurses have declared the use of a last name may place them in danger, but states this is a difficult claim to support.

Finally, the media frequently perpetuates the misappropriate use of the term *nurse* by referring to all nurse's aides, volunteers who do health-related work, and medical assistants as "nurses." Spear (2004) argues that this haphazard use of the title implies that nursing is not a profession, but instead is something that anyone can do. Spear goes on to say that if the title "nurse" continues to be used in such a cavalier fashion, nursing will continue to be regarded as a health service requiring little or no formal education.

Positive Talk by Nurses, About Nursing

Another strategy for improving the image of nursing is to change how nurses themselves talk about nursing to others. "I think one of the things we forget to tell nurses, especially the ones that work on units, is how important they are and how much of an impact they do make in everyday life" (Suzanne Begeny, in McPeck, 2004, p.18). Instead, nurses frequently bad-mouth the profession and discourage young adults from considering nursing as a profession. Therefore, nurses need to be more alert to how they discuss their work in public.

Nursing, like any other profession, has strengths and weaknesses. It is important, however, that nurses enjoy their work, whatever it might be. Nurses should not stay in jobs that make them unhappy because it demoralizes everyone around them. Whining and acting like a victim do little to improve the situation.

Bargagliotti (2002) suggests that many high school guidance counselors report having heard negative comments about nursing from their advisees. When asked where the students heard these comments, they often report that they heard them from close relatives who were nurses, but are not currently practicing. "When nurses wonder why they are not highly regarded by young people, they may want to consider how they are portraying their profession in casual conversation with others" (Bargagliotti, p. 36).

Fitzpatrick (2002, p. 6) concurs, arguing:

> *Every nurse controls the image of nursing. Each of us has a choice to make—in every encounter, with every word. Although advertisements and scholarships go a long way to attracting nurses, it's up to us to do the rest. "I" is for image, but it's up to you.*

Summer camps for youth interested in nursing are one way that nurses can tell a positive story about nursing to young people. Drenkard, Swartwout, and Hill (2002) describe a 1-week summer camp in which young people interact with nurses and learn more about nursing. This camp for seventh and eighth graders is directed at increasing awareness of traditional and expanded career opportunities in nursing, increasing outreach to males and culturally diverse student populations, advising students regarding prerequisite courses needed to obtain a nursing degree, and establishing a social forum in which students could relate and nurture an interest in a nursing career. In addition, students are given opportunities for "hands-on" skill building and they are introduced to the nursing process (Drenkard, Swartwout, & Hill).

Erickson et al. (2004) advocate classroom visits by nurse "ambassadors," job shadowing, and participation in "bring your child to work days" as additional ways nurses can be positive role models for their profession. In addition, Erickson et al. suggest that nurses should visit youth clubs and organizations such as Boy Scouts, Girl Scouts, and the Boys and Girls Clubs to talk with young people about the benefits and rewards of a nursing career.

The bottom line is that nurses must tell the public that nursing is an essential service with equal worth to other professions; that it can provide many services better than other health care personnel; and that nursing is often more cost effective than other disciplines. The public's demand for nursing likely rests on the demand nursing creates for itself in the public's eye.

Emphasizing the Uniqueness of Nursing

Another tactic nurses can use to improve nursing's image is not only to emphasize its unique combination of "caring" and "curing", but also to underscore the depth and breadth of the scientific perspective that underlies its practice.

Evidence-based practice and the application of best practice principles are an expectation for contemporary professional nursing practice. Nurses, then, must emphasize how clinical research and the use of current best evidence impact their decision making and the care they provide.

In addition, newer research on nursing sensitivity and nursing outcomes is able to clarify what it is that nurses do that makes a difference in patient outcomes; there is increasing recognition that patients get better as a result of nursing interventions, not despite them. Generally speaking, however, the public knows very little about the research base that drives high quality, evidence-based practice, and it is nurses who are in the best position to tell them about it.

*CONSIDER: "Until the public recognizes the value of nursing services to the extent that it recognizes the value of physician services, the image of nursing will not change substantially" (Schwirian, 1998, p. 38).

Participating in the Political Arena

The political process can influence nearly everything nurses do and every problem they confront each day (Want Safe Staffing?, n.d.). In addition, public opinion is often based on inaccurate images, and nursing is no exception. Participating in the political arena, then, becomes a powerful strategy for changing the public's image of nursing.

The reality, however, is that although the nursing profession has some strong professional organizations, of the approximately 2.6 million RNs, fewer than 7% are members of national nursing organizations (Beauregard et al., 2003). This limits the profession's ability to be a force in the political arena. In addition, many nurses know little about the political process or feel too overwhelmed by the daily demands of their job to become involved in addressing larger professional issues in the political arena. Some nurses just assume that the best interests of the profession are being guarded by some unknown force out there. Legislators wonder if inactivity means simply not caring or not having an opinion. The end result is that nurses are inadequately represented in the political arena, and another opportunity for nurses to be represented as knowledgeable, active participants in the health care system is lost.

Because the underlying causes of the profession's political inactivity are numerous, just as the strategies needed to address this issue are complex, it is only discussed briefly here. Instead, a separate chapter has been dedicated to more fully discussing the issue (see Chapter 22).

Corporate Initiatives and Coalition Efforts

Clearly, the efforts of individual nurses to date have not been adequate to make significant changes in the public's image of nursing. New efforts by major corporations and foundations, however, hold greater promise.

One major corporate initiative directed at creating a positive image of nursing was launched by Johnson & Johnson during the Winter Olympics in February 2002. This 3-year, $20 million initiative, the largest corporate contribution to date that exclusively promotes nursing as a career choice (Fitzpatrick, 2002), was called the *Campaign for Nursing's Future*. The campaign was directed at recruiting new nurses and nursing faculty, promoting opportunities in nursing, and increasing awareness of the value of the nursing profession in society and America's health care system (Nursing Shortage, 2002).

The campaign saluted America's nurses through television and print ads with phrases such as "Dare to care, dare to cry, dare to feel, dare to try"; "Nursing . . . building a better world"; and "Nursing . . . it's real" (Fitzpatrick, 2002). In addition, Johnson & Johnson launched a 30-second public service announcement, established a website, and distributed recruitment materials, including posters, brochures, and videos, to 20,000 high schools, 1,500 nursing schools, and several nursing organizations.

In addition, *Nurses for a Healthier Tomorrow* (NFHT), a coalition of 43 nursing and health care organizations that have banded together to address the nursing shortage and improve the attractiveness of nursing as a profession, was launched in 2001. Their activities have included a 30-second public service announcement, the establishment of a website, and the development of posters and recruitment materials (Ellis & Hartley, 2004). In addition, NFHT has launched a national advertising campaign titled "Nursing Education . . . Pass It On." The goal of this campaign is to increase the number of nurse educators. Members of the NFHT coalition are shown in Box 20.4.

BOX 20.4   Members of the Nurses for a Healthier Tomorrow Coalition (Elizabeth Dole and Luci Baines Johnson, honorary chairs)

Academy of Medical–Surgical Nurses
American Academy of Nurse Practitioners
American Academy of Nursing
American Association of Colleges of Nursing
American Association of Critical-Care Nurses, AACN Certification Corp.
American Association of Nurse Anesthetists
American College of Nurse Practitioners
American Hospital Association
American Nephrology Nurses Association
American Nurses Association
American Organization of Nurse Executives
American Psychiatric Nurses Association
American Public Health Association
American Red Cross

(box continues on page 408)

Professional Power

Members of the Nurses for a Healthier Tomorrow Coalition (continued)

American Society of PeriAnesthesia Nurses
Arthritis Foundation
Association of Academic Health Centers
Association of American Medical Colleges
Association of Pediatric Oncology Nurses
Association of periOperative Registered Nurses
Association of Women's Health, Obstetric and Neonatal Nurses
Center for Nursing Advocacy
Chi Eta Phi Sorority
Emergency Nurses Association
Health Occupations Students of America
Honor Society of Nursing, Sigma Theta Tau International
Hospice and Palliative Nurses Association
International Society of Psychiatric–Mental Health Nurses
National Association of Clinical Nurse Specialists
National Association of Neonatal Nurses
National Association of Orthopaedic Nurses
National Association of Pediatric Nurse Practitioners
National Association of School Nurses
National Coalition of Ethnic Minority Nurse Associations
National League for Nursing
National Organization for Associate Degree Nursing
National Student Nurses Association
Nurse Practitioner National Marketing Campaign
Oncology Nursing Society
Society of Otorhinolaryngology and Head–Neck Nurses
Society of Pediatric Nurses
Society of Trauma Nurses
U.S. Department of Veterans Affairs

Source: Nurses for a Healthier Tomorrow, n.d.

◗ CONCLUSIONS

From a sociological perspective, conflicting stereotypes of nursing have not served the nursing profession well, and a disconnect continues to exist between reality and public image. The greater public clearly doesn't understand what professional nursing is all about, and the nursing profession has done a poor job of correcting long-standing historically inaccurate stereotypes. As a result, the competence, skill, knowledge, and judgment of nurses are—as the word *image* suggests—only a reflection, not a reality (Sullivan, 2004, p. 45).

Despite the generous contributions of corporations such as Johnson & Johnson and the forward thinking of coalitions such as NFHT, the responsibility for nursing's image lies squarely upon the shoulders of those who claim nursing as their profession. Until such time as nurses are able to agree upon the desired collective image and are willing to do what is necessary to both tell and show the public what that image is, little will change. Derogatory stereotypes are likely to continue to undermine public confidence in and respect for the professional nurse.

1. Historically, images of physicians in the media have been more positive than those of nurses. Why? What factors have led to this difference?

2. Some nurses feel that no longer wearing white uniforms and caps has reduced the professionalism of nursing. Is how nurses dress an important part of public image? Would reverting to more traditional nursing attire improve nursing's public image?

3. Would you want your son or daughter to be a nurse? What have you told them about nursing that would either encourage or discourage them from doing so?

4. Who are the most well-known nurses currently depicted in the media (radio, television, movies)? Do their characters represent nursing stereotypes that have been discussed in this chapter?

5. What do you believe to be the greatest restraining forces that discourage nurses from interacting with the media? Is media training the answer?

6. The contributions of Johnson & Johnson to improve the image of nursing and increase recruitment into the nursing profession are unparalleled. Why would a corporation such as Johnson & Johnson be interested in this pursuit? Why did such an initiative not originate with a professional nursing organization?

7. Are nurses themselves confused about what shared image they want the American public to have of their profession?

REFERENCES

Aber, C. S. & Hawkins, J. W. (1992). Portrayal of nurses in advertisements in medical and nursing journals. *Image: Journal of Nursing Scholarship, 24*(4), 289–293.

Allen, D. (2004). No holds barred. *Nursing Standard, 18*(24), 24–26.

Bargagliotti, T. (2002). The contemporary image of professional nursing. In B. Cherry & S. R. Jacob (Eds.), *Contemporary nursing. Issues, trends & management* (2nd ed., pp. 26–49). St. Louis: Mosby.

Barnum, B. (1989). Nursing's image and the future. *Nursing & Health Care, 10*(1), 19–21.

Beauregard, M. A., Deck, D. S., Coughlin Kay, K., Haynes, J., Inman, R., Perry, M., et al. (2003). Improving our image a nurse at a time. *Journal of Nursing Administration, 33*(10), 510–511.

Boo! "ER"'s Abby Lockhart abandons nursing for medical school, as newcomer Samantha Taggart assumes lone nurse role. (2003). Center for Nursing Advocacy. Retrieved May 9, 2005, from http://www.nursingadvocacy.org/news/2003oct31_er.html.

Bridges, J. M. (1990). Literature review on the images of the nurse and nursing in the media. *Journal of Advanced Nursing, 15*(7), 850–854.

Christman, L. (1991). Perspectives on role socialization of nurses. *Nursing Outlook, 39*(5), 209–212.

Cunningham, A. (1999). Nursing stereotypes. *Nursing Standard, 13*(45), 46–47.

Curtin, L. (1994). 25 years: A slightly irreverent retrospective. *Nursing Management, 25*(6), 9–32.

Domrose, C. (2002). *Mending our image.* Retrieved May 9, 2005, from http://www.nurseweek.com/news/features/02-06/image.asp.

Drenkard, K., Swartwout, E., & Hill, S. (2002). Nursing exploration summer camp. *Journal of Nursing Administration, 32*(6), 354–362.

Ellis, J. R. & Hartley, C. L. (2004). *Nursing in today's world. Trends, issues, and management* (8th ed.). Philadelphia: Lippincott Williams & Wilkins.

Erickson, J. I., Holm, L. J., & Chelminiak, L. (2004). Keeping the nursing shortage from becoming a nursing crisis. *Journal of Nursing Administration, 34*(2), 83–87.

Fitzpatrick, M. A. (2002). "I" is for image. *Nursing Management, 33*(6), 6.

Gordon, M. (1998). *Nursing nomenclature and classification system development.* American Nurses Association Continuing Education Nursing Classification II. Retrieved May 9, 2005, from http://www.ana.org/mods/archive/mod30/cec2full.htm#article1.

Gordon, S. (2004). Coast to coast media friendly. *Nursing Management—UK, 10*(10), 9. Retrieved from Ebsco Host 1354–5760.

Huston, C. (unpublished). *Nursing stereotypes ingrained by second grade.*

International Council of Nurses. (2004). *Protection of the title "nurse."* Retrieved May 9, 2005, from http://www.icn.ch/pstitle99rev.htm.

Jones, J. M. (2002). *Effects of year's scandals evident in honesty and ethics.* Retrieved May 9, 2005, from http://www.gallup.com/content/login.aspx?ci=7357.

Kalisch, B. (2000). *The image of nursing. Evolution and revolution.* Presentation to Sigma Theta Tau International, Rho Chapter, University of Michigan. Retrieved May 9, 2005, from http://www.nursing.umich.edu/stti/news/Kalisch.html.

Kalisch, P. A. & Kalisch, B. J. (1982). Nurses on prime time television. *American Journal of Nursing, 82*(2), 264–270.

Kleinman, C. S. (2004). Understanding and capitalizing on men's advantages in nursing. *Journal of Nursing Administration, 34*(2), 78–82.

Leonard, D. J. & Iannone, J. M. (2000). Recruiting future nurses: A collaborative project. *Nursing Connections, 13*(3), 55–61.

Manthey, M. (1999). Nursing's image with the press. *Creative Nursing, 5*(4), 4–7.

Mason, D. J. & Buhler-Willkerson, K. (2004). Who's the RN? Identifying nurses simply by the patch. *American Journal of Nursing, 104*(4), 11.

McPeck, P. (2004). Can we fix it? *Nurseweek, 17*(5), 17–19.

Mills, A. & Blaesing, S. L. (2000). A lesson from the last nursing shortage: The influence of work values on career satisfaction with nursing. *Journal of Nursing Administration, 30*(6), 309–315.

Nevidjon, B. & Erickson, J. I. (2001). The nursing shortage: Solutions for the short and long term. *Online Journal of Issues in Nursing, 6*(1)a. Retrieved May 9, 2005, from http://www.nursingworld.org/ojin/topic14/tpc14_4.htm.

Nurses for a Healthier Tomorrow (n.d.). *Our members.* Retrieved May 9, 2005, from http://www.nursesource.org/members.html.

Nursing shortage: Johnson & Johnson campaign aims to increase awareness, generate interest. (2002). *Nursing Economics, 20*(2), 93–95.

Nursing stereotypes: Images that underestimate the profession. (n.d.). Retrieved May 9, 2005, from http://www.english.iup.edu/eaware/nursing/.

Pesut, D. (1999). Inquiry, insights, and history. Leadership and a spirit of service. *Journal of Professional Nursing, 15*(1), 6.

Procter & Gamble pulls offending ad. (2003). *Nursing, 33*(8), 35.

Rester, M. (November 18, 2003). Nurses fault television's 'ER' for portrayal of the profession. *The Miami Herald.* Retrieved May 9, 2005, from http://www.miami.com/mld/miamiherald/7300067.htm?1c.

Ryan, K. (n.d.). *Doctors and nurses.* Romantic Times Bookclub. Retrieved May 9, 2005, from http://www.romantictimes.com/f_reader/f3a_5.html.

Schwirian, P. M. (1998). *Professionalization of nursing. Current trends* (3rd ed.). Philadelphia: Lippincott

Sherman, G. (August 28, 2000). *Memo to Nurses for Healthier Tomorrow coalition members.* Retrieved May 9, 2005, from http://www.nursingadvocacy.org/research/lit/jwt_memo1.html.

Sigma Theta Tau International. (n.d.). *Benefits of nurses as sources.* Retrieved May 9, 2005, from http://www.nursingsociety.org/media/benefitsofnurses_sources.html.

Sigma Theta Tau International. (n.d.). *Woodhull study on nursing and the media.* Retrieved May 9, 2005, from http://www.nursingsociety.org/media/woodhullextract.html.

Spear, H. J. (2004). What does it take to be called a nurse? *American Journal of Nursing, 104*(5), 58.

Sullivan, E. J. (2004). *Becoming influential. A guide for nurses.* Upper Saddle River, NJ: Pearson Prentice Hall.

Summers, H. J. (2003). *E.R. (1994-present). Portrayal of nursing (2002–2003 season).* The Center for Nursing Advocacy. Retrieved May 9, 2005, from http://www.nursingadvocacy.org/media/tv/er.html#SeasonPortrayal.

Takase, M., Kershaw, E., & Burt, L. (2001). Nurse-environment misfit and nursing practice. *Journal of Advanced Nursing, 35*(6), 819–826.

Takase, M., Kershaw, E., & Burt, L. (2002). Does public image of nurses matter? *Journal of Professional Nursing, 18*(4), 196–205.

Want safe staffing? Get political! (n.d.). Massachusetts Nursing Association. Retrieved May 9, 2005, from http://www.massnurses.org/News/safestaff/videopage.htm.

Washington Post highlights center's "ER" campaign. (2003). Retrieved May 9, 2005, from http://www.nursingadvocacy.org/news/2003nov18_washpost.html.

Williams, S. (2001). Split decision. *NurseWeek, 2*(4), 20–21.

Young, L. (2002). *Stereotypes of male nurses live on.* Retrieved May 9, 2005, from http://www.hesta.com.au/content.asp?document_id=675.

BIBLIOGRAPHY

Berry, L. (2004). Is image important? *Nursing Standard, 18*(23), 14–17.

Campaign tagline tells young people: "Nursing. It's real. It's life." (2001). *South Dakota Nurse, 43*(3), 19.

Davis, C. (2004). Nurse? Two views: A case of mistaken identity. *American Journal of Nursing, 104*(5), 58–59.

Doolan, E. (2000). Nursing: Image, politics, and the media. *British Journal of Preoperative Nursing, 10*(9), 474–476.

Feldman, H. R. & Lewenson, S. (2000). *Nurses in the political arena: The public face of nursing.* New York: Springer.

Jinks, A. M. (2004). Angel, handmaiden, battleaxe or whore? A study which examines changes in newly recruited student nurses' attitudes to gender and nursing stereotypes. *Nurse Educator Today, 24*(2), 121–127.

Ogden, R. A. (2000). Nursing image more than what the doctor orders. *Imprint, 47*(3), 4, 14.

Pierce, S. (2002). Image of the nurse on Internet greeting cards. Oregon Health & Science University. School of Nursing. Nursing 470: Research in Nursing Practice Class Members. *Journal of Undergraduate Nursing Scholarship, 4*(1), 10.

Saver, C. (2000). Nursing image what meets the eye. . . . and more. *Imprint, 47*(3), 48.

Stern, E. A. (April 7, 2003). Capping nursing stereotypes . . . Editorial ("Caps off to nursing"). *Nursing Spectrum, 13*(7), 4–5.

Stewart, R. (2001). A negative nursing image. *Australian Nursing Journal, 9*(2), 4.

Summers, S. J. & Summers, H. J.(2004)Viewpoint. Media "nursing": Retiring the handmaiden: What viewers see on *ER* affects our profession. *American Journal of Nursing, 104*(2), 13.

Young, M. (2004). Nursing image . . . When perception is reality. *Imprint, 51*(3), 6.

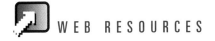 WEB RESOURCES

American Nurses Association: Planning a Career in Nursing	http://nursingworld.org/nursecareer/
Changing Image of Australian Nursing	http://www.ciap.health.nsw.gov.au/hospolic/stvincents/stvin99/Jacqui.htm
Looking for a Few Good Men	http://www.minoritynurse.com/features/nurse_emp/05-03-02a.html
Men in Nursing	http://www.hon.ch/News/HSN/516423.html
NurseWeek: A Few Good Men: Male Nurses Defy Stereotypes and Discrimination to Find Satisfaction in a Female-Dominated Profession	http://www.nurseweek.com/news/features/01-05/men.html
Nursing Stereotypes: Images That Underestimate the Profession	http://www.english.iup.edu/eaware/nursing/
Parent Times, The University of Iowa: Forget the Stereotypes: Nurses Explore New Fields	http://www.uiowa.edu/~ptimes/issues00-01/spring00-01/nurse.html
Regressive Nursing Stereotypes on a Major Network Soap Opera? No!	http://www.nursingadvocacy.org/news/2003oct24_cbs.html
Sigma Theta Tau, the International Honor Society of Nursing	http://www.nursingsociety.org
Stereotypes of Male Nurses Live On	http://www.hesta.com.au/content.asp?document_id=675

Advanced Practice Nursing: Challenges of Role Definition, Recognition, and Reimbursement

21

Margaret J. Rowberg

"The health system's increasing demand for front-line primary care, and the accelerating drive toward managed care, prevention, and cost-efficiency, are driving a need for nurses with advanced practice skills in this country" (American Association of Colleges of Nursing [AACN], 2004, para 17). As a result, there are currently almost 230,000 advanced practice nurses (APNs) in the United States. Of these, approximately 103,000 are nurse practitioners (NPs), 69,000 are clinical nurse specialists (CNSs), 14,600 are both nurse practitioners and clinical nurse specialists, 9,200 are certified nurse-midwives (CNMs), and 30,000 are certified registered nurse anesthetists (CRNAs) (American Nurses Association [ANA], 2004; AACN, 2004).

As a result of their advanced educational and clinical practice requirements, APNs have a greater scope of practice and more autonomy than registered nurses (RNs). Fifty states and the District of Columbia allow APNs to prescribe/furnish medications (Phillips, 2005). In addition, advanced practice nursing "involves critical decision-making on multiple levels that extends beyond the clinical setting" (Fields, 2000–2004, para 8).

Advanced practice nurses also usually earn higher salaries than RNs. In 2003, the average full-time salary for an NP was more than $69,000, although NPs who own their practices typically make almost $95,000 annually (Meyeroff, 2005). CNMs make approximately $60,000 to $90,000 a year and CNS salaries averaged almost $51,000 in the year 2000. The highest paid APN is the CRNA, whose average salary in 2001 was more than $116,000 (Meyeroff).

Even more impressive is the APN's impact on patient outcomes. Research suggests that APNs can provide 60% to 80% of primary care services as well as or better than physicians, and at a lower cost (ANA, 2004). This cost effectiveness reflects a variety of factors related to the employment setting, liability insurance, and the cost of education (ANA, 2004). In addition, the increased use of APNs has decreased infant mortality rates, cut inappropriate emergency department use, and increased immunization rates in children (Fields, 2000–2004).

The public has also responded favorably to APNs and to their characteristically longer visits with patients. "As APNs step out of the physicians' shadow and into increasingly responsible roles as health care providers, there is a heightened awareness of their value and skills, with some patients beginning to prefer the hands-on, unhurried care of the APN to that of their primary care physicians" (Hugg, 2002, para 5).

Despite these impressive numbers, much of the public is unclear regarding the role of APNs and their scope of practice. They also are unsure about their educational preparation or what the initials mean after the APN's name. They are also unclear if APNs are the same as physician assistants or other types of "physician extenders" or how their practice differs from that of a physician. Some people even erroneously believe that NPs are novices practicing to become licensed nurses. This confusion has resulted, at least in part, from nursing not clearly defining and delineating the roles of the APN. Even in the mid 1960s, De Young (1966) stated, "the public itself has not been able to identify differences" (p. 62) between the many individuals who provide care to patients. It is time to articulate, "what the professional nurse does" (p. 62). Unfortunately, 40 years later these comments still ring true for all levels of nursing.

Advanced practice nurses must face these issues head on. The roles of the APN must be defined and articulated to the public. In addition, shared nomenclature around job titles, professional credentials, and educational preparation must be pursued. Finally, the value of the APN in providing quality health care, not only in areas where other health care providers prefer not to tread, but also in mainstream America, must be better recognized.

This chapter will examine several of the critical issues facing APNs as they strive to become acknowledged as vital health care professionals in the 21st century. The challenges of defining the advanced practice role; of gaining recognition for the roles that nurse-midwives, clinical nurse specialists, nurse practitioners, and nurse anesthetists assume; of determining whether graduate and even doctoral degrees should be required for advanced practice nursing, and the issues surrounding reimbursement for the APN are discussed. The chapter concludes with a discussion of outcome studies that demonstrate the valuable contributions APNs make in our current health care system.

▶ ROLE DEFINITION: ADVANCED PRACTICE NURSING AND RELATED SPECIALTY AREAS

One of the first issues that surfaces in discussing advanced practice nursing is a lack of clarity regarding the definition of advanced practice nursing itself. The ANA (1996) defines APNs as registered nurses having "a high level of expertise in the assessment, diagnosis, and treatment of the complex responses of individuals, families, or communities to actual or potential health problems, prevention of illness and injury, maintenance of wellness, and provision of comfort" (p. 2). The complexities of this definition are not difficult to appreciate.

Hamric (1996) attempts to clarify this definition in her explanation: "Advanced practice nursing is the application of an expanded range of practical, theoretical, and research-based therapeutics to phenomena experienced by patients within a specialized clinical area of the larger discipline of nursing" (p. 47).

Unfortunately, Hamric's definition, while appropriate and accurate, loses clarity as a result of the complex terminology. A definition by the International Council of Nurses [ICN] (2003) is a bit clearer: "A nurse practitioner/advanced practice nurse is a registered nurse who has acquired the expert knowledge base, complex decision-making skills and clinical competencies for expanded practice, the characteristics of which are shaped by the context and/or country in which s/he is credentialed to practice" (para. 2). All of these definitions provide insight to the complexities of advanced practice nursing; however, the variety of role specialties encompassed by the term are not evident, and this is part of the reason so many people are confused.

*CONSIDER: If one looks at the medical profession, it seems evident that uncertainty does not exist for the public on the definition of a physician: A physician is a medical doctor. The public has a clear picture when hearing the "MD" acronym.

Currently, there are four identified areas of specialty practice in advanced practice nursing:

▶ Nurse practitioners
▶ Clinical nurse specialists
▶ Certified nurse-midwives
▶ Certified registered nurse anesthetists

While all these roles require specialization of knowledge and a high degree of practice autonomy, the roles themselves and their associated scope of practice differ greatly.

Nurse Practitioners

The California Association for Nurse Practitioners (CANP) (2004b) recently described NPs as: "advanced practice registered nurses licensed to provide healthcare independently, held to the same legal and ethical standard of care as physicians, with a commitment to giving personalized, quality health care to all" (para. 1).

The American Association of Nurse Practitioners [AANP] (2002a) describes nurse practitioners as APNs who "assess and manage both medical and nursing problems" (para. 4). In its scope of practice statement, AANP (2002b) delineates that NPs are "primary care providers who practice in ambulatory, acute, and long term care settings. According to their practice specialty, these providers offer nursing and medical services to individuals, families, and groups" (para. 1).

Clinical Nurse Specialists

The National Association of Clinical Nurse Specialists (NACNS) (2004) defines CNSs as nurses who: "independently provide theory and research-based care to clients in facilitating attainment of health goals, work with nurses to advance nursing practice to improve outcomes cost-effectively, and/or provide clinical expertise to effect system-wide changes in organizations to improve programs of care. The CNS is a licensed registered professional nurse who provides advanced levels of direct and indirect nursing care as defined by the state board of nursing. As such they assist other nurses and health professionals in both establishing and meeting the health goals of individuals and populations of patients" (NACNS, 2004, para 4).

Certified Nurse-Midwives

The American College of Nurse-Midwives (ACNM) (2004, para 2) defines CNMs as: "Individuals educated in the two disciplines of nursing and midwifery, who possess evidence of certification according to the requirements of the ACNM." Midwifery practice entails the "independent management of women's health care focusing particularly on common primary care issues, family planning and gynecologic needs of women, pregnancy, childbirth, the postpartum period and the care of the newborn."

Certified Registered Nurse Anesthetists

Finally, the Advanced Practice Special Interest Group (n.d., para 13) defines CRNAs as: "Advanced practice registered nurses who provide anesthesia and anesthesia related care. This care includes performance of pre-anesthesia preparation and evaluation; performance of anesthesia induction, maintenance and emergence; administration of local, regional and general anesthesia; establishing invasive monitoring; administering post-anesthesia care; the management of acute and chronic pain; and administration of clinical support functions."

D i s c u s s i o n   P o i n t

Given the diversity of these definitions and the roles identified, there is little surprise that the public lacks clarity regarding what is advanced practice nursing or what roles it represents. Is this a concern or should it be? Does this lack of clarity impact APN utilization or recognition?

Alphabet Soup—Clouding the Issue Further

FNP, APN, ANP, GNP, WHNP, PNP, ARNP, ACNP, CRNA, CNS, CNM, APRN . . . . To further cloud the issue, many APNs feel compelled to list every degree and/or certification after their names. While this may be an effort to increase credibility, it has only created more confusion for patients and providers alike. Each area of advanced practice nursing has its own unique set of educational and certification guidelines. CNSs and NPs are further defined into specific areas of focus. For example, although CNSs typically use a subtitle of CNS, NPs have routinely created a three-letter acronym to reflect their primary clinical focus. Consequently, one will find that family nurse practitioners are FNPs, pediatric nurse practitioners are PNPs, and so on.

Discussion Point

Should APNs have just one title and one set of letters to identify themselves? Do APNs do themselves a disservice by having multiple letters after their name or does it increase their status with the clients they serve?

A Name Is Just a Name?

One might argue, however, that having four major areas of focus—NP, CNS, CNM, and CRNA—does provide some clarity for the definition of advanced practice nursing. Keeping these four distinct titles provides the public and others in the health care system with a better understanding of the distinctness of APN roles but only if each is appropriately defined.

Historically, literature on advanced practice nursing suggested that NPs worked in primary care settings; CNSs were employed in acute care settings; CNMs delivered babies; and CRNAs worked in hospital operating suites. The reality, however, is that APN roles today are not so neatly proscribed. NPs often work at the bedside in acute care settings as more collaborating physicians request that they do hospital rounds, admissions, and discharges. CNSs are actively engaged in community and ambulatory care settings. CNMs provide a variety of maternal and child care services and in many cases, the agencies that employ CRNAs now extend beyond the hospital setting.

Does this variability complicate the definitions of advanced practice nursing or does it further exemplify the need to explain the similarities as well as practice differences in the roles? There are many opinions about this question. When asked the question "Would it be better to create one title that is all-inclusive?" Mary Knudtsen (personal communication, March 4, 2004), past president of the American College of Nurse Practitioners (ACNP), responded that nurse practitioners should eliminate all the categories of specialty and only put "NP" after their name with the area of board certification under the name. Physician-dominated groups, such as the American Academy of Family Physicians (AAFP) and the American Academy of Pediatrics (AAP), tried to simplify titles by grouping NPs with PAs calling them "midlevel providers" (MLPs), or worse, "nonphysician providers" (NPPs) or "nonphysician clinicians" (NPCs) (AAFP, 2004).

*CONSIDER: It is degrading and disrespectful to the nursing profession and all APNs to have another profession, particularly the medical profession, feel it has the right to choose a title for nonphysicians who are licensed and certified to provide health care.

The issue of credentialing letters is not likely to be solved in the near future. Barker (2000) suggests that "a nurse historian may well look back on this time period in a hundred years, viewing it . . . as a veritable semantic mine field and the current discourse on advanced practice as a rich source for analysis and deconstruction" (p. 89). He " ...challenges us all to reconsider the fundamental and often contentious question of what it means to be a nurse. Only with a sound understanding of what nursing is about can one begin to define what it means to be an expert or to provide 'advanced' nursing" (p. 90).

Barker goes on to ask, "When does advanced nursing practice become basic doctoring or something other than nursing? New roles must be integrated into nursing with a sound understanding of how such roles articulate with the philosophy and practice of nursing. Without starting from this position, nursing may be transformed into some form of super generic health worker, and the very things which lead nursing to be consistently rated by the public as the most trusted and respected occupational group may be lost" (p. 90).

The challenge remains as to how to develop an accurate definition of advanced practice nursing as well as an appropriate credentialing label for these dedicated health care providers. Although APN seems to be the acronym that is surfacing as the most acceptable idiom for advanced practice nursing, the issue remains that the public still does not have a clear understanding of its definition. It is paramount for all associations representing APNs to work together to develop terminology and definitions that are acceptable to the public and policymakers and that signify the role APNs assume in today's health care environment. Advanced practice nursing must clearly define its work to the public with a simple group of two or three letters if it expects to achieve the credibility that it struggles to have.

> ### Discussion Point
>
> Can advanced practice nursing associations work together collegially to create the needed terminology and definitions when nursing overall has had so much difficulty agreeing on key issues?

▶ ROLE RECOGNITION

Sometimes, "it seems as though advanced practice is synonymous with practicing behind the scenes" (Castner, 2001, p. 474). This is likely because advanced practice nursing was historically associated with caring for patients in rural, underserved areas as well as struggling to be recognized by insurance carriers as legitimate providers of care. Consequently, APNs have remained unknown to much of the public as well as many policymakers. Issues surrounding role recognition are related to confusion over the varied types of education, restrictions in scope of practice, and the lack of full prescriptive authority.

Education

Most education for APNs began out of necessity. Some of the first nurse anesthetists were recruited because physicians felt that women could adequately fulfill this role when other doctors did not want to accept the responsibility for anesthesia (Komnenich, 1998, p. 23). Consequently, much of the education for what have become advanced practice roles began in a manner, similar to that of registered nursing education: through hospital-based and hands-on training. Unfortunately nursing leaders did not encourage educational institutions to initiate graduate degree programs for advanced practice nursing until the mid-20th century with some certificate programs, particularly for midwifery and women's health NPs, still existing.

> *CONSIDER:* Is role confusion confounded because nursing has multiple methods for obtaining its education?

Advanced practice nurses are educated through a variety of programs, all with differing requirements. Of the four types of APNs, CNSs were the first to require education at the master's degree level (Komnenich, 1998, p. 27). In the 1970s, CRNAs began mandating baccalaureate or master's degrees (Komnenich, 1998, p. 25). Currently, CNMs are not required to have a master's degree. In fact, the Association of Certified Nurse Midwives (ACNM) has a position statement, written in 1992 but still current, which actually opposes mandating a master's degree for licensure (ACNM, 2003, para. 4).

Nurse practitioners are currently educated either through certificate programs or through universities that award a master's degree. Many of these programs are now assessing the need to elevate their programs to the doctorate level. Unfortunately, many currently practicing NPs and CNMs are only prepared at a certificate level. Authorizing certificate-prepared APNs to practice increases the likelihood that NPs will obtain their registered nurse education through a diploma program and then complete their NP or CNM education through a certificate program. Allowing certificate programs to continue is a disservice because it perpetuates the thinking that nursing, and advanced practice nursing specifically, does not have the same knowledge base as physicians and that APNs are not capable of providing the same level of care.

> *CONSIDER:* Not mandating that all APN specialties educate their students at the master's degree level opens the profession to questions by the public and policymakers about the level of expertise and critical decision-making done by these individuals.

The number of certificate programs has, however, decreased, as the culminating master's degree has become the norm. For example, in California, where an NP can still be licensed at the certificate level, there are 25 NP programs approved by the Board of Registered Nursing (BRN) with only 3 as certificate programs (California BRN, 2003).

The certificate programs that still exist, however, are at risk because NPs were required to have a master's degree in nursing, be nationally certified, and be recognized in their states as NPs on or after January 1, 2003 to obtain a Medicare personal identification number for the first time (AANP, 2002c). Exceptions were made for women's health NPs but they are to be master's prepared by 2007 to receive reimbursement from Medicare.

Discussion Point

How can the leaders in advanced practice nursing encourage a minimum of master's degree preparation without disenfranchising members who are not educated at that level?

The Clinical Practice Doctorate

Some nursing leaders have suggested that a master's degree may be inadequate for the scope of practice APNs are assuming. The AACN (2004) released its landmark position suggesting that a practice doctorate be adopted for APNs by 2015. A task force was convened and charged with assessing "the current status of clinical or practice doctoral programs, comparing various models, and making recommendations regarding future development" (para 1). The task force presented 13 recommendations for consideration to the AACN membership at the fall 2004 meeting. These 13 recommendations are listed in Box 21.1. In essence, the task force suggested that "the highly integrated health problems faced in the 21st century will be better served by clinicians who have the creativity and knowledge base...to create new models of delivery and that holders of the practice doctorate in nursing degree are expected to provide visionary leadership for the practice of nursing" (AACN, 2004, p. 11).

Furthermore, the task force posed that "given the tremendous time, credit and clinical experience required for master's degree APN programs, serious consideration should be given to moving toward the practice doctorate as the graduate degree for APN preparation...The challenge will be to identify, using an evidenced-based approach, the curricular standards associated with both master's and doctoral APN education and provide a seamless interface between educational programs" (AACN, p.13).

> *CONSIDER: AACN is recommending that nurse practitioner education be elevated to the doctoral level.

The controversy over the clinical practice doctorate will probably continue for many years but advanced practice nursing must reconsider what level of education is needed to adequately care for patients in today's health care system. Because NP programs struggle to include all current recommended content in the curriculum in a 2-year period, discussions are already occurring in regard to the need to extend programs to three years. If one considers that NP students already must achieve a bachelor of science in nursing degree, which takes a minimum of 4 years, and must then add another 2 to 3 years for attainment of a master's of science in nursing degree, requiring a doctoral degree for entry into advanced practice may create untold barriers to meeting the demand for health care providers, particularly in rural and other underserved areas. Requiring a doctorate, however, should reduce concerns by the medical community as well as the public regarding the ability of the APN to adequately care for patients. One must question, however, whether requiring a clinical doctoral degree is feasible in light of the ongoing nursing shortage, particularly for nurses prepared at the graduate level or higher.

Advanced Practice Nursing Competencies

To ensure consistency in education, the National Organization of Nurse Practitioner Faculties (NONPF) in partnership with the AACN developed competencies that cover education for adult, family, pediatric, gerontological, and women's health NPs (U.S. Dept. of Health and Human Services Health Resources Administration, 2002). These competencies are endorsed by the AANP (Towers, 2003) and the ACNP (ACNP, n.d.).

At the 2004 Master's Conference for the AACN in Phoenix, Arizona, there was extensive discussion about the multiple specialties within the advanced practice role that

BOX 21.1

AACN Recommendations on the Practice Doctorate

The Task Force recommends that

- The terminology, practice doctorate, is used instead of clinical doctorate.
- The practice-focused doctoral program is a distinct model doctoral education that provides an additional option for attaining a terminal degree in the discipline.
- Practice-focused doctoral programs prepare graduates for the highest level of nursing practice beyond the initial preparation in the discipline.
- Practice-focused doctoral nursing programs include seven essential areas of content.

The seven essential areas of content include:

1. Scientific underpinnings for practice;
2. Advanced nursing practice;
3. Organization and system leadership/management, quality improvement and system thinking;
4. Analytic methodologies related to the evaluation of practice and the application of evidence for practice;
5. Use of technology and information for the improvement and transformation of health care;
6. Health policy development, implementation and evaluation; and
7. Interdisciplinary collaboration for improving patient and population health care outcomes.

- Practice doctoral nursing programs should include development and/or validation of expertise in at least one area of specialized advanced nursing practice.
- Practice-focused doctoral nursing programs prepare leaders for nursing practice. The practice doctorate prepares individuals at the highest level of practice and is the terminal practice degree.
- One degree title should be chosen to represent practice-focused doctoral programs that prepare graduates for the highest level of nursing practice.
- The Doctor of Nursing Practice is the degree associated with practice-focused doctoral nursing education.
- The Doctor of Nursing degree title is phased out.
- The practice doctorate is the graduate degree for advanced nursing practice preparation, including but not limited to the four current APN roles: clinical nurse specialist, nurse anesthetist, nurse-midwife, and nurse practitioner.
- A transition period be planned to provide nurses with master's degrees, who wish to obtain the practice doctoral degree, a mechanism to earn a practice doctorate in a relatively streamlined fashion with credit given for previous graduate study and practice experience. The transition mechanism should provide multiple points of entry, standardized validation of competencies, and be time limited.
- Practice doctorate programs, as in research-focused doctoral programs, are encouraged to offer additional coursework and practica that would prepare graduates to fill the role of nurse educator.
- Practice-focused doctoral programs need to be accredited by a nursing accrediting agency recognized by the U. S. Secretary of Education (i.e., the Commission on Collegiate Nursing Education or the National League for Nursing Accrediting Commission).

Source: American Association of Colleges of Nursing, 2004. AACN draft position statement on the practice doctorate in nursing (pp. 5–15).

are being created by schools and universities. It appears that programs have had to focus on survival in these difficult economic times and so are creating new "specialities." It is paramount, however, for APN programs to develop strong curriculum that is consistent across programs and states.

Although core competencies have been developed, there is much room for interpreting these guidelines. Consequently, schools may have similar courses but the quality of those courses may vary greatly from one program to another. Because the public is unaware of these discrepancies, it depends on the regulating boards for the evaluation of all programs. In tough economic times, these boards have been stripped of needed funds and cannot always afford to monitor programs at the necessary level to ensure quality.

> * **CONSIDER:** In this time of critical nursing shortage and lack of nursing faculty, schools are creating new specialties in advanced practice nursing. Many of these specialties do not have certifying examinations or core competencies.

To overcome this dilemma, it is important that states require all programs grant a master's degree or higher and that all graduates obtain national certification. The public should not accept a lesser safeguard. If APNs are going to compete in today's health care environment, they must be educated at the master's level or higher. The CANP recently had a bill (A.B.2226 [Spitzer]) signed by the governor, which mandates a master's degree for nurse practitioners by 2008 (CANP, 2004a). The National Council of State Boards of Nursing (NCSBN) also promotes a master's degree in nursing or related field be required as minimum educational preparation (2002a, p. 4). This is additionally supported by the national certifying bodies, such as the American Nurses Credentialing Center (ANCC) (ANCC, 2003) and the AANP (AANP, n. d.) through their certification process, which mandates a master's degree to sit for the advanced practice examinations.

The time may come, too, in the not too distant future, when nursing schools may have to increase the length of advanced practice programs so that as science evolves, there continues to be sufficient basic instruction, particularly clinical hours, included in the curriculum. Specialization could then be an option as is seen in residencies for physicians. This will prevent the elimination or consolidation of key disease management courses that are vital to all basic knowledge.

In today's constantly changing health care environment, APNs must also have a basic understanding of business and technology. Tashakkori and Aghajanian (2000) discuss the importance of APNs having "the skills, credentials, and the knowledge in computer technology for communication, distance learning, diagnosis, and treatment" (p. 95). The NONPF (2002) has recommended increasing the business components in NP curriculum. Though each of these additions will place a burden on already overworked and underpaid faculty, advanced practice nursing must continually strive to maintain the quality it has worked so hard to achieve.

Discussion Point

Would extending the length of advanced practice nursing programs discourage nurses from seeking out these roles?

SCOPE OF PRACTICE: MEDICINE AND ADVANCED PRACTICE NURSING

Any discussion of role definition must include comments on scope of practice. Scope of practice in advanced practice nursing has been strongly influenced by its relationship with organized medicine. Physicians were the first health care providers to seek licensure by the states. Safriet (2002) states that, ". . . being first on the scene, physicians, perhaps understandably, swept the entire human condition within their purview" (p. 306). Safriet goes on to comment that since the physician's scope of practice was legally defined as "any activity directed at 'health or sickness,' especially if done for compensation" (p. 307), it created a hierarchy of care with physicians at the top. This authority was also construed to mean that physicians had the right to supervise all other health care providers, causing legislation to follow the same philosophy, to the detriment of the health care system.

As new groups, including APNs, emerged, and despite the evidence that each was well-educated in its particular field, existing law, social and economic forces, and a longstanding history of physicians defending their turf, prevented the creation of scopes of practice that accurately define the type of care being provided. If the right was obtained, it was usually only with some mandate on physician referral or supervision (Safriet, 2002).

Discussion Point

Should one profession have the right to mandate scope of practice for other professionals in related fields?

This paternalism is apparent in a statement released by the physician-dominated AAP regarding scope of practice issues in the delivery of pediatric health care. This policy commented that because "non-physician clinicians have succeeded in increasing their autonomy and scope of practice..." the AAP must adopt regulations that protect patient safety and ensure effective quality of health care for all infants, children, adolescents, and young adults" (AAP, 2003, p. 426). This is a rather presumptuous statement when it has been documented in several studies (Hooker & McCaig, 2001; Mundinger, et al., 2000) that APNs provide care equal to or better than physicians. The reality is that advanced practice nursing has not focused on expanding its scope of practice as the AAP policy statement implies; rather it has spent much energy on trying to more clearly define its roles.

CRNAs and CNMs have been fairly successful at defining their roles. CNSs and NPs have been less successful. According to Towers (2004), "NPs are recognized as primary care providers in statute or administrative rule in only twenty-six states" (p. 530). Eight states do not specifically mention nurse practitioners as providers (Towers, 2004).

An interesting but much needed change occurred, however, when the Joint Commission on Accreditation of Healthcare Organizations (JCAHO) included APNs in its standards as part of its "Shared Visions—New Pathways" initiative begun in 2002 (Towers, 2004). The new revisions incorporated the credentialing of APNs and PAs as part of the requirement for hospital accreditation. Although in existence for several years, in states where APNs are not recognized as providers, it remains to be shown whether JCAHO is enforcing this standard.

Safriet (2002) provides some practical guidance in this confused state of affairs. She discusses some of the needed changes that must occur if "nonphysician clinicians" are to survive. These include "greater consistency in scope of practice laws . . . with regulation as expansive as possible, consistent with safe and effective practice" (p. 323). "Increased flexibility in the regulatory process in order to facilitate the functional expansion of existing roles and the recognition of emerging roles, and . . . reform must explicitly acknowledge, and accommodate, existing and evolving overlaps among the professional competencies of various HCP (health care provider) groups" (p. 324).

Safriet (2002) goes on to state that: "by perpetuating a 'mine, and therefore not yours' practice culture, current laws erect, rather than remove, barriers to interprofessional collaboration, practice, and respect. They also continue to divert attention and resources from the business at hand: seeing to the well being of people who need health care. . . ." (p. 325).

Finally, Safriet (2002) provides an excellent discussion about APNs achieving equal status as providers when she states that:

> ▶ *. . . only physicians are free of the burden of having to reconcile their clinical abilities and their legal authority. That is they have a monopoly on authority, if not on ability. All others, including both long-established and emerging professions, must constantly choose between two unattractive alternatives: foregoing the safe practice of what they have been educated and trained to do, or risking legal sanction for stepping outside the boundaries of their legislatively-defined, static, circumscribed, and outdated scopes of practice. This double dichotomy– between legal authority and clinical ability and between physicians and all other HCPs -is the motive force behind the needless and never-ending legislative and regulatory battles that cripple our current system. Even more importantly, this double dichotomy means that the many qualified health care providers cannot give safe and effective care to people who want and need their services (p. 305).*

The key component heard throughout Safriet's writing is that laws must focus on clinical ability rather than physician dominance. Only through the assessment of the education and training of each provider can legislators decide whether a particular group provides safe and competent health care.

Phillips, Green, Fryer, and Dovey (2001) echo Safriet's concern in their assertion that "variations (in state regulations) exemplify and exacerbate a growing professional schism. Although many NPs and physicians enjoy successful collaboration, regulatory variations and the professional turf battles that cause this gap, threaten to make such collaboration more difficult" (p. 1325). They further comment "credible evidence showing that collaboration improves health outcomes for patients entreats the two professions to put cooperation before professional roles...A combined, sustained effort is urgently needed to permit new policies for redesigning and improving the U.S. health care system" (p. 1325).

Any fears that legislators may have in accepting the doctrine that APNs are held to the same standard as physicians should be allayed if they review and accept guidelines developed by the NCSBN. The NCSBN (2000) developed criteria for uniform advanced practice registered nurse licensure and authority to practice that could be adopted by state boards of nursing and would allow APNs to practice across state lines. At its delegate assembly in 2002, the NCSBN members voted to adopt this doctrine (NCSBN, 2002b).

BOX 21.2

General Purposes of the Advanced Practice Registered Nurse Compact

- Facilitate the states' responsibilities to protect the public's health and safety.
- Ensure and encourage the cooperation of party states in the areas of advanced practice registered nurse (APRN) licensure/authority to practice and regulation including promotion of uniform licensure requirements.
- Facilitate the exchange of information between party states in the areas of APRN regulation, investigation and adverse actions.
- Promote compliance with the laws governing APRN practice in each jurisdiction.
- Invest all party states with the authority to hold an APRN accountable for meeting state practice laws in the state in which the patient is located at the time care is rendered through the mutual recognition of party state licenses.

NCSBN, n. d., para. 2.

It builds upon the RN/LPN Licensure Compact adopted by the NCSBN in 1999 (NCSBN, 2000). The general purposes of the APRN Compact can be found in Box 21.2.

*CONSIDER: Scope of practice issues will continue as long as the medical profession is intent on controlling other providers. Perhaps, instead, it should be focused on the quality of health care being provided.

Prescriptive Authority

One of the most significant ongoing issues for advanced practice nursing is the right to prescribe medications. Depending on location, NPs and CNSs are permitted to write prescriptions but state law limits their autonomy. According to the most recent data for NPs and other APNs, only 13 states and the District of Columbia have full prescriptive authority (Phillips, 2005, p. 17). There are four states where NPs can prescribe medications but are not allowed to write prescriptions for controlled substances. Thirty-seven states still require some level of physician oversight (Phillips, 2005, p.17).

Discussion Point

Why is there such great variance among states in terms of prescriptive authority for APNs? What are the roots of this variance?

Towers (2004) relates that "the majority of the barriers to practice have roots in organized lobbying by certain parts of the medical community to limit the autonomy of APNs" (p.130). She further discusses that:

> *Confusion about the role and scope of practice of an APN through grouping of NPs, nurse-midwives, and PAs as "midlevel practitioners" has created problems for APNs. It is often assumed that the required supervisory arrangements*

for PAs is the same for NPs and nurse-midwives, so that policies related to practice, including prescriptive authority and ordering of medications for patients, are often based on statutes and rules governing PAs rather than the APNs (p. 131).

In a study conducted in Washington State on barriers to prescribing, Kaplan and Brown (2004) found that there were three recurring themes: physician concerns about liability, physicians choosing a different drug than the NP had selected, and physicians being reluctant to prescribe the drug selected by the NP. APNs must recognize these ongoing issues and begin the work needed to overcome these hurdles.

Florida is one state that continues an uphill battle toward prescriptive freedom. Although APNs in that state have the right to prescribe, they face daily fights with the Florida Medical Association on gaining the privilege to prescribe controlled substances. Unfortunately, the battle has been fought in the press, creating obvious confusion on the part of the public (R. Green, personal communication, March 25, 2004). The public does not understand the issues surrounding prescriptive authority and must rely on what it perceives as experts. Unfortunately, it perceives the experts as the physicians because APNs have not adequately educated the public on their role.

Similarly, in a study conducted in Georgia, it was concluded that APNs are "ordering medications appropriately without physician input" (Hodnicki et al., 2004, p. 24). Barriers persist because the physician must sign the prescription, causing increased wait time and delay of treatment (p. 23).

The public and the medical profession should feel confident that APNs have the educational background as well as the years of experience as registered nurses that provide the basis for prescribing accurately and safely. Only when APNs have full prescriptive authority, without the requirement of physician collaboration and/or supervision, will patients begin to understand the extent of their abilities to provide safe and competent care.

Reimbursement

Castner (2001) reports, "having the ability to bill places a value to our work" (p. 474). Obtaining the right to be reimbursed for services has been a long-fought battle for APNs. Robinson (2004) states, even though the "four advanced practice roles have been well established for decades, direct reimbursement for their services has been difficult to obtain"(p. 100). Earlier, Lindeke and Chesney (1999) reported that "despite increasing public acceptance of APNs, nurses continue to express frustration at being shut out of health systems and hindered by reimbursement barriers persistent in today's competitive managed care market" (p. 248). They found there were three recurring themes related to reimbursement. They were:

1. Lack of APN recognition by managed care organizations and third-party payers
2. Lack of APN knowledge and education relating to reimbursement
3. Difficulty in handling the rapid pace of change of reimbursement policies and procedures (p. 249)

Tashakkori and Aghajanian (2000) note that "The key point regarding reimbursement is for the state to recognize APNs' credentials, which are granted by the state board of nursing" (p. 94). In other words, it is critical for states to recognize the role that APNs play in the health care system.

One of the key areas APNs continually battle is in obtaining equal status as health care providers. Because many states do not recognize APNs as providers, it is difficult to obtain reimbursement for services. Many APNs have traditionally been employees of provider groups or individual physicians. Consequently, they are not identified as separate and distinct providers of excellent care. Lindeke & Chesney (1999) found that even when payers credential APNs, these APNs may not be given needed updates on reimbursement changes (p. 249), which places them at a disadvantage and makes them less effective in producing change.

In addition, many of the individuals who handle the billing for provider groups do not understand the regulations and do not bill for APN services. Usually they bill under the physician's name because all insurance companies do not pay at equal levels for both groups. Much of this misinformation occurs because Medicare allows two levels of reimbursement. Nurse practitioners can be reimbursed at 100% of physician rate if the physician is physically present in the office or clinic but this requirement also includes other restrictions that confine the APN's ability to function. These restrictions also include being limited to seeing patients with the same diagnosis in follow-up and not on an initial visit.

Reimbursement rates can be as much as 100% of physician rate if billed under the category of "incident to" (Lindeke & Chesney, 1999, p. 248), but requirements to obtain that level of reimbursement include the restrictions listed. Otherwise, NPs are reimbursed at 85% of the physician rate. Many NPs, medical groups and billing agents feel that this level reduces their income. Unfortunately, they do not understand that this method allows more flexibility since the restrictions are eliminated. Consequently, the system is a misunderstood process where few are clear in its methods. APNs must accept this challenge and take responsibility for educating themselves and their colleagues on this critical component of their practices.

Discussion Point

Should APNs be reimbursed at the same level as physicians if they are providing the same services with equal or better outcomes?

Linda Pearson (2004) discussed reimbursement issues in 2003 in the *Nurse Practitioner* journal (Box 21.3) and as Robinson (2004) states, "each year we can see the inconsistencies that exist between roles and within the same role, depending on the state in which the APN practices" (p. 107). Robinson noted multiple barriers for obtaining direct reimbursement. This long list can be found in Box 21.4.

It is vital, then, that third-party payers follow the lead of the Balanced Budget Act of 1997 and grant APNs direct reimbursement for their services without restrictions on location. This issue provides an opportunity for associations that represent APNs to come together to discuss these barriers and develop strategies that will create positive outcomes.

Clearly more work must be done before APNs achieve equal status as health care providers. The challenges of role definition, recognition, and reimbursement are significant but not insurmountable. Specific, targeted strategies for success will be needed (Box 21.5).

BOX 21.3

Research Study Fuels the Controversy

Legislation Affecting Scope of Practice

Published annually for 16 years, this legislative update contains the latest regulatory and statute updates for APNs in all 50 states (plus the District of Columbia). In addition, it presents a summary of legislation related to APN legal scope of practice (except the aspect of prescriptive authority) for the year 2003.

Study Findings

The year 2003 turned out to be quite positive for APNs. In 2003, compared with 2002, more states successfully broadened and expanded APN's legal, reimbursement, or prescriptive authority to practice. For example, in 2002, nine states expanded their legal authority in some way while in 2003, a total of 12 states expanded the legal authority area of their APN practice. In 2002, three states expanded some aspect of APN's reimbursement status, whereas in 2003, four states expanded APN's reimbursement abilities.

Similarly, six states expanded some aspect of an APN's prescriptive authority in 2003, while only three states did so in 2002. These continuing practice expansions help bring APNs closer to complete and fully autonomous practice.

The report concludes that practice barriers remain despite the countless studies that demonstrate that APNs deliver safe, cost-effective, patient-popular health care. The report argues that despite resistance and opposition from the American Medical Association, APNs, other health care professionals, and consumers should continue to introduce and support bills in state legislatures and in Congress that eliminate any and all forms of required physician collaboration or supervision over an APN. "Only then will APNs achieve the full professional autonomy they deserve" (p. 30).

BOX 21.4

Reimbursement Barriers for Advanced Practice Nurses

- Persistent opposition by physicians
- Exclusion of nursing nomenclature in the service classification codes
- Failure of managed care organizations and third-party payers to recognize APNs as providing reimbursable services
- Patient visits billed under physician provider number to ensure 100% reimbursement
- APNs lack of knowledge about reimbursement
- Lack of clarity regarding APNs and how they can be utilized in the provision of health care
- APNs having difficulty coping with rapid changes in reimbursement policies and procedures
- Governors being allowed to eliminate physician supervision requirements for CRNAs treating Medicare and Medicaid patients
- Image that CNMs are uneducated, unsafe, and practicing outside the system
- Restrictions on APNs on caring for certain groups such as workers' compensation
- Lack of consumer demand for APN services
- Division among APNs on scope of practice

Source: Robinson, 2004, pp. 107–112.

BOX 21.5

Strategies for Success for Advanced Practice Nurses

Advanced practice nurses should:

- Gain an understanding of business practices including budgets, organizational behavior, and leadership and management skills.
- Become actively involved in local, state, and national associations that represent the work of APNs.
- Vote, volunteer, and donate to local, state, and national politicians who support the personal and career goals of APNs.
- Volunteer to speak to consumer groups on health care issues.
- Develop collegial relationships with local physicians and discuss current issues impacting practice.
- Be educated on health care policy and be willing to voice opinions on its worthiness.

▶ OUTCOME STUDIES: VALIDATING THE WORTH OF ADVANCED PRACTICE NURSING PRACTICE

Many studies validate the contributions APNs make to quality health care. Bryan and Graham (2002) examined client satisfaction with care provided by APNs. "The average client satisfaction score for patients cared for by APNs was between 46.8 and 47.5 points" (p. 91) of a possible total of 50 points. The authors concluded that "consumer satisfaction benefits the individual client and provides important information for the health care payer. In addition, "measuring and reporting client satisfaction with care provided by APNs may increase the visibility and marketability of APNs" (p. 91).

Another study by Brooten et al. (2002) found that APN intervention "consistently resulted in improved patient outcomes and reduced healthcare costs across groups" (p. 369). In addition, "groups with APN providers were re-hospitalized for less time at less cost, reflecting early detection and intervention" (p. 369).

Another recent study discussed the need to compare the processes used in the delivery of care by APNs that "could be correlated with specific client outcomes" (Dontje, Corser, Kreulen & Teitelman, 2004, p. 63). The authors proposed a model that could be used as a framework for assessing NP practice and suggested that there are "four unique components of practice that differentiate primary care given by NPs from other health care practitioners" (p. 66). These processes as well as the potential outcomes are shown in Table 21.1. This latest data provide an opportunity for all APNs to assess their

TABLE 21.1   The MSU* Partnership Model of Nurse Practitioner Primary Care

Processes of Care	Potential Outcomes
Empowerment	Health-promoting behaviors
Continuity of care	Improved utilization of care
Shared decision making	Higher client satisfaction levels
Holistic care	Improved health status

*MSU: Michigan State University.
Source: Dontje, Corser, Kreulen, & Teitelman, 2004, pp. 66–68.

TABLE 21.2

Comparison of Advanced Practice Nurses

APN	Number	Education	Setting	Salary	Scope of Practice	Prescriptive Authority	Reimbursement
Nurse Practitioners	103,000	Master's degree required for certification; some certificate programs still exist	Primarily in physician practice and community clinics	$60,000 —$95,000 yearly	Not clearly defined; evolving	Some level in all states plus DC; only 12 states plus DC have full prescribing authority	Directly reimbursed by Medicare; private insurance varies by state
Clinical Nurse Specialists	69,000	Master's degree required	Hospitals, research facilities, clinics, long-term care facilities, private practices	$60,000 —$95,000 yearly	Defined	17 states grant some level of prescriptive authority	Directly reimbursed by Medicare; private insurance varies by state
Certified Nurse Midwives	9,200	68% have master's degrees but association does not mandate; four programs are post-baccalaureate	50% in physician practice or hospitals; other settings —birth centers, clinics, home births	$70,000 —80,000 yearly	Well-defined	48 states, DC, American Samoa, & Guam allow some level of prescriptive authority	33 states mandate private insurance reimbursement; 50 states mandate Medicaid
Certified Registered Nurse Anesthetists	30,000 (43% are men)	Master's degree required	Hospitals, outpatient surgery, physician practice, and all military and government facilities	~$100,000 yearly	Well-defined	Some authority depending upon state	Directly reimbursed by Medicare, state and federal programs; 22 states mandate private insurance reimbursement; 36 states reimburse for Medicaid
NP/CNS	14,600	See above					

Sources: Meyeroff, 2005; AACN, 2004; ANA, 2004; Phillips, 2005; Advanced Practice Special Interest Group, n.d.; NACNS, 2004; ACNM, 2004.

own practices and to "articulate the unique contribution of [clinical] practice" and "to better understand the complexities of their current and future practice" (p. 64). A comparison of the four types of APNs can be found in Table 21.2.

The literature is also clear that APNs are continuing to serve an underserved portion of the population. In a report released in June 2004 by Coffman, Quinn, Brown, and Scheffler (2004), which analyzed physician practice over the past 25 years in California, the "highest NP and PA-to-population ratios were found in the small, rural counties. This finding underscores the importance of these 'non-physician clinicians' in providing care in these areas" (p. 65). The researchers also found, when they compared patient care workforce-to-population ratios, which included active physicians, NPs, and PAs, that the role of the non-physician clinician was significantly important in those rural California areas (Coffman et al., 2004, p. 67). Coffman et al. concluded that "policymakers should take an active role in capitalizing on the skills and abilities of PAs and NPs" (p.73) by considering policies that may repay loans for students who are from and/or are willing to work in underserved areas as well as methods to increase the diversity of this workforce.

▶ CONTROLLING THE FUTURE OF ADVANCED PRACTICE NURSING

Schober (2004) points out that "nursing academics and leaders appear to lack consensus as to what advanced nursing practice really means, and at times support by nursing bodies is lacking as the roles develop. As a result, politicians, ministers of health, and policymakers worldwide have begun to venture forth to provide regulatory and credentialing advice" (p. 92). In many ways, this is unfortunate because it is nursing's responsibility to develop standards and regulations so that legislation can be proactively developed. Nursing leaders must accept this task so that the entire profession can move forward to claim its rightful position in the health care system. Nursing must define nursing before others take away the right to practice.

> *CONSIDER: Advanced practice nurses must understand the importance of joining the associations that represent them before the legislatures. Though nurses historically have not joined their professional organizations en masse, it is particularly significant for APNs to recognize the important work being done by these associations. APNs must have a voice in Congress as well as at the state and local level. There is power in that voice but only if the association can show that it represents significant numbers of APNs.

Although nurses have traditionally worked as employees, APNs must learn that they are developing a practice, the same as physicians develop a practice. To build a strong practice, APNs need to learn business practices such as budgeting and organizational behavior. It is vital that they study leadership theories and learn management skills. They must also focus on the power of the vote. They must support politicians who support APNs. Along with voting, it is very important to volunteer for those legislators' campaigns as well as support them with donations. Legislators listen to people who support them and can be swayed by three to four facsimile or e-mail comments. By voting, volunteering, and donating to politicians at all levels, APNs can influence change in the health care system.

Learning about health care policy and developing the willingness to speak out on important issues are also crucial. Advanced practice nurses should become familiar with the local media and welcome the opportunity to voice their opinions when discussions occur on health care issues.

Finally, APNs need to develop collegial relationships with local physicians so that each becomes educated on the other's practice issues. Usually physicians who know and work with APNs are supportive of their work and know the quality of care that they provide. These colleagues can then also be a voice within their own organizations when discussions turn to APNs and their roles.

At the organizational level, APN associations should create local, state, and national task forces that focus on the barriers to practice. These organizations must learn that the issues that separate them should be discussed privately because physicians, policymakers, and the public tend to dwell more on differences and dissension than on positive aspects. Internal battles should be fought in the conference room, not in front of the press or on the floor of the legislature. Groups can then present their united front to the world and help position APNs in their rightful place as qualified and competent health care providers.

Of equal importance is that individual APNs must learn the lessons of the past and develop the skills needed to survive as a vital constituent of the health care system in the 21st century. Strong leadership and much determination are key to walking the path to success but APNs have risen to the task throughout history and can achieve the success they desire today.

▶ CONCLUSIONS

There is little doubt that APNs make a valuable contribution in today's health care system. They provide care that, in most cases, achieves outcomes as good as or better than physicians and at a lower cost. They also continue to provide care in traditionally underserved areas that would otherwise have no primary health care.

Yet, APNs have many issues to resolve before they will have the recognition, status, and pay they deserve for the services they provide. Clarifying roles, creating common title nomenclature, and standardizing scope of practice nationally will be needed. In addition, APNs must determine what educational entry level is required to fulfill those role expectations. Finally, more studies are needed that examine APN practice and that demonstrate to other health care professionals, the public, and our policy making bodies that APNs consistently achieve quality outcomes in caring for patients in a multiplicity of settings.

All of these efforts will require collective action on the part of APNs and the professional organizations that represent them. It remains to be seen whether this is possible.

FOR ADDITIONAL DISCUSSION

1. What are some of the reasons advanced practice nursing has not clearly defined its roles?
2. How should APNs identify themselves? Is APN a clear and distinctive title?
3. Taking the many definitions discussed in this chapter, develop your own definition of advanced practice nursing. How does it compare to your classmates' definition?
4. Can an APN who is educated at the certificate level demand the same level of credibility as one with a master's or doctorate degree?

5. In today's litigious environment, is it legally sound for nurse-midwives to be educated at less than a master's degree?
6. How can the states come together to develop a uniform scope of practice that is clearly delineated for all APNs?
7. How can APNs effect change to the many laws that affect their right to practice?
8. What are the components of the APRN Compact adopted by the National Council of State Boards of Nursing? How can they be implemented? What states have achieved its purposes?
9. Why do you think defining the scope of practice has been so difficult for APNs?
10. What do you think are the concerns of physicians and other health care providers in allowing full prescriptive authority to APNs? How can those concerns be overcome?
11. Why are third-party payers so resistant to reimbursement to APNs?
12. How can APNs influence insurance companies to affect the needed change to full reimbursement without restrictions?
13. What do you see is needed for APNs to clearly define their roles, be recognized as key providers, and to receive full reimbursement for their services?

REFERENCES

Advanced Practice Special Interest Group. (n.d.). *Information on APRNs*. Certified Registered Nurse Anesthetist (CRNA). Retrieved May 9, 2005 from http://www.scnurses.org/A_P_SIG/aprns.asp#crna.

American Academy of Family Physicians. (2004). *Mid-level provider issues*. Retrieved May 9, 2005, from http://www.aafp.org/x19749.xml#x19767.

American Academy of Nurse Practitioners (n. d.). *Qualifications of candidates*. Retrieved May 9, 2005, from http://www.aanp.org/Certification/Qualification+of+Candidates.htm.

American Academy of Nurse Practitioners (2002a). *Nurse practitioners as an advanced practice nurse role position statement*. Retrieved May 9, 2005, from http://www.aanp.org/NR/rdonlyres/eap463m6vsieqvef-bthom5sfqrpxhwtqcrnjmiiw54cywbruf3oe44wm3kokmnpf5mrwithetrhcti/Position%2bStatement%2bNP%2bRole2.pdf.

American Academy of Nurse Practitioners. (2002b). *Scope of practice for nurse practitioners*. Retrieved May 9, 2005, from http://www.aanp.org/NR/rdonlyres/edhltucoxqd2xnrfwbve26d3cowleh5rqqcfmhlcoi3sp7ihpzxry7rdqtkezw5zvpggxsuc7z4iao/scope%2bof%2bpractice%2bv2.pdf.

American Academy of Nurse Practitioners (2002c). *Medicare update*. Retrieved May 9, 2005, from http://www.aanp.org/NR/rdonlyres/ejthcgzkld7ustki7v2a77rpaydvlli6vik7oxzvwzdt26uosirf3ertlpcgnptow46yghyp2xyarq753cejw7be2hc/Medicare+Update.pdf#search='must%20NPs%20have%20a%20masters%20degree%20medicare%20guidelines'.

American Academy of Pediatrics. (2003). Scope of practice issues in the delivery of pediatric health care. *AAP News 111*(2), 426–435. Retrieved from EBSCO Publishing.

American Association of Colleges of Nursing (last updated March 10, 2004). *Your nursing career: A look at the facts*. Retrieved May 9, 2005, from http://www.aacn.nche.edu/education/Career.htm.

American College of Nurse-Midwives. (2003). *Mandatory degree requirements for midwives*. Retrieved May 9, 2005, from http://www.midwife.org/prof/display.cfm?id=102.

American College of Nurse-Midwives (2004). *Position statement. Definition of midwifery practice*. Retrieved May 9, 2005, from http://www.acnm.org/prof/display.cfm?id=101.

American College of Nurse Practitioners. (1999). *HCFA's Final Rule on the Notice of Proposed Rule Making Regarding the Physician Fee Schedule / Year 2000, November 2, 1999*. Retrieved May 9, 2005, from http://www.nurse.org/acnp/medicare/hcfa.991102.shtml.

American College of Nurse Practitioners. (n.d.). Retrieved May 9, 2005, from http://www.nurse.org/acnp/facts/ed.position.shtml.

American Nurses Association. (1996). *Scope and standards of advanced practice registered nursing*. Washington, DC: American Nurses Publishing.

American Nurses Association (2004). *Celebrate national nurses week*. Retrieved May 9, 2005, from http://www.nursingworld.org/pressrel/nnw/nnwfacts.htm.

American Nurses Credentialing Center (2003). *Nurse practitioner certifications*. Retrieved May 9, 2005, from http://www.nursingworld.org/ancc/certification/cert/certs/advprac/np.html.

Barker, P. (2000). Advanced nursing practice: Experience, education and something else. *Journal of Psychiatric and Mental Health Nursing, 7*(1), 89–94.

Brooten, D., Naylor, M. D., York, R., Brown, L. P., Hazard Munro, B., Hollingsworth, A. O., Cohen, S. M., et al. (2002). Lessons learned from testing the quality cost model of advanced practice nursing (APN) transitional care. *Journal of Nursing Scholarship, 34*(4), 369–375.

Bryan, R. & Graham, M. (2002). Advanced practice nurses: A study of client satisfaction. *Journal of the Academy of Nurse Practitioners 14*(2), 88–92.

California Association for Nurse Practitioners (2004a). *AB2226 (Spitzer) passes out of committee.* Retrieved May 9, 2005, from http://www.canpweb.org/displaycommon.cfm?an=18.

California Association for Nurse Practitioners. (2004b). *NP fact sheet.* Retrieved May 9, 2005, from http://www.canpweb.org/displaycommon.cfm?an=1&subarticlenbr=3.

California Board of Registered Nursing. (2003). *Approved nurse practitioner programs.* Retrieved May 9, 2005, from http://www.rn.ca.gov/pdf/np-programs.pdf.

Castner, D. (2001). The "coming out" of the advanced practice nurse. *Nephrology Nursing Journal 28*(4), 474.

Coffman, J., Quinn, B., Brown, T., & Scheffler, R. (2004). Is there a doctor in the house? An examination of the physician workforce over the last 25 years in California. Berkeley, California: University of California, Berkeley, Nicholas C. Petris Center on Health Care Markets and Consumer Welfare.

DeYoung, L. (1966). *The Foundations of Nursing.* St. Louis: Mosby.

Dontje, K., Corser, W., Kreulen, G., & Teitleman, A. (2004). A unique set of interactions: The MSU sustained partnership model of nurse practitioner primary care. *Journal of the American Academy of Nurse Practitioners 16*(2), 63–69.

Fields, U. R. (2000–2004). *Meeting the needs: Advanced practice for nurses. MedCareers.* Retrieved May 9, 2005, from http://www.medcareers.com/resources/resource.asp?id=1093.

Hamric, A. A. (1996). Definition of advanced practice nursing. In Hamric, A., Spross, J., & Hanson, C. (Ed). *Advanced nursing practice*: *An integrative approach* (2nd ed.). Philadelphia: W. B. Saunders.

Hodnicki, D. R., Dietz, A., McNeil, F., & Miles, K. (2004). Medication-ordering patterns of advanced practice nurses in Georgia, 2002. *The American Journal for Nurse Practitioners 8*(1), 9–12, 15–18, 23–24.

Hooker, R. S. & McCaig, L. F. (2001). Use of physician assistants and nurse practitioners in primary care, 1995-1999. *Hospital Quarterly 5*(1), 32–36. Abstract retrieved May 9, 2005, from PubMed database.

Hugg, A. (2002). *The choice is yours.* Retrieved May 9, 2005 from http://www.nurseweek.com/news/features/02-05/apn.asp.

International Council of Nurses. (2003). *Definition and characteristics of the role.* Retrieved May 9, 2005, from http://www.aanp.org/inp%20network/practice%20issues/role/%20definitions.asp.

Kaplan, L. & Brown, M. (2004). Prescriptive authority and barriers to np practice. *The Nurse Practitioner 29*(3), 28–29, 32–35.

Komnenich, P. (1998). The evolution of advanced practice in nursing. In Sheehy, C. M. & McCarthy, M. C. (Eds). *Advanced practice nursing* (pp. 8–46). Philadelphia: F. A. Davis.

Lindeke, L. & Chesney, M. (1999). Reimbursement realities of advanced nursing practice. *Nursing Outlook 47*(6), 248–251.

Meyeroff, W.J. (2005). *Advance your nursing career. Monster Feature Reports.* Retrieved May 9, 2005, from http://featuredreports.monster.com/nursing04/advanced/.

Mundinger, M., Kane, R., Lenz, E., Totten, A., Tsai, W., Cleary, P., Friedewald, W., Siu, A., & Shelanski, M., et al. (2000). Primary care outcomes in patients treated by nurse practitioners or physicians. *Journal of the American Medical Association 283*(1), 332–351.

National Association of Clinical Nurse Specialists. (2004). *Model rules and regulations for CNS title protection and scope of practice.* Retrieved May 9, 2005, from http://www.nacns.org/updates/model_language.pdf.

National Council of State Boards of Nursing. (2000, August). Proposed *Uniform Advanced Practice Registered Nurse Licensure/Authority to Practice Requirements.* Retrieved May 9, 2005, from http://www.ncsbn.org/pdfs/aprnsupportingpaper.pdf.

National Council of State Boards of Nursing. (2002a). *Regulation of advanced practice nursing 2002 national council of state boards of nursing position paper.* Retrieved May 9, 2005, from http://www.ncsbn.org/pdfs/APRN_Position_Paper2002.pdf.

National Council of State Boards of Nursing. (2002b). *NCSBN delegates vote on significant actions at delegate assembly 2003.* Retrieved May 9, 2005, from http://www.ncsbn.org/pdfs/2002_DA_Recommendations.pdf.

National Council of State Boards of Nursing. (n. d.). *Advanced Practice Registered Nurse Compact.* Retrieved May 9, 2005, from http://www.ncsbn.org/pdfs/APRNCompact.pdf.

National Organization of Nurse Practitioner Faculties. (2002). *Nurse practitioner primary care competencies for specialty areas: Adult family, gerontological, and women's health.* Retrieved May 9, 2005, from http://www.nonpf.com/finalaug2002.pdf.

Pearson, L. (2004). Sixteenth annual legislative update. *Nurse Practitioner, 29*(1), 26–51.

Phillips, R. L., Green, L. A., Fryer, G. E., & Dovey, S. M. (2001). Trumping professional roles: Collaboration of nurse practitioners and physicians for a better U.S. health system. *American Family Physician 64*(8), 1325.

Phillips, S. (2005). Seventeenth Annual Legislative Update. *The Nurse Practitioner 30*(1), 14–17.

Robinson, K. (2004). Payment for advanced practice nursing services: Past, present and future. In L. Joel (Ed.), *Advanced practice nursing: Essentials for role development* (pp. 99–121). Philadelphia: F. A. Davis.

Safriet, B. (2002). Closing the gap between can and may in health-care providers' scopes of practice: A primer for policymakers. *Yale Journal of Regulation 19*(2), 301–333.

Schober, M. (2004). Global perspective on advanced practice. In L. Joel (Ed.), *Advanced practice nursing: Essentials for role development* (pp. 73–96). Philadelphia: F. A. Davis.

Sheehy, C. M. & McCarthy, M. C. (1998). *Advanced practice nursing.* Philadelphia: F. A. Davis.

Tashakkori, Z. & Aghajanian, A. (2000). Reimbursement issues in advanced practice nursing: An overview. *Medsurg Nursing 9*(2), 93–96.

Towers, J. (2004). Advanced practice nurses and prescriptive authority. In L. Joel (Ed.), *Advanced practice nursing: Essentials for role development* (pp. 122–135). Philadelphia: F. A. Davis.

U.S. Department of Health and Human Services Health Resources Administration Bureau of Health Professions Division of Nursing (2002). *Nurse practitioner primary care competencies in specialty areas: Adult, family, pediatric, and women's health.* (HRSA Publication No. 00-00532P). Rockville, MD: Author.

BIBLIOGRAPHY

Brown, M. & Draye, M. (2003). Experiences of pioneer nurse practitioners in establishing advanced practice roles. *Journal of Nursing Scholarship 35*(4), 391–397.

Cole, F. (2003). Emergency care advanced practice nursing in the US: An overview. *Emergency Nurse 11*(5), 22–25.

Donnelly, G. (2003). Clinical expertise in advanced practice nursing: A Canadian perspective. *Nurse Education Today 23(3)*, 168–173.

Evitts, E. (2004). Rx: Nurse practitioners. *John Hopkins Nursing 2*(1), 14–19.

Hanson, C. & Hamric, A. (2003). Reflections on the continuing evolution of advanced practice nursing. *Nursing Outlook 51*(5), 203–211.

Jenkins, M. (2003). Toward national comparable nurse practitioner data: Proposed data elements, rationale, and methods. *Journal of Biomedical Informatics 36*(4–5), 342–350.

Joel, L. (2004). *Advanced practice nursing essentials for role development.* Philadelphia: F. A. Davis.

Mundinger, M. (2002). Twenty-first-century primary care: New partnerships between nurses and doctors. *Academic Medicine 77*(8), 776–780.

Mundinger, M. (1999). Can advanced practice nurses succeed in the primary care market? *Nursing Economics, 17*(1), 7–14.

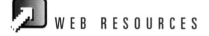

WEB RESOURCES

American Academy of Nurse Practitioners	http://www.aanp.org
American Academy of Pediatrics	http://www.aap.org
American Association of Nurse Anesthetists	http://www.aana.com/
American College of Nurse-Midwives	http://www.acnm.org/
American College of Nurse Practitioners	http://www.nurse.org/acnp/index.shtml
American Nurses Association	http://www.nursingworld.org/
Association of American Colleges of Nursing	http://www.aacn.nche.edu/
California Association for Nurse Practitioners	http://www.canpweb.org
National Association of Clinical Nurse Specialists	http://www.nacns.org/
National Organization of Nurse Practitioner Faculties	http://www.nonpf.com/
NP Central	http://www.npcentral.net/

Nursing and Public Policy: Getting Involved

Catherine J. Dodd

22

M any of the preceding chapters in this book discussed policy issues affecting the nursing profession. For example, mandatory overtime, staffing ratios, whistle-blower protection, and the treatment of chemically impaired nurses have all been addressed recently in the health care policy arena. Indeed, nurses have long been involved in shaping public policy. Some of the earliest policy debates in nursing were about the "training" of nurses. Subsequent debates centered on both the process for licensing nurses as well as the appropriate scope of their practice. State legislatures responded and adopted licensure laws relating to the practice of nurses and the protection of the public. Today these laws define the scope of nursing practice as distinctly separate from medicine and inclusive of responsibilities independent of medicine.

> ***CONSIDER:** Nursing's involvement in policy and politics has resulted in state nurse practice acts that allow many things, including autonomy of practice, reimbursement for advanced practice nurses (APNs), and limitations on the ability of hospitals to force nurses to work overtime.

In addition, policy debates regarding nursing shortages and working conditions have occurred every decade of nursing's policy history. Often these debates have centered on whether policy should be shaped by collective bargaining or by legislation and/or regulation.

Participating in shaping public policy is an essential part of professional nursing practice because public policy shapes the environment in which nurses provide care and determines the kind of care nurses are permitted to provide. This chapter defines public policy, explains the policy process and the role of politics in that process, and demonstrates how policy and politics are inextricably linked. Kingdon's three streams metaphor, a systems model, stages of nursing's political development and a continuum of political involvement are introduced to conceptually explore the relationship between politics and policy and to examine how nurses participate in both.

In addition, this chapter identifies nursing leaders who were pioneers in public policy, traces nursing's involvement in key policy/political debates throughout the 20th century, and explores contemporary issues currently being debated in the political arena. Finally, because politics is part of every organization and a part of government at every level, the political skills necessary for nurses to protect their practice, their profession, and the patients entrusted to their care are identified. In addition, the chapter discusses actions nurses may take to increase their influence in public policy.

▶ DEFINING POLITICS AND POLICY

Defining terms helps to clarify the relationship between politics and policy. Definitions of *politics* include the "art or science of government or governing, the activities or affairs engaged in by a government, politician or political party, the methods or tactics involved in managing a state or government, intrigue or maneuvering within a political unit or group in order to gain control or power, and internally conflicting relationships among people in a society" (*American Heritage Dictionary of the English Language,* 2000).

While this chapter focuses on policy and politics of government, many of the principles are applicable to non-governmental institutions and organizations as well.

Indeed, politics is part of all organized human activity; any group of two or more individuals has to establish how to make decisions that require common action and how to resolve conflicts. Ellis and Hartley (2004, p. 70) define politics as "the way in which people in any society try to influence decision making and the allocation of resources." Because resources (money, time, and personnel) are limited, it is necessary to make choices regarding their use. There is no perfect process for making optimum choices, because whenever one valuable option is chosen, usually some other option must be left out.

In contrast, *policy* has been defined as "a plan or course of action, as of a government, political party, or business, intended to influence and determine decisions, actions, and other matters" (The American Heritage Dictionary of the English Language, 2000). The word policy is Greek in origin and is linked to citizenship. In government, it comes from the relationship of citizens to one another in public. Timus (as cited in Mason, Leavitt, & Chaffee, 2002, p. 23) defines policy as "principles that govern toward a given ends." Another definition describes policy as "an authoritative decision made in the legislative, executive, or judicial branches of government that are intended to direct or influence the actions, behaviors, or decisions of others" (Longest as cited in Harrington & Estes, 2004).

Discussion Point

How great an impact does politics have on policy at the institutional level? At the governmental level? Are politics typically considered before policy development begins at both levels?

DEFENSE, DOMESTIC, AND FOREIGN POLICY

At the federal level, the United States Congress and the president make policy in three major areas: defense, domestic, and foreign. Health-related policies can be found in all three areas. Health-related *defense* policies include what kinds of health care the military and their families will receive, and whether or not weapons of mass destruction (such as the nuclear weapons recently approved by Congress) will be used by the United States. *Domestic* policy refers to policies such as whether children's vaccinations will be paid for in the public health budget, or what services are included in Medicare, the health insurance plan for the elderly. Health is also a major part of our *foreign* policy. Congress decides whether to assist other nations with preventing HIV/AIDS or in providing family planning and nutrition assistance to developing countries.

*CONSIDER: Nurses serving in the military are affected by *defense* policy, nurses working to improve health in developing countries are affected by *foreign* policy, and nurses working within the health care system anywhere in the United States are affected by *domestic* policy. The president and Congress decide how many of our tax dollars to spend on defense, foreign aid and domestic health care. If more is spent on one, less is available for the others, unless taxes are increased.

POLICIES AND VALUES

Policy involves the setting of goals and priorities by a society, or an organization and the decisions about how and what resources should be used to achieve those goals. Thus, policies reflect the values and beliefs of the leaders of society and/or organizations who make the policies (Mason et al., 2002).

> ***CONSIDER:** Policy always has a moral dimension because it relates to decisions about how to act toward others.

Frequently, female policy makers, regardless of their political party, have tended to promote policies that address social issues such as family medical leave, childcare, and domestic violence (Mason et al., 2002). Similarly, policies developed by nurses have frequently shown a strong belief in the importance of assisting people to care for themselves despite their illness or disability and this belief has distinguished nursing from other professions (Gebbie, Wakefield, and Kerfoot, as cited in Mason et al., 2002). Caring, whether it be for families, for patients or for the environment is a value central to nursing and to women (Mason et al., 2002). Unfortunately it is not a value that receives much attention by institutions and government policy makers. Nurses have had some success at the state and federal level at moving such a policy agenda forward; however, if nurses want policies that reflect nursing's values, then nurses must get involved in the policy process that makes decisions on which policies to adopt, and that requires involvement in politics.

Discussion Point

What values are reflected in state nurse practice acts that limit the autonomy of the advanced practice nurse in prescribing? Similarly, what values are reflected in state policies that allow chemically impaired nurses to participate in diversion programs rather than face disciplinary proceedings?

CONCEPTUALIZING POLITICS AND POLICY DEVELOPMENT

Although there are many models for conceptualizing politics and policy development, only four are presented in this chapter: 1) Kingdon's Streams of Policy Development, 2) a systems model approach to policy making, 3) Cohen et al.'s Stages of Political Development, and 4) Mason, Leavitt, & Chaffee's (2002) Continuum for Political Development.

Kingdon's Three Streams of Policy Development

Kingdon posits that there are *three streams* that determine why some problems are chosen over others for policy development (Sabatier, 1999) (Box 22.1). The three streams are the *problem stream*, the *political stream*, and the *policy stream*. These three streams often flow endlessly without converging, but when the streams come together, a window of opportunity opens to move an agenda, to legislate or to regulate policy solutions to problems.

BOX 22.1	The Three Streams of John Kingdon's Streams Metaphor

1. **Problem:** embodies the process of problem recognition
2. **Policy:** embodies the formulation and refining of policy proposals, as responses to problem recognition
3. **Politics:** considers the associated benefits and costs to subgroups of the population and the degree of external pressure the legislator feels to take action

The *problem stream* includes what are defined as problems, indicators of a problem, and the social construction of problems. It also includes how problems come to the attention of policy makers, such as in the form of causal stories or personal experiences. For example, U.S. Rep. Caroline McCarthy, a licensed practical nurse, ran for Congress after her husband and child were shot on the New York subway and she wanted to pass gun control legislation.

Another example of the problem stream coming to the attention of legislators is the current nursing shortage. Legislators have had to take note of the shortage as a result of constituent complaints, an increasing number of medical errors, and high nursing vacancy rates. In addition, television and newspapers abound with stories of poor patient care due to the shortage of nurses.

Dodd also emphasizes the significance of the problem stream in her *Ten Universal Commandments of Politics for Nurses* (Box 22.2). The first commandment states that the personal is political, and that each of us is just one personal or social injustice away from being involved in politics (Harrington & Estes, 2004, p. 19).

Kingdon's second stream is the *policy stream*. Ideas that are potential policy solutions are considered based on their "technical feasibility and value acceptability" (Sabatier, 1999, p. 76). The reality is that policy makers are presented with many problems and it is impossible to address all of them. Policy makers, then, must set an agenda that reflects their values and select problems to focus legislation or regulatory action on that fit their priorities. Because policy makers want to be successful (determines reelection and job security), most avoid introducing legislative or regulatory proposals that are unlikely to pass and or to be implemented.

439

BOX 22.2	Ten Universal Commandments of Politics for Nurses

1. The personal is political. Each of us is just one personal or social injustice away from being involved in politics.
2. Friends come and go but enemies accumulate.
3. Politics is the art of the possible. . . majority rules.
4. Be polite, be persistent, be persuasive, be polite.
5. Ignore your mother's rule. Talk to strangers.
6. Money is the mother's milk of politics.
7. Negotiate visibility. Take credit, take control.
8. Politics has a "chit economy." So keep track.
9. Reputations are permanent.
10. Don't let 'em get to ya.

Source: Dodd, C. as found in Harrington, C., & Estes, C.L. (2004). Making the political process work. *Health policy: Crisis and reform in the U.S. health care delivery system* (4th ed.). Boston: Jones and Bartlett Publishers.

For example, a policy to resolve the nursing shortage by reestablishing hospital-based nursing diplomas is unlikely to be pursued because technically, hospitals are no longer set up as nursing schools, and because nursing education outside the hospital has become more highly valued and accepted by society. Another example might be when Rep. McCarthy was not successful in banning guns, because Americans value the "right to bear arms" as protected by the second amendment of the U.S. Constitution. She was successful, however, in leading the fight to at least temporarily pass a ban on assault weapons (legislation passed in 1993 and made effective for 10 years, expired in September 2004), because Americans value their safety. Technically, banning assault weapons provided the safety and protected the value of the second amendment.

Discussion Point

California is currently the only state that has enacted minimum licensed staff to patient ratios in acute care hospitals and this passed only after vigorous opposition from the state hospital association. Is this an issue most state legislators would be eager to take on? Is such an issue "technically feasible and value acceptable"?

The political stream is the third and final stream. Politics, according to Kingdon, describes an environment that includes 1) the national mood–what the public sentiment is on issues, 2) support or opposition of *interest groups*, and 3) legislative or executive branch turnover accompanied by a change in political ideology and values (Sabatier, 1999). In other words, the political stream looks at associated benefits and costs to subgroups of the population and the degree of external pressure the legislator feels to take action.

An example of a strong *political stream* occurred when support from the public, professional nursing, and consumer and hospital organizations came together to help fund the *Nursing Education Act*. In contrast, the ban on assault weapons met with opposition because of the change of national mood, the turnover of Congress and the White House to Republican rule, and the powerful interest group of the National Rifle Association.

The significance of interest groups as part of the political stream cannot be underestimated. Indeed, throughout history, ideological *interest groups* have shaped social change. Interest groups provide politicians with one of three resources essential for their success (reelection). The first, and sometimes seemingly most important, is money; the second is the ability to mobilize voters; and the third is image. It is this image enhancement that may be most significant for nurses in terms of legislative interest. Clearly, having the support of nurses improves a candidate's image.

Historically, nurses have ranked high in public opinion polls and the public believes the endorsement of nurses demonstrates a candidate's integrity. After September 11, 2001, the importance of nursing's endorsement took second place only behind firefighters and it has been in first place every year since then. Nursing is a profession of more than 2 million members nationally. When divided by 435 congressional districts nationally, there are approximately 5,000 registered nurses (RNs) per congressional district who can and have mobilized voters.

A strong political stream, however, is not enough. Convergence of the three streams is required. Nursing and the professional organizations that represent nursing (interest groups) in the legislature at the state and federal levels, then, have repeatedly worked to achieve this degree of stream convergence in public policy decisions related to health care. For example, in the 1990s, during the Clinton Administration, the rising costs of health care, President Clinton's personal respect for nurses (his mother was a nurse anesthetist who worked in rural Arkansas), and pressure from nursing organizations created an opportunity to add nurse practitioners and clinical nurse specialists as providers under Medicare.

Another example of stream convergence was medical errors, workplace injuries and mandatory overtime. Public awareness of rampant medical errors were the subject of the Institute of Medicine report *To Err is Human* during President Clinton's administration (Kohn, Corrigan, & Donaldson, 2000). Nursing organizations collected data and proposed that mandatory overtime contributed to medical errors and injuries in the workplace (the idea/policy proposal stream) (ANA, 2001b, ANA, 2001c). Combined with public awareness (stream one), ideas/policy proposals (stream two), and the ideological support of the Clinton administration for nursing combined with nursing and labor interest group pressure (stream three), the Department of Labor promulgated regulations limiting overtime and budgeting funding for occupational health needle safety training. In this instance, the idea/policy stream combined with the political stream comprised the interest groups of nursing and labor combined with an administration (president) whose ideology embraced labor and nursing.

During the first 3 years of President George W. Bush's administration, however, the overtime regulations were overturned and needle safety training was curtailed. This was an example of the (third) political stream. The ideological shift and the powerful hospital interest group lobby succeeded in overturning the regulations and cutting the budget.

> ***CONSIDER:** Nursing interest groups have seized the public's frustration with rising health care costs and promoted policies that emphasized the cost-effectiveness of advanced practice nurses (stream one—conditions + stream two—ideas/policies). President Clinton supported this idea and included APNs in his Medicare budget (stream three—political change in values).

System Model Approach to Analyzing Policy Making and Interest Groups

A more traditional/ approach to analyzing policy making is a systems-based model that considers policy making in sequential stages. It is much like the nursing process: *assess, plan, implement, evaluate, assess again.* In a policy system, a problem is identified and put on a policy agenda, a policy is developed, adopted, implemented, evaluated and terminated and either extended, modified or terminated and the cycle begins again (Mason et al., 2002).

Critics of the systems model approach suggest that the model fails to consider that the elected government's policy agenda rarely, if ever, reflects a consensus. In the past two decades the country has become more and more divided on a partisan and thus philosophical basis of how best to govern (Cook, 2004). Critics argue that the systems analysis of policy development leaves out the influence of interest groups whether they are nursing organizations or oil companies. It would be like using the nursing process for diabetic teaching of an adolescent without taking into consideration that the patient might not follow their diet because their peer group is eating fast food everyday after school.

In contrast, policy development, adoption and implementation, and politics are inextricably linked in Kingdon's model and the political environment in which policy is formed is considered. Nursing can play a role in all three of Kingdon's policy streams that create windows of opportunity: for example nursing professional organizations and unions raise public awareness about the quality of care, or lack of access to care. Professional nursing organizations and unions develop ideas and propose policies to solve problems of worker safety, health and safety or quality of care. Nursing professional organizations and unions are interest groups that lobby and engage in political action to influence policy.

In all of these examples, nursing is acting as an "interest group." The unique thing about nursing as an interest group is that when nurses advocate for nurses and nursing, patients and the public get better care. Political action is a key part of "interest group" action. Interest groups do more than support or oppose policies; they help elect the policy makers via grassroots campaign activity and raising money for campaigns.

Stages of Political Development

Another model used to explore nursing's development in politics and the policy arena was described by Cohen, Mason, Kovner, Leavitt, Pulcini and Sochalski (cited in Mason et al., 2002, p, 7). Cohen et al. identified four stages of political development in nursing. *Stage One: Buy In* occurred when the profession began to promote the political sensitivity of nurses to injustices or changes needed in the policy arena. *Stage Two: Self-Interest* occurred when the nursing profession began to develop its identity as a special interest and crystallized its uniqueness as a political voice. *Stage Three: Political Sophistication* began when nurses began to be recognized by policy makers and health care leaders as having valuable perspectives and expertise in health policy. The final stage, *Stage Four: Leadership* indicates that nursing has developed its own political identity as exemplified by setting the agenda for change.

Cohen et al. argued that nursing has only begun to enter this final phase. In this phase, nursing will set the agenda for health policy and that agenda will include issues beyond those traditionally defined as relevant only to nursing. Thus, nurses become the initiators of critical health care policy. Cohen et al. concluded that the move to this stage must be deliberately pursued if the perspective and values of nursing are to help reshape our health care system.

> *CONSIDER: Nursing has the potential to hold a significant leadership position in policy and politics. At least some groups within nursing have already developed a political identity and set an agenda for change.

Continuum of Political Involvement

The final conceptual model used here to explore nursing's involvement in policy and politics is that of a continuum. Continuums for political involvement extend from no involvement in politics to that of extreme activism. Individuals move up and down these continuums throughout their lives in response to intrinsic and external motivators, time and energy resources, and situational opportunities and needs.

Mason et al. (2002) identified such a continuum with their description of *Nurse-Citizens, Nurse-Activists,* and *Nurse-Politicians* (pp. 42–43). This work is similar to that of Kalisch and Kalisch (1982) who described *spectator activities, transitional activities,* and *gladiatorial activities* (p. 316). Another continuum that has been identified is that of people *who make things happen, people who watch what's happening,* and *people who wonder what's happened.* For example, nurses who wonder *what's* happened vote occasionally, or not at all; they are not involved in improving the workplace or their community. Nurses who *watch* things happen, are spectators; they expose themselves to political stimuli, they are members of their union, they vote, sometimes they wear buttons or put bumper stickers on cars, they participate in community activities that are personally important to them like parent–teacher organizations or homeowners associations.

> ┌ ***CONSIDER:** There are people who make things happen, people who watch what's happening, and people who wonder what's happened! ┐

Nurses who *make* things happen fall into three categories: professionals, leaders, and political change agents. Professional nurses vote in every election and stay informed regarding issues affecting the health care system. They participate in their union, or speak out about working conditions and quality of care. They participate in their professional organization, know who their local, state and federal elected officials are and communicate with them regarding issues of concern.

Nurse leaders are active members of nursing organizations that are political; they are active members of a political party and attend political meetings, forums and rallies; they help register people to vote; they contribute and raise money for causes and campaigns AND to nurses' political action committees (PACs) that are concerned about access to quality nursing care; they lobby elected and appointed officials on issues of concern to the profession; they write letters to the editor of professional journals and newspapers; they participate in coalitions; they encourage the participation of other nurses; they mentor future leaders.

Finally, nurse political change agents are nurse leaders who use their nursing expertise to enact and implement policies that enhance access to quality health care including nursing care; they seek appointments or assist other nurses and friends of nursing in securing appointments to governing boards in the public and private sector; they are active members of political parties, they query candidates about their positions on health care and assist with fundraising for candidates that support nurses and nursing; they seek elected and/or appointed office and continue to identify themselves as an RN; they work on staffs of elected/appointed officials; they extend their policy influence beyond the health system to the community and the globe.

▶ ROOTS OF INVOLVEMENT IN POLICY AND POLITICS: EARLY 1900s

Nursing has a long history of involvement in politics and policy development. At the end of the 19th century, nursing alumnae associations, motivated by the need for "standardization in nurse training schools, as well as by the need to protect the public from poorly trained nurses," came together to establish "standards of nursing education and nursing practice and to promote the general welfare of nurses" (Flanagan, 1976, p. 27).

Nursing Alumnae Associations

The *American Nurses Association* (ANA) was founded by these alumnae associations. Almost immediately after this founding, the United States engaged in the Spanish American War, requiring a nursing workforce to care for the wounded and those who had yellow fever, typhoid and other communicable diseases. *Isabel Hampton Robb*, ANA's first president, sought to influence the Secretary of War and the Surgeon General to insist that the nurses needed for the war be trained and offered to organize them, but was unsuccessful. Both trained and untrained nurses were recruited and sent to the battlefield without any system of care or triage by skilled nurses.

After the war, a special committee of nurses formulated the *Army Bill for Nurses*. Congress initially failed to enact the legislation; however, the policy/idea had become popular, and in 1901 the *Army Reorganization Act* included an army nurse corps under the direction of a "graduate nurse" (Flanagan, 1976). Indeed, in 1900, Robb called for a complete system of registration for nurses and state nurses associations began to lobby for registration.

Nursing Leaders as Public Policy Pioneers

There are numerous nursing leaders who served as pioneers in public policy formation in the early to mid-1900s. Only a few are presented here, as is the area of policy they were most noted for. Yet their stories are similar; all of them shared passion, courage, and perseverance. They also all shared a commitment to collective strength. These same attributes are recognized in nursing policy activists today (Box 22.3).

Lavinia Dock: Organizing Nurses for Social Awareness

At the 1904 convention, Lavinia Dock, a founder of the ANA and the first to donate money to establish the *American Journal of Nursing* that same year, stated that it was

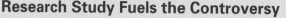

BOX 22.3

Research Study Fuels the Controversy

Political Competence

This phenomenological study used narratives from six politically expert nurse activists to examine the concept of *political competence*. Political competence was defined as the skills, perspectives, and values needed for effective political involvement within nursing's professional role.

> Warners, J. R. (May 2003). A phenomenological approach to political competence: Stories of nurse activists. *Policy, Politics & Nursing Practice, 4* (2), 135–143.

Study Findings

Six themes emerged from the analysis of the lived experiences of the six activists. They included nursing expertise as valued currency, opportunities created through networking, powerful persuasion, commitment to collective strength, strategic perspectives, and perseverance. All six themes were represented in almost all of the interviews and the author concluded that political competence was not about demonstrating one or several of these behaviors. Instead, it appeared to be a "wholistic enterprise requiring the whole package" (p. 142). Each identified theme was a necessary, but not sufficient, ability in political competence.

The findings, while not generalizable to the total population, concluded that nurses who aspire to be more effective in political contexts should consider the behaviors described in the narratives of these seasoned activists and explicitly explore their use in their practice and professional lives. The author concluded with an assertion that more and more practitioners, educators and leaders need to hone and express their political competence if nursing's collective political development is to be advanced.

essential that nurses exercise social awareness. As a result, delegates to the ANA convention that year considered social (policy) issues of the time including child labor, women's suffrage and sex education.

Lillian Wald: Public Health and Child Welfare

Lillian Wald, one of the founders of the ANA, exemplified involvement in social change, community leadership and in politics. She was born to a family of Jewish scholars and rabbis. She graduated nursing school and entered Women's Medical College in New York to become a doctor. During her first year of medical school, she volunteered to teach hygiene to immigrant women in a school on Henry Street.

She quit medical school and in 1893, she and a classmate, Mary Brewster moved to the lower east side neighborhood to provide nursing care in the community (American Association for the History of Nursing [AAHN], 2004). A friend and philanthropist, Jacob Schiff and Mrs. Solomon Loeb agreed to fund Wald and Brewster's purchase of a house on Henry Street. This house became the *Henry Street Settlement* and is considered the founding place for public health nursing. Neighbors came to the house for help with their health, housing, employment and educational needs.

Wald was also concerned about the living conditions of the neighborhood and the lack of safe places for children to play. She helped found the *Outdoor Recreation League*, which worked to gain attention for the need for public parks and which raised funds for what would become the first municipal playground in New York City.

Fortunately, Wald's concern for children at the time was shared by many wealthy charity leaders. During the 1890s, close to 250 new orphanages were incorporated. Vast numbers of children were working in factories. Wald believed that the government needed to protect children and that child labor should be abolished. In 1904, she participated in a meeting with President Theodore Roosevelt lobbying for the creation of a national *Children's Bureau*. However, the powerful industrialist lobby made up of the wealthy factory owners who used child labor was successful in tabling the legislation through their lobbying and political support of legislators (JWA-Lillian Wald, 2004).

However, as an example of how Kingdon's first stream (the conditions that are defined as problems sometimes come to the attention of policy makers through personal experiences), one of President Roosevelt's close friends was James West, who was an orphan himself. West joined Wald and others in 1909 to host a national Conference on Children drawing over 200 leaders from all over the country. The publicity created a public sentiment largely among women of all classes, that child welfare must be put on the national policy agenda.

Kingdon's third stream, politics, resulted in the creation of the *Children's Bureau* in 1912 (Krain, n.d.). Wald was appointed to New York's Immigration Commission in 1908 by Governor Hughes after he visited the Settlement House. Wald's efforts resulted in a report that called for improved living and working standards for workers and their families. The report led to the formation of a *State Bureau of Industries* in New York. Kingdon's three streams again appeared to prevail: conditions—of immigrant workers, idea/policy—need for government regulation, and politics—Wald's relationship with the governor.

By 1909, Wald convinced Metropolitan Life Insurance Company that protecting the health of employees was good for business and they funded nurses from Henry Street to care for their sick policy holders, who were employees of companies insured by Metropolitan Life. The *Henry Street Visiting Nurses Society* began with 10 nurses in 1893. By 1916, it had 250 nurses and was serving over 1,300 patients a day in their homes. Wald convinced the New York Board of Education to hire a nurse in 1902 and so began school nursing in the United States. She also lobbied successfully to change divorce laws so that abandoned spouses could sue for alimony and she assisted the Women's Trade Union League in protecting women from "sweatshop working conditions" (NAHC, 2004).

In 1912, Wald founded the *National Organization for Public Health Nursing.* She was also part of the peace movement against World War I (WWI) and for that was cited as an "undesirable" citizen. In spite of this, she served as chairperson of the Committee on Community Nursing of the American Red Cross and worked with the International Red Cross in the campaign to fight the flu epidemic of 1918 (JWA-Lillian Wald, 2004). Wald was also active in the suffrage movement and believed women should have the right to vote and to be involved in politics.

Wald was also active in nursing at the local, national, and international level. At her insistence, Columbia University appointed the first professor of nursing at a U.S. college or university. She was among the founders of the International Council of Nurses in 1899. Wald's nursing leadership also demonstrated that policy and politics are linked, and that nurses must be active beyond their immediate workplace but also in the community, in business, and in government.

Margaret Sanger: Birth Control

Among the many nurses whose training included a rotation through the Henry Street Settlement, was Margaret Sanger. Sanger witnessed maternal and infant mortality resulting from uncontrolled fertility in the neighborhoods of the Lower East Side of New York city. She cared for women suffering from self-induced abortions and was motivated to make birth control available to women. In 1912, she began writing a column on sex education titled "What Every Girl Should Know," but it was soon censored (Steinem, 2004).

In 1914, Sanger was indicted for violating postal "Comstock" laws after disseminating contraceptive information. She jumped bail and fled to England. She returned to the United States and continued to promote access to birth control throughout her life. She opened a clinic in New York with her sister Ethel Byrne and was jailed, only being released after a hunger strike. She smuggled contraceptive diaphragms from Europe, she founded the *National Committee on Federal Legislation for Birth Control,* and the *American Birth Control League*, which became the *Planned Parenthood Federation of America.*

In 1965, after years of effort, the Supreme Court decision *Griswold v. Connecticut* made birth control legal for married couples. Sanger died shortly thereafter (Margaret Higgins Sanger, 1999). Here again, Kingdon's stream took some time to come together: first conditions had to be compelling—maternal and infant mortality caused by lack of spacing pregnancies and poverty. Then the political stream converged with the women's movement and women demanding that they be able to control their pregnancies. Finally, policy change occurred with the legalization of birth control.

Martha Minerva Franklin: Segregation and Discrimination

Martha Minerva Franklin was another public policy pioneer nurse in the early 20th century. She founded the *National Association of Colored Graduate Nurses* (NACGN) in 1908, with the fundraising assistance of Lillian Wald and Lavinia Dock, who mailed letters to over 1,000 nurses (ANA Hall of Fame, n.d.). The NACGN was formed because many states barred Black nurses from membership in State Nurses Associations. Segregation and discrimination kept nursing education and hospitals separate.

NACGN was instrumental, however, in political lobbying efforts to integrate Black nurses into the armed services during World War II. In 1951, the NACGN merged with the ANA (Flanagan, 1976). Today the *National Black Nurses Association* exists as one of over 70 national nursing organizations, some organized around clinical issues, some relating to ethnicity, some relating to religious beliefs.

D i s c u s s i o n   P o i n t

Can you identify nurses today who are demonstrating the same degree of risk-taking in attempting to influence nursing/health care policy as Dock, Wald, Sanger, & Franklin did in the early 20th century? If so, who are they and what causes are they championing? If not, why not?

NURSING, PUBLIC POLICY, AND POLITICS: MID-TO LATE 1900s

World War II

War has always impacted nursing. In January 1945, President Roosevelt proposed the induction of every registered nurse between the ages of 18 and 45 years into the land and naval forces. ANA lobbied to amend the legislation to provide for the "commissioning" of nurses and for deferments for teachers and supervisors that were essential on the home front. In addition, ANA suggested that credit be given to the states for voluntary recruitment, that a commissioned nurse corps be established by the Veterans Administration with the same benefits that were applied to the military, and that the draft be voluntary. ANA also lobbied for the protection of nursing standards and education at accredited schools, and for prohibition of discrimination based on race, color, creed, or sex.

All of ANA's conditions were accepted except the voluntary recruitment. Instead, Congress agreed to implement mandatory enlistment only if voluntary enlistment failed to meet needed quotas. Final action on the bill was tabled because of changes in the events of the war (Deloughery, 1998; Flanagan, 1976).

D i s c u s s i o n   P o i n t

Wars have played an important role in nursing history and in nursing's involvement in politics. Are nurses highly visible in any current conflict/war worldwide? Are you aware of any current legislative efforts that are being driven by nursing's involvement in such conflicts?

Effecting Social Change

Historically, nursing leaders have participated in many efforts to bring about social change. The efforts of nurse leaders in the suffrage movement have already been discussed. Nurse leaders in the early 20th century were also integrally involved in passing socially-focused legislation that outlawed child labor and provided protection for women abandoned by their husbands.

Nursing was also at the forefront and lent integrity at the time to the civil rights movement. During the civil rights movement, poll taxes and literacy tests were made illegal. In addition, Blacks voted for the first time and the politicians they elected passed laws to eliminate discrimination based on race. Nursing was one of the first professions to eliminate segregation; however, educational opportunities remain out of reach for many students of color today and nursing's responsibility to ensure that the face of the profession reflects the faces of those entrusted to our care still requires much work.

Nursing did not formally participate in the "peace movement," however, it was a movement that brought an end to the Vietnam War after the voting age was reduced to 18 years and young men voted against the draft. The women's movement emerged in the 1970s, and some nursing leaders participated in that movement as well. Nursing and teaching were professions almost exclusively made up of women and employment ads were separated for men and women.

In 1974, the American Nurses Association set up a special account to help pass the equal rights amendment to the constitution. ANA joined the national boycott and moved its convention to a state that had ratified the amendment. The amendment failed ratification by the states. The women's movement continued and nursing and teaching were often used as examples of professions requiring a significant amount of knowledge and skill for which compensation fell far below male-dominated jobs requiring the same levels of knowledge and skill, or "comparable worth." Nursing also became involved in the effort to establish *comparable worth* in employment settings during the 1970s. During this time, women were often paid less for the same work men did. Many states passed "comparable worth laws" during the 1970s, supported by state nurses associations. During the 1980s and beyond, nurses throughout the country went on strike to achieve wages of "comparable worth." Nursing's involvement in the women's movement as its own interest group working in coalition with other women's interest groups strengthened the women's movement.

National Health Insurance and Recognition of Nursing's Impact

National health insurance and efforts to increase access to health care have also been recurrent political and policy issues for nursing. Indeed, nursing leaders such as Lillian Wald, Lavinia Dock, and *Annie W. Goodrich* supported the first unsuccessful platform for national health care proposed by Theodore Roosevelt in 1912. In fact, some critics labeled Goodrich and Wald *socialists* at the time, as a result.

The next proposal for national health care came during Franklin Delano Roosevelt's administration. It was made by *Frances Perkins*, the first female cabinet member to serve as Secretary of Labor. Perkins headed up a committee on economic security during the Great Depression that recommended both income security (social security) and health security. The American Medical Association (AMA), however, opposed national health care insurance and mounted a successful grassroots campaign to discredit a government-sponsored and regulated health system.

Roosevelt abandoned the linkage of health insurance to the social security provisions because he did not want to jeopardize the New Deal programs, which included social security (Corbin, 1993), but he did promise to consider it in his next term. However, Roosevelt died in 1945 and was succeeded by Harry Truman. When Truman ran for his first full term as president, he promoted a prepaid medical insurance plan financed by increasing the social security tax. Again, the AMA opposed these efforts and likened national health coverage to the totalitarianism in [Nazi] Germany (Corbin, 1993).

The ANA, the National League for Nursing Education, and the National Organization for Public Health Nursing however, supported Truman's proposals (Kalisch & Kalisch, 1982).

In 1948, Truman won his first full term as president on a platform promoting universal health coverage, a comprehensive benefit package including prescription drugs, dental coverage, and nursing home care. However, just before the 1950 congressional election, the AMA again waged a successful campaign by assessing each of their members $25 to fund a program designed to "educate" physicians and the public throughout the country about the dangers of socialized medicine, and conspired against candidates for congress who supported Truman's plan. The AMA spent over $4.5 million dollars to defeat this health reform because there were not enough members elected to Congress in 1950 who supported Truman's plan.

National Health Insurance was an idea that lost its attraction in the 1950s, despite the fact that families were losing their life savings and being forced into poverty by costly hospitalizations while science and technology promised to save lives (*a.s.a.p.*, 1993). Again, applying Kingdon's perspective, this occurred because only one of the three criteria was met: conditions—the rising costs of medical care, the idea/policy had significant support; however, the politics—the opposition from powerful interest groups, the AMA, and organized labor who used health coverage as a tool to recruit members made it impossible to pass national health reform (*a.s.a.p.*, 1993). This is an early documented example of grassroots political activity by a group of health professionals (the AMA) directly in the electoral (political) process.

Yet efforts to create national health insurance did not die. In 1974, the ANA continued its historic support of national health insurance, and adopted a resolution supporting national health insurance with the intent to increase nursing's participation in the policy debate. The resolution stated that a national health insurance program should be implemented that would "guarantee coverage for all people for the full range of comprehensive health services" and that nursing care should "be a benefit of the national health insurance program." The resolution also said that data systems necessary for effective management of the national insurance program should be in place to "protect the rights and privacy of individuals" and that nurses should be designated "as health providers in all pending or proposed legislation on national health insurance" (Flanagan, 1976, pp. 670–671). This was an example of the nursing profession's foresight: to cover all people, to protect privacy, to include nurses as essential providers. Indeed, the legislative agenda of the ANA has included all of these principles in subsequent health care legislation.

In follow-up, in 1978, the first Black president of ANA, *Barbara Nichols*, was asked to testify on behalf of Senator Edward Kennedy's *Health Care for All Americans Act*. Television coverage of major issues meant that the organizations selected to testify had to have the trust of the public, and nursing was held in high regard. President Nichols not only advocated for access to comprehensive health services for all, she specifically mentioned mental health services and nursing care in all settings. She insisted that we needed a health system and not a medical system. The AMA opposed the measure. It failed by only a few votes and no major health legislation has passed since that time.

*CONSIDER: The ANA was selected to testify at key hearings on national health insurance, amplifying nursing's voice on television to households throughout the country advocating for comprehensive health coverage, including nursing care in all settings for all Americans.

The ANA has remained active, however, in advocating for access to quality affordable health care. ANA and NLN drafted *Nursing's Agenda for Health Care Reform* (ANA, 2001a), which emphasized the cost effectiveness of using the appropriate provider in the appropriate place at the appropriate level of care. An example of this tenet was public health nurses providing primary care screening in community-based settings. More than 70 nursing specialty organizations signed onto the agenda so that nursing could speak with one voice about health care reform.

President Bill Clinton was elected in 1992 with the support of the ANA and he promised to reform the health care system and to include nursing as part of the solution. Nurse leaders were a part of the task force that developed the *Health Security Act*. This legislative proposal was opposed by the insurance industry, the pharmaceutical industry, and the AMA.

In 1994, these powerful well-financed interest groups successfully worked to defeat any member of Congress who supported reform. Unfortunately, the proposal was completed and introduced after the 1994 elections and the members of Congress who supported it had lost their elections. So, like President Truman, President Clinton lost the majority he needed in Congress to pass health care reform.

Discussion Point

Why would the insurance industry, the pharmaceutical industry and the AMA work together to defeat the *Health Security Act?* What motives may they have shared?

Nursing and Collective Bargaining

Another area nurses were actively involved in politics and policy in the mid- to late 1900s was in determining eligibility for nurses to participate in collective bargaining. For the most part, nurses had little opportunity to participate in the decision making regarding their working conditions in the early to mid-1900s. In 1935, the *Wagner-Connery Labor Relations Act* passed as part of the New Deal. This act guaranteed the right of employees to organize, form unions, and bargain collectively with their employers (see Chapter 17). It assured that workers would have a choice on whether to belong to a union or not, and promoted collective bargaining as the major way to ensure peaceful industry-labor relations.

The act also created a new National Labor Relations Board to arbitrate deadlocked labor–management disputes, guarantee democratic union elections, and penalize unfair labor practices by employers (*Brain.com*, 2004). Health care workers were not at that time included as protected workers; however, they were permitted to organize under this law (Foley, 2002).

Nursing struggled with whether collective bargaining was consistent with professional ethics and whether collective bargaining should be controlled by professional societies or unions. ANA asserted that nurses had the "right and responsibility to promote and protect their economic security" and "to participate actively in determining the conditions of employment which directly affect them" and that included: "the freedom of association," "unified action through organization." The ANA Board of directors in 1938 advised that nurses carefully evaluate the benefits of union membership before joining.

In 1946, after WWII, the ANA established a *Committee on the Employment Conditions of Nurses* because of the persistence of poor salaries and difficult working conditions. The ANA House of Delegates endorsed legislation promoting the 8-hour day, 40-hour workweek for all nurses and the California Nurses Association negotiated their first hospital contracts. That same year, ANA affirmed that state nurses associations should represent nurses in collective bargaining. However, in 1947, Congress passed the *Taft–Hartley Amendments* to the *Wagner Act* and exempted the nonprofit health care industry from governance under the National Labor Relations Act (NLRA). It would be 27 years until 1974 that those amendments were repealed with ANA participating in that political debate (Flanagan, 1976).

Emergence of Medicare and Medicaid

After several draft proposals, Medicare, medical insurance for those older than age 65 and Medicaid, medical insurance for the poor, were passed in 1965 as part of President Lyndon Johnson's dream of a *Great Society*. The AMA initially opposed Medicare and Medicaid and lobbied successfully for compromises to charge "usual" or "customary fees for services," which were included in the bill. Their position changed, however, when doctors realized they would be paid for all their care by the government, without government interference. Not surprisingly, just as Medicare and Medicaid passed, yet before "usual and customary" were defined, physician fees increased dramatically, so physician fees started out higher in the new government-funded Medicare and Medicaid systems than they were before their passage because the government was paying the bills (*a.s.a.p.*, 1993).

The AMA and other health care PACs have continued to strongly support Medicare and Medicaid since these programs began. Physicians and the health insurance industry, which stood to reap billions of dollars, made combined contributions of $48,616,570 to congressional campaigns and national political party soft money accounts during July 1, 1985 through June 30, 1995 to overhaul Medicare (Common Cause News, 1995). In addition, the 73 health care companies approved to administer the new Medicare drug discount card programs gave President George W. Bush and congressional conservatives a total of more than $5 million in hard money, soft money, and PAC contributions between 2000 and 2004 (Paying to Play, 2004). The Center for American Progress suggests that the Bush administration has overlooked the fact that 20 of the 73 contributors (almost one-third) have been involved in fraud charges because of their financial ties to the Bush presidential campaign (Paying to Play, 2004).

Managed Care

Health Maintenance Organizations (HMOs) were also a product of the early 1970s and thus a part of nursing's policy agenda. HMOs as then designed, would provide insurance on a "capitated" basis, or per capita per month rather than per procedure (fee for service). The goal was to keep members healthy so they would not require costly hospital care (Corbin, 1993). The ANA supported HMOs under public or nonprofit organizations.

President Nixon reluctantly signed the *Nurse Training Act of 1971* in which Congress authorized $855 million for 3 years. Unfortunately, because of the costs of the Vietnam War, the president's budgets in 1972 and 1973 fell far below the amount authorized by Congress in 1971. Congress added the funding back in and Nixon vetoed the appropriation bill. In 1974, the president cut the nursing appropriation from $160 million to $49 million. Lobbying efforts by ANA and National League for Nursing convinced Congress to continue to fund the *Nurse Training Act* at the 1973 level despite the president's cuts.

Nursing Political Action Coalitions

The year 1974 brought new election laws allowing for contributions by PACs. The laws limited the amount an individual could contribute to a campaign, and allowed groups to contribute up to $5,000 per election. Nurses contributing small amounts individually could not compare to what physicians gave; however, together, they could contribute to a PAC and give $5,000. N-CAP, the *Nurses Coalition for Action in Politics* (the precursor of the ANA PAC), was created by the ANA to establish political power through endorsement of candidates and political contributions. The slogan "1 in 44" was worn on buttons when nurses visited their legislators to point out that 1 in 44 registered women voters was a RN.

When President Gerald Ford vetoed the *Nurse Training Act of 1974* and attempted to eliminate the scholarship and student loan programs for nursing, ANA lobbied Congress and passed legislation extending the Nurse Training Act, which included, for the first time, funding for advanced practice nursing. President Ford vetoed the bill and ANA mounted a nationwide lobbying effort. Congress overrode the veto with many more than the two-thirds votes required (Kalisch & Kalisch, 1982). Again, a convergence of Kingdon's streams can be identified: a problem of not enough nurses and a powerful political interest group of nurses!

▶ NURSING IN CONTEMPORARY POLITICS AND POLICY

There are many contemporary issues that nursing is discussing in the political arena and at the policy table. Environmental health, the current nursing shortage, and access to health care, are among the most pressing.

Environmental Health

As we begin a new century, an international "environmental health" movement is taking hold in an effort to protect the public from harmful manmade toxins. Anderko (2003) details a list of manmade diseases that have arisen from declining environmental health conditions and advocates for political advocacy in uncovering and tracking this health problem. For example, nurses are currently involved in drafting legislation to decrease the use of polyvinylchlorides (soft plastics) in hospitals because of their known carcinogenic effects. Nurses are also working in neighborhoods (like Lillian Wald) to insist on cleaning up toxins and to make safe places for children to play. Nurses as a powerful, respected, and sophisticated interest group must be a part of future social movements to increase access to quality, affordable health care and to make the world a safer place for all people. Jennings (2003, p. 3) articulately stated that nurses must raise their consciousness about their "professional responsibility to be informed and to join hands with communities as they put in place strategies to mitigate the devastating effects of environmental toxins and pollutants."

Nursing Shortage

This century will experience the greatest nursing shortage in history. The last generation of women to enter the profession (the Baby Boomers) will retire between 2015 and 2025 and the nursing education system does not have the resources in terms of faculty or funding to replace them. Many hospitals in the United States have already begun "poaching" or recruiting from other English-speaking countries around the world that have their own nursing shortage for similar reasons to ours (Health Resources and Services Administrations, 2000). See Chapters 5 and 6 for further discussion of these issues.

Access to Health Care

The number of people in the United States without health coverage grows annually. The high unemployment rate contributes to the number of uninsured, and the rising cost of care results in employers dropping coverage. The Institute of Medicine found overwhelming evidence that the uninsured receive poor health care, if they receive care at all. The uninsured are less likely to receive preventive and screening services; therefore, serious diseases are detected later. The IOM estimated that 20,000 people die each year because they are uninsured (Cutler, 2004). People of color comprise a higher percentage of these mortality statistics. Lack of health insurance is one factor in explaining why people of color rank the lowest on key health status indicators. Three-fourths of the 23 million uninsured in communities of color in the United States lived below 200 percent of the federal poverty level of $37,670 for a family of four in 2003 (Lillie-Blanton & Hoffman, 2005).

More than 50 million Americans rely on Medicaid for their health care. The greatest number of people relying on Medicaid are poor families with children; however the majority of Medicaid dollars are spent on the elderly and disabled—particularly on care provided by for-profit nursing homes. Medicaid pays for two-thirds of all nursing home residents in the country (Editorial: Medicaid Reform, 2005). The number of people requiring nursing home care will increase every year, and cuts in Medicaid funding will result in less care for the most frail in nursing homes. Medicaid spending has increased 65 percent in the last five years. The federal government pays, on average, 57 cents out of every dollar Medicaid spends, and the states pay the balance. President Bush's 2006 budget cuts Medicaid funding to the states.

Per capita, the United States has the most expensive health care system in the world, yet the United States ranks in the lower one-half of health outcome measures internationally—barely higher than Turkey, Mexico, Poland, Hungary, and Korea. The U.S. ranks highest in diabetes mortality. Americans pay 40 percent more per capita than Germans do for health care but received 15 percent fewer real health resources, with much of the money often spent on high-cost, high-tech treatments for preventable diseases.

Nurses must be involved in policy debates to ensure that health care reform addresses cost, quality, and access simultaneously, and preserves the notion that health care is a right and not a privilege.

Professional Organizations or Unions? Who Best to Represent Nursing's Interests?

Whether or not professional nursing and nurses should be involved in politics should not be in question today. Nurses have been involved in politics since the beginning of the profession and will continue to be because they bring a perspective closest to the patient/public. The key question then is "who should speak for nursing?" Foley (2002) asks: Are unions who have multiple groups to represent and multiple agendas the best prepared to represent the profession? Or should it be professional organizations, who are concerned with all aspects of nursing and only nursing?

The proliferation of nursing specialty organizations and unions all claiming to represent "nursing" sometimes jeopardizes nursing's effectiveness because different nursing organizations bring different messages to elected officials. Elected officials tend to listen to the people who help elect them, so whichever nursing organizations are most active in political campaigns through contributions and through grassroots activity (usually only important in first few elections because of the power of incumbency) are the organizations that will be heard.

As more and more nurses are represented by unions, unions are often the voice of nurses in the nation's capitol. It is essential for nurses to be involved in all organizations that represent nurses especially those with PACs because "money talks." Contributing to candidates that promote nursing's agenda to improve the quality of health care is important. It is unfortunate that campaigns are expensive, but it costs money to buy television ad time and to mail literature to people's homes. Professional nurses must make things happen or they will find themselves not only wondering what happened, but complaining about it.

> ***CONSIDER:** Of the 252 candidates endorsed by ANA-PAC for election to the 106th Congress, 88% won their elections (ANA, 2000).

Aligning with a Political Party

Nurses naturally work to effect policy in the workplace but often fail to realize that the work they do and the environment in which it is done is controlled by the government. So, nurses must be involved beyond the private sector if they are to affect change. To do so requires nurses to examine their own values and pick a political party that reflects their views and become involved.

From a health perspective, the primary difference between the two major parties in the United States is that *Democrats* typically favor "public" systems with taxpayers funding access to health services with a guaranteed benefit package and price controls. Criticism of this philosophy is that price regulation will stifle innovation and quality and taxpayers should not have to pay for the ills of others.

Republicans tend to favor a market strategy in which consumers will make choices based on cost and quality within private systems, and that with consumers making market choices, competition will keep prices down. The major criticisms of this strategy are that education and health do not behave like traditional market systems and that market mechanisms in health care yield an advantage to the more affluent and healthier people as well as for providers, suppliers, and insurers. In this system, the financial burden for the sick, disabled, and uninsured is left to the public (government) sector. The public risk pool, or the group of people being cared for by the public sector, is more costly than if the risk were spread among the entire population (Evans, as cited in Harrington & Estes, 2004). The reality is that nurses aren't born Republicans or Democrats and party affiliation is often a reflection of core personal values. It is important, then, to have nurses as leaders in both political parties.

Discussion Point

Do your personal beliefs about health care align more closely with traditional Democratic or Republican party values?

Getting Involved

The message throughout this chapter has been that nurses need to be increasingly involved in both politics and public policy. A good place for most nurses to increase their involvement is to join a professional organization that is politically active. Nurses can also become better informed about current issues by consulting the web sites of these professional organizations (see "Web Resources" at the end of this chapter). Nurses can also check the status of federal and state legislation online.

Other actions that nurses can take to increase their influence in politics and health care policy are shown in Box 22.4. The first of these is to get more involved in electing candidates they want to win. This requires that nurses be knowledgeable regarding the candidates and what values they stand for. It is politically smart for nurses to pick candidates that have a good chance of winning and who share nursing's values. The nurse who works for a losing candidate risks alienating the winner. In races where the candidate is an incumbent and is in a district where they are likely to be reelected, candidates still need help. Specific activities that might be undertaken to support such a candidate include telephone banking, precinct walking, fundraising, letters to the editor, and publicly supporting the candidate in public forums, including other organizations in which you participate.

> ***CONSIDER:** Working together, speaking with one strong voice, nurses are a powerful political force.

Actions that nurses can take to increase their influence in policy setting are also shown in Box 22.4. Again, becoming involved in a professional nursing organization and being informed head the list. Nurses must also know the legislator who represents them. District office staff usually handle "constituent case work" dealing with local, state, or federal agencies. For example, if someone has a problem with the post office, or if he or she is a veteran and cannot get benefits, they would seek help from their U.S. congressional member's district office. The *district chief of staff* is often the only "policy person" in the district. The Capitol office deals with legislation (bills) and policy issues. Staff are key in getting access to your legislator so the politically astute nurse is polite and respectful in dealing with these individuals.

Finally, nurses who want to increase their influence in policy should write their legislative representatives regarding health care issues (Box 22.5). Letters should arrive before any proposed legislation (bill) is heard in committee because key decisions on proposed legislation are made in committee. Bills that have a financial impact are heard in a policy

---

BOX 22.4 Actions Nurses Can Take

To Influence Politics
- Be knowledgeable and get involved in campaigns (the earlier the better).
- Assist candidates in winning the endorsement of key organizations that you may be involved in, such as nursing organizations, parent–teacher organizations, neighborhood organizations.

To Influence Policy
- Be a member of a nursing organization that influences policy at the local, state and federal level.
- Be informed. Subscribe to electronic listservs of elected officials that you agree with and compare the record of your officials.
- Get to know your elected officials.
- Write lobbying letters.
- Write letters to the editor.
- Participate in coalitions of organizations.

BOX 22.5

Sample Lobbying Letter

[1]Lillian Wald, RN, BSN
5 Henry Street
New York, New York 00251

[2]The Honorable Harry Nemo
Member, U.S. House of Representatives
House Office Building
Washington DC, 20015

[3]RE: SUPPORT for HR 1435

[4]Dear Representative Nemo,

[5]I am a Registered Nurse and I have worked in the area of home health care for over five years. In the past two years more and more of the elderly patients I care for have had to be readmitted to the hospital shortly after being discharged from the hospital because they are not taking their prescribed medications.

As you know, H.R. 1435 would provide a guaranteed, affordable prescription drug benefit within the Medicare program. Currently, despite many drug coverage programs for seniors, many remain unaffordable.

[6]It will save costly hospitalizations to provide needed prescription drugs at affordable costs to seniors. Please support H.R. 1435 and please advise me of your current position on this bill. Sincerely,

[7]Lillian Wald, RN, BSN

1: Include your address
2: Address properly (most elected and appointed officials are addressed as "the Honorable")
3: State what the letter is regarding
4: Use their office title in the salutation
5: State your credentials and experience/belief/position
6: Urge support/opposition, ASK for a response with their position
7: Sign letter

committee and a financial committee. Some bills are assigned to two or more committees. This is often a tactic used to defeat the bill before it comes to the floor. If your legislator is not on the committee, write to the Committee Chair at the Committee Office Address. If you write to a legislator who does not represent you (you do not reside in their district or capital address) he/she is unlikely to respond to your communications because you are not one of their constituents. It is good to send a copy of the letter with a brief cover letter to your legislator urging their support when the bill comes before them on the floor (if bills pass out of committee, they go to the "floor" or the entire house of the legislature). If your legislator supports your position on legislation, *SEND A THANK YOU NOTE*! Thank you notes tell legislators you are watching what they are doing.

▶ CONCLUSIONS

In 2001, the ANA called together all the nursing specialty organizations in a *Call to the Profession* to begin a dialogue on collaboration and to develop *Nursing's Agenda for the Future*. Ten domains of mutual efforts were identified and legislative and regulatory activities were one of them. ANA argues that it is essential that nursing speaks with one voice to be heard (ANA, 2003).

So the question is "what should nursing say?" At a time when the country is deeply divided along party lines, nurses must speak for the clients they serve. Nurses are "stakeholders" in what happens in health care (access, insurance coverage, cost, research) in the workplace (staffing levels, safety, scope of practice, autonomy, working conditions), in the economy (unemployment's effect on mental and physical health and access to care, funding for Medicare and Medicaid), in international trade issues (foreign nurse licensure, importation of less expensive prescription drugs) and in the environment (preventing illness caused by pollution). That is, nurses are directly affected by the outcome of countless policies that are enacted or regulated.

There are many levels of political involvement and many spheres in which nurses can be influential, both public and private. Nurses can influence policies in the workplace (both public and private) and the community (both public and private). They can also influence policy within professional organizations (private) and within, the government (Mason et al., 2002). The bottom line is that they must accept a responsibility to be involved in some way.

Pierce (2004, p. 115) perhaps said it best:

> *For the nursing profession to flex its collective political muscle and get involved with the redesign of the nation's health care system, we have to use our leadership to get the professional organizations to think and act collaboratively and to deliver a clear and strategic message to lawmakers.*
>
> *As nurses, as voters, and as constituents, we must be a part of the solution. Our elected officials truly want to know what nurses think and it is our obligation as professionals and as citizens to let them know. Our patients and the American public trusts nurses and are counting on us to advocate on their behalf.*

FOR ADDITIONAL DISCUSSION

1. Are nongovernmental and governmental politics more alike than not? If not, how do they differ? If so, how are they alike?
2. Why do you believe nursing was the first profession to eliminate segregation?
3. What are the most significant nursing issues being debated in the policy arena today?
4. With such limited membership in ANA, will nurses ever have a political power base that is representative of their voting block size?
5. Why are so many nurses reluctant to become active in the political arena? Do they lack the skills to do so? The confidence? Do nurses perceive a lack of congruity between professional behavior and politics?
6. With the AMA typically being far better represented than the ANA in legislative lobbying, is nursing's risk of being dominated by medicine greater than ever?
7. How well informed are most legislators about contemporary health care and professional nursing issues?
8. What do you believe will be the next "great" policy issue affecting nursing, to be debated in the political arena?

REFERENCES

American Association for the History of Nursing [AAHN] (2004) *Gravesites of prominent nurses: Lillian D. Wald*. Retrieved from http://www.aahn.org/gravesites/wald.html.

American heritage dictionary of the English language. *Policy, definition (2000)*. Retrieved June 27, 2005 from http://dictionary.reference.com/ search?q=politics.

American Nurses Association (2000). *ANA-PAC endorses Hillary Clinton for U.S. Senate*. Retrieved June 27, 2005 from http://www.ana.org/pressrel/2000/pr0208.htm.

American Nurses Association. (2001a). *Nursing's agenda for health care reform*. Washington, D.C.

American Nurses Association. (2001b). Analysis of American nurses association staffing survery. Retrieved from www.nursingworld.org-staffing-ana-pdf.pdf.

American Nurses Association. (2001c). Health and safety survey. Retrieved June 27, 2005 from www.nursing-world.org/surveys/hssurvey.pdf.

American Nurses Association. (2003). *Nursing's agenda for the future.* Washington, DC.

ANA Hall of Fame: Martha Minerva Franklin. (n.d.) Retrieved June 27, 2005 from http://www.nursingworld.org/hoh/ franmm.htm.

Anderko, L. (2003). Protecting the health of our nation's children through environmental health tracking. *Policy, Politics & Nursing Practice, 4*(1), 14–21.

a.s.a.p. (1993). Washington, DC: Families USA.

Brain.com. (2004). *National Labor Relations Act.* Retrieved June 27, 2005 from http://www.classbrain.com/art-teenst/publish/ article_122.shtml.

Common Cause News (1995). *Politically insured: Doctor recommended.* Retrieved June 27, 2005 from http://www.ccsi.com/~comcause/news/medical.html.

Cook, C. (2004). *The Cook political report.* Retrieved May 10, 2005, from http://www.cookpolitical.com.

Corbin, D. (1993). *A history of health care reform: Six decades of debate.* Washington, DC.

Cutler, D.M. (2004). *Your money or your life.* Oxford, New York: Oxford University Press.

Deloughery, G. (1998). *Issues and trends in nursing.* St. Louis: Mosby.

Editorial: Medicaid reform: The next big thing. (March 3, 2005) *The Economist.* Retrieved 5/8/05 from http://www.economist.com/world/na/displayStory.cfm?story_if=3723112.

Ellis, J. R. & Hartley, C. L. (2004). *Nursing in today's world: Trends ,issues and management.* (8th ed.). Philadelphia: Lippincott Williams & Wilkins.

Flanagan, L. (1976). *One strong voice.* Kansas City, MO: American Nurses Association.

Foley, M. (2002). Collective action in health care. In D. J. Mason, Leavitt, J. K., & Chaffee, M. W. (Ed.), *Policy and politics in nursing and health care* (pp. 387–397). Philadelphia: W. B. Saunders.

Harrington, C. & Estes, C. (Eds.). (2004). *Health policy: Crisis and reform in the U.S. health care delivery system* (4th Ed.). Boston: Jones and Bartlett.

Health Resources and Services Administration [HRSA] (2000). *The national sample survey of registered nurses.*

Jennings, C.P. (2003). A fond Forwell to Managing Editor Many Chaffee Politics Nursing Practice. 2003;4:3

JWA- Lillian Wald-outdoor recreation league, New York Immigrant Commission, Nursing Insurance Partnership, Federal Children's Bureau, House on Henry street, red scare resistance (2004) Retrieved May, 10, 2005, from http://www.jwa.org/exhibits/wov/wald/lw5.html.

Kalisch, B. & Kalisch, P. (1982). *Politics of nursing.* Philadelphia: Lippincott.

Kohn, L., Corrigan, J., & Donaldson, M. (2000). *To err is human: Building a safer health system.* Washington, DC: National Academy Press.

Krain, J. B.(n.d.). *Lillian Wald.* Retrieved May, 10, 2005, from http://www.jewishmag.co.il/51mag/wald/lillianwald.htm.

Lillie-Blanton, M. & Hoffman, C. (2005). The role of health insurance coverage in reducing racial/ethnic disparities in health care. Health Affairs *24*(2), 398–408

Margaret Higgins Sanger. (1999). Retrieved May, 10, 2005, from http://search.eb.com/women/articles/Sanger_Margaret_Higgins.html.

Mason, D. J., Leavitt, J. K., & Chaffee, M. W. (Eds.). (2002). *Policy & politics in nursing and health care* (4th ed.). Philadelphia: W. B. Saunders.

National Association for Home Care [NAHC]. (2004). *History of home health.* Retrieved.

Page, A. (2004). Keeping patients safe: Transforming the work environment for nurses. In IOM (Ed.), *Crossing the quality chasm* (vol. 435): National Academies.

Paying to play: Health care companies, campaign contributions and Medicare drug discount cards (June 1, 2004). Center for American Progress. Retrieved from http://www.americanprogress.org/site/pp.asp?c=biJRJ8OVF&b=84766.

Pierce, K. M. (2004). Insights and reflections of a congressional nurse detailee. *Policy, Politics & Nursing Practice, 5*(2), 113–115.

Sabatier (Ed.). (1999). *Theories of the policy process.* Boulder, CO: Westview Press.

Steinem, G. (2004). *Margaret Sanger.* Retrieved from http://www.time.com/time/time100/leaders/profile/sanger3.htm.

Warners, J. R. (2003). A phenomenological approach to political competence. Stories of nurse activists. *Policy, Politics & Nursing Practice, 4*(2), 135–143.

BIBLIOGRAPHY

Belcher, D. (2003). Nurses making a difference. Bridging the gap between nurses and the media: The grassroots Center for Nursing Advocacy. *American Journal of Nursing, 103*(5), 130.

Beu, B. (2003). Health policy issues. Organizing and energizing the grass roots. *AORN Journal, 78*(6), 1011–1013.

Brekke, M. (2004). Grassroots efforts do change policy. *Beginnings, 24*(3), 5.

Brown, T. M. & Fee, E. (2004). Voices from the past. Peace and feminism. *American Journal of Public Health, 94*(1), 34.

Des Jardin, K. E. (2001). Political involvement in nursing—politics, ethics, and strategic action. Second article in a two-part series. *AORN Journal, 74*(5), 613–615, 617–618, 621–626.

Evans, C. H. & Degutis, L. C. (2003). What it takes for Congress to act. *American Journal of Health Promotion, 18*(2), 177–181.

Franko, F.P. (2001). Health policy issues. Further debating the issue of political action committees. *AORN Journal, 74*(2), 236, 239, 241–242.

Gonzales, R. & Meehan-Hurwitz, J. (May 2004). The politics of caring. Tips for political action. *American Journal of Nursing, 104*(8), 30.

Gordon, S. & Buresh, B. (2001). *From silence to voice.* Canadian Nurses Association. Now distributed by Cornell University Press, New York.

Harrris, E. (2004). Nurses making an impact through grassroots advocacy. *Michigan Nurse, 77*(1), 10.

Hughes, F. A. (2002). Role of the government chief nurse in policy and the profession. *Nursing and Health Policy Review, 1*(2), 93–101.

Jennings, C. P. (2004). Political elections shaping health policy. *Policy, Politics & Nursing Practice, 5*(1), 3–4.

Jennings, C.P. (2000). Up close and personal. Meeting our nurse legislators: U.S. Representative the Honorable Lois Capps, 22nd Congressional District of California. *Policy, Politics, & Nursing Practice, 1*(1), 52.

Kitchen, L. (2004). To impact political policy, first prepare. *Nursing Management, 35*(1), 14–15.

Olson, L. L. (2004). Politics, health policy, and ethics: Is there a relationship? *Chart, 100*(7), 9–10.

O'Sullivan, A. (2004). Mentoring students for political action. *Chart, 100*(7), 8–9.

Phillips, R. C. (2003). The legislative process. The ABCs of lobbying. *AAACN Viewpoint, 25*(6), 6–7.

Shamian, J. & Griffin, P. (2003). Translating research into health policy. *Canadian Journal of Nursing Research, 35*(3), 45–52.

Trossman, S. (2004). Political action, anyone? *American Journal of Nursing, 104*(7), 73–74.

Warner, J. R. (2003). A phenomenological approach to political competence: Stories of nurse activists. *Policy, Politics & Nursing Practice, 4*(2), 135–143.

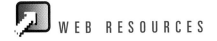

WEB RESOURCES

Academy of Medical Surgical Nurses (AMSN) Official Position Statement on Political Awareness for the Registered Nurse	**http://www.medsurgnurse.org/**
American Nurses Association	**http://www.needlestick.org/gova/federal/ legis/109/legreg109.pdf**
American Public Health Association	**http://www.apha.org/**
ANA State Government Relations	**http://www.nursingworld.org/gova/ state.htm**
Federal Election Commission. (November 2003). Pacronyms.	**http://www.fec.gov/pages/pacronym.shtml**
Government Affairs: American Nurses Association	**http://www.nursingworld.org/gova/**
How a Bill Becomes a Law (narrative)	**http://thomas.loc.gov/home/ lawsmade.toc.html**
How a Bill Becomes a Law (pictorial)	**http://www.leginfo.ca.gov/bil2lawd.html**
Letters to a Legislator (Tips)	**http://www.arcwa.org/ hottipsletterstolegislators. htm**
Letters to Legislators (Adapted from League for Women Voters, American Nurses Association Voter materials)	**http://nursing.boisestate.edu/nursb434spring/ letters.htm**
Library of Congress: Meta-Indexes for State and Local Government Information	**http://www.loc.gov/global/state/ stategov.html**
Nurses for a Healthier Tomorrow	**http://www.nursesource.org/members.html**
Nurses: Money to Congress (2004)	**http://www.opensecrets.org/industries/ summary.asp?Ind=H1710**
Nursing World: Reading and Reference Room	**http://www.nursingworld.org/readroom/**
Registered Nurses Association of Ontario (RNAO)— compares the platforms of the three main political parties to RNAO's Commit to Health, Health Care & Nurses	**http://www.rnao.org/policy/ platform_ comparison.asp**
Understanding and Influencing the Legislative Process: Society of Gastroenterology Nurses and Associates, Inc.	**http://www.sgna.org/Resources/guidelines/ guideline10.pdf#search='Understanding%20 and%20Influencing%20the%20Legislative%20 Process%20nursing'**

Nursing's Professional Associations

Marjorie Beyers

N
ever underestimate the importance and power of nursing's professional associations. Whether you are a member or not, professional associations are of value to nurses and to the profession. These associations promote the development of leaders and advancement of nursing practice. They provide valuable resources for both nurses and the public and they serve as forums for communication with consumers, business, industry, and government on matters affecting nursing and nursing practice.

Clearly, professional nursing associations are an integral part of the culture of nursing as evidenced by the number of associations today. The Encyclopedia of Associations lists almost 300 nursing associations worldwide. Of these, over 40 associations represent countries other than the United States. The remainder are based in the United States, although many have international ties (Hunt, 2004). Thirty-seven associations serve the nursing home specialty. The remaining 200 or so associations are named for a clinical specialty group, a type of service, such as long-term care; policy interests or functions, such as education, administration or clinical practice role; or a cultural background such as native Alaskan nurses. A listing of many of these nursing associations is in the Web Resources section located at the end of this chapter.

For many professionals, membership in their professional association is meaningful. There is a dearth of information, however, about the numerous professional nursing associations that exist today, what populations they serve, how their purposes overlap and differ, and what benefits result from that membership. One must question whether professional associations in nursing are more alike than different and what criteria separate one from the other. Little is known about why some of these associations were formed in the first place, what sustains them over time and how these associations are being impacted by changes in society as well as the contemporary economic and political environment. Similarly, systematic thinking about the future needs of the nursing profession and of nurses individually is lacking. This information is essential to shaping the future of professional nursing associations.

Discussion Point

What is the rationale for the professional association's continuing existence?

This chapter introduces the association as an organizational entity and explores the role professional associations have played in the nursing profession's history and their potential for becoming a significant force for shaping the future of the profession. The vital role of members in association work and contemporary challenges faced by professional nursing associations are discussed. Finally, the future of professional associations is examined in response to societal, economic and health care changes.

▶ THE GROWTH OF PROFESSIONAL ASSOCIATIONS

Professional associations have evolved over hundreds of years. Their history reflects the natural tendency of people to join together for a common purpose, the development of commerce and industry and the political and societal realities of achieving public recognition and prestige. The impetus for the development of many professional associations was and continues to be public safety and welfare. The growth of professional associations reflects the often chaotic progress toward recognition of a given profession by society.

*CONSIDER: The professions of law, medicine and the clergy were among the first to be recognized by professional associations, followed over time by a multitude of other groups.

Professional associations as we know them today began to take shape during the time of the industrial revolution. This time was characterized by the emergence of trade associations, guilds and professional associations that reflected changes in society. Essentially these groups served a dual but interrelated purpose of recognition; people were concerned about the quality of the goods and services they consumed and "professionals" were seeking public recognition for their work. Professional associations recognized and met both these needs.

▶ THE FORMATION AND WORK OF NURSING'S EARLY PROFESSIONAL ASSOCIATIONS

There are few, if any, studies of the role professional nursing associations have played in the development of nursing as a profession. Such studies would most likely reveal that nursing has achieved national and international recognition as a result of leaders working together through the structure of associations in the late 19th and early 20th centuries (Box 23.1).

Associations have long been integral to world cultures and societies as evidenced by historical texts, historical novels, family legend, and lore. In the late 18th and 19th centuries, associations generally served the interests of the elite; the landowners, wealthy merchant, and other influential people. A wealth of information on "secret

---

BOX 23.1 | Milestones for Professional Nursing Associations

1893: American Society of Superintendents of Training Schools for Nurses (forerunner to the National League for Nursing (NLN) is chartered.
1897: Nurses' Associated Alumnae of the United States and Canada, forerunner to the American Nurses Association (ANA) is chartered.
1899: International Council of Nurses is chartered.
1900: American Journal of Nursing is chartered.
1903: First Nurse Practice Acts are passed in the United States.
1908: National Association of Colored Graduate Nurses is founded (became part of ANA in 1951, making ANA one of the first national associations to declare membership open to all ethnic groups).
1911: Nurses Associated Alumnae of the United States and Canada is renamed ANA.
1912: Society of Superintendents of Training Schools for Nurses is renamed. The National League for Nursing Education (NLNE). It assumes functions of other associations and becomes the organization known as the National League for Nursing in 1952.
1922: Sigma Theta Tau is founded; it becomes the International Honor Society of Nurses in 1985.

Source: Adapted in part from Cherry & Jacob, 2002, p. 4.

societies" and private clubs further illustrates how people with common interests and affluence joined together to set their own agenda. During the end of the 18th century and beginning of the 19th century, associations flourished. Associations were the vehicle used by the growing number of scholars, trade groups, and individuals with common economic interests to advance their work within the social structure. Nursing associations in the United States have their roots in this movement, which was closely tied to the emancipation of women.

Reading the history of professional nursing associations engenders respect for the nursing leaders who shaped the profession of today. There is ample evidence that nursing leaders were driven by a common cause, clear direction for action, and passion for achieving the goals to advance the profession for the benefit of the public and of nurses. The work of what we know now as the American Nurses Association, the National League for Nursing, and the International Council of Nurses resulted from collaboration toward a common goal. A brief overview of the origins of each follows.

National League for Nursing

The National League for Nursing (NLN) began its legacy as the Society of Superintendents of Training Schools for Nurses, formed in 1893. Renamed the National League for Nursing Education in 1912, a new association, the National League for Nursing was formed in 1952 as a result of the reorganization of nursing's major professional associations (Spaulding & Notter, 1965, p. 335; Henderson & Nite, 1978, p. 73). From the outset, NLN's mission has been advancing nursing education.

American Nurses Association

The history of the American Nurses Association (ANA) began with a convening of alumnae groups led by nurses from Bellevue, the Illinois Training School, and Johns Hopkins, in the 1880s. These alumnae groups adopted the constitution and bylaws for a new organization, the Nurses Associated Alumnae of the United States and Canada, in 1897. Charter alumnae groups included Bellevue Hospital Training School; New York Hospital Training School; and Brooklyn Hospital Training School in New York City; the Farrand Training School; Harper Hospital, Detroit; the Garfield Hospital Training School in Washington, DC; the Illinois Training School; Cook County Hospital, Chicago; Johns Hopkins Training School, Baltimore; the Massachusetts General Hospital Training School, Boston; the Philadelphia Training School and The University of Pennsylvania Training School in Philadelphia; and two schools from Canada.

The *American Journal of Nursing* was established in 1900 as the official journal of the association. In 1911, the association was renamed as the American Nurses Association (ANA), which continues to be the official name. The ANA began its collective bargaining activities in the 1940s.

International Council of Nurses

The early development of the ANA and the NLN was influenced by the women's movement at the turn of the last century. The June 1899, meeting of the *International Congress of Women*, held in London, was particularly notable for nurses. At this meeting, nurses from around the world attended and American nurse leaders, along with leaders from Great Britain and Germany founded the International Council of Nurses (ICN). What is now the ANA was both a charter member and constituent member of the ICN. The ICN focused its energy on the organizational development of nurses throughout the world.

Ethel Gordon Fenwick, the first president of the ICN strongly believed that nurses should step forward to guide their own destiny. Her tireless work for the profession is documented in the literature. Typical of her addresses is this excerpt from the public address she presented in Buffalo, New York, in 1901. In this address she said,

> *Every country needs practice curriculum, examinations, a uniform system of nursing education and uniform statement of qualification ... registration essential to practice ... to protect the public" (Fenwick, 1901).*

▶ SHAPING THE NURSING PROFESSION

Nurse leaders in the United States, led by the National Associated Alumnae of the United States and Canada and the Society of Superintendents of Training Schools for Nurses, created the template for nursing's development in the United States. The three main prongs for development of the profession were uniform education, standards of practice and regulation of the profession. In keeping with the spirit and strategy of the ICN, to achieve a legal basis for nursing in every country throughout the world, nurse leaders in the United States began work to achieve licensure for nurses in every state. This work to develop *nurse practice acts* in every state took place concurrently with similar development in many countries throughout the world. Nursing was not alone in this effort. Many other professional groups were also seeking licensure in the United States and the District of Columbia.

> ***CONSIDER:** The connection between professional competence and licensure in the early 20th century was considered a modern notion.

Imagine the passion and energy it took to convince members of the nursing profession, the public and legislators that licensure was important for the profession and the public. It took almost 20 years for every state to pass nurse practice acts. The first was passed in North Carolina in 1903. All states had a nurse practice act by 1923. Nurse leaders collaborated on defining the profession, achieving legal recognition of the profession and establishing a culture for professional nursing which has continued to the present time. Nursing continues to benefit from this work to establish nurse practice acts, mandatory licensure, the development of standards for nursing education and practice, and promulgation of nursing's *Code of Ethics*.

Early nursing associations not only worked together to build the base for recognition of nursing as a profession, but also acted as stewards of the profession. Nursing's professional associations were viewed as resources to advance the profession. In addition to the ANA and the NLN, several other nursing associations were formed by the 1940s. Nurse leaders, cognizant of the role of associations to serve nurses commissioned the Raymond Rich Associates to study what nurses needed from their professional associations. Changes in society and in health care delivery were considered.

The *Rich Report* recommendations led to reorganization of the professional nursing associations formed between 1892 and 1949. The rationale for the reorganization was that larger associations with more assets and capability could advance the profession better than any one of the participating associations and groups could, working singly. In this reorganization, the ANA continued with its mission to advance and support the profession. The National League for Nursing Education (NLNE) became a new organization, The National League for Nursing (NLN). The new NLN absorbed the education functions and related functions of the National Organization for Public Health Nursing, the Association of Collegiate Schools of Nursing, the Joint Committee on Practical Nurses and Auxiliary Workers in Nursing Services, the Joint Committee on Careers in Nursing and the National Committee for the Improvement of Nursing Service and the National Nursing Accrediting Service (Raymond Rich Associates Report, 1946; Henderson & Nite, 1978). The reorganization of nursing's professional associations is testimony to the wisdom and vision of the early leaders as they focused on how best to advance nursing practice and the environment for practice.

> **Discussion Point**
>
> Imagine a world without any professional nursing associations. In this world, how are standards of education and practice, regulation of the practice and advancement of nursing knowledge achieved?

▶ DEVELOPMENT OF SPECIALTY NURSING PROFESSIONAL ASSOCIATIONS

While the ANA the and NLN concentrated on shaping the nursing profession as a whole, a number of nurses formed associations to meet their practice related needs. The *American Association of Industrial Nurses*, which traces its origins to 1915, is one of the oldest specialty nursing professional associations. Many other specialty nursing groups established professional nursing associations in the 1950s. Among these associations were the American Association of Nurse Anesthetists established in 1952, the Association of Operating Room Nurses formed in 1957, The American College of Nurse Midwifery formed in 1955, the National Association for Practical Nurse Education and Service (NAPNES) established in 1941, the National Federation of Licensed Practical Nurses formed in 1949 and both the Catholic and Lutheran Nursing Groups (Spaulding & Notter, 1965).

Nursing Professional Associations in the Last 50 Years of the 20th Century

During the early years of the 20th century, most nurses could name the professional nursing associations and could articulate their mission, services to members and their contribution to the nursing profession. The focus was on establishing nursing as a profession. The number of nursing professional associations continued to grow. By the 1950s, there was some concern about how to bring these associations together in an effort to strengthen nursing and to unify the voice of nursing. Virginia Henderson observed that "Proliferation of organizations is so marked that only through some federation of organizations could unity be achieved" (Henderson & Nite, 1978, p. 73). However, the focus had changed from concentration on the nursing profession to advancing nursing and nurses.

The proliferation of nursing associations has occurred naturally. Reasons for this proliferation are not fully understood, but it can be speculated that contributing factors were development of specialization in health care following World War II, the growing number of nurses and the expansion of hospitals. The value of associations to the public may also have been a factor. By the second half of the 20th century, associations were an accepted way for professional, business- and industry-related groups to gain recognition and acceptance of their work by the public. It stands to reason that nurses would develop and use professional nursing associations for this purpose.

Discussion Point

How important are relationships among professional associations within health care to the work of nurses in health care?

It would be informative to study the patterns of association development in nursing, the reasons why there are so many specialty nursing associations, and their value to the profession. It could be postulated that these associations grew because of several factors. Among them might be the growing complexity of nursing practice, the expanded and more differentiated knowledge base for each nursing specialty, the influence of collegial relationships with physicians and other health professionals, and the growing demand for ensuring practice qualifications through certification. Some nursing professional associations had their origins as nursing sections in physician associations such as the Association of Women's Health, Obstetric and Neonatal Nurses, which evolved as a separate association to provide education, certification and support for nursing practice in collaboration with other health professionals.

Each nursing professional association has its own valued history and traditions and plays an important role in advancing nursing practice. Members participating in their respective associations adopt a code of ethics, develop standards of behavior and practice, and establish designations of competency designed to serve the public and to achieve recognition. Certification supported by education, mentoring, and networking is a valued service of most specialty nursing associations. Associations also provide opportunities for leadership development through volunteer leadership roles. Most associations hold conventions, annual meetings, or both, provide educational programs and develop tools and resources to support and advance the practice of nursing. Another function of associations is to advocate for the practice of nursing with the public, government, and within health care. Major categories of professional association services are shown in Box 23.2.

It can be posited that the proliferation of nursing associations was inevitable in the culture of the United States. Associations can be viewed as a cultural phenomenon

BOX 23.2 Major Categories of Professional Association Services

Professional Development including networking; publications such as newsletters, journals, and multimedia materials; educational programs; conferences and conventions; information and resources, such as tools and issue papers; credentialing and socialization.

Advancing the Profession through activities including research, establishing standards of practice, designations and productivity and ethics for the profession.

Policy and Advocacy including government relations, liaisons with related and influential groups, legislative advocacy to provide the resources and support for professional practice and the appropriate environment for practice.

and nursing was probably influenced by this. Therefore, to better understand nursing associations it is useful to review a perspective of associations in general. Insights on what the public has grown to expect of associations and what members expect follow.

The Public and Professional Associations

Professional associations serve members whose common bond is their profession and are formed, at least in part, to enhance the professional status of members. The public depends on associations as a way to reach members, to learn about standards of practice or to become informed about matters within the association's expertise. The mutual interdependency of professional associations and the public is grounded in trust. The professional association, through the collective work of its members, is expected to define and promote standards of behavior and practice.

[***CONSIDER:** The public expects the association to be informed about practice.]

Disseminators of Information

As a source of information about standards of practice and qualifications of persons engaged in the practice, associations are viewed as credible sources of information about services needed by the public. They advocate for the public served, identifying and resolving issues surrounding practice, which can be raised by members, leaders, or the public. When called for, the association takes action to enhance the profession by establishing relevant standards, laws, and rules and regulations. This action may involve changing or eliminating practices that are harmful or no longer useful and involves cooperation with other groups that impact or influence the practice, the laws and regulation. The focus on the action is to protect the public safety and welfare.

Advocacy, Integrity, and Competency

Nurses, as members, also have expectations from their professional nursing associations. The fact that there are so many nursing associations is evidence that they are of value to nurses who form them, establish the mission and who participate in the association activities. Associations as we know them today, advocate for their members. Some view this advocacy role as protecting the "property rights" of members to practice their profession. A counter view is that associations enhance the ability of members to fulfill their professional role with integrity. Generally, their mission is to identify issues and resolve problems affecting the profession, to promote professional development and provide services useful to members. Joining a professional nursing association enables nurses to use the services that association provides to enhance their ability to practice with integrity and competency.

Nurses, like members of other professional associations, value membership in their professional association because it conveys professional status, a willingness to uphold the standards of the profession and a vested interest in the issues and concerns the professional association takes on for benefit of the members. Credentials are valued in this society. For nurses, the credentials include licensure, certification, formal and continuing education, experience and participation in community or professional activities. Resumes often include a section for "professional development" or "professional accomplishments." The public often looks for the professional membership credential when seeking services and may view this membership as a seal of approval or as a mark of professionalism.

The Vital Role of Members

Associations exist because of members. Members have many opportunities for leadership development within associations. Because most associations do their work through task forces, committees and groups and because they rely on members for information about

BOX 23.3

Self-Evaluation: Professional Association Involvement

- Do you belong to one or more professional associations? In nursing? In other areas?
- Do you participate in activities or use services of professional nursing associations? Do you ever visit the websites?
- Do you subscribe to e-news?
- Do you attend meetings, conventions or educational programs?
- Do you behave as a loyal member by being informed regarding issues?
- Do you share your opinions and concerns with leaders?

trends in practice, changes in competencies and other aspects of the practice role, members have great influence in the direction associations set for their work. To be an effective member, one must know about the association, understand the issues and concerns the association faces, keep informed about new events and happenings, participate in association programs and projects, and contribute to the association through volunteer activities.

The first step is the decision to join an association. A self-evaluation regarding professional association involvement is included in Box 23.3. Once a decision is made to join an association, members must then decide their level of involvement in the selected association.

There are four ranges of member involvement. *First level* involvement includes becoming a member and participating in meetings, conventions, educational programs, or using products and services. *Second level* involvement entails engagement in projects or programs. *Third level* involvement requires a time commitment such as appointment to committees or a leadership role in a major activity. *Fourth level* involvement engages members in leadership roles as an officer, committee chair, spokesperson, or other type of engagement that relies on the member's expertise and talent of leaders. All members contribute to the association by participating in surveys for member input, selection of leaders, and member recruitment and retention.

Recruitment and retention of members is guided by member input. Most associations routinely survey members to learn why they joined the association, what motivates their continued membership, what type of programs and services they need to support and advance their practice and whether their expectations of the association are being met. Such surveys inform association leaders in the process of strategic planning. Member participation in these surveys is essential to develop realistic future goals. Being informed about the survey results also helps members understand how their association is responding to member needs and values.

One of the most important roles of members is to understand what associations are, how they function and how to participate in ways that make a difference. Members seek value from professional associations but have a role to ensure that the association has the capability to produce that value. Typically nursing professional associations are voluntary not-for-profit organizations formed to advance the profession. The key relationships of these associations are relationships between and among members and relationships between the association and external groups such as other nursing associations, related health care associations and the public. An overview of associations follows.

The Organization of an Association

Associations are legal entities and as such are "democratic" organizations. The organizational structure of associations embodies volunteer leadership and depending on the size and resources, paid staff to manage the association's business. The size of the association influences the level of staff and volunteer involvement. Larger associations typically have more staff structure than smaller associations. Both volunteer leadership and staff manage the business of the association, work with members to identify issues, develop positions and insights about the issues for public discussion, conduct meetings, engage members in forming and adopting resolutions that affect practice, plan and provide programs and services and are accountable to the members.

*CONSIDER: Member involvement is critical to maintaining relevant agendas for associations.

First, associations must sustain sufficient numbers of members to represent their interests and influence within the profession and in the public arena. Monitoring membership numbers, trends in membership, and member demographics is essential for membership associations. Second, associations must maintain interaction with members to keep members up-to-date on change and to learn about their needs for programs and services. Maintaining interaction with members is more complex for associations with chapters or other forms of local or regional divisions that may be separate but related associations. In this situation, the interaction has two focal points, the chapter and the member. Third, associations must support visionary leaders. Members have an accountability to identify and select and elect leaders capable of visioning the future and leading the association.

Most associations establish membership requirements in keeping with their mission, to define eligibility and types of membership. Multiple categories of membership enable an association to engage more people in association activities. Types of membership categories may include *Full, Associate, Affiliate, Honorary, Organizational*, or *Liaison*. Each association defines criteria for the rights and responsibilities of each type of membership. Generally full members have access to all programs and services and may vote. Associate members may have access to selected programs and services as do affiliate members. Honorary members are selected and recognized for their contributions to the association and to the profession. Organizational members may represent a partnership or relationship tied into the core functions of the association. Liaison members may have access to information and none or limited member privileges.

Associations with chapters or other types of divisions may have dual membership. The point of joining the association may be the local chapter or the national or international association. In some cases members have the option of joining only the national or only the local association.

Membership categories are tied to the association's revenue base and to the association's public agenda to foster working partnerships with companies and related businesses with mutual concerns and interests. Boxes 23.4 to 23.6 identify types of membership for three professional nursing associations.

*CONSIDER: Associations achieve power that is more than the sum of members, but they depend on collective action of members and respected leaders to gain recognition and influence.

The work of associations is similar to the work of most businesses in that each association has a charter, a mission and legal status in the state in which it resides. Most associations are not-for-profit organizations and as such are eligible for tax-exempt status, an important consideration in association finance. Associations do pay tax on their for-profit ventures, which are separated from their mission-specific activities. There are different types of tax-exempt codes that determine what the association may or may not do, such as accepting grants and becoming involved in political campaigns, to retain its tax-exempt status. Associations may create separate organizations, such as foundations for these purposes.

BOX 23.4

Membership Structure of the American Nurses Association

- Functioned as the Nurses Associated Alumnae before 1887
- Founded as the Nurses Associated Alumnae of the United States and Canada in 1887
- The American Journal of Nursing was founded in 1900
- Renamed, The American Nurses Association in 1911
- Established the American Nurses Foundation in 1955

Mission

The ANA is the only full-service professional organization representing the nation's 2.7 million registered nurses (RNs) through its 54 constituent-member associations. The ANA advances the nursing profession by fostering high standards of nursing practice, promoting the economic and general welfare of nurses in the workplace, projecting a positive and realistic view of nursing, and by lobbying the Congress and regulatory agencies on health care issues affecting nurses and the public.

Members

ANA Constituent Members
There are 54 constituent nurses associations which include the 50 states, the District of Columbia, Guam, the Virgin Islands, and the Federal Nurses Association.

Associate Organizational Members
- Center for American Nurses
- United American Nurses, AFL-CIO

Organizational Affiliates
- American Association of Critical Care Nursing
- American Association of Nurse Anesthetists
- American Psychiatric Nurses Association
- Association of periOperative Registered Nurses
- Association of Rehabilitation Nurses
- Association of Women's Health, Obstetric & Neonatal Nurses
- Emergency Nurses Association
- National Association of Orthopaedic Nurses
- Oncology Nursing Society
- Society of Otorhinolaryngology and Head–Neck Nurses

Direct Individual Members
Currently RNs who live or practice in the following states can join under this category: Missouri, New Hampshire, New Mexico, Oklahoma, Pennsylvania, Rhode Island, Utah

Individual Affiliate Members
ANA recognizes that you may not be able to afford full membership in ANA but still want to support the important work ANA does on behalf of the profession and access ANA's Members Only. Individual Affiliate members receive access to the Members Only website of NursingWorld.org and receive some discounts. They have no voting rights in ANA.

Related Entities
- American Nurses Credentialing Center
- American Nurses Foundation
- American Academy of Nursing

BOX 23.5

Membership Structure of Sigma Theta Tau International, Honor Society of Nursing

Established in 1922 by six students from the Indiana University Training School for Nurses in Indianapolis, Indiana, Sigma Theta Tau's charter members were Mary Tolle Wright, Edith Moore Copeland, Marie Hippensteel Lingernan, Dorothy Garrious Adams, Elizabeth Russell Belford, Elizabeth McWilliams Miller and Ethel Palmer Clarke, advisor.

The Sigma Theta Tau International (STTI) Foundation for Nursing was created in 1993. Its purpose is to raise money to support programs and initiatives of STTI.

Mission

Through global linkages, STTI, the honor society of nursing, strives to support nurses and the profession to enhance the health of all people. The honor society values the diversity of knowledge, experience, culture and beliefs of other health care organizations and believes that working together can make the most impact on health care issues.

Membership

Individual member: selected based on high levels of achievement in scholarship, leadership, research, or practice. Seeks individuals who have demonstrated a commitment to nursing excellence.
Organizational affiliate: legal organizations whose purposes, goals, and initiatives are consistent with and supportive of STTI's purposes, goals, and initiatives.

Purpose of Organizational Affiliate Program
The honor society's organizational affiliates program seeks to create a formal relationship with other nursing and health care organizations. . . .

- Strengthen nursing and/or health care through knowledge dissemination, education, research, leadership, and scholarship
- Support learning and the professional development of nurses
- Make a difference with a positive impact on health-related issues

Source: Honor Society of Nursing, Sigma Theta Tau International 2005. *Homepage.* Retrieved January 27, 2005 from *http://www.nursingsociety.org/index.html.* Reprinted with permission.

The Internal Revenue Service provides information outlining criteria for each of the different types of tax exempt status. There are 27 designations of tax-exempt status, set forth in the 501(c) section of the 1986 tax code (Internal Revenue Service, 2003a). Generally, nursing professional associations have 501(c)(3) status, which includes religious, charitable, educational, scientific, and literary associations or those with selected social missions. Labor organizations engaged in educational activities to improve conditions of work, to improve products and efficiency have the 501(c)(5) designation. Tax-exempt status generally prohibits involvement in political action and campaigning, but does allow associations to engage in lobbying or advocacy related to their exempt purposes (Internal Revenue Service, 2003b). Many states also have requirements for registration by associations to maintain their tax-exempt status.

Bylaws establish the governance structure including board membership, committees and meetings and staff accountabilities. Governance responsibilities are set forth in job descriptions. Board members are stewards of the association and their functions typically include oversight of performance including audits, decision making regarding membership eligibility, dues structure, policy, strategic direction, budget approval and

Membership Structure of the National League for Nursing

- Formed in 1893 as the American Society of Superintendents of Training Schools for Nursing for the purpose of establishing and maintaining a universal standard of training
- Named the National League for Nursing Education in 1912
- Renamed the National League for Nursing in 1952
- Established the National League for Nursing Accrediting Commission in 1997

Mission

To advance quality nursing education that prepares the nursing workforce to meet the needs of diverse populations in an ever-changing health care environment.

Membership Categories

- Constituent leagues
- Individual membership
- Agency, schools of nursing members
- Health care agency members
- Allied/public agency members

Source: National League for Nursing, 2005. *Homepage*. Retrieved January 27, 2005 from *http://nln.org/*. Reprinted with permission.

board development. Accountability of the board for keeping the association's bylaws up to date, ensuring financial stability with appropriate investment plans and budgets, and developing and implementing the strategic plan for the work of the association is shared with the staff.

The mission and goals of the association impact the type of member eligibility established. Nursing associations range from the most exclusive membership to the most inclusive membership. Sigma Theta Tau International and the American Academy of Nursing are examples of exclusive honor societies or associations that limit membership to those selected through an established process. Some nursing associations limit membership to registered nurses with credentials in a specialty field of practice. Others limit membership to registered nurses. An example is the State Nurses Association. Some associations with broad-based membership have subsidiaries or sections dedicated to nurse members. A few professional nursing associations have more inclusive membership. The NLN is an example of an association with the more inclusive membership eligibility. In the reorganization of the professional associations in the 1950s, NLN was designated as the association with personal membership open to the public. As shown in Box 23.6, one of the NLN membership categories is personal membership, which does not require the registered nurse credential.

Members of the association also have a responsibility to be informed about the association's activities and to participate in keeping the association up-to-date. Nursing associations, like all types of organizations, are dynamic, influenced by internal and external forces. The development of many associations over time is marked by structural changes, renaming or reorganization. Many of these changes are driven by member concerns and actions.

For example, the ANA recently restructured the organization in response to member perceptions about internal conflict within the ANA. Two organizations emerged in the restructuring, The Center for American Nurses (CAN), and the United American Nurses (UAN), AFL/CIO. CAN, a 501(c)(6) organization formed in 2003, is an ANA affiliate that promotes and supports nurses and nursing in the workplace through noncollective bargaining. UAN, also an affiliate of AFL/CIO in its Department for Professional Employees, was launched in 2004 and provides workplace advocacy and collective bargaining (Box 23.4).

Some associations are long-standing and others have a shorter life cycle. Nursing specialty associations formed because of a shared common bond in practice, and are most likely to be affected by changes in care such as new knowledge or technology which significantly impacts the practice. As practice changes, some associations find new partners for collaboration. An example is the new Alliance for Nursing Informatics formed in 2004. Nurses from 18 associations with more than 2,000 members who work in information technology joined to form this Alliance for Nursing Informatics to collaborate on public policy and to set common standards and disseminate best practices. Some practice areas, especially technologically dependent ones, may be eliminated because of new technology or new modes of treatment. Others, such as Space Nursing, emerge in accordance with new discoveries and new practice venues.

▶ CHALLENGES FOR CONTEMPORARY PROFESSIONAL ASSOCIATIONS IN NURSING

Key among the challenges nursing professional associations face in the 21st century are membership, finance, the short life-cycle of information, changes in nursing practice, diversity, and an unknown future.

Membership

Membership is a particular challenge in the 21st century. A pertinent question for associations is, "Will nurses continue to value membership in their professional association?" Although most associations survey their own membership, this author could find no national independent study of the extent to which nurses join professional associations and how many nurses belong to more than one professional association.

> ***CONSIDER:** In changing times, association member needs and values are impacted by numerous forces.

The importance of such research cannot be over- or underestimated. Indeed, a study by White & Olson (2004) of the association of Rehabilitation Nursing and four other specially nursing organizations, identified multiple reasons for both joining and declining membership in these associations (Box 23.7). Such research informs leadership about the member's perceptions of the association's value to their practice, their satisfaction and loyalty to the association, and the critical issues facing members in their practice as well as ways to further the association's well-being.

> ***CONSIDER:** Conventional wisdom derived from previous studies indicates that there are "joiners" and "nonjoiners," but the reality is that the majority of registered nurses are not dues-paying members of one or more professional associations.

Box 23.7

Research Study Fuels the Controversy

Why Nurses Join Specialty Organizations

This descriptive research study, with a convenience sample of 81 participants from the *Association of Rehabilitation Nursing* and four other specialty nursing organizations, used mailed surveys, telephone surveys, and questionnaires to examine why nurses join specialty nursing organizations and what changes would be necessary to increase membership. Herzberg's motivational theory was applied as the conceptual framework.

White, M. J., & Olson, R. S. (2004). Factors affecting membership in specialty nursing organizations. *Rehabilitation Nursing, 29(4),* 131–137.

Study Findings

The most frequent reasons given by study participants for joining a professional organization were to increase knowledge, benefit professionally, network, and earn continuing education units. Reasons given for not choosing to participate were family responsibilities, lack of information about these organizations, and lack of time.

Membership is always a key concern in professional associations because the credibility and influence of professional associations depends on membership numbers. A few of nursing's professional associations have exclusive, limited membership, but most depend on membership campaigns and aggressive marketing to sustain membership. Some associations strive to increase membership by changing eligibility requirements, taking care to gain member support for the changes. Associations need members to serve members, to be influential in practice and effective in public relations. The integrity of associations is threatened when membership numbers decline.

Some experts referring to the "new social order" argue that professional associations have declining membership numbers because they tend to continue to be traditional, bureaucratic organizations that are preoccupied with sustaining the status quo. Such preoccupation may impede openness to learn about changing member needs and to respond appropriately, to design innovations required to meet these needs. On the other hand, members may value the traditions and rituals of associations related to their heritage and past practices. Visionary leadership and active participation of members are needed to keep the association relevant.

Discussion Point

Will the majority of professional health-related associations begin to merge and partner in significant ways in the next 20 years? If so, what is the potential impact on the nursing profession?

Finance

Membership is directly related to an association's finances. Many professional nursing associations are stretched to sustain resources for programs and services. Some associations are now sharing services, to share costs with others. Others strategies to use resources prudently include joining coalitions or groups for shared programs and services, linking with other groups to develop and promulgate policy, participating in shared advocacy and legislative advocacy, merging to reduce overhead and establishing new financial and budgeting policies to increase flexibility.

Many associations, rather than increase dues, meet their resource needs through investments, fees for services, and margins on major events such as conventions and educational programs. Advertising fees for promotions on websites and in journals, and participation of vendors in meetings and conventions are another source of revenue. Development of Foundations and solicitation of funding for member services is yet another approach as is embarking on earned revenue ventures. The trend to increase income through revenue-producing ventures was examined by Foster and Bradach, 2005. Noting that there is a growing perception that nonprofit leaders must become entrepreneurial to become self-sustaining, these authors concluded that there is little likelihood that these earned income ventures will be successful. They recommend that any new earned income ventures be evaluated according to the contribution they make toward the nonprofit's mission (Foster & Bradach).

New demands on associations to adopt new communications technology, however, often require large outlays of capital. Considering these outlays necessary to attract and retain members, many associations are seeking creative ways to finance the changes while continuing important programs such as advocacy and legislation. Valued as one of the most important services associations provide, advocacy and legislation do not produce revenues. Therefore, associations are reaching out to external groups and influential persons in business and industry to gain support for their activities.

Discussion Point

What business approaches would be most effective for professional nursing associations to ensure continuation of essential services and to develop useful innovations?

Communication: The Short Life Cycle of Information

Associations have historically been valued for their thoughtful and reliable communications on important matters requiring expertise, peer review and testing for reliability. This professional communication, however, has been influenced by the rapid production of knowledge, increasing acceptance of short-lived ideas and information and the shortened lifecycle of information. Members now expect rapid communication, immediate feedback, and prompt resolution of problems and issues.

Many associations now have websites, online directories, chat rooms, and other Internet devices to facilitate member interaction online. Many produce CDs and web resources to share proceedings of meetings and conventions. However, the rapid production and dissemination of new knowledge goes beyond these efforts and often involves capital expenditures for research and development, costly production and staff training, or adding additional staff. In an era of instant messaging, on-the-spot global reporting and unfettered transmittal of information, associations are challenged to develop new communication strategies. Production of association issue papers, educational materials, and other information typically involves member input and review and time-consuming processes to ensure reliability. Generating new knowledge and managing instant transmission of knowledge is, however, important for associations to retain their position as expert sources of knowledge.

Members will seek the most convenient, reliable source of information. Associations now compete with Internet communications from many sources accessible by members. It is possible that some nurses may be lured away from association membership by their effective use of new technology. Those who have successfully used a search engine to rapidly and independently obtain reliable information on a multitude of topics may also be open to finding new networks with immediate entry that do not entail paying dues or attending to the requirements of professional associations for membership.

Discussion Point

Associations looking to the future must ask: Will members value their associations if they continue along the path of traditional rules of order, procedures and protocols?

Changes in Nursing Practice

Nursing practice is changing. Many nurses now participate in multidisciplinary care teams. Their practice colleagues are more diverse. Their practice issues now extend beyond the nursing component of care, and they value networking with team members from a variety of disciplines. Chat rooms and new types of affinity groups and even new associations are forming around issues and topics of common concern that go beyond a given profession. The American Association of Critical Care Nurses recognized this phenomenon early and expanded their membership beyond nurses.

*CONSIDER: Associations of the future are challenged to respond to the complex issues of multidisciplinary practice and issues surrounding the new environment for practice.

This challenge involves supporting the domain of nursing practice concurrently with supporting inter-professional interchange, in a straight-forward manner. It can be projected that in the future, interdisciplinary groups will work together to deal with issues and resolve problems they experience in today's integrated management and clinical systems, regulation and legislation. Will these nurses continue to participate in nursing's professional associations? Or will nursing's professional associations be challenged to adapt to a new reality of partnerships, alliances, membership eligibility, and services?

As nursing practice changes, so do nurses' preferences for networking. Networking has been a mainstay of associations. Meeting colleagues, listening to respected leaders, and exchanging business cards are networking devices related to educational programs, conventions, and association gatherings. The Internet now allows nurses to exchange ideas and meet colleagues at any time without travel expenses, from the comfort of the computer. Some associations, anticipating that networking practices are changing, are exploring how these changes affect the way they provide member services. Will members continue to value the association for personal contacts? Associations have many questions about how people are learning to network and share and about the value of networking to members. Will members want to come to meetings when they can review the proceedings online after the meeting? Or will they want informal groups and small convenings?

Association literature suggests that associations will need to become more flexible and more integrated to accommodate these anticipated changes in member preferences. Traditional associations may have difficulty adjusting to the new environment, in which distinction among official meetings, conferences, and journals (all marks of an effective association), is blurred by instant communication systems and rapid exchange of information in cyberspace.

To remain viable, associations must focus on understanding member needs, on balancing traditional attitudes and practices with contemporary ways of managing and interacting, and on prioritizing use of resources. As nursing roles change and expand, member needs will change. Balancing current programs and services with emerging expectations involves establishing a new way of approaching the business of associations. Some associations are enlisting participation of members with particular expertise to create the vision and plan for the future. Others are reaching out to other associations to share learning and to fill in gaps. Many associations have already begun to refocus services, becoming brokers for communication, mentoring, and professional dialogue.

The new demands on nursing's professional associations are beginning to change the perspective of "competitor." Previously, competitors have been other nursing and practice-related associations. Competitors, instead of having name recognition and elegant structure, may be flexible, open to experimenting with new approaches and focused on member loyalty to services rather than to associations. Members and association leaders are now challenged to remain focused on their mission, their membership, and their services to make wise decisions about how to use and shape their resources for now and the future.

Discussion Point

What should professional nursing associations do now to better understand networking, the motivation to network and methods for effective networking?

What steps should nursing's professional associations take to keep pace with changing networking needs of members?

Diversity

As the population becomes increasingly diverse, associations are challenged to ensure that their membership is representative of the cultural diversity of members. Representation of current and potential members is an aspect of an association's mission. It is also a strategic imperative. Definitions of diversity include age, gender, ethnicity, race, physical ability, religion, socioeconomic status, and geographic distribution.

Outreach to potential members to increase the association's diversity, although a simple strategy on the surface, can be complex. To be effective, the association's policies and practices must reflect the diversity of its members. Staff and volunteer leadership, member involvement, programs, and services often need to be changed or adapted to

BOX 23.8

Strategies for Achieving Diversity in Professional Associations

- Governing boards commitment to diversity demonstrated in behaviors
- Allocation of funds to support activities to increase diversity
- Policy statements encompassing the vision and goals for diversity
- Goals and objectives for achieving diversity in the association's strategic plan
- Materials and tools to promote diversity among members
- Staff selection and staff development to promote diversity
- Management practices to promote involvement of diverse staff in all activities
- Outreach to diverse groups to gain support and mentors for diversity
- Evaluation and measurement of objectives to increase diversity

reflect the diversity of the membership. For some associations, movement toward greater diversity is a giant step, for others a natural evolution. Some of the strategies commonly used by professional associations to increase diversity are shown in Box 23.8.

THE ASSOCIATION FOR THE FUTURE

Associations are thoughtful organizations that follow structured patterns to elect officers, develop agendas, to study problems and issues, to obtain member responses to findings and recommendations, and then to transmit the final draft of the information to members and to the public. As cultures evolve and societal, economic, and political structures and mores change, one must question the future viability of associations. Clearly, technology, the increasing complexity of issues, innovation, and societal changes are forces that impact professional associations. Associations are challenged to be relevant to changing member needs. Those associations that remain understandable to members and dedicated to meeting members' needs will find ways to implement innovations while upholding their values. The relevant associations will be the most likely to survive in the face of generational gaps and changing values (Judge, 1979).

Reinvention for Relevance

To remain relevant, it is predicted that many associations will recreate themselves to be viable organizations in a rapidly changing world. These recreated associations will be characterized by the ability to identify and resolve issues with a short life cycle, and to change from a structured control and command pattern to become flexible organizations able to meet demands in a changing world. The culture and work of the association may change dramatically to reflect emerging cultures of work and of the profession as well as changes in organizations. Some associations are expected to become hybrids, blending the best of the old and the new to remain relevant to members and to the public.

Are nursing's professional associations the appropriate group to move nursing into its future? Insights gleaned from Hackman's (2002) study of the role of professional associations in the Baltic are helpful in exploring the usefulness of associations for nursing's future in this country. Hackman's work indicates that professional associations contribute to the integration of regional "elites" that eventually influence national political action. The association shapes the culture through cultural orientation, relationships, shared traits, and common purpose to achieve unity. Associations that build trust and communication among members are capable of defining ways to move the agenda and to achieve support toward change have the potential to influence. Associations, then, develop a culture and, in turn, influence the cultures in which they function.

Culture of the Future

Applying this study to nursing, nursing associations have a role in shaping the future culture of nursing. Building on the legacy of the past and the template for nursing's development established by early leaders, nursing associations have the capability to influence the cultures in which nurses function. Nursing has a valued legacy of shaping the future for the profession. Great strides have been made to achieve recognition of nursing as a profession and of nurses as professionals. The first half of the 20th century focused on the solidifying the profession in society. The second half of the 20th century focused on expanding nursing capability to provide patient care. Which association or group of associations will step forward to identify the focus and lead the journey of the 21st century?

It is difficult to imagine a future so different from the present experience. However, change is inevitable and forecasting the direction of change is difficult. A first step is collaboration among nursing's professional associations to develop an awareness of forces that impact future nursing practice and the profession. Nursing associations have already established collaboration. Ten associations are organizational affiliates of the ANA (Box 23.4). The newly formed Nursing Organizations Alliance holds promise for courageous leadership for nursing. The Alliance was formed by vote of two nursing coalitions: The National Federation of Specialty Nursing Organizations and the Nursing Organizations Liaison Forum. The future agendas of the collaborative groups have the potential for confronting the future well before it can be understood through experience.

Using the template established by early nursing leaders, the ANA is another association with potential to forge into the future. The ANA is the U.S. member of the ICN and is generally considered the representative of the nation's nurses in matters affecting the solidarity of the profession and professionalism. As such, the ANA has the public recognition essential to shape the future. Consider how powerful the ANA could be if the nation's 2.6 million nurses supported common policy initiatives for the future of the profession.

Public Involvement

Because nursing is integral to society, the public must be involved in shaping nursing's future. Creating an agenda to inform the public and to gain support for the future is critical to advancing the profession. Nursing's influence relies on the support of every nurse and on the capability for effective communication between nursing and the public. Each nursing association has its circle of influence within health care and in the public arenas. The Internet is proving to be an effective way to communicate with many audiences and may be an important link in nursing's communication with the public but it must be managed. As an experiment, put "nursing" in a search engine and analyze the results. The number of results is overwhelming. A first step in preparing for the future could be codification of references about nursing to facilitate effective web searches. A collaborative website, "*All About Nursing,*" could explain the codes and could be linked to all associations, schools of nursing, and related sites.

Hybrid associations would logically be crafted from changes in practice. In nursing, these associations would find ways to support nurses in maintaining their strong professional identity, their understanding and commitment to the profession while also supporting their capability to practice in integrated management and clinical patient care services. The hybrid association would grow from one that formerly concentrated on nursing to concentrate on teamwork, bridging territorial domains and recognizing issues and challenges of integrated systems.

Recreating professional associations can be considered a journey to the future. This journey begins with creating and sharing a vision of the future that is then continuously reinterpreted to evolving realities as change takes place. Once a vision is in place, other steps fall into place more naturally but not always easily.

New Initiatives

Types of initiatives associations will undertake on this journey include evaluation of the complexity of nursing practice, needs of nurses, the environment for practice, and nursing roles in health care delivery. Involvement of key stakeholders to grapple with key issues, make recommendations, and deliberate on action plans is important to the success of the endeavor. Preparing nurses and others for potential changes paves the way for action, especially when changes involve experimentation and some risk-taking. Intentional outcomes center on serving members within the constraints of the available resources through increasingly flexible and adaptable associations.

The journey is fueled by communication among members and between the association and the public. Understanding the nature and intent of change facilitates participation and support. Keeping in touch with members and the public paves the way for difficult decisions or radical change. If nurses examined their needs for nursing associations of the future, would they recommend radical change? Some may believe that steps should be taken to reduce the redundancy of association functions. For example, does the profession need more than one association to accredit nursing programs? To provide certification for nurses? Or would one strong association serve the profession and the public better? Others believe that the "redundancy" provides necessary competition and responsiveness to members.

Unification: A Radical Change?

Yet another radical change would be creating a manageable unifying body that engenders cooperation of all nursing associations to identify issues for the profession as a whole and to develop an action plan involving all. The proliferation of nursing associations in the 20th century may be viewed as a strength. Each of these associations must, of necessity, focus on its own mission, but has an important role to play in shaping the nursing profession. To create a unifying body of nursing associations, nursing must transcend some of the current issues. For example, because the ANA is perceived as a union, employers of nurses often see membership in the ANA as a conflict of interest. The ANA has responded to this concern as well as its internal issues presented by state nurses associations with non-collective bargaining by restructuring the organization. Will the ANA or CAN emerge as the national leader toward the future of nursing?

Discussion Point

Would it make any difference to you personally and professionally if the multitude of professional nursing associations did not exist?

Many association experts predict that a new social order for professional associations is inevitable. Nursing's professional associations would be impacted by a new social order. Members aware of the importance of value will look for evidence of performance outcomes, the effectiveness of political and legislative advocacy and collaboration to advance the profession and patient care. Demonstrating value is a key to future success of any association. This value is demonstrated by the design of future plans and initiatives, enhanced capability to meet new demands, and elegant communication on issues, change and outcomes.

Discussion Point

What steps should professional nursing associations take now to develop new approaches to become the association that provides evidence-based performance reports to demonstrate value to members?

Research Needed

There is a dearth of information, however, about nursing's professional associations. Nursing would be well served by establishing a research agenda to investigate the role of associations now and in the future to inform initiatives to shape the future of the profession. A starting point for developing research questions follows:

- What populations are served by nursing associations?
- What populations do these associations serve?
- To what extent are the purposes of the associations the same, different?

- What are the benefits of associations to nurses? To the profession?
- What factors influenced the proliferation of nursing associations?
- What sustains associations over time?
- How are associations impacted by society, economic and political forces?
- What factors influence changes in associations? Mergers? Disbanding?
- What are the future needs of the profession?
- How should the profession structure itself to meet these needs?
- What role should associations have to advance the future of the profession?

To shape the future of nursing associations, there is a need to establish an evidence base for nursing associations. As mentioned previously, associations are shaped and sustained by societal, political, and economic forces. Nursing associations are influenced by these forces and particularly by changes in health care, where change is now the norm. Research is needed to understand how these forces will impact the nursing profession and nursing associations. At issue is designing the most appropriate venue to advance nursing, to protect the public, sustain the public recognition for the practice of nursing and to sustain the profession. Strategies for continuing to advance the profession of nursing, whether led by associations or others, take time to formulate and longer to implement. Research is needed to inform these strategies.

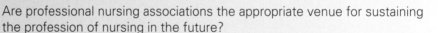

Discussion Point

Are professional nursing associations the appropriate venue for sustaining the profession of nursing in the future?

CONCLUSIONS

Associations are integral to the cultures of work and society as we know it today. Associations serve members by engaging them in leadership initiatives and providing member services such as education and credentialing, initiatives to advance the profession, and advocate for the profession and the health needs of the public. Legislative advocacy and policy development entail strong ties with influential persons and groups. Association work is informed by interaction with members and the public, and by research. Support is facilitated by public relations to transmit information to members.

Nursing leaders are challenged by future demands and current resources. More than 100 years ago, nurses with vision and passion were defining professionalism for nurses and designing strategies to achieve public recognition for nursing practice, to protect public safety and welfare, and to improve health. Is it time to reexamine their template for nursing's development, to evaluate the relevance of current definitions and strategies, and to reflect on what nursing's professional associations contribute to the profession. Have nursing's professional associations become so embedded in the culture that nurses find it difficult to look beyond the present to envision and shape the future?

A century ago, nurse leaders struggling to gain recognition for nursing as a profession created associations that served the profession. Their passion has been relegated to the history books. The profession they shaped has become pluralistic, diffuse, and uncertain of its future. The profession is being impacted by an emerging new social order. The new environment is replete with opportunities and venues for nurses with energy and commitment to meet their needs for professional development, support, and networking. One hundred years from now, what will nurse leaders write about the nurse leaders and the professional nursing associations of this century?

FOR ADDITIONAL DISCUSSION

1. Do most registered nurses relate more directly to their work place than to professional nursing associations on matters pertaining to the advancement of the nursing profession and protection of the public?
2. Some people join professional associations, others do not. What motivates registered nurses to participate in and become active in their professional association?
3. Should nurses, through professional associations take responsibility for regulating the profession? Or is regulation a matter for the public domain?
4. What measures would be effective to engage every registered nurse in activities that protect the public welfare and ensure quality nursing care in the policy and legislative arenas? Can this effort be accomplished without professional nursing associations?
5. What alternatives are there to professional nursing associations to provide professional nurses with opportunities to network, socialize, and grow in their profession outside the workplace?
6. Are associations so embedded in society that they will continue to exist even in the new social order? Will associations with redundant functions join to provide accreditation of educational programs, certification for nurses?
7. If you were to establish a professional nursing association today, what would you state as the mission and strategic direction for that association?
8. What research is imperative to better understand the role of professional nursing associations designed to meet member needs in the future? Who should conduct this research and how should the findings be used?
9. How can nurses capitalize on their resources to examine the nursing profession of the future from a worldview perspective, to develop approaches and strategies to sustain nursing in the future? Can professional nursing associations play a part in this activity?
10. How can professional nursing associations become flexible and responsive to changing member values and needs? To new ways of providing members with information and resources to support their work?

REFERENCES

American Nurses Association (2005). *ANA Nursing World homepage*. Retrieved May 11, 2005, from http://nursingworld.org/.

Cherry, B. & Jacob, S.R. (2002). *Contemporary nursing. Issues, trends, & management* (2nd ed). St. Louis: Mosby.

Fenwick, E. G. (1901). *The organization and registration of nurses*. Paper presented at the 3rd Quinquennnia Meeting of the International Council of Nurses held in Buffalo, New York. From the Proceedings, International Council of Nurses, 1901, p.336.

Foster, W. & Bradach, J.(2005). Should nonprofits seek profits? *Harvard Business Review, 83*(2), 92–100.

Hackman, J. (2002). *Voluntary associations and region building. A post-national perspective on Baltic history, Center for European Studies Working Paper Series, 105*. Presented at the German Study Group at CES.

Henderson, V. & Nite, G. (1978). *Principles and practice of nursing*, (6th ed., pp. 70–75). New York: Macmillan.

Hunt, K. N. (Ed.) (2004). *Encyclopedia of Associations, An Associations Unlimited Reference* (41st ed.). Farmington Hills, Michigan: Gale Publishing.

Internal Revenue Service. (2003a). *Publication 557, Tax-exempt status for your organization.* Retrieved May 10, 2005, from http://www.irs.gov/publications.

Internal Revenue Service. (2003b). Department of the Treasury: *IRS issues guidelines for tax-exempt groups engaged in public advocacy* IR-2003-146. Retrieved May 10, 2005, from http://www.irs.gov.

Judge, A. (1979). *The associative society of the future.* Paper presented to a panel on "Cumulation in international relations: Transnational relations" at the 20th annual convention of the International Studies Association, Toronto. Retrieved May 10, 2005, from http://www.laetusinpraesens.org/docs/assfut.php.

National League for Nursing (2005). *Homepage.* Retrieved May 10, 2005, from http://nln.org/.

Raymond Rich Associates report on the structure of organized nursing (1946) *American Journal of Nursing, 46*(10), 648–661.

Sigma Theta Tau International Honor Society of Nursing (2005). *Homepage.* Retrieved May 10, 2005, from http://www.nursingsociety.org/index.html.

Spaulding, E. K. & Notter, L. (1965). *Professional nursing.* Philadelphia: JB Lippincott.

The ALLIANCE. Nursing Organizations Alliance (2004). *Homepage.* Retrieved May 10, 2005, from http://nursing-alliance.org/.

BIBLIOGRAPHY

Center for American Nurses (2004). *Prairie Rose, 73*(1), 10.

Center for American Nurses becomes independent organization. (2003). *American Nurse, 35*(4), 17.

Chwedyk P. (2004). Vital signs. NCEMNA expands its activities, launches Web site and scholarship program. National Coalition of Ethnic Minority Nurse Associations. *Minority Nurse,* 6.

Dickinson, T. (2003). Treasurer's message. Are professional nursing organizations important? *Urologic Nursing, 23*(1), 8.

Directory of certifying organizations (2004). *Critical Care Nurse, AACN Critical Care Careers 2004,* 39–40.

Fontaine, D. (2003). Powerful partnerships achieve nursing's greatest outcomes. *Nursing Management, 34*(5), 6.

Gilmore, V. (2003). Outlining the activities of the National Nursing Organisations. *Australian Nursing Journal, 10*(8), 15.

Guide to specialty certification organizations (2004). *Nursing. CareerDirectory,* 42–43.

Kennedy, M. S. (2004). AJN reports. A banner year: the Center for American Nurses notes achievements. *American Journal of Nursing, 104*(9), 26.

Mason D. J. (2004). The Nursing Organizations Alliance: A new coalition provides hope for nurses' collective power. *American Journal of Nursing, 104*(2), 25–26.

Mason, D. J. (2003). AJN reports. History being made: The inaugural meeting of the Nursing Organization Alliance. *American Journal of Nursing, 103*(1), 25.

New international alliance of LP/VNs, RPNs and enrolled nurses. (2004). *Journal of Practical Nursing, 54*(2), 2.

Nursing specialty organizations (Part 2). (2004). *American Journal of Nursing, Career Guide 2004,* 71–73.

Seifert, P. C. (2003). Forging a nursing alliance — leading beyond your comfort zone: the creation of an organization of organizations. *SSM, 9*(6), 14–17.

Sullivan, E. (1999). President's message. Peer support, collaborations build strong nursing societies. *Reflections, 25*(4), 3.

Vale, D., Schmidt, S., Mills, E., Shaw, T., Lindell, A., Thomas, C., & Tuchfarber, A. (2003). A collaborative effort between nurse leaders to address the hospital nursing shortage. *Nursing Leadership Forum, 8*(1), 28–33.

Wardell, L., White, C., & Fitzgerald, G. (2003). Professional nursing organizations: What nurses want. *AXON, 25*(2), 8–9.

White, M. J. & Olson, R. S. (2004). Factors affecting membership in specialty nursing organizations. *Rehabilitation Nursing, 29*(4), 131–137.

Wolf, P. (2003). Guide to nursing organizations. *Nursing Management, 34*(11), 40, 43–44.

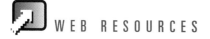 WEB RESOURCES

This resource lists nursing associations from a web search conducted in 2004. National associations in the United States of America were selected. If the association was listed only as international, the international resource was used. The list includes about half of the nursing associations listed in the *2004 Encyclopedia of Associations.*

Academy of Medical-Surgical Nurses   http://www.medsurgnurse.org/cgi-bin/WebObjects/AMSNMain.woa

Academy of Neonatal Nursing LLC   http://www.academyonline.org/

Aerospace Nursing Association	http://www. Aerospacenursingsociety .org/
Air and Surface Transport Nurses Association	http://www. astna.org/
American Academy of Ambulatory Care Nursing:	http://www. aaacn.inures.com
American Academy of Nursing	http://www.nursingworld.org/aan/
American Academy of Nurse Practitioners	http://www.aanp.org/
American Academy of Pain Management	http://www.aapainmanage.org/
American Assembly for Men in Nursing	http://www.aamn.org/
American Assisted Living Nurses Association	http://www. alnursing.org/
American Association for Continuity of Care	http://www.continuityofcare.com/
American Association for the History of Nursing	http://www.aahn.org/
American Association of Colleges of Nursing	http://www.aacn.nche.edu/
American Association of Critical Care Nursing	http://www.aacn.org/
American Association of Legal Nurse Consultants	http://www.aalnc.org/
American Association of Managed Care Nurses	http://www.aamcn.org/
American Association of Neuroscience Nurses	http://www.aaan.org/
American Association of Nigerian Nurses	http://www.aangnurse.org/
American Association of Nurse Anesthetists	http://www.aana.com/
American Association of Nurse Assessment Coordinators	http://www.aanac.org/
American Association of Nurse Attorneys Inc.	http://www.taana.org/
American Association of Occupational Health Nurses	http://www.aaohn.org/
American Association of Office Nurses	http://www.aaow.org/
American Association of Spinal Cord Injury Nurses	http://www.aascin.org/
American College of Nurse Midwives	http://www.midwife.org/acnm.org/
American College of Nurse Practitioners	http://www.nurse.org/acnp/
American Forensic Nurses	http://www.amrn.com/
American Health Information Management Association	http://www.ahima.org/
American Heart Association Council on Cardiovascular Nursing	http://www.americanheart.org/
American Holistic Nurses Association	http://www.ahne.org/
American Medical Informatics Association	http://www.jamia.org/
American Nephrology Nurses Association	http://www. anna.nurse.com/
American Nurses Association	http://www.nursingworld.org/affil/
American Nursing Informatics Association	http://www.ania.org/
American Organization of Nurse Executives	http://www. aone.org/
American Pediatric Surgical Nurses Association	http://www.apsna.org/
American Psychiatric Nurses Association	http://www.apna.org/
American Radiological Nurses Association	http://www.arna.net/
American Registered Professional Nurse Association	http://www.mwankd.net/ARPNA/
American Society of Heart Failure Nurses	http://www. aahfn.org/
American Society of Ophthalmic Registered Nurses	http://www.webeye.ophth.uiowa.edu/asorn/
American Society of Pain Management Nurses	http://www.aspmn.org/
American Society of PeriAnesthesia Nurses	http://www.aspan.org/
American Society of Plastic & Reconstructive Surgical Nurses	http://www.aspsn.org/
American Surgical Nurses Association	http://www.pdcnet.com/APSNA.html
Anthroposophical Nurses Association of America	http://www.artemmisia.net/anaa/
Association for Child & Adolescent Psychiatric Nurses, Inc. (A division of the International Psychiatric-Mental Health Nurses)	http://www.ispn-psych.org http://www. acapn.org/
Association of Black Nursing Faculty in Higher Education Inc. Journal	http://www.tuckerpub.com/
Association of Clinicians for the Underserved	http://www.clinicians.org/
Association of Community Health Nurse Educators	http://www.uncc.edu/achne/
Association of Legal Nurse Consultants	http://www.aahc.org/
Association of Neonatal Nurses	http://www.nann.org/
Association of Nurses in AIDS Care	http://www. anacret.org/
Association of Pediatric Oncology Nurses	http://www.apon.org/
Association of periOperative Registered Nurses	http://www.aorn.org/
Association of Rehabilitation Nurses	http://www.rehabnurse.org/
Association of State and Territorial Directors of Nursing	http://www.astdn.org/
Association of Women's Health, Obstetric & Neonatal Nurses	http://www.awhonn.org/
Commission on Graduates of Foreign Nursing Schools	http://www.cgfns.org/

Council on Cardiovascular Nursing	http://www.americanheart.org/
Council on Graduate Education for Administration in Nursing	http://www.ibiblio.org/cgean
Dermatology Nurses Association	http://www.dna.inurse.org
Developmental Disabilities Nurses Association	http://www.ddna.bluestep.net/
Emergency Nurses Association	http://www.ena.org/
Home Health Care Nurses Association	http://www.hhna.org/
Hospice and Palliative Nurses Association	http://www.hpna.org/
Infusion Nurses Society	http://www.insnec.org/
Interagency Council on Information Resources for Nurses	http://www.nursingcenter.com/people/nrsorgs/icirn/page1.html/
International Association of Forensic Nurses	http://www. forensicnurse.org/
International Nurses Society on Addiction	http://www.intsna.org/
International Society of Nurses in Genetics Inc.	http://www.Creighton.edu/isong/
International Society of Psychiatric Mental Health Nurses	http://www.ispn-psych.org/
Intravenous Nurses Society	http://www.ins1.org/
Midwest Nursing Research Society	http://www.mnrs.org/
Minority Nursing Associations	http://www. minoritynurse.com/
National Alaska Native American Indian Nurses Association	http://www.nanaina.com/
National Association for Associate Degree Nursing	http://www.noadn.org/
National Association for Practical Nurse Education & Service	http://www.napnes@bellatiantic.net
National Association of Clinical Nurse Specialists	http://www.nacns.org/
National Association of Directors of Nursing Administration in Long Term Care	http://www.nadona.org/
National Association of Hispanic Nurses	http://www.thehispanicnurse.org/
National Association of Neonatal Nurses	http://www.nann.org/
National Association of Nurse Massage Therapists	http://www.tranquilmoment.com/
National Association of Nurse Practitioners in Reproductive Health	http://www. ahrp.org/
National Association of Orthopaedic Nurses	http://www.orthonurse.org/
National Association of Pediatric Nurse Associates & Practitioners	http://www. naon.inures.com/
National Association of Pediatric Nurse Practitioners	http://www. napnap.org/
National Association of School Nurses	http://www.nasn.org/
National Organization of Nurse Practitioner Faculties	http://www.nonpf.com/
National Black Nurses Association	http://www. nbna.org/
National Coalition of Ethnic Minority Nurse Association	http://www.ncemna.org/
National Council of State Boards of Nursing	http://www.ncsbn.org/
National League for Nursing	http://www.nln.org/
National Nursing Staff Development Organization	http://www.nnsdo.org/
National Organization of Nurse Practitioner Faculties	http://www.nonpf.com/
National Student Nurses Association	http://www.nsna.org/
Navy Nurse Corps Association	http://www.nnca.org/
North American Nursing Diagnosis Association International	http://www.nanda.org/
Nurse Healers Professional Association International	http://www.therapeutictouch.org/
Nurse Organization of Veterans Affairs	http://www.vanurse.org/
Nursing Organizations Alliance	http://www. nursing-alliance.org/
Nurses Christian Fellowship	http://www.intervarsity.org/
Oncology Nursing Society	http://www.ons.org/
Pediatric Endocrinology Nursing Society	http://www.pens.org/
Philippine Nurses Association of America Inc.	http://www.pnaaO3.org/
Respiratory Nursing Society	http://www.respiratorynursing society.org/
Sigma Theta Tau, the International Honor Society of Nursing	http://www. stti.upui.edu/
Society of Gastroenterology Nurses and Associates Inc.	http://www.signa.org/
Society of Otorhinolaryngology and Head-Neck Nurses	http://www.sohnnurse.com/
Society of Pediatric Nurses	http://www.pedsnurses.org/
Society of Urologic Nurses & Associates Inc.	http://www.suna.org/
Society for Vascular Nursing	http://www.sunnet.org/

Society of Trauma Nurses	http://www.traumanursessoc.org/
Space Nursing Society	http://www.geocities.com/
Transcultural Nursing Society	http://www.tcns.org/
Uniformed Nurse Practitioners Association	http://www.unpa.org/
Wound, Ostomy & Continence Nurses Society	http://www.wocn.org/

Index

Page numbers followed by letters *b, f,* and *t* indicate boxes, figures, and tables, respectively.

Index

509